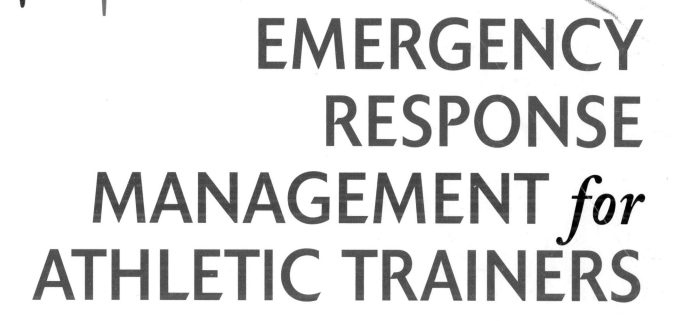

EMERGENCY RESPONSE MANAGEMENT *for* ATHLETIC TRAINERS

MICHAEL G. MILLER, EdD, ATC, CSCS
Professor and Program Director
Graduate Athletic Training Education
Department of Health, Physical Education, and Recreation
Western Michigan University
Kalamazoo, Michigan

DAVID C. BERRY, PhD, ATC, EMT-B
Associate Professor and Program Director
Undergraduate Athletic Training Education
Crystal M. Lange College of Health & Human Services
Department of Kinesiology
Saginaw Valley State University
University Center, Michigan

 Wolters Kluwer | Lippincott Williams & Wilkins
Health

Philadelphia • Baltimore • New York • London
Buenos Aires • Hong Kong • Sydney • Tokyo

Acquisitions Editor: Emily Lupash
Product Manager: Andrea M. Klingler
Marketing Manager: Christen Murphy
Designer: Doug Smock
Photographer: Zolton Cohen Incorporated
Compositor: Aptara, Inc.

First Edition

Library of Congress Cataloging-in-Publication Data

Miller, Michael G., 1968-
  Emergency response management for athletic trainers / Michael G.
Miller, David C. Berry. – 1st ed.
      p. ; cm.
  Includes bibliographical references and index.
  Summary: "This is a comprehensive emergency trauma management text specifically for athletic trainers and athletic training students that addresses the cognitive and psychomotor skills taught in traditional first aid courses (community first aid, first responder, emergency medical technician, and professional rescuer CPR) and discusses specific athletic training emergency trauma skills outlined in the educational competencies set by the Board of Certification (BOC). It is a resource to help readers develop concepts and instruction on current techniques used in the recognition and management of athletic trauma identified in the NATA Educational Competencies. Within each chapter there will be a mix of cognitive knowledge addressing theory and demonstration of the psychomotor skill. Each chapter is designed to account for multiple learning styles, incorporating didactic, visual, and kinesthetic learning where appropriate"–Provided by publisher.
  ISBN 978-0-7817-7550-2 (pbk. : alk. paper) 1. Sports medicine. 2.
Emergency medical services. I. Berry, David, 1971- II. Title.
  [DNLM: 1. Athletic Injuries–therapy. 2. Athletic
Injuries–diagnosis. 3. Emergencies. 4. Emergency Treatment. QT 261]
  RC1210.M4945 2011
  617.1'027–dc22

                                                              2010026568

DISCLAIMER

Care has been taken to confirm the accuracy of the information present and to describe generally accepted practices. However, the authors, editors, and publisher are not responsible for errors or omissions or for any consequences from application of the information in this book and make no warranty, expressed or implied, with respect to the currency, completeness, or accuracy of the contents of the publication. Application of this information in a particular situation remains the professional responsibility of the practitioner; the clinical treatments described and recommended may not be considered absolute and universal recommendations.

The authors, editors, and publisher have exerted every effort to ensure that drug selection and dosage set forth in this text are in accordance with the current recommendations and practice at the time of publication. However, in view of ongoing research, changes in government regulations, and the constant flow of information relating to drug therapy and drug reactions, the reader is urged to check the package insert for each drug for any change in indications and dosage and for added warnings and precautions. This is particularly important when the recommended agent is a new or infrequently employed drug.

Some drugs and medical devices presented in this publication have Food and Drug Administration (FDA) clearance for limited use in restricted research settings. It is the responsibility of the health care provider to ascertain the FDA status of each drug or device planned for use in their clinical practice.

To my family and friends: your support, guidance, love, and friendship will always be cherished!

—Mike

To my family: Leisha, Tyler, and McKinley—thank you for allowing me the opportunity to explore life and for sharing in my journeys. I am grateful for your patience, encouragement, and especially the many sacrifices that you made during this venture. Finally, to my parents, without whom none of what I do would be possible. Your encouragement and infinitesimal wisdom that you instilled from the beginning has allowed me to achieve all that I set out for. Thank you!

—David

Shari Bartz, PhD, ATC, CSCS
Department of Movement Science
Program Director, Undergraduate Athletic Training
Grand Valley State University
Allendale, Michigan

Joel Beam, EdD, ATC
Program Director, Undergraduate Athletic Training
Univeristy of North Florida
Department of Clinical and Applied Movement Sciences
Brooks College of Health
Jacksonville, Florida

Michelle Cleary, PhD, ATC
Department of Kinesiology and Rehabilitation Science
Program Director and Clinical Education Coordinator
University of Hawaii—Manoa
Honolulu, Hawaii

Jeffrey Grunow, MSN, UT EMT-P, NREMT-P
Chair
Department of Emergency Care Rescue
Weber State University
Ogden, Utah

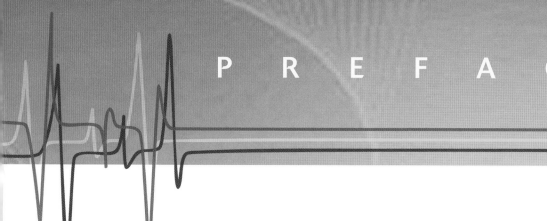

Certified athletic trainers are qualified and appropriately credentialed health care professionals qualified in the domains of injury prevention, recognition, evaluation and immediate care, rehabilitation and reconditioning of injuries and illnesses, and the administration of health care systems. Although most injuries and illnesses that are sustained by athletic participants are not life threatening, catastrophic injuries can and do occur. Certified athletic trainers must be properly trained in prehospital care and equipped to handle any emergency trauma and medical situation that arises whether on the athletic field or in an outpatient rehabilitation setting.

In our inaugural text, *Emergency Response Management for Athletic Trainers,* we provide students with both the theoretical and practical knowledge of prehospital emergency trauma and medical techniques as well as overall emergency management for injuries and/or illnesses commonly seen when working with diverse patient populations. Though this text is best suited for entry-level athletic training students, the information presented may also be useful for practicing certified athletic trainers as a means to refresh their emergency response cognitive knowledge and psychomotor skills.

When creating this text, we incorporated the most current evidence-based science and practice recommendations (from NATA Position Statements) for assessing and managing a variety of non–life-threatening and life-threatening trauma and medical situations. However, emergency cardiovascular care and first aid skills are currently re-evaluated every 5 years in collaboration with the International Liaison Committee on Resuscitation and organizations such as the American Heart Association and American Red Cross to ensure current emergency care procedures are effective. When inconsistencies arise between our text and the current science (e.g., NATA Position Statements), defer to the most current scientific evidence for proper assessment and treatment guidelines.

ORGANIZATION

The cognitive knowledge and psychomotor skills necessary when dealing with an emergency trauma and/or medical situation requires certified athletic trainers to recognize, evaluate, intervene, and provide follow-up care based on a variety of factors. The recognition and management of some athletic injuries and illness does not differ from other athletic heath care team members' protocols (e.g., emergency medical service), but athletic trainers must possess a unique set of educational competencies and proficiencies that have not been adequately addressed in current emergency management texts. Traditional first aid textbooks are geared toward the general public and are limited in their scope of practice, whereas pure emergency trauma and management texts (which provide very useful information) are geared to toward the scope of practice for Emergency Medical Technicians, Advanced Emergency Medical Technicians, and paramedics and in some cases contradict protocols established by certified athletic trainers. Therefore, creating a comprehensive emergency trauma management textbook for certified athletic trainers to address the cognitive and psychomotor skills taught in traditional first aid courses (community first aid, emergency medical responders, emergency medical technician, and professional rescuer CPR) while discussing specific athletic training emergency trauma skills as outlined in the educational competencies will serve as a blueprint to bring together knowledge and psychomotor skills that may be taught in a variety of courses.

As an educational tool used in the classroom, *Emergency Response Management for Athletic Trainers* will be a resource to develop concepts and instruction on current techniques used in the recognition and management of athletic traumas and medical emergencies identified in the National Athletic Trainers' Association Educational Competencies.

The goal when writing this text was to follow a logical order in the development of cognitive knowledge and psychomotor skills. Where appropriate and feasible, we have provided photos, figures, skill boxes, and algorithms to enhance your knowledge and understanding of a wide variety of topics and techniques. The text is divided into three major sections, each of which is comprised of several chapters focusing on general knowledge, skill techniques, and suggested management strategies for emergency situations in the athletic environment.

Section I, Preparing for an Emergency, introduces professional responsibilities, terminology, and strategies for the certified athletic trainer when preparing for and responding to an emergency situation. In Chapter 1, the relationship and roles and responsibilities of the emergency medical team and athletic trainer are discussed providing in-depth knowledge and examples of how the interactions between both parties can function as a "whole" during an emergency situation. In Chapter 2, we discuss the "well-being" of the certified athletic trainer and how personal and philosophical aspects of emergency trauma affects the care of the athlete. In addition, strategies on how to cope with personal and professional issues that occur in emergency situations are emphasized. Chapter 3 provides an overview of a certified athletic trainer's professional, legal, and moral obligations when rendering care to an injured individual during an emergency situation. The goal of Chapter 4 is to review the development of Emergency Action Plans as it pertains to emergency situations at various athletic venues along with the focus of implementation of these plans when/if an emergency situation arises. Finally, Chapter 5 reviews the basic anatomical systems of the body that should be reviewed before proceeding to the other section of the text. Although not all inconclusive, Chapter 5 is meant to supplement past anatomy and physiologically courses or act as an introductory to the human body if the reader's knowledge is limited.

Section II, Emergency Medical Care Assessment, is the first section of the text in which basic emergency management techniques are utilized. In Chapter 6, many ambulatory techniques are discussed and demonstrated to provide a means to get the inured individual to either a safe environment to render care or to the athletic training or medical facility for appropriate follow-up medical care. Chapter 7 discusses how to properly recognize, mange, and dispose of potentially infectious materials according to recommended guidelines. We felt this chapter was needed in the text because many emergency situations involve injuries or situations where blood or other fluids are present. Chapter 8 explains the appropriate steps for the assessment of the scene of a trauma or medical emergency. These include surveying the scene, conducting a primary and secondary assessment, and how to perform and an on-going assessment of an injured individual throughout the management and transportation processes. Chapter 9 focuses on the proper methods and techniques for assessing the vitals of an ill or injured individual during an emergency.

Section III, Emergency Management, is the major emphasis of the book. Our goal was to provide the cognitive knowledge and psychomotor skills necessary for managing a variety of medical emergencies encountered at any athletic venue or other work settings where a certified athletic trainer is employed. Chapter 10 begins by discussing the proper management of breathing emergencies. Chapter 11 examines the use of different adjunct breathing devices such as an oropharyngeal airway, suction, and supplemental oxygen. Although some aspects of this chapter may not comply with individual state practice acts, the importance of understanding how to use and/or assist other trained medical personnel may be paramount during an emergency situation. Chapter 12 focuses on the most current techniques and procedures of emergency cardiac care, CPR, and AEDs. In Chapter 13, we concentrate on the recognition and management steps for providing care in persons who developed shock. Chapters 14 and 15 provide an in-depth look at how to recognize and manage various injuries and illnesses throughout the body. These chapters specifically focus on step-by-step details with numerous figures and skill sets to enhance the learning and comprehension of the skills presented. Chapter 16 focuses on the skills and techniques necessary for immobilizing various injures of the body with multiple illustrations. Chapter 17 concentrates on the management of head and spine injuries with emphasis placed upon helmet and shoulder pad removal techniques. In Chapter 18, the recognition and management of athletes exposed to various environmental hazards are presented. Chapters 19 and 20 review information and skill techniques for emergency management of general medical conditions and allergic reactions to various poisons or triggers found in the environment.

FEATURES

This text has several features that are crucial for the delivery of the content.

Before You Begin – Each chapter begins with a series of questions that serve as a chapter overview. The questions are meant to determine current knowledge or experience before reading the presented materials. After reading the chapter, the goal is to reread each question and determine if your answer changed based on what you learned.

Nomenclature – Found immediately after the Before You Begin, this section highlights some of the important chapter terminology with layman definitions. Though the list is not all conclusive, the terms listed will assist you in understanding the meanings and context for which the terms were derived.

Voices from the Field – These boxes allow practicing certified athletic trainers to introduce the course content in each chapter. We choose individuals with a variety of backgrounds to provide insight or personal experiences either for a subset of the content found within the chapter or the importance of comprehending all the chapter information.

Current Research Boxes – While writing this text, we tried to include all the latest research or standard clinical practices. However, in certain chapters, we felt it was important to highlight some important research topics to further expand your depth and breadth of knowledge about the subject matter. In many cases, you will read about previous research that was the impetus for current practices.

Breakouts – These boxes provide a bit more in-depth information about material presented in the chapter.

Signs & Symptoms – These boxes list signs and symptoms of various conditions to help the reader learn how to recognize various conditions.

Highlights – These boxes provide extra, interesting comments about topics discussed within the text.

Scenarios – At the end of each chapter, we provided several scenarios, when applicable, based on some of the important content found in the each respective chapter. The scenarios are meant to incorporate many of the techniques or knowledge discussed into a problem-solving approach. Each scenario encapsulates many management techniques or stimulates thought about how you would handle emergency situations if they should present in an athletic training setting.

ADDITIONAL RESOURCES

Emergency Response Management for Athletic Trainers includes additional resources for both instructors and students that are available on the book's companion website at thePoint.lww.com/MillerBerry.

Instructors

Approved adopting instructors will be given access to the following additional resources:

- Test questions
- PowerPoint lecture outlines
- Image bank
- Answers to Scenarios

Students

Students who have purchased *Emergency Response Management for Athletic Trainers* have access to the Skills from each chapter in PDF form, for use when practicing and studying the skills presented.

In addition, purchasers of the text can access the searchable full text online by going to the *Emergency Response Management for Athletic Trainers* Web site at http://thePoint.lww.com. See the inside front cover of this text for more details, including the pass code you will need to gain access to the Web site.

Emergency Response Management for Athletic Trainers was created and developed to provide students with both theoretical and practical knowledge of prehospital emergency trauma and medical techniques as well as overall emergency management for injuries and/or illnesses com-

monly seen when working with diverse patient populations. Please take a few moments to look through this User's Guide, which will introduce you to the tools and features that will enhance your learning experience.

Chapter Outcomes open each chapter and present learning goals to help you focus on and retain the crucial topics discussed in each chapter.

The **Nomenclature** section highlights key terms and definitions that are presented in the chapter. The key terms listed are bolded throughout the chapter for easy reference.

Before You Begin questions allow you to quiz and challenge your current knowledge before you begin reading the chapter. Review the questions again after reading the chapter and determine if your answer has changed based on what you've learned.

SECTION II · Emergency Medical Care Assessment

CHAPTER 6

Transportation and Ambulatory Techniques

CHAPTER OUTCOMES

1. Identify the proper mechanics for lifting and transporting an athlete.
2. Recognize when situations arise that require an athlete to be moved or transported.
3. Explain moves and transports to be done by one athletic trainer and by two or more athletic trainers.
4. Identify standard and fabricated equipment used to transport or move athletes.
5. Identify moves or drags using the athlete's torso or limbs.
6. Explain the various water rescues with or without emergency equipment.
7. Describe ambulatory aids and transport techniques for athletes with a lower extremity injury.

NOMENCLATURE

Ambulate: to walk, having only one foot leave the ground with each step
Axilla: armpit
Greater trochanter: the large eminence located approximately 1 cm lower than the head of the femur and a little to the side and back of the upper femur

Popliteal fossa: the space behind the knee joint
Power grip: also known as the supinated grip or underhand grip, palms facing up and knuckles facing down
Tandem: together, as in a group of persons working together, not necessarily in line

BEFORE YOU BEGIN

1. How would an athletic trainer ambulate an injured athlete off the field?
2. When should an injured athlete be moved off the field or away from the playing environment?
3. Should equipment lifts ever be used in the athletic training setting?
4. Should an athletic trainer be knowledgeable about removal techniques for athletes in water environments?

75

Voices from the Field boxes highlight the perspectives of individuals from a variety of backgrounds, providing their insights or personal experiences around the content found within the chapter.

Voices from the Field

Safe and effective movement of an injured athlete requires training and technical skill development in a variety of situations to avoid aggravating the injury. The athletic trainer must be able to make quick decisions about the severity of the injury and condition of the athlete, whether there is an emergent need for removal from the environment, time until emergency medical transportation arrives, the equipment accessible for effective rescue and movement, and the number of people that are trained to assist. Once the decision to move an injured athlete takes place, the athletic trainer must choose which technique is going to be implemented to get the athlete to a safer location for further evaluation.

Knowing the different techniques available and the biomechanics of performing them is important for the protection of the athlete as well as the safety of the athletic trainer. The athletic trainer must be able to select the appropriate technique for the environmental condition (e.g., heat, cold, rain, snow), physical location (e.g., gym, field, pool), and the athlete's condition (e.g., conscious or unconscious, head or back injury, medi-

cal emergency). The athletic trainer needs to be competent in a variety of single athletic trainer moves to accommodate a variety of athlete sizes, situations, and conditions. In addition, the athletic trainer must know how to perform and instruct others in assisting with carries, lifts, and equipment rescues requiring more than one person to safeguard the athlete.

Communication is critical when transferring the athlete to the emergency medical services, hospital personnel, or other allied health professionals. Using appropriate medical terminology is essential to enhancing the credibility of the athletic trainer's assessment of the athlete's condition and expediting the care given to the injured athlete.

Helen M. Binkley, PhD, ATC, CSCS*D, NSCA-CPT*D
Associate Professor
Department of Health and Human Performance
Director, Undergraduate Athletic Training Program
Middle Tennessee State University
Murfreesboro, Tennessee

Current Research boxes highlight important research that was impetus for current practices to help expand your depth and breadth of knowledge.

Current Research
Efficacy of Face Shields

An examination of the effectiveness of three commonly used face shields found that all three tested demonstrated adequate delivery of the recommended **tidal volume** (0.5 to 0.6 L) according to the current American Heart Association standards,[13] American Society for Testing and Materials,[12] and the European Resuscitation Council.[14] Another study examining three methods of ventilation by lay responders found that mouth-to-face shield ventilations generated a mean tidal volume of 694 mL, which is higher[15] than current recommendations. Airflow resistance has also been reported with face shields, increasing the difficulty of ensuring adequate ventilations.[13]

Breakouts provide a bit more in-depth information about material presented in the chapter.

Breakout

Assessing Cardiac Distress Using OPQRST
OPQRST is a mnemonic often used in emergency medicine to help guide the S (signs and symptoms) of the SAMPLE history by allowing the athletic trainer to ask certain pertinent questions about the individual's condition. OPQRST stands for:

- Onset—When did the problem start?
  - Angina pectoris usually occurs at times when the heart requires large amounts of oxygen, as during physical or emotional stress, after a large meal, or with sudden fear. As the demands for oxygen diminish, so does the pain.
  - Heart attacks can occur during periods of increased oxygen demand as well when no increased demands are placed on the heart.
- Provocation—What makes the symptoms better or worse?
  - If an individual took his or her prescribed medication, such as nitroglycerin, has it helped to alleviate some of the discomfort?
  - Positioning may increase or decrease symptoms.
- Quality—What does it feel like? Can you describe the pain and/or symptoms?
  - Angina pectoris presents with a crushing or squeezing pain that normally subsides with 3 to 8 minutes.
  - Heart attacks present also present with a crushing or squeezing sensation that does not changes with each breath. Remember that about one third of individuals experiencing a heart attack may not report any chest pain at all.
- Radiation—Where do you feel your pain? Does it travel to another location of your body?
  - Heart attacks often present with referred pain or discomfort in lower jaw, neck, and arm (normally the left side), abdomen, and/or back.
- Severity—How bad is it on a scale from 0 to 10? Zero being no pain and 10 being the worst pain ever experienced.
- Time—Has there been a change in the pain or symptoms over time?
  - Heart attacks do not resolve ... last from 30 minutes to several hours.

Signs & Symptoms boxes list these for various conditions.

Signs & Symptoms
Abdominal Injuries Requiring Referral

- Diffuse or localized quadrant pain
- Pain or difficulty breathing
- **Hematuria**
- Inability to urinate
- Uncontrolled external hemorrhage
- Abnormalities or absence of abdominal/bowel sounds
- Abnormal vital signs
- Rigidity of abdominal and/or back musculature
- Point or rebound tenderness in quadrants
- Abnormal percussion sounds
- Signs of shock

Highlights provide extra, interesting comments about topics discussed.

Highlight
Administering Nitroglycerin and Aspirin during a Cardiac Emergency

Evidence suggests that the administration of chewable aspirin (acetylsalicylic acid, 325 mg) in the pre-hospital setting is safe and that the earlier aspirin is given, the greater the reduction in risk of mortality.[51] Individuals with a history of aspirin allergy or signs of active or recent gastrointestinal bleeding should not be given aspirin.[52] However, **do not delay** providing care while waiting to administer aspirin.

Individuals with a known cardiac condition may have a prescription for nitroglycerin. It is most commonly used in the treatment of angina[25] and is administered either orally (**lingually**), by placing a pill under the tongue, or by using a liquid spray format. Nitroglycerin acts by dilating the blood vessels (i.e., the coronary arteries), allowing more blood to flow to the heart, while reducing its workload. Occasionally, an individual may have a nitroglycerin patch to prevent attacks of angina.[25] An individual who is conscious, has a prescription, and is exhibiting signs and symptoms of a cardiac emergency should be encourage to administer his or her medication as long as he or she is hemodynamically stable (systolic blood pressure above 90 mm Hg, pulse rate between 50 and 100 beats per minute,[52] with no signs of increased cranial pressure, and no history of the use of Viagra or similar medications. The nitroglycerin should take effect within a couple of minutes; however, if there is no relief of chest pain after 5 minutes, the individual may use another dose, up to three total doses. Be sure to document the individual's response to the medication and the number of doses, as EMS will need this information when they arrive on scene.

Remember, *always to consult* your individual state laws and practice acts, facility policy and procedure manuals, and/or standing medical orders to determine how and when these medications can and should be administered during a cardiac emergency situation.

Skills provide a step-by-step breakdown of techniques and procedures, providing written instructions and four-color photos for each step.

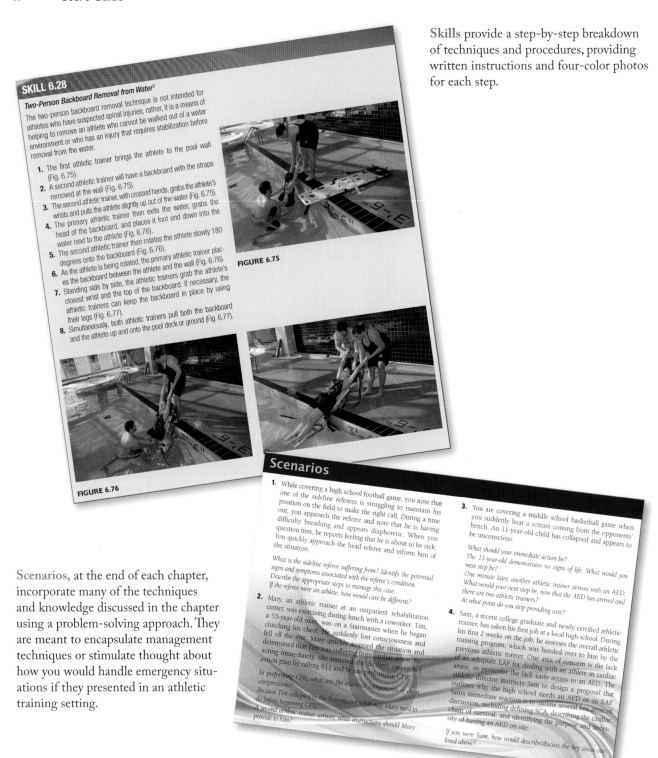

SKILL 6.28

Two-Person Backboard Removal from Water[2]

The two-person backboard removal technique is not intended for athletes who have suspected spinal injuries; rather, it is a means of helping to remove an athlete who cannot be walked out of a water environment or who has an injury that requires stabilization before removal from the water.

1. The first athletic trainer brings the athlete to the pool wall (Fig. 6.75).
2. A second athletic trainer will have a backboard with the straps removed at the wall (Fig. 6.75).
3. The second athletic trainer, with crossed hands, grabs the athlete's wrists and pulls the athlete slightly up out of the water (Fig. 6.75).
4. The primary athletic trainer then exits the water, grabs the head of the backboard, and places it foot end down into the water next to the athlete (Fig. 6.76).
5. The second athletic trainer then rotates the athlete slowly 180 degrees onto the backboard (Fig. 6.76).
6. As the athlete is being rotated, the primary athletic trainer places the backboard between the athlete and the wall (Fig. 6.76).
7. Standing side by side, the athletic trainers grab the athlete's closest wrist and the top of the backboard. If necessary, the athletic trainers can keep the backboard in place by using their legs (Fig. 6.77).
8. Simultaneously, both athletic trainers pull both the backboard and the athlete up and onto the pool deck or ground (Fig. 6.77).

FIGURE 6.75

FIGURE 6.76

Scenarios

1. While covering a high school football game, you note that one of the sideline referees is struggling to maintain his position on the field to make the right call. During a time out, you approach the referee and note that he is having difficulty breathing and appears diaphoretic. When you question him, he reports feeling that he is about to be sick. You quickly approach the head referee and inform him of the situation.

   What is the sideline referee suffering from? Identify the potential signs and symptoms associated with the referee's condition. Describe the appropriate steps to manage this case. If the referee were an athlete, how would care be different?

2. Mary, an athletic trainer at an outpatient rehabilitation center, was exercising during lunch with a coworker. Tim, a 55-year-old man, was on a Stairmaster when he began clutching his chest. He suddenly lost consciousness and fell off the unit. Mary quickly assessed the situation and determined that Tim was suffering from cardiac arrest. Reacting immediately, she initiated the facility's emergency action plan by calling 911 and began performing CPR.

   In performing CPR, what are the essential components of chest compressions?
   Because Tim collapsed by the Stairmaster, what may Mary need to do before beginning CPR?
   A second athletic trainer arrives, what instructions should Mary provide to him?

3. You are covering a middle school basketball game when you suddenly hear a scream coming from the opponents' bench. An 11-year-old child has collapsed and appears to be unconscious.

   What should your immediate action be?
   The 11-year-old demonstrates no signs of life. What would you next step be?
   One minute later, another athletic trainer arrives with an AED. What would your next step be, now that the AED has arrived and there are two athletic trainers?
   At what point do you stop providing care?

4. Sam, a recent college graduate and newly certified athletic trainer, has taken his first job at a local high school. During his first 2 weeks on the job, he assesses the overall athletic training program, which was handed over to him by the previous athletic trainer. One area of concern is the lack of an adequate EAP for dealing with an athlete in cardiac arrest, in particular the lack early access to an AED. The athletic director instructs Sam to design a proposal that outlines why the high school needs an AED or an EAP discussion, including defining SCA, describing the cardiac chain of survival, and identifying the purpose and necessity of having an AED on site.

   If you were Sam, how would describe/discuss the key areas outlined above?

Scenarios, at the end of each chapter, incorporate many of the techniques and knowledge discussed in the chapter using a problem-solving approach. They are meant to encapsulate management techniques or stimulate thought about how you would handle emergency situations if they presented in an athletic training setting.

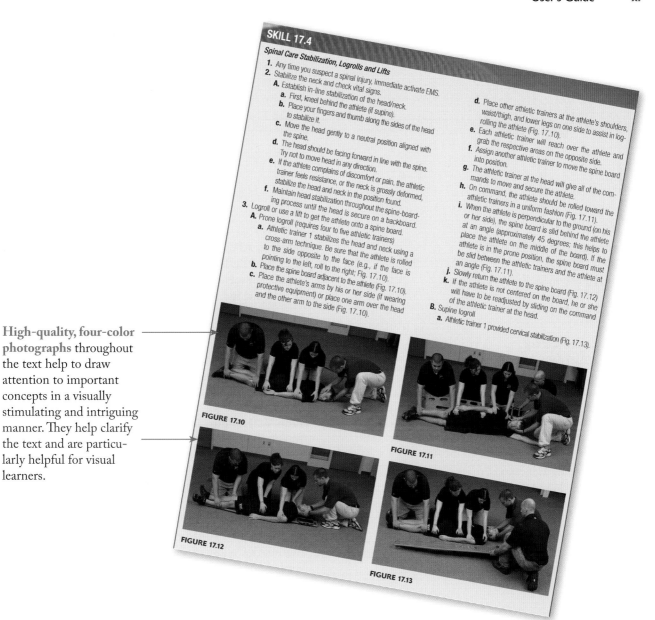

SKILL 17.4

Spinal Care Stabilization, Logrolls and Lifts

1. Any time you suspect a spinal injury, immediate activate EMS.
2. Stabilize the neck and check vital signs.
   A. Establish in-line stabilization of the head/neck.
      a. First, kneel behind the athlete (if supine).
      b. Place your fingers and thumb along the sides of the head to stabilize it.
      c. Move the head gently to a neutral position aligned with the spine.
      d. The head should be facing forward in line with the spine. Try not to move head in any direction.
      e. If the athlete complains of discomfort or pain, the athletic trainer feels resistance, or the neck is grossly deformed, stabilize the head and neck in the position found.
      f. Maintain head stabilization throughout the spine-boarding process until the head is secure on a backboard.
3. Logroll or use a lift to get the athlete onto a spine board.
   A. Prone logroll (requires four to five athletic trainers)
      a. Athletic trainer 1 stabilizes the head and neck using a cross-arm technique. Be sure that the athlete is rolled to the side opposite to the face (e.g., if the face is pointing to the left, roll to the right; Fig. 17.10).
      b. Place the spine board adjacent to the athlete (Fig. 17.10).
      c. Place the athlete's arms by his or her side (if wearing protective equipment) or place one arm over the head and the other arm to the side (Fig. 17.10).
      d. Place other athletic trainers at the athlete's shoulders, waist/thigh, and lower legs on one side to assist in logrolling the athlete (Fig. 17.10).
      e. Each athletic trainer will reach over the athlete and grab the respective areas on the opposite side.
      f. Assign another athletic trainer to move the spine board into position.
      g. The athletic trainer at the head will give all of the commands to move and secure the athlete.
      h. On command, the athlete should be rolled toward the athletic trainers in a uniform fashion (Fig. 17.11).
      i. When the athlete is perpendicular to the ground (on his or her side), the spine board is slid behind the athlete at an angle (approximately 45 degrees; this helps to place the athlete on the middle of the board). If the athlete is in the prone position, the spine board must be slid between the athletic trainers and the athlete at an angle (Fig. 17.11).
      j. Slowly return the athlete to the spine board (Fig. 17.12).
      k. If the athlete is not centered on the board, he or she will have to be readjusted by sliding on the command of the athletic trainer at the head.
   B. Supine logroll
      a. Athletic trainer 1 provided cervical stabilization (Fig. 17.13).

FIGURE 17.10

FIGURE 17.11

FIGURE 17.12

FIGURE 17.13

High-quality, four-color photographs throughout the text help to draw attention to important concepts in a visually stimulating and intriguing manner. They help clarify the text and are particularly helpful for visual learners.

STUDENT RESOURCES

Inside the front cover of your textbook, you'll find your personal access code. Use it to log on to http://thePoint.lww.com/MillerBerry—the companion Web site for this textbook. On the Web site, you can access various supplemental materials available to help enhance and further your learning. These assets include the Skills from each chapter as well as the fully searchable online text.

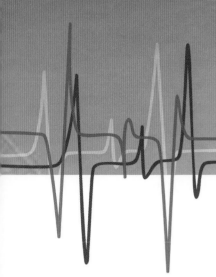

Jay M. Albrecht, PhD, ATC
Assistant Professor
Health, Nutrition, & Exercise Sciences
North Dakota State University
Fargo, North Dakota

Nicole Baker-Cosby
Professor/Assistant Athletic Trainer
Kinesiology
Point Loma Nazarene University
San Diego, California

Rebekah R. Bower, MS, AT, ATC
Education Coordinator
Athletic Training Education Program
Wright State University
Dayton, Ohio

Anthony Breitbach, PhD, ATC
Assistant Professor/Director
Athletic Training Education Program
Saint Louis University
St. Louis, Missouri

Lisa M. Cantara, MS, ATC, CSCS
Athletic Trainer
Athletics
Siena College & Thomas Nicolla Consulting Services
Albany County, New York

Brian K. Farr, MA, ATC, LAT, CSCS
Director, Athletic Training Education Program
Kinesiology & Health Education
The University of Texas
Austin, Texas

Jolene Fisher, MS, ATC, AT/L
Assistant Professor
Health Sciences
Whitworth University
Spokane, Washington

Dan Fox, ATC, FF, EMT-B
Head Athletic Trainer
Indiana University – Purdue University Fort Wayne
Fort Wayne, Indiana

Pat Graman, ATC
Director
Athletic Training Program
University of Cincinnati
Cincinnati, Ohio

Hugh W. Harling, EdD, LAT, ATC
Athletic Trainer
Athletic Training Education Program
Methodist University
Fayetteville, North Carolina

Birgid Hopkins, MS, ATC
Director of Sports Medicine
Merrimack College
North Andover, Massachusetts

Chris Hummel, MS, ATC
Clinical Assistant Professor/Athletic Trainer
Exercise and Sport Sciences
Ithaca College
Ithaca, New York

Mark R. Lafave, PhD, CAT (C)
Associate Professor/Chair
Certified Athletic Therapist
Physical Education & Recreation Studies
Mount Royal University
Calgary, Alberta

Eric Lehnert, MS, ATC, EMT-CC
Certified Athletic Trainer
Athletics
Stony Brook University
Stony Brook, New York

William T. Lyons
Head Athletic Trainer
Kinesiology & Health Promotion
University of Wyoming
Laramie, Wyoming

Melissa Marty
Instructor
Kinesiology
Midwestern State University
Wichita Falls, Texas

Chris Moss
Instructor
Athletic Training
Lincoln Memorial University
Harrogate, Tennessee

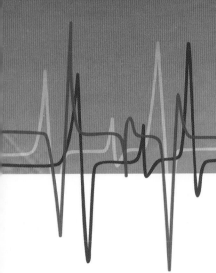

ACKNOWLEDGMENTS

The authors would first like to thank chapter contributors: Dr. Joel Beam, Dr. Michelle Cleary, Dr. Shari Bartz, and Jeffrey Grunow, MSN, UT EMT-P, NREMT-P, for their expertise in the subject matter. We also would like to thank LIFE EMS for the use of their ambulance and emergency equipment for photos used throughout the book. We also thank all support staff of LIFE EMS for their time and assistance.

We would also like to thank our Product Manager, Andrea Klingler, for her hard work and tireless efforts in producing this text. We express our sincere appreciation to the additional members of the publishing team at Lippincott: Emily Lupash, Acquisitions Editor; Jennifer Clements, Art Director; Sara Krause, Artist; and Doug Smock, Design Coordinator. Finally, we would like to thank all of the reviewers for their insight and suggestions; our professional and personal colleagues; and past students for their support.

Michael G. Miller
David C. Berry

CONTENTS

CHAPTER • 1

The Certified Athletic Trainer and Emergency Medical Services: Understanding Roles and Responsibilities

CHAPTER OUTCOMES

1. Describe the development of the Emergency Medical Services (EMS) system.

2. Discuss how the EMS system functions as part of an integrated health care system.

3. Identify the 10 standard components of an EMS system.

4. Identify the components of the chain of survival and the athletic trainer's role within this chain.

5. Identify and describe the four levels of EMS training.

6. Identify the skills an athletic trainer can expect in an emergency situation from each of the four levels of EMS providers.

7. Define medical oversight.

8. Discuss the types of medical oversight that may affect the medical care provided by a first responder.

9. Identify and describe the four types of EMS agencies.

10. Identify and describe the activation of the EMS system, including on-field standby coverage, traditional activation, and aeromedical EMS.

11. Discuss the roles of the on-field physician and sports medicine physician and how medical care may be affected by EMS providers and athletic trainers.

12. Identify and discuss the athletic trainer's professional behaviors, characteristics, scope of practice, and responsibilities during an emergency situation and as part of the EMS system.

13. Identify and discuss the need for developing professional relationships with local EMS providers.

NOMENCLATURE

Advanced emergency medical technician (AEMT): having completed the next to highest level of the United States Department of Transportation (DOT) EMS training, AEMTs provide basic and limited advanced emergency medical care and transportation for the critical and emergent patient who accesses EMS

Advanced life support (ALS): implies that an EMT is capable of performing ALS skills as either an AEMT or paramedic commonly referred to simply as a paramedic or medic

Basic life support (BLS): is a specific level of prehospital medical care provided by trained responders, including EMTs, in the absence of advanced medical care. BLS consists of a number of fundamental lifesaving techniques focused on the airway, breathing, and circulation (the ABCs) of prehospital emergency care

Cardioversion: restoration of the heart's rhythm to normal by electrical countershock

Citizen responder: an individual capable of identifying different types of emergencies and of providing supportive care until professional help arrives. The citizen responder recognizes an emergency, decides to act, calls 911, and provides bystander care until help arrives

Chain of survival: this term refers to a series of actions that, when put into motion, reduce the mortality associated with injury or illness. Like any chain, the chain of survival is only as strong as its weakest link. The four interdependent links in the chain of survival are early access, early cardiopulmonary resuscitation (CPR), early defibrillation, and early advanced care

CombiTube: an airway management device inserted blindly into an patient; it is designed to seal off the laryngopharynx from the oropharynx and esophagus

Critical: quality, state, or degree of being of the highest importance

Cricothyrotomy: an emergency procedure performed by a paramedic where an incision is made through the skin and cricothyroid membrane to secure a patient's airway during certain emergency situations

Endotracheal (ET) intubation: passage of a tube through the nose or mouth into the trachea for maintenance of the airway during anesthesia or for maintenance of an imperiled airway

Enteral: within or by way of the intestine or gastrointestinal tract (e.g., a feeding tube)

Emergency medical dispatcher (EMD): a professional telecommunicator, tasked with the gathering of information related to medical emergencies as well as the provision of assistance and instructions by voice prior to the arrival of EMS; an EMD is also responsible for the dispatching and support of EMS resources responding to an emergency call

Emergency medical responder (EMR): having completed the lowest level of U.S. DOT EMS training; EMRs, using minimal equipment, initiate immediate lifesaving care to critical patients who access the EMS system

Emergency medical technician (EMT): having completed next to last level of U.S. DOT EMS training, provides basic emergency medical care and transportation for critical and emergent patients who access the emergency medical system

Hypoglycemia: an abnormally low concentration of glucose in the circulating blood, or low blood sugar

Intravenous line: an apparatus designed to introduce medication and fluid directly into a patient's venous system

Intubation: insertion of a tubular device into a canal, hollow organ, or cavity; specifically, passage of an oro- or nasotracheal tube for control of pulmonary ventilation

Intraosseous injection: introduction of medication or fluid into the bone marrow

Laryngoscope: a flexible, lighted tube inserted through the mouth into the upper airway; used to look at the inside of the larynx

Medical emergency: an illness such as diabetes, myocardial infarction, seizure, syncope, or stroke that causes an interruption, cessation, or disorder of bodily functions, systems, or organs

Medical oversight: the process by which a physician directs the care given by out-of-hospital providers to ill or injured athletes

Nasogastric: pertaining to or involving the nasal passages and the stomach, as in nasogastric intubation

Offline (indirect) medical direction: a type of medical oversight where medical control includes education, protocol review, and quality improvement of emergency care providers

Online (direct) medical direction: a type of medical oversight where the physician speaks directly with EMS providers at the scene of an emergency

Packaging: the act of securing a patient for transport via EMS

Paramedic: having completed the highest level of DOT EMS training, a paramedic possesses the complex knowledge and skills necessary to provide patient care and transportation

Parenteral: by some other means than through the gastrointestinal tract; referring particularly to the introduction of substances into a patient by intravenous, subcutaneous, intramuscular, or intramedullary injection

Percutaneous cricothyrotomy: an emergency surgical airway procedure on the neck to open a direct airway through an incision in the trachea. It may also be accomplished by inserting a 14-gauge IV cannula

Protocols: standard procedures followed when providing care to a patient during a trauma or a medical emergency

Standing orders: protocols issued by the medical director allowing specific skills to be performed and/or specific

medications to be administrated in certain situations by a trained provider

Trauma: an injury, normally as a result of physical or mental experience

Sublingual: below or beneath the tongue

Tracheobronchial: relating to both trachea and bronchi

BEFORE YOU BEGIN

1. Define EMS. How does EMS differ today as compared with when it was established in the late 1960s?

2. Describe the chain of survival. How does an athletic trainer function within this system?

3. Identify and describe the four levels of professional training within EMS. Whom would you rather have on scene for an athlete with a femoral fracture, and why?

4. Define medical oversight. What is the difference between online and offline medical oversight? As certified athletic trainers, do we have medical oversight?

5. Identify and describe the four different types of EMS agencies. Which one does your institution routinely use? Do you see an advantage of one over another?

6. What are some of the professional behaviors and characteristics required of an athletic trainer during an emergency injury or illness situation?

7. What are some steps an athletic trainer can employ to develop better professional relationships with EMS providers?

Voices from the Field

Collegiate Perspective

Professional longevity allows one to be able to succinctly appreciate the advances that have occurred in the last 46 years with respect to immediate emergency care of those participating in sporting activity.

The 1963 collegiate sports care scene was generally not privy to CPR trained full-time or student athletic trainers. Emergent situations were handled by a call for an ambulance from a local hospital. Over the ensuing years, I was involved in four episodes in which a participant succumbed during a collegiate sporting activity, including two National Collegiate Athletic Association (NCAA) football players, a spectator at an indoor track meet, and an on-the-field football official.

Would the above outcomes be different in today's atmosphere of emphasis on the multiple modes of emergency care? Perhaps not, but, emergency room survival data, combined with hundreds of press reports, would strongly suggest that the presence of a certified athletic trainer greatly

enhances the chances of recovery of a person in respiratory or cardiac distress.

Today's athletic training education programs have successfully raised the bar with respect to the skills of recognizing life-threatening injuries (e.g., a ruptured spleen and head trauma). Briefly said, if you are an athletic trainer at the secondary or higher education level, you can bet the farm that you *will* be faced with a life-threatening situation during your career.

A old sports saying is apropos: "You play like you practice." Preparation can be a life-or-death matter.

Clint Thompson, MA, ATC, Semiretired
Head Athletic Trainer at Michigan State University
Colorado State University Truman State University
  (ATEP Director)
National Athletic Trainers' Association Hall of Fame
  Class of 2004

Professional Sports Perspective

The emergency medical care of injuries is a vital component of the athletic trainer's repertoire of skills in the field. Although these skills are not called upon on a daily basis, preparation and the proper execution of emergency care is critical to the health and future well-being of our patients. Whether those patients are our athletes, coaches, or other staff members, a number of emergencies can occur, and we must be prepared to administer effective treatment while working in conjunction with other health care providers.

Our staff has had to provide care for a number of injuries that have occurred during the course of a football game. From concus-

sions and dislocated joints to fractured bones and ruptured ligaments, several athletes over the years have presented with injuries that required emergency care. Likewise, coaches and staff members may have pre-existing medical conditions that we have not been informed of. One year, before the start of a playoff game, a staff member at the stadium collapsed while performing his pregame duties. He then had a seizure and subsequently went into cardiac arrest in a nearby hallway. We were called to the scene outside the locker room and attended to him immediately. We effectively revived him after using the athletic training automated external

Professional Sports Perspective *(Continued)*

defibrillator (AED), which we always have on hand. Without our training and the necessary medical attention, this staff member could have suffered fatal consequences.

It is in these instances that the athletic trainer must be proficient in emergency medical techniques and understand the role he or she plays as part of the emergency medical team. As stated, these skills are not called upon on a daily basis, but they should be learned, practiced, and perfected in an effort to provide the best possible care when the time arises. Whether

it's on a field with thousands of fans watching in the stadium—and millions more on television—or in a small hallway in your athletic facility, your emergency medical skills and management techniques can help save and protect many lives.

Corey A. Oshikoya, M.Ed., ATC, CSCS
Assistant Athletic Trainer
Denver Broncos Football Club
Englewood, Colorado

Emergency Medical Services Perspective

In many communities across America, emergency medical providers are working to build a comprehensive emergency medical system. This system is made up primarily of public safety agencies all working together to improve response times and patient care during medical and trauma emergencies.

These systems involve EMS agencies; local fire departments; city, county, and state law enforcement agencies; area hospitals; air medical services; lay athletic trainers; and local medical direction.

An important component of the EMS system and a discipline that is often excluded is the certified athletic trainer. These professionals are the first responders to many types of medical and trauma emergencies at athletic events held by high schools, colleges, universities, and communities. Certified athletic train-

ers are trained in CPR, basic life support, the use of AEDs, and the management of potential spinal cord injuries. Athletic trainers should be part of the comprehensive EMS system in every community. They should be invited to join all activities of the EMS system, from training sessions to interaction with local medical direction, and should truly be utilized as a first response professionals. Athletic trainers are also a great resource for training other first responders within the system in identifying and treating sports-related injuries.

James A. Judge II, BPA, CEM, EMT-P
Executive Director
Lake Sumter Emergency Medical Services (EMS)
Mount Dora, Florida

It would be great if, during an athletic practice/event or while working with a postoperative total knee replacement, a certified athletic trainer did not have to worry about injuries or illnesses or the "what ifs." This is never really the case, though. In fact, as an allied health care provider and holders of the ATC credential from the Board of Certification (BOC) (Omaha, Nebraska), we are required to demonstrate proficiency in the immediate care domain as outlined by the BOC's *Role Delineation Study*.[1] As certified athletic trainers, we can handle many emergent situations on our own; however, there may come the time when local Emergency Medical Services (EMS) need to be summoned, often to assist in employing lifesaving techniques to reduce morbidity and the incidence of mortality, prevent exacerbation of non–life-threatening condition(s) in order to reduce morbidity, and facilitate the timely transfer of care of our athletes for conditions beyond the scope of practice of the athletic trainer by implementing appropriate referral strategies to stabilize and/or prevent exacerbation of the condition(s). Whether you are the host team's athletic trainer or visiting team's athletic trainer, pre-event investigation and collaboration with the local EMS agencies will prove advantageous in the event that you should have to work with the local EMS system.

However, as athletic trainers, do we really understand how an EMS systems works? Even if we know we need advanced medical care, do we know what level of EMS responders we actually need and what they can perform once on site? Did you know that there are actually four types

of EMS agencies you have to interact with? What about your role as an athletic trainer: what are your responsibilities, and how does this influence your professional behaviors? To assist you in understanding these questions, this chapter discusses the following concepts: (a) understanding the EMS system, including the **chain of survival**, EMS personnel levels of training and competencies, and types of EMS agencies; (b) activation of EMS; (c) the role of the on field physician; and, finally and most important, (d) the professional behaviors, characteristics, scope of practice, and responsibilities of a certified athletic trainer as part of the EMS system.

UNDERSTANDING THE EMS SYSTEM

A certified athletic trainer rarely works in an emergency medical vacuum while covering an athletic practice or event. At the scene of a **trauma** (injury) or **medical emergency** (illness) or subsequent to a 911 call, designated (statutory) community responders (i.e., police and fire and rescue) will minimally be your "cavalry" and most likely be those responsible for assisting in care of or transporting your athlete to higher medical care. With this in mind, there are several important emergency care questions an athletic trainer must answer, including (a) "What is EMS?" (b) "What is the certification level of EMS emergency care personnel responding to my event?" and (c) "How do I, as a certified athletic trainer, function when working with EMS?" The level of certification of the EMS provider will also dramatically impact the knowledge, skills, medications, and critical thinking expectations that will be available at your incident when EMS arrives and should also be factored into the equation when requesting EMS.

History of the EMS System

Many would be surprised to know that since 1970, the principal party responsible for Emergency Medical Services in the United States has been the National Highway Traffic Safety Administration within the U.S. Department of Transportation (DOT).[2] Although at first glance this may seem odd, in the late 1960s, returning Vietnam veterans were appalled that trauma patients whom they could have saved during the war—using military medics, helicopters, and Mobile Army Surgical Hospitals (MASH) units—were dying on American highways in automobile accidents. In 1966 the report *Accidental Death and Disability: The Neglected Disease,*[3] often referred to as the *White Paper,* spawned the birth of the EMT, primarily to treat trauma cases on the growing highway systems. This paper identified accidental injury as the leading cause of death among persons between the ages of 1 and 37 and fourth leading cause of death among persons of all ages. Even today, unintentional injury is still the leading cause of death in persons 1 to 37 years of age, with motor vehicle accidents accounting for 58.5% of the 292,763 fatalities that occurred between 1999 and 2006 in the United States.[4] This high rate of accidental deaths during the 1960s was compounded because, in most cases, ambulance services were inappropriately designed, ill equipped, and staffed with inadequately trained personnel; in fact, at least 50% of the nation's ambulance services were being provided by 12,000 morticians.[3] Accordingly, the report sparked the American health care system and Congress to address an injury epidemic that was then considered "the neglected epidemic of modern society" and "the nation's most important environmental health problem."

The *White Paper* report made 29 recommendations to improve out-of-hospital or prehospital care for injured patients; 11 of these were specifically related to the current EMS system. Congress responded to the report by establishing the National Highway Safety Act of 1966, which mandated the newly formed U.S. DOT, a subsidiary to the National Highway Traffic Safety Administration (NHTSA), to develop minimal standards for the provision of out-of-hospital care for accident victims, including program implementation and the development of standards for provider training. By 1969, the first recognized EMT training program was established.[2]

The 1970s saw significant growth in federal funding for the development of regional EMS agencies and the development of emergency medicine as a medical specialty. By 1980, there were four national categories of EMS certification levels: First Responder (most recently referred to as Emergency Medical Responder), EMT-Basic (EMT-B), EMT-Intermediate

(EMT-I), and EMT-Paramedic (EMT-P, or just Paramedic). However, since each state certifies or licenses its providers and may have additional requirements for each level, these 4 levels of emergency medical providers soon splintered into 38 state-specific levels of certification. Although each state justified its individual need for specificity, so many certification levels made reciprocity between states a nightmare for the emergency medical provider wishing to relocated to a new state. For example, several states allow an EMT-B to start an **intravenous (IV) line** at a scene. Other states allow the EMT-B to perform blind airway insertions with a device similar to a **CombiTube.** Furthermore, several states allowed **endotracheal intubation.** In addition, mainstream television has muddied the identity of these professionals, calling all EMS personnel "medics," very similar to what we as athletic trainers face with the term "trainer."

EMS therefore looked toward the various levels of defined nursing practice, that of Nurse Assistant (CNA), Practical Nurse (LPN), Registered Nurse (RN), and Nurse Practitioner (NP). EMS then followed a similar pattern and developed for the DOT–NHTSA an EMS scope of practice that included Emergency Medical Responder, Emergency Medical Technician, Advanced Emergency Medical Technician, and Paramedic. Each level of certification or licensure varies significantly in skills, practice environment, knowledge, qualifications, services provided, risk, and level of supervisory responsibility, autonomy, and judgment/critical thinking. Because recognizing the capability of EMS responders who may respond to an athletic event is absolutely critical to an athletic trainer, the detailed DOT–NHTSA scope-of-practice definitions for each level provider are discussed further on.

The EMS System Today

Today, EMS is an intricate system, with each component (community and medical resources) serving an essential role to coordinate a seamless system of emergency medical care for ill and injured individuals, including the athletes under the care of an athletic trainer. EMS providers, like certified athletic trainers responding to an athletic emergency, do not work in a vacuum or in isolation. Rather, the EMS system is an integrated system working with many other services and systems in order to maintain and enhance the health and safety of the community, operating between health care providers (e.g., certified athletic trainers) and public health and public safety (i.e., police and fire and rescue)[5] (Fig. 1.1).

According to the NHTSA Office of EMS, the mission of EMS is to "reduce death and disability by providing leadership and coordination to the EMS community in assessing, planning, developing, and promoting comprehensive, evidence-based emergency medical services and 911 systems."[6] Interestingly enough, given our technological age, the activation of EMS and its associated medical resources still relies on the public, as they are often the first to identify public health problems, issues, and emergencies.[5] The ability to identify public health problems, issues,

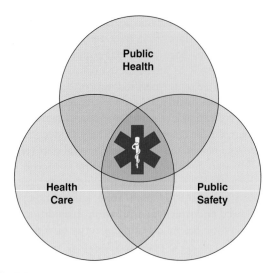

FIGURE 1.1   EMS as part of an integrated health care system.

and emergencies by the public often triggers the chain of survival, which is a series of events that, when implemented, increase the likelihood of survival for an ill or injured athlete and is an essential component of any successful EMS system (Fig. 1.2).

Chain of Survival

Recognition and Activation of EMS   Critical to this chain is the immediate recognition and initial care provided by a **citizen responder.** In the case of an athletic event or in the outpatient rehabilitation setting, the athletic trainer will typically be responsible for the recognition of said emergency. Depending upon the emergency action plan, the athletic trainer or a designated representative will then access EMS. Activation of EMS typically occurs through the use of the 911 (or another designated number in other communities), which connects the caller directly with an **emergency medical dispatcher** (EMD). An EMD is a professional telecommunicator responsible for gathering emergency medical information, dispatching EMS, and assisting the caller when necessary (Fig. 1.3). During this period, what is communicated to the EMD is critical. More information on this is presented further on.

Emergency Medical Responder   The next link in the chain of survival is first-responder care. This care is normally provided by the first person arriving on scene with medical training higher than that of a citizen responder, such as an

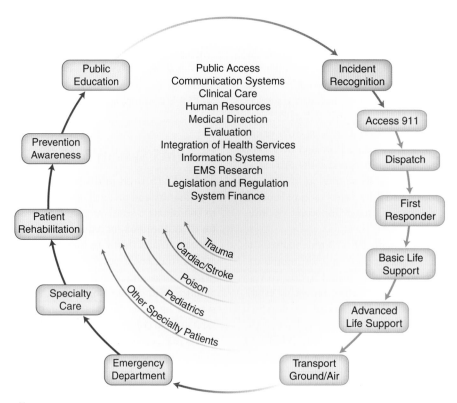

FIGURE 1.2   The Emergency Medical System. The large circle represents each system element as it is activated in response to an incident. The brown-arrowed elements within the circle represent the specialty care areas within EMS. The list within the circle represents the elements acting "behind the scenes" to support the system. In order to be "ready every day for every kind of emergency," an EMS system must be as comprehensive as the one pictured above. Developing and maintaining such a system requires thoughtful planning, preparation, and dedication from EMS stakeholders at the local, state, and federal levels.[5]

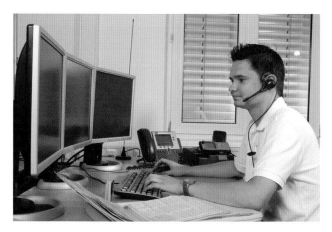

FIGURE 1.3 Emergency medical dispatcher.

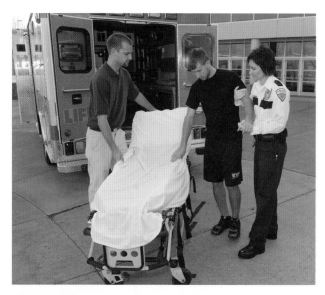

FIGURE 1.5 Athletic trainer working with EMS to package an injured athlete.

EMR. Again, in athletics or in the outpatient rehabilitation setting, the athletic trainer will normally fill this role, as he or she typically has a duty to act in the situation and normally has the required minimal equipment to provide such care (Fig. 1.4).

Advanced Out-of-Hospital Care   The arrival of EMS personnel at any level to provide out-of-hospital or prehospital care is the next link in the chain. The initial care provided at this time may be classified as **basic life support** (BLS) or **advanced life support** (ALS), depending on the training of the EMS personnel, structure of the EMS agency in the community, and the information provided to the EMD during activation of 911. Regardless of the level of training of the EMS personnel, their immediate role once on scene will be to reassess the athlete and begin and maintain appropriate care until the he or she can be packaged and transported to the hospital (Fig. 1.5).

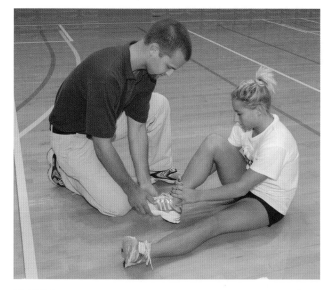

FIGURE 1.4 Athletic trainer as an emergency medical responder.

Hospital Care   Hospital care includes immediate care provided by emergency room physicians, nurses, x-ray technologists, and many other individuals. Their role is to provide care to stabilize the ill or injured athlete and determine what type of medical specialty, facility, or center is most appropriate for this individual. In some situations an athletic trainer will work directly with the hospital staff, particularly in situations requiring the removal of athletic equipment.

Rehabilitation and Prevention   The final step in the chain can be collapsed into athlete rehabilitation and prevention. These are two of the main functions of an athletic trainer. In these links, the athletic trainer's goal is to return the athlete to his or her preinjury/illness state in order to return to play or allow for a return to activities of daily living (Fig. 1.6). The goal is to also educate the individual and develop strategies to prevent a recurrence of the injury or illness. This is often accomplished using a team approach, which may involve other health care professionals such as an exercise physiologist, nutritionist, massage therapist, and physical therapist, to name just a few.

The unique difference between EMS and an athletic trainer is the degree of the athletic trainer's involvement in this chain of survival. Whereas EMS provides a critical link, athletic trainers have the unique opportunity to be involved in almost every facet of the chain. From recognition to assisting BLS to rehabilitation, athletic trainers must have a clear understanding of how each link in the chain of survival functions in order avoid professional conflicts and expedite the return to normal function of the athlete.

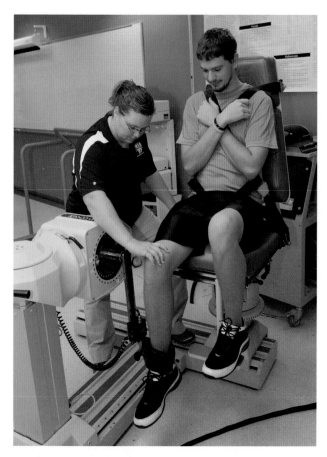

FIGURE 1.6   Athletic trainer rehabilitating an injured athlete.

EMS Program Administration

Finally, the EMS system, regardless of its location or structure, is evaluated based on 10 criteria established by the U.S. DOT–NHTSA. These 10 components are used primarily in administrating an EMS system and measuring the effectiveness of the existing and proposed EMS programs.

Breakout

The 10 standard components of an EMS system include the following:

1. Regulation and policy
2. Resource management
3. Human resources and training
4. Transportation equipment and systems
5. Medical and support facilities
6. Communications systems
7. Public information and education
8. Medical direction
9. Trauma system and development
10. Evaluation

EMS LEVELS OF PROFESSIONAL TRAINING

As a certified athletic trainer, you will often be the individual to recognize an incident (injury or illness) when working with athletes, activate EMS according to the emergency action plan, and assist EMS personal once they have arrived on scene. Activation and arrival of EMS does not mean that an athletic trainer should automatically relinquish care to the EMS personnel. Instead, both professionals should cooperate, playing to each other's scope of practice and strengths, to manage the emergency situation appropriately. To do this, athletic trainers must understand the scope of practice and capability of the four types of EMS responders (Table 1.1).

Emergency Medical Responder (EMR)

The EMR was formerly known as first responder. The primary focus of the EMR is to initiate immediate lifesaving

TABLE 1.1	Summary of EMS Personnel Professional Training	
Level	**Training**	**Function**
EMR	DOT lowest level of EMS training, requires 50–60 hours of training.	Initiates immediate lifesaving care with minimal equipment to critical patients who access the EMS system.
EMT	Next to last level of DOT EMS training, requires 120+ hours of training.	Provides basic emergency medical care and transportation for critical and emergent patients who access the EMS system.
AEMT	Next to highest level of the DOT EMS training, requires 300–400 hours of training.	Provides basic and limited advanced emergency medical care and transportation for the critical and emergent patient who accesses the EMS system.
Paramedic	DOT Highest level of EMS training, requires 1,000–1,500 hours of training.	Possesses the complex knowledge and skills necessary to provide patient care and transportation using basic and advanced equipment for the critical patient who accesses the EMS system.

DOT = Department of Transportation.

care to critically injured patients who access the EMS system.[7] This individual (e.g., police, firefighters, lifeguards, athletic trainers, ski patrollers, industrial response team members) possesses the basic knowledge and skills necessary to provide lifesaving interventions while awaiting additional EMS response and to assist higher-level EMS personnel at the scene as well as to perform basic interventions with minimal equipment. They function as part of a comprehensive EMS response team and require medical oversight. One eligibility requirement for licensure at this level is successful completion of an accredited EMR training program[8] offered by organizations such as the American Red Cross (Washington, DC) or individual state offices of EMS. An athletic trainer can expect an EMR to perform skills related to airway and breathing emergencies, pharmacological intervention, and medical and trauma care. However, many athletic trainers, based on their level of training and scope of practice (as defined by individual states), can provide the same level of care as an EMR. In some cases, additional training may be required.

Breakout

Psychomotor Skills of an EMR

Airway and breathing emergencies	○ Insertion of the oropharygeal airway (OPA) or nasopharygeal airway (NPA).
	○ Use of positive-pressure ventilation device such as a bag-valve-mask (BVM).
	○ Ability to suction the upper airway using manual suction devices.
	○ Provide supplemental oxygen therapy (via cannula, resuscitation mask, BVM, nonrebreather mask).
Pharmacological interventions	○ Administer "patient assist" or over-the-counter medications with appropriate medical oversight, including:
	○ Unit dose autoinjectors for the administration of lifesaving medications intended for self or peer rescue in hazardous situations (e.g., Epi-Pen, MARK I, etc.)
	○ Metered dose-inhaler for the administration during respiratory distress, particularly during an asthma attack
	○ Oral glucose for the administration for a hypoglycemic athlete
Medical/cardiac care	○ Competent usage of an AED
Trauma care	○ Manual stabilization of suspected cervical spine injury
	○ Manual stabilization of extremity
	○ Bleeding control
	○ Emergency (rescue) moves

EMRs can be of great assistance under the direction of a higher medical authority. An athletic trainer should remember that this level of EMS provider care *does not* provide "back of the ambulance" care, such as transportation of the ill or injured. This is the function of an EMT. It should also be noted that even though an athletic trainer may consider himself or herself an EMR, because the skills of an EMR and certified athletic trainer are very similar, some states in fact do regulate the scope of practice and require certification or licensure to practice as an EMR. Athletic trainers may therefore have to refrain from using this title until he or she meets the certification or licensure requirements of state where he or she works.

Emergency Medical Technician (EMT)

The EMT was formerly known as the emergency medical technician–basic. The primary focus of the EMT is to provide basic emergency medical care and transportation for critical and emergent patients who access the emergency medical system.[7] This individual possesses the basic knowledge and skills necessary to provide patient care and transportation. EMTs perform interventions with the basic equipment typically found on an ambulance (i.e., patient litter [gurney], oral and nasopharyngeal airways, electric suction, bag-valve-mask device, and medical oxygen).

Eligibility requirements for licensure at this level include successful completion of an accredited EMT course, normally offered as a college/university class or through the local EMS system.

Breakout

Psychomotor Motor Skills of an EMT

Airway and breathing	○ Use of positive-pressure ventilation devices such as manually triggered ventilators or automatic transport ventilators
	○ Ability to suction the upper airway using mechanical suction devices
Pharmacological interventions	○ Administer "patient assist" or over-the-counter medications with appropriate medical oversight, including:
	○ Aspirin for chest pain of ischemic origin
	○ Activated charcoal for poisonings
	○ Nitroglycerine for chest pain
Trauma care	○ Application and inflation of the pneumatic antishock garment (PSAG) for fracture stabilization or hypoperfusion
	○ Application of a traction splint for stabilization of a femoral fracture
	○ Application of a short board for immobilizing an athlete in a seated position

The EMT is a link from the scene to the emergency health care system and should have the final say on how the athlete should be transported.[9] Since all EMS personnel levels "build" upon the one previous, an athletic trainer can expect performance of these *additional* skills by an EMT.

As a general rule throughout the nation, all ambulances making emergency response calls will have at least one EMT to provide patient care at the scene and en route to the hospital. EMTs make up the largest group of EMS providers in the nation.

Advanced Emergency Medical Technician (AEMT)

The AEMT was formerly known as the emergency medical technician–intermediate. The primary focus of the AEMT is to provide basic and *limited* advanced emergency medical care and transportation for the critical and emergent patient who accesses the EMS.[7] Like EMRs and EMTs, AEMTs function as part of a comprehensive EMS response team under medical oversight and may be requested by on-scene EMTs depending upon the status of the athlete. AEMTs perform interventions with the basic and advanced equipment (e.g., vital sign monitoring equipment and glucometer) typically found on an ambulance.

Eligibility requirements for licensure at this level include successful completion of an accredited EMT course, normally offered as a college/university class or through the local EMS system.

The AEMT is also a link from the scene to the emergency health care system. AEMTs perform lower-risk, high-benefit advanced skills that can be performed safely in an out-of-hospital setting with medical oversight and limited training. As stated above, all EMS personnel levels "build" upon the one previous; thus an athletic trainer can expect performance of these *additional* skills by an AEMT.

The AEMT can be of significant value to the athletic trainer in an emergency situation. A person with this level of EMS training is fully capable of handling an athlete suffering from sudden cardiac arrest. In the event of exercise-induced asthma (EIA), **hypoglycemia,** severe dehydration, and the need for pain management from injury, early scene intervention by an AEMT can make a huge difference in patient outcomes.

Paramedic

The paramedic was formerly known as the emergency medical technician–paramedic. Today's paramedic is an allied health professional (often with an associate's degree) whose primary focus is to provide advanced emergency medical care for critical and emergent patients who access EMS.[7] This individual possesses the complex knowledge and skills necessary to provide patient care and transportation. Paramedics function as part of a comprehensive EMS response team under medical oversight. Paramedics perform interventions with the basic and advanced equipment (e.g., laryngoscopes and bone IV insertion) typically found on an ambulance (Fig. 1.7).

Breakout

Psychomotor Motor Skills of an Advanced EMT

Airway and breathing	◦ Insertion of airways *not* intended to be placed in the trachea (i.e., CombiTube, King, and pharyngeal-tracheal lumen [PTL]) ◦ **Tracheobronchial** suctioning of an already **intubated** patient
Assessment	◦ Utilizes enhanced techniques, such as evaluating lung sounds, using vital sign monitoring equipment and glucometer
Pharmacological interventions	◦ Establishes and maintain peripheral intravenous (IV) access ◦ Establishes and maintain **intraosseous** (IO) access in a pediatric patient ◦ Administers nonmedicated IV fluid therapy ◦ Administers **sublingual** nitroglycerine to a patient with chest pain of ischemic origin ◦ Administers subcutaneous or intramuscular epinephrine to a patient in anaphylaxis ◦ Administers oral glucose to a hypoglycemic patient ◦ Administers intravenous dextrose 50% (D50) to a hypoglycemic patient ◦ Administers metered-dose inhaler to a patient with difficulty breathing or wheezing ◦ Administers a narcotic antagonist to a patient suspected of narcotic overdose ◦ Administers nitrous oxide for pain relief

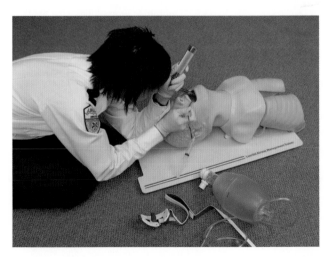

FIGURE 1.7 Psychomotor skills of a paramedic.

Breakout

Psychomotor Motor Skills of a Paramedic

Airway and breathing	○ Performs **endotracheal (ET) intubation**
	○ Performs **percutaneous cricothyrotomy**
	○ Inserts a **laryngoscope**
	○ Uses a crycothyrotomy set to perform a **cricothyrotomy**
	○ Decompresses the pleural space
	○ Performs gastric decompression
Pharmacological interventions	○ Inserts intraosseous (IO) catheters
	○ Competently operates a manual external defibrillator (MED) vs. an automated external defibrillator (AED)
	○ Administers approved **enteral** and **parenteral** prescription medications (varies by agency, nominally 25–35 different medications)
	○ Accesses indwelling catheters and implanted central IV ports for the administration of fluids and medications
	○ Administers medication by IV infusion
	○ Maintains an infusion of blood and blood products
Medical/cardiac care	○ Performs **cardioversion**, manual defibrillation, and transcutaneous pacing
	○ Inserts a bone (IV) insertion device
	○ Performs gastric decompression using a **nasogastric** (NG) tube

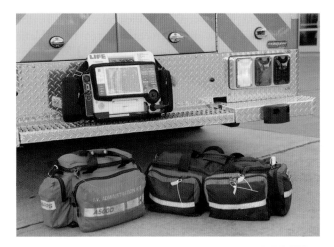

FIGURE 1.8 Paramedic emergency response equipment.

Eligibility requirements for licensure at this level are extremely rigorous, often including successful completion of a nationally accredited paramedic program at the certificate or associate's degree level, owing to the extensive, complex decision-making and emergency skills required.

The paramedic is the final and most qualified link from the scene to the EMS system. As with other level of EMS training, the paramedic's skills "build" upon the one previous; thus an athletic trainer can expect performance of these additional skills by a paramedic.

The paramedic is the highest-level EMS provider and has a very ample tool box to bring to the athletic event (Fig. 1.8). Most paramedic-level agencies allow the use of analgesics such as morphine, fentanyl, and nitrous oxide. Additionally, many agencies carry a steroid such as methyprednisolone, which could be advantageous as a treatment option for spinal cord injuries.[10–13] Since the medications carried by individual EMS agencies may vary greatly, athletic trainers and their team physicians should ask for a medication list or set of treatment protocols as part of pre-event collaboration to establish what will be on site during an emergency.

MEDICAL OVERSIGHT

The explanation, above, of the different levels of EMS providers, employs the term "medical oversight." Throughout the nation, medical oversight for prehospital emergency responders is provided by a duly licensed physician who directs the care given by out-of-hospital providers to ill or injured athletes. These physicians give direction to EMS providers using both on- and offline procedures. This is similar to many athletic training practice acts that require a certified athletic trainer to be overseen by a qualified medical provider, normally a medical doctor or in some cases a dentist.

In **online (direct) medical direction,** an EMS provider is able to contact medical command and discuss the situation at hand in real time. Real-time discussions are normally accomplished by two-way radios and portable phones. Perhaps in the future, online medical direction will include text messaging. With online medical control, the athletic trainer may be able to speak with a physician if required.

Offline (indirect) medical direction is provided using treatment **protocols** and **standing orders.** Treatment protocols are written guidelines that that define the scope of prehospital care for an EMS provider. These protocols are usually developed by an advisory group and EMS medical director. An EMS provider must follow the protocols unless advised otherwise by online medical direction. Standing orders are more specific than protocols and can be quite detailed by procedure. They provide the "safety net" to the ALS provider in the event that online communications should fail.

The athletic trainer should recognize that EMS providers cannot deviate from treatment protocols or standing orders without permission from medical control. In the event that there is a disagreement between the athletic trainer and the local EMS personnel, the local EMS protocols and standing orders will typically "trump" any decision unless online medical control is contracted. In the event that medical disagreement becomes disorderly, law officers are instructed to support and protect local EMS personnel and protocols. Thus, proper planning and a cooperative understanding of each profession's scope of practice, protocols, and standing orders is warranted.

UNDERSTANDING THE EMS AGENCIES

Now that we've discussed the various personnel levels that may respond to an ill or injured athlete, a review of the structure under which these personnel work is in order. Throughout the country there tend to be four basic EMS agency models that have their own unique characteristics and idiosyncrasies. These models include (a) volunteer, (b) public services (police and fire), (c) other governmental services, and (d) private for-profit agencies (Table 1.2).

Volunteer EMS Agencies

Volunteer EMS agencies are very prevalent throughout the nation, particularly in small towns and rural communities. Trained and certified just as the fully paid organizations are, volunteer agencies tend to respond to lower volumes of emergency calls and are a cost-effective way for communities to have locally based EMS.

The staffing makeup of volunteer EMS services has both advantages and disadvantages. Volunteer agencies may include AEMTs and paramedics, but typically they are primarily staffed by EMTs. Most volunteer agencies respond using pager-type systems; thus response times to the scene can vary greatly as compared with those of a public agency.

However, volunteer agencies, because of strong community pride, are often willing to "sit standby" at an athletic event for no compensation or only a nominal donation. In

the event of an illness or injury, this can be a significant time saver for the athletic trainer, resulting in decreased time to transport. It is also an excellent public relations tool for the community as well as the athletic trainer. This type of relationship helps to open the line of communication between professionals (EMS and athletic trainers) and may allow a greater level of professional cooperation and mutual understanding of each other's scope of practice. The two major disadvantages of a volunteer EMS standby is that, in a small community, the crew may know or, worse yet, be related to an ill or injured athlete; also, in some cases, they may be unavailable for a period of time when they are responding to another call.

All things considered, if a volunteer group offers to sit standby at your event, collaborate with the crew and accept this as a true bonus.

Public EMS Agencies

The second most prevalent type of EMS agency structure tends to be the public services sector, most often the fire service or police/sheriff organization. Although law enforcement EMS is a very small segment in the nation overall, the full-time, paid fire agencies have assumed provision of EMS services in larger towns and cities. Fire service agencies are almost always staffed with EMTs, and a large number of communities have "gone ALS" and have one or more AEMTs or paramedics on all response vehicles. Fire service–based EMS response may include an EMS fire apparatus (no transport capability), ambulance, or paramedic quick response vehicle. These vehicles tend to be placed in fixed fire stations.

The upside to this system is that paid responders are ready to respond quickly; the downside is they have to be summoned and respond to the emergency situation. Depending upon other system needs at the time of the call, you may not get the vehicle from the geographically closest station. Since every fire-based system in the nation has individual variations of standard operating procedure, it is not practical to discuss them in this chapter. However, the athletic trainer is encouraged to make contact with the

TABLE 1.2	Summary of EMS Agencies
Volunteer	Comprises members of the local community; tends to be staffed mostly by EMTs.
Public service	Tends to be the public services sector, most often the fire service or police/sheriff organizations. Staffed by EMTs, with most communities having one or more AEMTs or paramedics to provide ALS.
"Other government" model	The public utility model EMS system is designed for situations where the government regulates and oversees system performance and contractors are held accountable to meet or exceed performance requirements under penalty of removal and the possible imposition of fines. Performance contracts are generally very strict in terms of response times to critical calls.
Private	For-profit organizations. Staffed using a mixed crew of two EMTs and/or one EMT and an AEMT and/or paramedic.

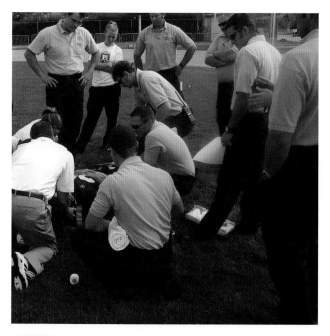

FIGURE 1.9   Pre-event meeting to review policies and procedures.

EMS captain or chief and discuss and establish policy and procedure guidelines for the management of the ill or injured athlete. To alleviate any conflicts during an emergency situation between the athletic trainer and EMS system, yearly training should be conducted to review the policies and procedural guidelines, protocols, and standing orders; familiarize the crew with the facility; and establish a personal relationship with the crews (Fig. 1.9). Depending upon its resources, a fire agency may dedicate a transport or nontransport EMS unit to an event (generally for a fee), assign an EMS unit to an event subject to call, or respond under 911 response request only.

"Other Government" Model

Similar to the public service model is the "other government" model. This has typically been called the "third service" version, because police and fire are considered the first and second public services in a community. Like fire agencies, third service agencies are supported though governmental funding and tend to hire full-time employees. Sometimes a government body will contract with a private agency under a stringent franchise agreement to provide EMS services.

Although both public service and governmental services utilize full-time employees, there tend to be significant differences. Whereas fire agencies tend to work out of fixed stations, there is a greater tendency for third services to use system status management. System status management uses computer projections to move an EMS vehicle to an opportune location based on previous call history and time of day. Although this system is extremely effective in reducing call times, if the dispatch center is unaware of an athletic event,

it could mean that the geographically closest vehicle may not be dispatched, since historically no calls occur at the stadium 99% of the year.

EMS staffing for third service agencies (governmental) is variable and is dependent upon the needs (and pocketbook) of the community. For the most part, EMS responds in ambulances that may have a mixed crew of two EMTs and/or one EMT and an AEMT and/or paramedic. Many agencies place two paramedics on each ambulance. As in the case of the fire model discussed above, the athletic trainer should discuss event needs with the EMS agency manager or supervisor. Depending upon resources at these agencies, the EMS agency may be able to dedicate an EMS unit to an athletic event, assign an EMS unit at your athletic event subject to call, or send a unit under 911 response request only.

Private Agencies

The last agency type is private. Needless to say, the bottom line of a private agency is to at least break even and hopefully make a profit. That being said, do not assume that private agencies skimp on vehicles, equipment, personnel, and procedures. In fact, many private agencies are leaders in EMS since they can maneuver more quickly and are less restricted than government-based organizations. Many private EMS providers have achieved national accreditation.

Almost all private industry responses are in ambulances that may have a mixed crew of two EMTs and/or one EMT and an AEMT and/or paramedic. Many private agencies also place two paramedics on each ambulance. Private EMS agencies vary greatly as to what they can provide to an athletic event and at what cost. As in the case of the fire and other government models discussed above, the athletic trainer should clarify event needs with the EMS agency's corporate manager or operations supervisor and establish policy and procedure guidelines for the management of the ill or injured athlete. To alleviate any conflicts between the athletic trainer and EMS system during an emergency situation, yearly training should occur to review the above policy and procedure guidelines, familiarize the crews with the facility, and establish a personal relationship with the crews. As stated previously, private agencies may dedicate an EMS unit to an athletic event (most likely with a charge), assign an EMS unit at your athletic event subject to call, or send a unit under 911 response request only.

ACTIVATION OF EMS

As discussed, EMS in the United States tends to be provided using four models: volunteer, public service (police and fire), other governmental, and private. All models will respond to a 911 emergent request, no questions asked; however, the greatest variation occurs as to the availability of or willingness to provide "dedicated, on-field" standby coverage.

With operator-assisted telephone service yielding to dialing in the late 1950s, numerous emergency phone numbers came into play. This situation was confusing for both local residents and travelers because it was difficult to remember multiple seven-digit phone numbers. In 1968, American Telephone and Telegraph (AT&T) borrowed from the Canadian system and spearheaded 911 as the national emergency phone number. Nearing the 1980s, enhanced 911 (E-911) was created. Thus, when someone dialed 911, a physical address was automatically associated with the calling party's telephone number and then routed the call to the most appropriate Public Safety Answering Point (PSAP) for that address. Additionally, the caller's address and information was displayed to the PSAP call taker immediately upon call arrival.

It should be noted that cell phones, voice-over Internet protocol (VOIP), iPhones, Blackberries, and so on are not physically connected (hard-wired) to the E-911 system. Although calls made from these devices *will* reach a 911 call center, they may not reach the closest or correct municipality. Additionally, physical addresses will not be computed but may be represented as a GPS location based on call triangulation. Should you fail to connect to the correct 911 center (PSAP), **stay on the line,** as you will be transferred to the correct location. Wireless communication poses a vexing problem to the Federal Communications Commission (FCC), which is currently being addressed.

On-Field Standby Coverage

"On-field standby" coverage should certainly be the gold standard. Every second an athlete lies on a field or court may seem like a minute to the spectators but feels like an hour to the athlete.

Within all reasonable considerations, including but not limited to financial resources, event managers and athletic trainers should strive for the gold standard of on-field standby coverage, particularly for high-risk athletic events

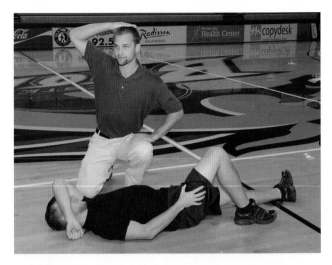

FIGURE 1.10   On-field communication signal with EMS.

such as football, ice hockey, and rugby. On-field EMS coverage allows for a response time of less than 30 to 60 seconds[14] in the event of an emergency.

When on-field standby coverage is utilized, it is imperative for the athletic trainer to establish a line of communication—a mechanism to activate EMS—and determine who exactly should be on the field during an injury or illness. Not every injury or illness will require the activation of EMS. In fact, if EMS were to walk onto the field or court for every injury or illness, administrators, coaches, athletes, and spectators might begin to question the role and competence of athletic trainers. However, when a genuine emergency situation occurs, a simple hand to the head (Fig. 1.10) should be all that is necessary to activate standby EMS coverage.

Traditional Activation of EMS

Although on-field EMS standby should be the gold standard, particularly for high-risk athletic contests, the reality is that this does not occur regularly. Activation of EMS

Highlight

"Golden Hour" and "Platinum 10"

Dr. R. Adams Cowley, through painstaking work, recognized that definitive surgical care had to be delivered quickly, generally within an hour. He has been quoted as saying, "There is a 'golden hour' between life and death. If you are critically injured you have less than 60 minutes to survive. You might not die right then; it may be three days or two weeks later—but something has happened in your body that is irreparable." The U.S. military and trauma centers around the world have embraced this concept for nearly 40 years.

With their strong embrace of the "golden hour" concept, EMS providers had to find a way to operate more efficiently during the first 30 minutes after an incident. In the average urban environment, EMS arrives on the scene in 8 to 10 minutes, with transport time to a medical facility also being 8 to 10 minutes. In doing the math, that leaves approximately 10 minutes for scene time. Thus, out of the golden hour, the "platinum 10" is the maximum amount of time the EMS team should normally be at a trauma scene. From this genesis, the term "load and go" supplanted "stay and play."

normally occurs through the use of the local 911 or EMS system (check your local area to determine how EMS is actually contacted), which connects the caller directly with an EMD. **What you communicate to the 911 dispatcher regarding the incident is critical!**

It is very common for EMS dispatch services to utilize a concept of "priority reference dispatch protocol." Similar to the system status management of ambulances, covered above, the EMD, using carefully scripted questions, determines what type of EMS response is needed and/or is available. If the scripted questions are answered in a very basic manner, a standard ambulance with two EMTs may be displaced to the emergency. If the questions are answered with attention to **criticality** (i.e., quality, state, or degree of being of the highest importance), the caller will receive a "higher" level of response including AEMTs and paramedics.

Although we do not advocate jimmying the system, sprinkling key words of criticality, such as "chest pain," "suspected paralysis," or "difficulty breathing" most likely will garner higher-level EMS personnel including AEMTs or paramedics. In some systems, 911 dispatch is authorized to place an aeromedical helicopter (see below) on standby based upon the dispatch protocol.

Although it is assumed that most athletic events will be held within reasonable proximity to a community medical facility, the type and level of specialized care provided at such facilities may vary greatly. Most community hospitals are capable of handling extremity trauma and standard medical issues such as dehydration, diabetes, and respiratory or cardiac emergencies. However, in the event of spinal cord or head injury or other significant trauma or medical illness, a specialty or tertiary care facility may be in the best

---

Highlight

Land-Zone Procedures in Working with an Aeromedical Helicopter

Safety

Call helicopter through the appropriate agency with the following information:

- **Location:** Cross streets, LAT/LONG coordinates, and prominent features.
- **Communication:** Call-back number, radio frequency (statewide, etc.), and call sign of landing zone (LZ) command. Designate one person to coordinate, set up, and communicate.
- **Weather:** Low ceilings, poor visibility, icing, high wind.
- **Patient status:** Number, condition, age, mechanism, hazards.
- **Landing zone:** The preferred LZ is 100 by 100 feet.

Setup

Set up the landing zone as follows:

- **Size:** 100 by 100 feet.
- **Level:** Select a landing area as level as possible (minimal slope).
- **Landing surface:** Hard surface, grassy, hard-packed snow (avoid loose dirt, dust, power snow).
- **Clear overhead:** Free of overhead obstructions (wires, antennas, poles).
- **Clear area:** Area is clear of debris, large rocks, posts, stumps, vehicles, people, animals, and other hazards.
- **Mark area:** Clearly mark using five weighted cones, flares, or beacons: one at each corner of the LZ and one on the side that the wind is coming from.
- **Select alternate landing zone:** Plan for alternate LZs (pilot may determine LZ to be unsafe).
- **Hazardous materials (HAZMAT):** Always inform pilot and medical crew of HAZMAT. In selecting a LZ, find a site at least 1/4 to 1 mile *upwind* from the accident, depending on the type and amount of materials involved. Avoid low areas where vapors may collect. Patient must be removed from the hot zone. All patients must be decontaminated *prior* to flight.

Other Issues

The following must be considered when determining and working with an **aeromedical landing zone:**

- Maintain radio contact at all times until helicopter has landed, loaded, and departed the area.
- Approach angles over obstacles should be less than 20 degrees.
- Always keep landing zone clear of people and other potential hazards.
- Approach from 3 and 9 o'clock positions only (side of helicopter).
- Night landing zones always require good communications, lighting, and alertness.
- Set up night landing zone with five flares or other secured lights. One flare should be on the side that the wind is coming from.
- If no flares are available, mark with strobes or other light systems.
- If no other portable lights are available, cross headlight beams into the wind at the center.

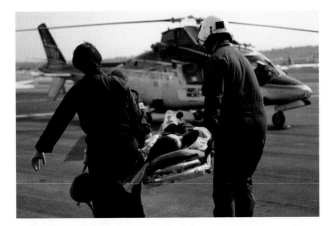

FIGURE 1.11   Aeromedical helicopter.

interest of the injured athlete. The major issue for the athletic trainer is to ascertain the name of the facility, distance to that facility, and available options for transportation to the facility.

This is why making contact with the local EMS system and receiving facility is imperative, as it allows the athletic trainer to ask questions such as the following:

- What are the normal protocols for spinal cord or head injury?
- Do they transport to the local medical facility and then arrange for retransport by ground or helicopter ambulance?
- Do they make a direct ground transport run to the specialty facility?
- Do they have a helicopter respond to the scene and transport directly to the specialty facility?

Since there are numerous variations to specialty care transport, these issues should be fleshed out prior to the event and any potential injury.

Aeromedical EMS

As discussed previously, on-field EMS standby should be the gold standard. Aeromedical helicopters (Fig. 1.11) are often aligned with large medical centers and have names and logos prominently emblazoned on them. If an athletic event is large and has significant media coverage, some aeromedical providers may consider redeploying a "ship" to your location if the location has space for the flight to land. It doesn't hurt to ask!

ON-FIELD PHYSICIANS AND EMS

The last area to explore is the concept of "physicians on the field." EMS personnel will tell you that this is either a blessing or a curse. Physicians on the field may be part of the

sports medicine medical staff responsible for the health and welfare of the athletes or, worse yet, a "Good Samaritan" who comes out of the stands.

Sports Medicine Physician

As a member of the sports medicine medical staff, a physician (depending on medical specialty) is usually a blessing (Fig. 1.12). This type of physician normally has a vested interest in the program and has assisted the athletic trainer in developing a chain of command in emergency situations, established and defined a working relationship with the EMS system and the athletic trainer, planned and trained with the EMS system and athletic trainer for emergencies during games and practices, and can provide medical oversight for clinical policies and procedures that may arise during an emergency (e.g., concussion management, sudden cardiac arrest, transport decision).[15] The law in most states allows a duly licensed physician *of that state* to assume and direct patient care at the scene with one important caveat: once such a physician has assumed responsibility, *he or she must accompany the patient and EMS to the hospital.*

Certainly, having a preplanned physician on location is preferable, but remember—the physician in question **must** be licensed to practice medicine in the state of the event. EMS personnel, particularly AEMTs and paramedics, are generally not authorized to accept medical orders from physicians licensed out of state. Should the visiting team physician be from out of state, preplanning with the in-state physician will allow him or her to review what medications may be available based on local protocol and to work collaboratively with the in-state physician endorsing the medical orders to the EMS personnel. Again, the key here is pre-event planning and communication with all involved parties.

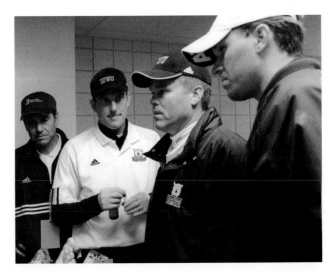

FIGURE 1.12   Developing a positive relationship with the team physician.

Other Physicians

There are two worst-case scenarios we must now discuss. First, if an unknown physician shows up unannounced and second, if the physician is a relative. When a physician or "doctor" shows up unannounced, an element of chaos has been injected to the situation. Coaches, athletic trainers, and EMS personnel have now lost the preplanning time to check licensure and medical specialty training. Without prior vetting, it is hard to gauge the emergency care capability of a dermatologist or proctologist, let alone a dentist or veterinarian. Strange things can and *do* happen on EMS calls! In this situation it is best for the EMS personnel and athletic trainer to work cooperatively to minimize the activities of these Good Samaritans and to implement the already established and rehearsed emergency action plan.

The second case arises when a physician or other medical personnel related to a player arrives on the filed or sideline. This creates a very delicate situation. It is widely known in the medical community that emotional involvement with the situation does not always make for sound decision making, especially during a crisis. Most EMS personnel will not accept any type of medical orders or directives from a relative other than a parent. However, to make lemonade out of lemons, medical information obtained from these medical providers can be an asset.

The best way to handle this situation is to respect the reported medical background of such individuals but keep them in bystander status. You may have to use escalating tactics to keep intrusions down to a minimum, such as starting with a simple "please step back" to asking a uniformed officer to intervene. Public relations considerations are key! Although your first duty and that of the EMS personnel is to help the athlete, remember that there is an audience watching that may not understand what is happening on the field or sidelines with an emotional relative.

THE ATHLETIC TRAINER AS PART OF THE EMS SYSTEM

The majority of this chapter up to this point has focused extensively on the EMS system, particularly the history, levels of provider training, types of agencies, and activation of EMS. The question you are probably asking is why? How does this benefit me as an athletic trainer? Why do I need to understand the EMS system? The answer is simple: without EMS, we would be unable to stabilize and transport critically ill or injured athletes, and all too often we fail to address the impact EMS has as part of an athlete's advanced out-of-hospital care and as a member of the sports medicine health care team.

We now change our focus and examine how the athletic trainer functions as part of the EMS system. Specifically, we address the professional behaviors, characteristics, scope of practice, and roles and responsibilities of an athletic trainer in dealing with an emergency injury or illness.

Professional Behaviors, Characteristics, Scope of Practice, and Responsibilities

As alluded to throughout this chapter, athletic trainers play a critical role in the increasing the likelihood of survival during an emergent emergency situation. And although an athletic trainer may not be certified or licensed as an EMR, his or her scope of practice as defined by the *Board of Certification Role Delineation Study*[1] and/or state practice act(s) allows many athletic trainers function in a similar capacity. Thus, athletic trainers do share many of the same personal characteristics and professional roles and responsibilities as EMS personnel.

Professional Behaviors and Characteristics

Emergency situations do not occur when no one is looking and many athletes do interact with athletic trainers during an emergency. Therefore, an athletic trainer's professional behaviors and characteristics often influence the how athletes and other health care professionals perceive us as allied health care providers. These professional behaviors and characteristics have been adapted from the foundational behaviors outlined by the *Foundation of Professional Behaviors* found in the Athletic Training Educational Competencies, 4th ed,[16] and includes the following:

1. *Primacy of the athlete:* In emergency situations, the athlete should be the primary focus of the athletic trainer. This is not the time for personal or professional conflicts with EMS personnel; rather this should be a time when the best available health care should be available for the athlete. This is also the time when an athletic trainer may need to be the advocate for his or her athlete, ensuring that a certain level of care is provided by the most qualified individual(s).

2. *Team approach to practice:* Athletic trainers and EMS personnel must begin to dialogue and interact prior to an emergency situation in order to recognize their respective, unique skills and abilities and understand each other's scope of practice (Fig. 1.13). Being able to "take charge" of an emergency situations is a personal quality required of an athletic trainer. However, once EMS personnel arrives, these different health care providers must work together seamlessly. This helps to reduce an individual's anxiety and fears during an emergency situation and allows all parties to maintain the highest standard of athlete care,[17] thus ensuring positive athlete outcomes.

3. *Legal practice:* Athletic trainers must demonstrate the ability to practice athletic training competently and ensure an optimal level of fundamental emergency care to an ill or injured athlete while adhering to the specific

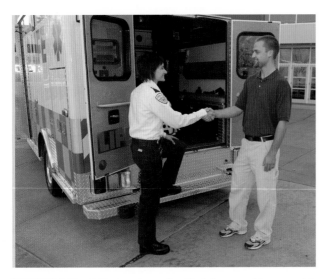

FIGURE 1.13 Athletic trainers should dialogue and interact with EMS before the event to understand each other's scope of practice.

guidelines associated with one's scope of practice. Performing emergency techniques or skills outside of one's scope of practice not only puts the athletic trainer at risk for legal actions but, more importantly, also places the athletic trainer ahead of the needs of his or her athlete, thereby jeopardizing the administration of necessary lifesaving care.

4. *Advancing knowledge:* Emergency medicine is constantly evolving, and remaining up to date on the body of knowledge is critical. This serves not only to maintain the highest standard of care but also to demonstrate to other health care providers that athletic trainers are competent in this regard. The foundation for best practice is the use of evidence-based medicine.

5. *Cultural competence:* Athletic trainers work with diverse patient populations, and advanced-out-of-hospital providers may also demonstrate such diversity. This takes a variety of forms, including emergency medicine philosophies. Thus, athletic trainers must demonstrate knowledge, attitudes (pleasant demeanor), behaviors (a certain level of self-confidence, desire to work with people, emotional stability), and skill to achieve optimal athlete outcomes and positive working relationships.

6. *Professionalism:* The remaining behaviors and characteristics fall under the heading of professionalism. Athletic trainers must be able to demonstrate a certain level of honesty and integrity in interacting with EMS personnel and athletes. When interacting specifically with athletes during an emergency, controlling one's fears, remaining physically and mentally fit, exhibiting compassion and empathy, and maintaining a professional appearance are all skills aimed at achieving optimal athlete outcomes. In interacting specifically with EMS personnel, being able to demonstrate effective interpersonal communication skills is essential.

Breakout

At the time of printing of this text, athletic trainers were working under the performance domains outlined by the BOC Role Delineation 5th Edition. However, the BOC is currently working on validating the sixth edition of Role Delineation, which will be in effect from 2011 to 2016. Therefore, in 2011, be sure to visit the BOC's website for an updated statement outlining the role of the athletic trainer as it relates to immediate medical care.

Scope of Practice and Professional Responsibilities

Athletic trainers are typically responsible for all phases of an athlete's health care. This includes (a) prevention of injuries and illness; (b) clinical evaluation and diagnosis; (c) immediate care; (d) treatment, rehabilitation, and reconditioning; (e) organization and administration; and (f) professional development. The roles and responsibilities or scope of practice of an athletic trainer is defined by the *Board of Certification Role Delineation Study*, 5th edition (BOC study),[1] state practice act(s) (which may trump the BOC study), and, in certain situations, an individual's practice setting.

Scope of Practice Performance Domain III of the BOC study outlines the knowledge and skills needed by an athletic trainer to provide immediate care in an emergency injury or illness situation independent of the athletic trainer's practice setting. The current scope of practice as defined by the BOC study is divided into five specific task statements with multiple knowledge of (cognitive) and skill in (psychomotor) statements.

It should be noted that 48 of the 50 states do have some form of regulation (i.e., licensure, certification, or registration) that governs the practice of athletic training.

The task statements are as follows:

1. Employ lifesaving techniques through the use of standard emergency procedures in order to reduce morbidity and the incidence of mortality.
   a. Athletic trainers must demonstrate knowledge of items such as normal and compromised human anatomy and physiology, common life-threatening medical situation, appropriate management techniques for life-threatening conditions, emergency action plans, federal and state occupational, safety, and health guidelines, standard protective equipment and removal devices and procedures, and appropriate use of emergency equipment and techniques (e.g., AED, CPR masks, and BP cuff).
   b. Athletic trainers must demonstrate skills in implementing emergency action plan(s), performing CPR techniques and procedures, removing protective equipment and using removal devices, using emergency equipment, implementing immobilization and

Breakout

According to the BOC, "State law delineates the scope of practice and requirements for the legal practice of athletic training. Scope of practice can vary from state to state. State regulation always takes precedence over certification standards."[21] And although many states have used the BOC studies in establishing the specific scope of practice of the athletic trainer, regulations can and do vary from state to state. Therefore, prior to beginning any employment as an athletic trainer, you would be prudent to contact the regulatory agency of the state in which you intend to practice. A listing of these agencies can be found on the BOC's website by doing a web search using the URL search phrase "Board of Certification, Inc.—State Regulatory Agencies."

transfer techniques, managing common life-threatening emergency situations/conditions, transferring care to appropriate medical and/or allied health professionals and/or facilities, measuring and monitoring vital signs.

2. Prevent exacerbation of non–life-threatening condition(s) through the use of standard procedures in order to reduce morbidity.
   a. Athletic trainers must demonstrate knowledge of items such as normal and compromised human anatomy and physiology, common non–life-threatening medical situations, appropriate management techniques for non–life-threatening conditions, emergency action plans, federal and state occupational, safety and health guidelines, standard protective equipment and removal devices and procedures, and pharmacological and therapeutic modality usage for acute conditions.
   b. Athletic trainers must demonstrate skills in implementing emergency action plan(s), using standard medical and emergency equipment, removing protective equipment and using removal devices, implementing immobilization and transfer techniques, managing common non–life-threatening emergency situations/conditions, transferring care to appropriate medical and/or allied health professionals and/or facilities, applying pharmacological and therapeutic modalities, and determining appropriateness for return to activity.
3. Facilitate the timely transfer of care for conditions beyond the scope of practice of the athletic trainer by implementing appropriate referral strategies to stabilize and/or prevent exacerbation of the condition(s).
   a. Athletic trainers must demonstrate knowledge of items such as emergency action plan(s), conditions beyond the scope of the athletic trainer, roles of medical and allied healthcare providers, and common

management strategies for life- and non–life-threatening conditions.
   b. Athletic trainers must demonstrate skills in implementing emergency action plan(s), recognizing acute conditions beyond the scope of the athletic trainer, communicating with other medical and allied healthcare providers, and Managing life-threatening and non–life-threatening conditions until transfer to appropriate medical providers and facilities.
4. Direct the appropriate individual(s) in standard immediate care procedures using formal and informal methods to facilitate immediate care.
   a. Athletic trainers must demonstrate knowledge of items such as roles of individual members of the medical management team, components of the emergency action plan(s), and effective communication techniques.
   b. Athletic trainers must demonstrate skills in communicating effectively with appropriate individuals, implementing the emergency action plan(s), educating individuals regarding standard emergency care procedures.
5. Execute the established emergency action plan using effective communication and administrative practices to facilitate efficient immediate care.
   a. Athletic trainers must demonstrate knowledge of items such as emergency action plan(s), communication techniques, and pertinent administrative practices.
   b. Athletic trainers must demonstrate skills in communicating effectively with appropriate individuals, identifying the need to implement the emergency action plan(s), implementing the emergency action plan(s), and implementing relevant administrative practices.

Professional Responsibilities   Athletic trainers, like other EMS personnel, will also have several specific responsibilities upon arriving at the scene of an emergency. How an athletic trainer immediately responds will ultimately determine the athlete outcomes. Some of these responsibilities include the following:

1. Ensuring safety for yourself, fellow athletic trainers and EMS personnel, bystanders, and athlete, in this order. Although athletic trainers do not share the same scene hazards (e.g., fire, explosion, crime) as EMS, making sure it is safe to enter a scene and limiting who has access helps prevent any additional injuries.
2. Gaining access to the athlete. An athlete's protective equipment such as football helmet, shoulder pads, and bracing are the concern here. It is difficult to evaluate a knee with a hinged knee brace in place or to ventilate a comprised airway when a football or ice hockey helmet is still in place. Being prepared with the proper knowledge and equipment to remove these items is a must.

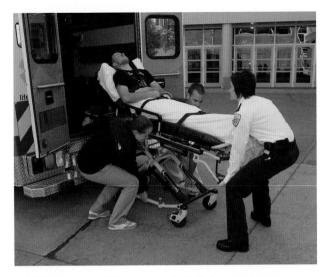

FIGURE 1.14 Collaborating with EMS during an emergency.

3. Athlete assessment to identify life-threatening conditions. After ensuring scene safety, assessment of life-threatening conditions that could compromise the airway, breathing, and circulation is critical. This should be followed by more thorough evaluation to identify conditions that could become life-threatening.

4. Initial athlete care is based on assessment findings based on one's scope of practice.

5. If warranted, provide any ongoing assessment and continuing care until the arrival of additional EMS resources.

6. Collaborate with and assist EMS personnel in providing care according to your scope of practice. Assisting with the additional care may include **packaging,** transporting, and unloading the athlete at the receiving facility (Fig. 1.14). This will be dependent upon the guidelines established prior to an emergency situation.

7. Participation in record keeping/data collection as per institution/local/state/federal requirements.

Developing Professional Relationships with EMS Providers

Finally and most important is liaising with and developing professional relationships with EMS providers and public safety officers. As previously mentioned, athletic trainers and EMS personnel have to work together as a cohesive team to provide seamless emergency care. An emergency situation is not the time or place to debate emergency care philosophy, become territorial, or undermine the scope of practice of either profession. Establishing a positive, good working relationship is critical to having a successful experience with EMS. And this must really be established prior to an emergency. Because EMS systems are responsible for a community and an athletic trainer is responsible for a very different clientele, the athletic trainer should initiate a dialogue between the two groups early on, prior to any emergency situations.

The following outlines several strategies an athletic trainer may choose to employ to improve athletic training–EMS relationships.[17–20] These include:

1. Introducing yourself to the local EMS personnel before the start of an athletic season and scheduling a meeting to share your emergency action plans as well as protocols for different emergency situations. Establish ahead of time who is most qualified to transport an athlete with a suspected cervical spine injury from the playing field. Should an athletic trainer immediately transfer to EMTs or paramedics the medical care of *all* injured athletes requiring EMS transport to a hospital? If an on-field physician is present, who will be the ultimate authority? In one study, EMS directors who had preseason meetings with an athletic trainer had a significantly better perception of the athletic trainer's ability to handle emergency situations than did those who did not have preseason meetings.[20]

2. When EMS personnel are scheduled to work an athletic event, the first conversation should not take place over a spine injured athlete. Take a few minutes and introduce yourself before the start of the event, discuss the emergency plan and location and type of emergency equipment available, and clarify any signals or other methods of communication to be used to activate EMS (Fig. 1.15). If an on-field physician is present, include him or her in the conversation and establish the chain of command.

3. Notify EMS personnel well in advance of all scheduled dates and times of athletic practices and competitions.

4. Provide directions and maps of athletic practice and competition venues and location of medical equipment at these facilities.

5. Invite the EMS personnel to spend some time in the athletic training room and/or observing practices or games.

6. Spend time riding along with the EMS personnel in order to better understand their perspective on emergency medicine.

7. Provide in-service training for local EMS agencies on athletic equipment (specifically football equipment) and

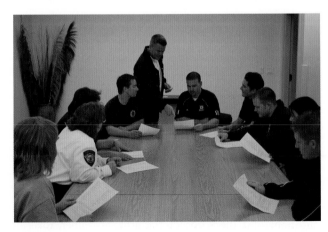

FIGURE 1.15 Preparing for an athletic event.

Scenarios

1. Before the beginning of the fall athletic season your athletic director approaches you regarding EMS coverage for varsity football games. He states that he was able to get a great deal this year. Turns out his next-door neighbor is an EMT for the local volunteer agency and that his son plays for the team. Your response is not what he expected and he questions your disapproval.

   Describe the disadvantages of having the local EMS volunteer agency sit and cover the football game. Could there be disadvantages to having a parent on the EMS scene?
   Discuss the other possible coverage options available to an athletic trainer.

2. While you are working in an outpatient rehabilitation facility, a 65-year-old male patient lapses into cardiac arrest. Your immediate response to the situation is to summon 911.

   Of the different types of EMS providers, who is best equipped to handle this situation and why?
   How can you ensure that this level of training will be the first to arrive on the scene?

3. You are sitting at lunch with a coworker, having an enjoyable afternoon discussing the athletic trainer as part of the EMS system. Your coworker believes that once EMS arrives, the athletic trainer should completely relinquish his or her duties to the EMS. However, you believe this is inappropriate, and your discussion eventually leads to what really is an athletic trainer's scope of practice related to emergency medical care.

   Identify and discuss an athletic trainer's scope of practice during an emergency situation. If and when should an athletic trainer relinquish all his or her duties to the EMS service?

4. While you are covering a high school baseball game, one of the parents in the crowd begins to scream. You realize that her 11-month-old infant is in respiratory distress. You arrive at the mother's side and note that the infant is blue and unresponsive. Your immediate reaction is to begin an initial assessment and to tell someone to call 911. A bystander calls on his cell phone.

   Your action, according to the chain of survival, would be known as what?
   What are the remaining components of the chain of survival?
   How does the chain of survival differ for an athletic trainer and an EMS provider? In summoning 911, what is the difference between using a land line and cell phone?

how to handle the challenges (e.g., facemask removal) it poses during patient care. Be sure to include any known on-field physicians and consider opening the training to the physicians and nurses at the receiving facilities.

8. Offer the opportunity for EMS personnel to provide in-service training on how they are required to handle certain situations in emergency care.

9. After an emergency situation does occur, schedule a meeting with the EMS personnel/service and perform a debriefing or critical-incident review session to determine what went well and what calls for improvement.

10. If the time and opportunity arises, complete at least the EMT certification. See what it is like on the other side of the fence!

WRAP-UP

Clearly, injuries and illnesses do not occur in a vacuum or when no one is watching. Athletic trainers and EMS personnel also do not work in a vacuum or when no one is watching. In fact, it is just the opposite; we must rely on each other's knowledge and skill to increase positive athlete outcomes. As athletic trainers, we take great pride in establishing positive working relationships with our team physicians, nutritionists, strength coaches, etc., yet we do a poor job of understanding and interacting with EMS professionals.

Why? Probably because we only call on them two or three times a year. However, this is probably the most important of all times to have a positive working relationship.

This chapter has provided a general overview of the EMS system; chain of survival; EMS personnel levels of training and competencies; types of EMS agencies; activation of 911 calls; the role of the "physician on the field"; and the professional behaviors, characteristics, scope of practice, and responsibilities of a certified athletic trainer as part of the EMS system. The name of the game is pre-event planning and understanding each profession's scope of practice. No matter what level of EMS responder has been assigned to your event, it's imperative that you create the opportunity to introduce yourself to the EMS crews who will be at your location. The moments you take to review basic procedure, communication styles, and "rules of engagement" will pay multiple dividends in the event that you should have to work together during a trauma or medical emergency.

REFERENCES

1. Board of Certification. *Board of Certification Role Delineation Study.* 5th ed. Omaha, NE: Board of Certification; 2004.

2. National Highway Traffic Safety Administration. The history of EMS at NHTSA. U.S. Department of Transportation. Available at: http://www.ems.gov/portal/site/ems/menuitem.5149822b03938f65a8de25f076ac8789/?vgnextoid=782a10d898318110VgnVCM1000002fd17898RCRD. Accessed August 21, 2009.

3. Committee on Trauma and Committee on Shock DoMS, National Academy of Sciences, National Research Council. *Accidental Death and Disability: The Neglected Disease of Modern Society.* Washington, DC: National Academy Press; 1966.

4. Centers for Disease Control and Prevention. Web-based Injury Statistics Query and Reporting System (WISQARS) (Online): 10 leading causes of death, United States, Ages 1–37. Available at: http://www.cdc.gov/injury/wisqars/index.html. Accessed August 21, 2009.

5. National Highway Traffic Safety Administration. What is EMS? Available at: http://www.ems.gov/portal/site/ems/menuitem.5149822b03938f65a8de25f076ac8789/?vgnextoid=9990f44e90578110VgnVCM1000002fd17898RCRD. Accessed August 12, 2009.

6. National Highway Traffic Safety Administration. Traffic Safety. United States Department of Transportation. Available at: http://www.nhtsa.dot.gov/portal/site/nhtsa/menuitem.2a0771e91315babbbf30811060008a0c/;jsessionid=EJkeuZcjL2N3I95QImc8jCou5J4yJ7hkHsZCt3OFRVOkucvrD3ei!. Accessed August 21, 2009.

7. National Highway Traffic Safety Administration. National EMS Scope of Practice Model. In: Services NHTSA-EM. Washington, DC: U.S. Department of Transportation; 2007.

8. National Highway Traffic Safety Administration. National Emergency Medical Services Education Standards: Emergency Medical Responder Instructional Guidelines. In: Services NHTSA-EM. Washington, DC: U.S. Department of Transportation; 2009.

9. Prentice WE. *Arnheim's Principles of Athletic Training.* 13th ed. Boston: McGraw-Hill; 2009.

10. Lee H, Cho D, Lee W, Chuang H. Pitfalls in treatment of acute cervical spinal cord injury using high-dose methylprednisolone: A retrospect audit of 111 patients. *Surg Neurol.* 2007;68(Suppl 1:):S37–S41; discussion S41–S32.

11. Bracken M. Pharmacological intervention for acute spinal cord injury. *Cochrane Rev.* 2001(1).

12. Cass D, Dvorak M, Fewer D, et al. Steroids in acute spinal cord injury. *Can J Emerg Med.* 2003;5(1):7–9.

13. Tsutsumi S, Ueta T, Shiba K, Yamamoto SKT. Effects of the Second National Acute Spinal Cord Injury Study of high-dose methylprednisolone therapy on acute cervical spinal cord injury: Results in spinal injuries center. *Spine.* 2006;31(26):2992–2996; discussion 2997.

14. Pinderski C, Dunham SF. Bringing emergency services to the event: The Champ Car experience. *Curr Sports Med Rep.* 2008;7(3):144–148.

15. Fu F, Tjoumakaris P, Buoncristiano A. Building a sports medicine team. *Clin Sports Med.* 2007;26:173–179.

16. National Athletic Trainers' Association. *Athletic Training Educational Competencies.* 4th ed. Dallas: National Athletic Trainers' Association; 2005.

17. Potter BW. Developing professional relationships with Emergency Medical Services providers. *Athl Ther Today.* 2006; 11(3):18–19.

18. Tolbert RS. Emergency planning for H.S. athletics. *Coach & Athletic Director.* 10 2004;74(3):58–59.

19. Courson R, Henry GR. Communication: The critical element in emergency preparation. *Athl Ther Today.* 2005;10(2): 16–18.

20. Biddington C, Popovich M, Kupczyk N, Roh J. Certified athletic trainers' management of emergencies. *J Sport Rehabil.* 2005;14(2):185.

21. Board of Certification. State regulation. Board of Certification. Available at: http://www.bocatc.org/index.php?option=com_content&task=view&id=113&Itemid=121. Accessed August 21, 2009.

The Well-Being of the Athletic Trainer

CHAPTER OUTCOMES

1. Identify the difference between good and bad stress.
2. Understand how burnout occurs.
3. Recognize the various signs and indicators of stress in an individual.
4. Identify key components of stress management.
5. Understand how critical incident and crisis stress differ from daily stress.
6. Recognize the types of crises or critical incidents that an athletic trainer may encounter.
7. Recognize common reactions to critical incidents.
8. Identify basic crisis intervention/early psychological intervention skills.
9. Identify indicators that require referrals to mental health providers/next level of care.
10. Understand the steps involved in the referral process.
11. Recognize the need for self-care for one's stress levels.

NOMENCLATURE

Burnout: a reaction to chronic stress involving negative interactions between environmental and personal characteristics, leading to decreased productivity and performance[1-4]

Crisis response: an individual's acute response to an incident where his or her psychological homeostasis is disrupted, usual coping strategies are ineffective, and signs of significant distress, impairment, and dysfunction appear[5,6]

Critical incident: an incident that falls outside of one's normal day-to-day experiences, has the potential to cause significant levels of distress, and can exceed one's normal coping skills[5,7]

Critical incident stress management (CISM): a comprehensive, integrated, multicomponent crisis intervention system[5,7]

Debriefing and defusing: "Debriefing" can refer to many things; in this chapter we're referring to psychological critical incident stress debriefings (CISDs), specifically using the CISM or the "Mitchell model." These are both components of the CISM system and are structured small group meetings intended to help decrease stress, provide an opportunity for ventilation, promote learning about normal stress responses, provide education on coping skills, and allow for triage for further services and referrals to other levels of care[7]

NOMENCLATURE *(Continued)*

Distress: bad stress

Eustress: good stress

Stress: a state of physiological arousal that helps one respond to threatening or demanding situations, either actual or perceived[8]

Stressor: any event acting as a stimulus that places demands upon a person, group, or organization and brings about a stress response[8]

BEFORE YOU BEGIN

1. What are the key components of managing stress?
2. How does the well-being of the athletic trainer relate to his or her ability to identify and manage stress?
3. Describe the basic crisis intervention/early psychological intervention skills of which an athletic trainer should be aware.
4. What is the difference between stress management and crisis management?
5. How can athletic trainers prepare themselves for crisis or critical incident situations?
6. Describe how the athletic trainer's self-care differs from the care that he or she will use in crisis situations with athletes.

Voices from the Field

A role that I did not audition for or want, I hold a resume of tragedy during my life from the Marshall airplane crash, losing a player in my arms on the field, and dealing with losses of lives involving team members, shootings, and pipe bombs. Death has been my constant companion throughout my career as an athletic trainer. I would hope that no one has to get acquainted with "my companion," and yet it is likely that you will experience tragedy and loss during your lifetime at some level. Preparation for tragic events is key; however, no one can be totally prepared until such a tragedy occurs. Preparedness also means practice each step of emergency procedures regularly so that, no matter how scared you are when faced with these situations, you can still perform your duties as if it's second nature. When the initial trauma and action have ended, you will feel exhausted, numb, and on some occasions, second guessing yourself.

There is another component so often overlooked with tragedy that any athletic trainer must anticipate and immediately address. In the days, months, and years that follow, the well-being of you and others associated with a loss of life must be carefully considered early on. I suffered from PTSD for 30 years after the Marshall tragedy. It took me 30 years to get the help I needed. I waited far too long to deal with my grief and my loss. With proper counseling the grieving process is a vital step in "transcending through tragedy" with grace and peace and some level of closure.

Mark J. Smaha, MS, ATC
NATA Past President
NATA Hall of Fame
MJS Communications
Keyport, Washington

As a primary health care provider, the athletic trainer is responsible for overseeing the well-being of the athletes and clients being served. Athletes, by the nature of competition, face high levels of stress on a daily basis, whether striving for a personal best, a college scholarship, or a place on an Olympic or professional team. Athletic trainers must also be prepared to deal with their own daily stresses: having all athletes taped, treated, and ready for practice on time; having to stay at work late several nights in a row, keeping them away from family; and holding daily meetings with coaches to talk about the status of injured athletes. In addition to the daily **stressors,** athletic trainers must be prepared to handle crises faced by the individuals they serve; for example, the elite track athlete who suffers a third-degree hamstring strain, the professional bull rider who suffers a shoulder dislocation, and

the industrial worker who has recently had a limb amputated while working on the line. Each of these situations could potentially be career-ending. It is the responsibility of the athletic trainer not only to treat the physical injuries but also to address and be aware of the emotional component of these injuries. Keep in mind that the principles of self-care are not dissimilar to those used with the clients being served, and self-care is often talked about in conjunction with the care of others. As you read this chapter, you will see that the focus is not on the individuals that athletic trainers will treat but rather on the athletic trainers themselves.

Some topics in this chapter may cause you stress and be of a difficult nature; however, it is important even now to find ways to manage the discussion of such topics so that, when you're faced with them in real-life situations, you will be better prepared to deal with them. Although this chapter does discuss the concept of crisis intervention, its main purpose is to raise awareness; it should not be considered a substitute for formal training in crisis intervention, nor should it replace the need for mental health consultation.

ALL IN A DAY'S WORK

Every day we go to our jobs expecting a fairly routine schedule, seeing the same people, filling out the same paperwork, and feeling safe and comfortable. However, at any moment that next phone call or red-flagged urgent e-mail can alter all of that and change our day from a routine to a chaotic one. How might your job change if you were informed that:

- A sudden death has taken the life of an athlete on the field in front of team members, friends, family, and your local community.
- A close friend, colleague, or the school's beloved coach has been killed in a car accident on the way to a game.
- A student you recently worked with committed suicide over the weekend.
- During a preparticipation physical examination, you notice several bruises on one of your female athletes, leading you to suspect that she has recently been assaulted.

How are you feeling right now, after reading this? A little stressed? These are certainly not aspects of your job that you were expecting to experience, but they end up being real possibilities; in many cases, you may be the one people look to for support. These situations push the limits of emotional and physical health for athletes, coaches, support staff, family, and friends as well as your limits as the athletic trainer. It is the role of the athletic trainer to triage the situation, be knowledgeable about appropriate referrals, and have an action plan in the event that any incident builds up into a crisis. However, above all, at the end of the day, what are you, the athletic trainer, doing to take care of yourself? This section discusses the often-neglected well-being of the athletic trainer, whose professional focus is on taking care of others.

This chapter focuses on the identification and management of stress, whether day to day or in crisis situations. In addition, strategies for managing emergency situations and their emotional impact are covered, including when to refer to trained mental health professionals. Information is also provided to assist athletic trainers in finding help for themselves in situations of daily stress as well as crisis. It is important to note that the well-being of athletic trainers depends on recognizing the signs of their own personal stress and applying the same intervention and referral strategies that they would apply to their athletes.

WHAT IS STRESS?

Stress is a part of our daily lives; it is not something we can escape but rather something we must embrace, harnessing the energy and benefits it can bring. Stress in moderation can brings us benefits; for many people, it adds motivation, excitement, and new adventures to their lives. However, if not managed and controlled, stress can have a profound impact on many aspects of our lives both acutely and chronically. It is important to remember that stress is in the eye of the beholder. Stress occurs because something is seen as a potential challenge or threat at some level. What one individual may consider stressful or a crisis, another may not. Examples of stressful situations for the athletic trainer may include pressure to return a player a week after suffering a grade III MCL sprain or having to diagnose a condition on the field in front of a large crowd. Other examples could include communicating with an overbearing coach (Fig. 2.1) or having to tell a coach that a star player has suffered a

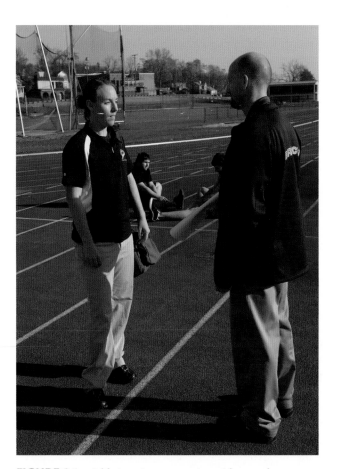

FIGURE 2.1 Athletic trainer conversing with a coach.

season-ending injury. Examples of situations that can cause stress are limitless. It is the threat or worry of the threat—for example, from making a wrong diagnosis or being let go from your job—that triggers a "fight-or-flight" response in our bodies. The fight-or-flight response results in changes that help us "get the job done." It also functions to protect us from the threat, whether real or perceived. All of the stresses around the athletic trainer can eventually begin to take their toll; thus, it is important to know how to manage your own stress.

When we go into this fight-or-flight mode, our bodies respond to the stress in order to promote survival; that is, our bodies increase strength, endurance, and sensory perception of the environment and initiate other physiological, emotional, and behavioral reactions. The sympathetic and parasympathetic nervous systems help our bodies respond to and recover from crisis. The sympathetic nervous system automatically aids us in this fight-or-flight reaction because, in emergencies, we don't want to have to think of how we want our bodies to react to protect us but rather for our bodies to react as quickly as possible to keep us safe. Our bodies aid in our survival by increasing heart rate, blood pressure, and breathing; dilating our pupils; increasing perspiration; constricting our blood vessels; and decreasing digestive processes.[9] The parasympathetic nervous system does the opposite, by helping us slow down these responses and return to a more normal, homeostatic state, which is also a survival mechanism.[9] Although we need the work of the sympathetic nervous system to help us survive the acute crisis period, we also need the parasympathetic nervous system to help bring us back to a calmer state that will allow our bodies to recover and rest. Failure to achieve these calmer and relaxed periods can lead to chronic health and even emotional issues.

Good Stress

Good stress, or **eustress,** helps to motivate and add "zip" to our lives. Without this good stress to help us better ourselves, meet new people, earn a paycheck, or tackle new challenges, we'd probably get little done and have dull lives. For the athletic trainer, the confidence gained from the pressure to return a player to competition in a short time after a serious injury can also be considered a positive outcome to stress if successful. Eustress helps us to improve and achieve better performance by increasing energy, motivation, endurance, concentration, and strength. Generally this type of stress is not harmful to our bodies because it is acute in nature. Through our actions and events, we "burn it off" and allow ourselves to return to a more relaxed state until we're faced with another stressful situation. However, if we're constantly in this increased state of stress and/or quickly encounter another stressful situation, lower levels of good stress can begin to have negative impacts and lead to bad stress, also known as **"distress."** An example of this may be the athletic trainer who faces multiple athletic injuries to be rehabilitated in a single season (Fig. 2.2). The level of stress experienced by the athletic trainer is often related to the stress experienced by the clients they serve: the athletes and coaches.

Signs & Symptoms

Sympathetic Versus Parasympathetic Response

Sympathetic Responses

- Increased heart rate
- Increased blood pressure
- Increased respiratory rate
- Dilated pupils
- Increased perspiration
- Constriction of blood vessels
- Decreased digestive processes

Parasympathetic Responses

- Decreased heart rate
- Decreased blood pressure
- Decreased respiratory rate
- Decreased body temperature
- Dilation of blood vessels
- Increased digestion

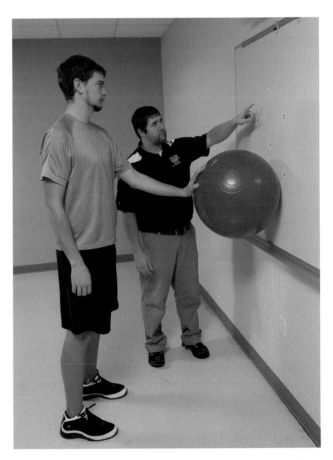

FIGURE 2.2 Athletic trainer conducting rehabilitation with an athlete.

Breakout

Sources of Stress for the Athletic Trainer

- Overload of work
- Low pay
- No or limited health or other benefits
- Limited opportunities for advancement
- Uncertain future about job
- Uncertainty about what one's job actually entails
- Little or no feedback
- Administrative hassles
- Having the responsibility for the life, health, or safety of another person
- Traumatic or critical incidents

Breakout

Sources of Stress for the Athlete

- Starting position on the team
- Pressure from parents
- Losing a position on team
- Injury
- Grades
- Eligibility
- Scholarship
- Relationships
- Home life
- Pregnancy
- Drug testing
- Coach and colleagues

Bad Stress

The opposite of eustress is distress, or bad stress. This occurs when the negative effects of stress start to outweigh the benefits. Distress may happen gradually through several small stressful situations building up and having a cumulative effect, as discussed above; from several large events occurring simultaneously; or from one large enduring event. Stress can be interesting in this respect: an individual may have faced the same situation (or one similar to it) over and over again with little negative impact, but then he or she suddenly has a greater reaction.

Several factors affect the way in which we respond to a stressor: how well we normally cope with daily stressors in our lives, how likely this current stressor is to affect us negatively, what else is currently going on in our lives, the resources we have to cope with the current stressor, and our current overall physical and emotional health. If we're currently dealing with several stressors that are either happening simultaneously or overlapping, with little time to relax and recover from an earlier stress, it is highly likely that we will experience negative impacts. Negative impacts may include decreased performance and inability to effectively deal with the current stressors or any subsequent events in the near future.

Because of their numerous responsibilities, it becomes important for athletic trainers not only to develop a personalized plan for balancing and managing their own daily stressors but also to have appropriate workplace policies and procedures in place to respond to various types of crises and other situations that can occur outside of their daily routine.

Knowing that there are resources and a plan to aid in emergencies can help reduce stress among athletic trainers. It is also important to realize that athletes' stress can begin to impact the athletic trainer's own stress level. Failure to recognize such causes of stress can lead to **burnout.**

Burnout

If high levels of stress are not mitigated, they begin to take a toll on an individual's physical and emotional well being. When the benefits that were once evident at the lower levels of stress are no longer present and actually decrease drastically, the stage is set for burnout. This becomes evident as the individual shows a marked decrease in attitude, motivation, and energy levels; he or she may also show apathy and increased exhaustion, which may generalize to other aspects of his or her life. For many people, being able to recognize the signs of burnout and take time away from the tasks or stressors (e.g., vacation, long weekend, taking on a new project, shifting attention to something else for a while, etc.) may be all that is needed. However, where this has become a recurring pattern, the change may not be so simple; larger lifestyle changes may be required due to the physical and emotional stress that has occurred.

Current Research

The Multiple Roles of the Athletic Trainer

Research on role orientation hierarchy among athletic trainers at the collegiate and university levels[10] indicates that they are often pulled in many directions at once, including clinical work, faculty responsibilities, commitments to research, teaching, service, continuing education, student advising, administrative duties, and responsibilities to professional organizations.

Consider, for example, a certified athletic trainer who has accepted a position at a high school with the understanding that her day starts at 2:00 P.M. and ends when the events of the day are over; many times 10:00 P.M. Initially she finds this acceptable. But after time, especially if the athletic trainer is married and has a family, the toll of missing family activities, such as seeing her child in a student play or athletic event, may start to take an emotional toll on the athletic trainer and on the family relationship. The motivation to go to work may be lost or reduced. This pattern may be compounded by low pay at the high school level. Eventually the high school athletic trainer may change her career path in order to adjust to her new life priorities and reduce stress. Therefore, she will look for positions that allow her to have more time with her family.

Athletic trainers are faced with stress on many levels. Their well-being is dependent upon reducing the amount of bad stress and maintaining an acceptable level of good stress, thus hopefully reducing or preventing the likelihood of burnout. Acceptable levels of stress differ for each individual based upon his or her level of tolerance. To avoid burnout, athletic trainers must be able to identify their own symptoms of stress, find their levels of tolerance, and learn ways to manage their stress.

SYMPTOMS OF STRESS

Traumatic and even everyday stress can affect individuals across various dimensions of their lives. These dimensions are physical, emotional, behavioral, cognitive, and spiritual; they also involve relationships.[7,11–16] Even under low levels of stress, symptoms may be apparent; however, they can have a compounding effect as they increase. It is important to remember that not everyone will react the same way to stress and that different symptoms may be present. For example, not all of these will be apparent in a given individual, and even specific ones such as loss of appetite and poor sleep may vary. An individual may experience better or worse eating or sleeping patterns depending on his or her personal traits as well as the nature and intensity of the stressors. The athletic trainer should look for the symptoms listed below and be prepared to seek additional support.

Physical

The following physical symptoms are common and should be looked at collectively with the other dimensions listed. It is also important to differentiate between injuries and stress symptoms. These include increased heart rate, increased breathing, increased blood pressure, headaches, changes in sleep patterns, increased or decreased appetite, fatigue/exhaustion, increased or decreased activity level, muscle tension, teeth grinding, increased startle responses, pacing, finger or foot tapping, *chest pains, collapse, loss of consciousness, blood in vomit, urine, stool, sputum, numbness/paralysis (especially in the arm, leg, or face), inability to speak/understand.**

Emotional

Emotional symptoms of stress include depression, anxiety, feeling hopeless or helpless, fear, guilt, crying spells, excessive worrying, loss of interest in activities or life events, mood swings, lack of motivation, feeling easily frustrated, emotionally numb, angry, or short-tempered—also having nightmares, *thoughts or ideas of suicide, homicide, or self-harm, panic attacks, severe depressive symptoms (i.e., not wanting to get out of bed, not eating, not caring for self).**

Behavioral

Behavioral symptoms include increased withdrawal and isolation; increased impulsiveness/risk taking; increased alcohol, drug, or tobacco use; family and relationship strain; *increased violence/fights; physically or emotionally abuse of others; decreased personal hygiene or concern for physical safety; self-medicating (i.e., overuse of prescription medications of one's own or those of others, over-the-counter medications such as sleeping medications).**

Cognitive

Cognitive symptoms include difficulty concentrating, making decisions, memory, solving problems; forgetfulness, poor creativity, confusion, focusing only on things related to the stressor, obsessiveness, perfectionism, racing thoughts, negative attitudes/self-talk, negative self-perceptions, sensory distortion, *paranoia, hallucinations, delusions, disabling guilt, persistent hopelessness/helplessness, persistent diminished problem solving or concentration.**

Relational

Relational symptoms include distrust of people, self-isolation, lowered sex drive, lack of intimacy, lashing out, resentment, intolerance, decreased contact/connection with friends, and "using" people.

---

*The symptoms in italics are all severe levels of symptoms that require referral to a higher level of professional care. Severe physical symptoms need a medical referral and workup prior to being seen by a mental health professional. All others should be seen by a mental health professional, preferably someone with training, experience, and potential access to a referral network for emergency mental health services and evaluations. In some areas, this may have to be done at a hospital emergency department. Your team, agency, and staff should research such services in your area and have a plan and policy in place of how to refer to or access their services.

Spiritual

Spiritual symptoms include anger at one's spiritual faith or higher power, loss of direction, apathy, loss of meaning, emptiness, withdrawal from one's practice of faith, challenging one's beliefs, overcompensating for one's faith and practice (e.g., increased practice of faith, such as going to church daily, preaching to everyone, and other suddenly increased spiritual behaviors), *cessation of the practice of faith, religious hallucinations or delusions** (this may involve certain cultural influences or traditions, which can be confused with more severe symptoms).

STRESS MANAGEMENT

There is no magical formula or one plan that solves every problem of managing stress. Stress management requires a holistic, whole-person approach. It is important to keep in mind that what may work for a colleague may not work for you. A colleague may take a week-long trip to the mountains while you take short day trips or just add an extra day to your weekend. You may find that playing hooky for a day to do something you've wanted to do for a long time is more relaxing than a long trip.

While learning even a few strategies can provide some relief and help, often it is examining multiple aspects of one's life (exercise, diet, relationships, etc.) that leads to the greatest success. The athletic trainer must be knowledgeable about stress management techniques not only for his or her athletes but also for his or her own personal well-being. This may be applied on a day-to-day basis to handle stress, from the everyday variety to major crisis events. Everyday stress management techniques that help to calm and relax one's body and mind are very helpful. This can be done by learning skills such as diaphragmatic breathing, yoga, meditation, progressive muscle relaxation, and imagery (Fig. 2.3). These help to calm down physical responses to stress, which often helps with other responses such as racing thoughts and difficulty concentrating. While most of these skills are often easy enough to learn and do on a daily basis, regular practice is encouraged in order to manage everyday levels of stress, which ultimately helps individuals cope with more stressful crisis situations.

Higher-level strategies such as time management and assertiveness challenge the way we think and perceive events in our lives and are effective for the more pervasive and larger life stressors we may encounter. This awareness of stress management strategies will also provide the tools to assist athletic trainers in their professional roles as caretakers on a daily basis. When a crisis occurs, having awareness of these stress management skills and strategies will help one better cope with the increased and possibly traumatic stress associated with a given event.

Although the strategies mentioned above may help an individual after a crisis, it is difficult to teach some of these skills to people who haven't already learned them or become

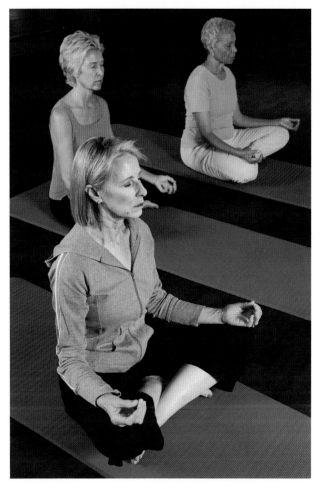

FIGURE 2.3 Yoga for relaxation.

proficient with them. In a crisis situation, other more practical strategies, such as those listed below, may better help the athletic trainer to cope.[7,12,14,15]

Helpful Tips for Stress Management

Physical exercise/movement: Keep a normal workout routine and don't forget about doing it. If you don't already have a routine, begin some type of physical movement/activity even if it is only mild to moderate (always consult with a physician prior to initiating an exercise program). Movement can be a great stress management tool.

Keep busy with a normal routine: Keep busy and don't sit around dwelling on the events. Keeping to your normal routine helps with this and helps one to realize that things can return to normal again after a crisis. It may also help to prevent avoidance of things related to the event.

Normal reactions to an abnormal event: Recognize you are going to show and feel common reactions to stressful situation and that you're not going crazy. It is important to use your clinical judgment and skills to assess and be aware of more concerning reactions (see the more severe reactions noted above) and know when to refer to a higher level of care (even for yourself).

Talk: Talk to people you trust and spend time with them. If you're not the talking type, then consider keeping a journal or writing letters. The important thing is to get your feelings out in some way that is safe for you. With online journaling, it is important to watch what is made "public" versus what is kept private (e.g., rants about coaching staff or individuals), which could come back to haunt/hurt you and cause more stress.

Know that it's OK to feel bad: Watch out for thoughts such as "suck it up," "toughen up," or not showing feelings or emotions.

Know that it's OK to take time for yourself: Do healthy things for yourself that feel good or are pampering. Don't make any big life-changing decisions (e.g., large purchases, changing jobs, moving, quitting the team).

Take control: You may feel out control because of something that has happened, so try to take control over your life, even if this seems to involve relatively small decisions (i.e., taking a full lunch break, not staying late at work, talking to friends, etc.).

Practice good nutrition; be sure to eat: Eat well-balanced, regular meals, and drink good fluids (i.e., water, juices), even if you're not feeling hungry or thirsty. Because of its stimulant properties, monitor and moderate your caffeine intake.

Focus on regular sleep and rest periods: Even if you don't feel like it, be sure to get enough rest and a good night's sleep.

Don't increase your use of alcohol or other substances: While this may not be the healthiest lifestyle or stress management choice you have, it is also probably not the time to stop or make significant changes in usage.

Know your resources: Have referral and resource information readily available. Know if you have employee assistance programs or other employee benefits to assist with your own personal wellness and self-care.

Many of these may sound like commonsense things to do for someone in a stressful situation, and they are. The problem is that because of the stressful situation you may forget these basic tips. Keep in mind that we're not thinking as clearly as we should during periods of high stress or crisis and in general may not think to use our normal coping strategies. It's helpful to remind ourselves of these strategies. As you apply these strategies, it is a good idea to ask yourself if they are effective or if the symptoms are getting worse both over time and/or in spite of their use. In these cases, it is important to consult with appropriately trained mental health professionals for further evaluation.

CRISIS MANAGEMENT

Now that we've talked about everyday stress, let's talk about getting yourself prepared to deal with those situations—both large and small—that can really strain your daily routine: crises and emergencies. Although you've probably been trained well to deal with physical and medical emergency situations, you've probably not thought much about the emotional side of these events. No two crises are exactly alike, and you will need to adapt all of the following points to your specific situation. The more you practice and exercise your plans and procedures to address emergencies and crises, the better prepared you will be. Although there are different types of crisis intervention models, there are common points and recommendations around the use of early psychological intervention (EPI).[17] Providing EPI and crisis intervention strategies for emotional support can be seen as similar to responding to a medical emergency.[11] Lay persons can learn basic first aid and cardiopulmonary resuscitation and provide these services until emergency medical services arrive to administer a higher level of care and transport to more advanced treatment in the hospital setting. Similarly, in their professional roles and working with their clients or athletes, athletic trainers will assess the situation, provide emergency emotional support, and refer to the next level of care—such as outpatient counseling or, in more severe cases, inpatient psychiatric care. For this to occur, the athletic trainer must first be able to recognize the difference between indicators of normal stress and severe stress (as discussed earlier in this chapter) and the importance of having a referral process for advanced psychological consultation and care. Where this becomes more complicated is with self-recognition and care. When a crisis situation occurs, further emphasis needs to be placed on taking care of yourself, even though your focus may be on taking care of others. The key to good emotional crisis management is having a good base in stress management. If you don't take care of your own emotional health first, you may have problems with the level of care you are able to provide to your clients.

The following paragraphs focus on the application of the **critical incident stress management** (CISM) model. This model is designed to assist you in managing the emotional aspects of crisis situations. Other models may address the mental and emotional health aspect of crisis management; however, CISM was created with an original focus on high-risk emergency personnel such as law enforcement, fire personnel, and emergency medical professionals.[8]

Critical Incident Stress Management Model

The CISM model is an integrated, multicomponent, comprehensive system of care for those in crisis, including components for group crisis intervention, individual crisis intervention, and peer support (see www.icisf.org for a

Breakout

Consensus Document: Recommended Components of EPI

1. Preincident training
2. Incident assessment and strategic planning
3. Risk and crisis communication
4. Acute psychological assessment and triage
5. Crisis intervention with large groups
6. Crisis intervention with small groups
7. Crisis intervention with individuals, face to face, and hotlines
8. Crisis planning and intervention with communities
9. Crisis planning and intervention with organizations
10. Psychological first aid
11. Facilitating access to appropriate levels of care when needed
12. Assisting special and diverse populations
13. Spiritual assessment and care
14. Self-care and family care, including safety and security
15. Postincident evaluation and training based on lessons learned

current listing of training opportunities).[5,7] Particularly important benefits of this model are that it allows the non–mental health professional trained in this model to work with trained mental health professionals to provide crisis emotional support and provides a common language to use in addressing intervention strategies. Whether you choose to be trained in CISM or another type of crisis intervention, the important thing is to have an understanding of a model of crisis intervention that will allow you to feel comfortable in providing assistance to those in crisis, including yourself.

In 2005, several organizations that provide emotional support in times of disaster convened a group of experts to examine key components of EPI outlined in the *Early Psychological Intervention Points of Consensus* document.[17] These recommended components, which are included in the CISM model, can also be applied to situations faced by the certified athletic trainer, who plays a part in the overall continuum of care for an individual's emotional well-being.

SCENARIO

You are working at a university as the head athletic trainer. You receive a call at 4:00 A.M. from the local trauma center in a rural county more than 400 miles away. You were notified that about an hour earlier the men's and women's basketball team bus ran off the road during a severe snow storm. Initial reports from the scene indicate that six individuals died at the scene; two more died in the hospital's emergency department, and all of the remaining 32 team members are being treated for various injuries, including several that are life-threatening, requiring emergency

surgery. You know that those on the bus included players, managers, coaching staff, and your assistant athletic trainer. At this time, the hospital is unable to identify those who have died or what level of treatment is required by the rest. The state police ask that no one attempt to travel to the area for the next 24 hours because of the worsening weather and travel conditions. They inform you that they will be back in touch within the next several hours with more information.

Application of CISM Components for EPI

Based on the information given, this scenario has the strong potential of being a **critical incident** to you as the athletic trainer, as well as to victims, families, friends, and university staff due to the number of people impacted, the extent of injuries, loss of life, etc. Using concepts from CISM, let's examine how you may apply some of the recommended components of EPI to the scenario.

A. **Preincident Training and Planning** (which may include a crisis communication plan, phone trees, and crisis team procedures—e.g., how they can assist, crisis team members and roles, survival tips on aftermath, etc.)   After reading this scenario, you may be wondering, What do I do? What is my role? What role do others play? How do we respond? These are all questions that may already be answered for you. One way to be prepared both individually and organizationally is to have an emergency plan in place. These type of plans address how to help to prepare, respond, and promote recovery for all types of crises and emergencies in a variety of domains, including the emotional well-being of those affected. This training helps you, your staff, and your athletes better prepare to handle not only emergencies and crises but also day-to-day stress. For many individuals, an understanding of their roles or how they fit into a larger plan allows them to feel more confident and less anxious in these types of situations. This approach can also include policies and procedures to help identify personnel and understand roles in an emergency, which helps to reduce anxiety and stress by providing knowledge and structure to situations that are often confusing and unstructured. In this example, there are some interesting and challenging factors that will have to be assessed and planned for: a mass casualty situation, multiple deaths, distance, current lack of information from an initial report, and one factor that can't be ignored—media, press, and other forms of rapid to immediate communication (e.g., cell camera/video phones, text messaging, etc.). As the athletic trainer, your role may be to assist in contacting or providing support to family members or speaking to medical professionals in other locations. One other aspect of preincident training and planning is how well you manage your stress on a day-to-day basis. This may include learning and practicing your own stress management techniques as well as passing along stress management tips to those you work with.

B. **Incident Assessment and Strategic Planning**   This step is often not taken in isolation. Most groups, organizations, and teams will probably have a **crisis response** or management team or at least more than one individual assessing the situation to determine the best course of action. Your role in this group may be limited or you may be one of the key players, depending on your group's structure. This will be discussed in your preincident training and practice. An important thing to remember is to not overlook the emotional needs of those around you, their families, and also yourself. You should consult with your prearranged psychological resources at times like this. You're likely to share information with your psychological resources to help determine appropriate levels of emotional support. Because of the sensitive nature of this medical information, confidentiality should be maintained by all team members involved. In addition, in situations where there have been reported deaths, the athletic trainer must understand that everyone has an individualized response to death and must be prepared for multiple reactions, including anger, self-blame, and denial. In this scenario, you will need to identify the unique factors of this incident with your planning:

1. You have an incident that occurred 400 miles away that you won't have access to for the next 24 hours.
2. Since families can't get to their loved ones, where are they likely to go? Will your school provide a central meeting place for them and support services once they arrive? What if the families are located across the state or even country? How will you provide information and services to them?
3. What type of crisis counseling and other support services will you have to provide or arrange for your own staff over the next 24 hours while they wait for news updates, work with families, or take phone calls from parents, friends, and the media?
4. What services will you have to provide for those not directly involved? Other teams? Classmates? Friends? Significant others? Do they need more information and support?

C. Risk and Crisis Communication

Your emergency plan should identify someone to serve as a public or media relations person who has knowledge in this area and will likely take over communications with the public (at the university level, this is often the sports information director). However, as mentioned earlier, it is important to realize that with today's technology, it may be hard to stay ahead of the flow of information, rumors, and speculation. With crisis communication, it is important to provide timely and accurate information. It is also important to respect a family's desire to receive information before it reaches the general public and the media. This is another part of the plan that should be practiced before it's needed. Also a part of emergency preparation in this area would be to have documents or files on resources, healthy coping strategies, self-care information, typical reactions, and so on ready to be printed and distributed. These documents could be "fill-in-the-blank"

templates that you have prepared to be used in a variety of situations and then customized for the particular situation at hand. A good suggestion is to have not only electronic versions of these documents as part of your plan, which could be printed anywhere, but also hard copies that could be duplicated in case computers are not readily available.

D. Acute Psychological Assessment and Triage

This can be done by looking at the key indicators mentioned earlier. These should be used to determine if symptoms are improving or worsening. In addition, it is necessary to assess if individuals need referral to higher levels of care. In this example, during the following 24 hours, this would likely occur with staff, other students, and family members who are gathering for more information. Although you may have psychological support services at your school during this time, it is unlikely that these professionals would be able to see or notice everyone. So they would look to you and other staff members to help identify those experiencing more severe reactions and to make referrals. A benefit of preincident training and large group meetings soon after critical incidents is that people can receive practical self-care tips and also learn to identify more severe signs of distress in themselves and others. You will also be assessing larger needs and working with your psychological resources to determine what other parts of the CISM model may be needed and when (i.e., large group meetings, small group crisis interventions, one-on-one crisis intervention, and so on).

E. Crisis Intervention with Large Groups

Early on, disseminating information to various larger groups will be important not only from a crisis communication/information point of view but also from an educational and self-care perspective. In CISM, crisis management briefings (CMBs) help to accomplish this by organizing a structured "town meeting" format to provide facts and self-care information as well as to dispel rumors.[7] In this scenario, setting up this type of meeting early, perhaps the first thing the next morning at a scheduled time so family and friends can attend, may be a good plan. Your group may also consider using the latest technology to help disseminate the information to those who are too far away to attend or can't attend because of other circumstances. Your role in this may be as one of the experts sharing your area of knowledge. As with all CISM regarding psychological issues, stress reactions, and respond to immediate emotional needs.

F. Crisis Intervention with Small Groups

Small-group crisis interventions can take on different formats and consist of different stages. In CISM there are two main types of small-group interventions—**debriefing** and **defusing**.[7] "Debriefing" can refer to many things; in this chapter we're referring to psychological critical incident stress debriefings (CISDs), specifically using the CISM or the Mitchell model. These are structured small-group meetings that are intended to decrease stress, provide an opportunity for ventilation, and learn about normal stress responses. Defusing is a small-group crisis intervention that is arranged shortly after a critical incident, focusing on providing an opportunity to supply information and education and to normalize responses. Both interventions provide education about stress and coping skills and assess for further needs for services or referrals. It may be recommended that one or both be used depending on your earlier assessment and what strategies and interventions are chosen to be most appropriate. Mental health professionals will work with you to assess not only which interventions to use but also their timing and who may be appropriate to lead them or participate in them. Again, in delivering these services, the CISM model calls for a mental health professional to be present, although other non–mental health professionals who have been trained in the model may help to co-lead the group.

G. Crisis Intervention with Individuals, Face to Face, and Hotlines
One-on-one crisis intervention is probably the most widely used EPI skill, not only in a scenario like this, but also in everyday professional life. At any time, you could be talking to an athlete who is going through a crisis in their life. Knowing how to be able to sit down, listen, support, and recognize the need to refer them to more professional care is critical. While this may seem routine, don't minimize the effect that this has on you as the primary care giver. Larger crises, like that in the scenario, will impact individuals emotionally not only immediately, but for weeks, months, and sometimes years to come. It is important to remember and plan for this long-term emotional impact for not only your athletes, but also yourself as anniversary dates of important events (i.e., graduation, opening day, etc.) occur.

H. Crisis Planning and Intervention with Communities
Looking at how an incident will affect the larger community is important. In this scenario the community is the university and those on the campus. It is also important to know how the incident could affect the surrounding town or city. With other types of teams, perhaps those of a high school or middle school, even if you and your staff are not directly providing support to the larger community, it may be necessary to work with your local mental health professionals and other support agencies.

I. Crisis Planning and Intervention with Organizations
As mentioned above, with communities, it will be important to look ahead in your planning process to determine how a crisis on your team or within your school or agency may affect other organizations around you and to consider how they may be brought in to help. Contact organizations such as your local American Red Cross ahead of time to find out what resources they can provide and how access them; this will be key to the successful implementation of your plan.

J. Psychological First Aid
Depending on the crisis management model you choose to follow, there may be differ-ent protocols for the implementation of psychological care. Generally, psychological first aid (PFA) is parallel to medical first aid[11] in that it gives those who are trained a basic awareness of emotional or stress signs and symptoms that must be watched for and when to refer to the next level of care. Also, like medical first aid, PFA may provide suggestions on how to help those with less severe stress symptoms. Various versions of this training are available. The American Red Cross (www.redcross.org) offers one version through many of their local community chapters for volunteers working in disaster situations.

K. Facilitating Access to Appropriate Levels of Care when Needed
A time of crisis is not the time to learn about resources in your area. As you would learn about medical resources and specialties in your area when you take on a new job, you should do the same for mental health services. Develop resources and referrals for more critical issues like crisis and inpatient care in addition to outpatient counseling services, including specialists for everyday types of mental health services (e.g., anxiety, depression, eating disorders, etc.). A good emergency plan would include what your crisis resources are and how to access them in times of emergencies. In this scenario, either early on when you may be talking to individuals who have lost someone in the incident or later, once the injured athletes return back to campus, you will be assessing individuals who may need more intense counseling services. Having an immediate referral system in place either on site or in the community will facilitate these referrals.

L. Assisting Special and Diverse Populations
As part of your planning, it is important to identify the diverse populations that may require services. This may include making sure that services are delivered in a way that is accessible to all who may seek them (e.g., providing for family meetings in rooms that are physically accessible, sign language interpreters if a family member is hearing-impaired) or having services translated into other languages. Planning for access to follow-up care if needed should also be completed (e.g., counselors who may speak languages other than English). Modes of transportation should be physically accessible and language translators available if your school decides to transport family members to the area of the crash to be reunited with hospitalized loved ones.

M. Spiritual Assessment and Care
It is important to address the spiritual needs of those involved in the crisis and to plan for variety in the levels of needs. Some individuals may not want any spiritual care and may even be offended if it is offered. Others may desire spiritual support but want it from their own faith, which may not be dominant in your community or organization. In this case you may need to assist in making these connections. In this scenario, especially because of the deaths, it is likely that you will have a memorial service. It is important to recognize that different

religions have different ceremonial practices, and every effort should be made to respect and involve the varying wishes of the families that have lost a loved one.

N. Self-Care and Family Care, Including Safety and Security

Self-care is the focus of this chapter; we've discussed it a great deal, but to reiterate once again, it is important to take care of yourself. This is just as important as addressing the self-care of your staff, their families, your own family, and the families of those who have experienced a loss or tragedy in the crisis. This component is critical to many groups. In some cases self-care may include not only information about common signs and symptoms of stress and strategies to help manage the stress but also safety and security issues (for example, the family members who are coming to your school to await news and information about their loved ones should be allowed to enter and leave the school and gather in an area protected from the media, so that they are not swarmed or bombarded with cameras in their faces while they are concerned for loved ones). Starting with you: it is important to address self-care issues such as eating during the day, getting rest, and even how to go home at night. Helping your family to understand what you're going through with all of the stress and informing them about how they can assist during this time will be useful to them.

Self-care of your staff and colleagues is also important. Make sure they stick to schedules to get rest, food, and go home to focus on themselves and their families. Not only is getting food vital but so is getting the right food (i.e., healthier alternatives to caffeine, high-sugar foods, etc.). It is also essential to help their families by understanding the stressful days their spouse, parent, or significant others may be experiencing and how to support them when they come home. You can also share with family members the signs of stress and resources that are available to your staff for counseling and follow-up if needed.

The families of those involved in the crisis will also need much the same information and support as discussed above, including food, rest, water, and so on. Safety and security concerns should also be addressed. In this case, safety and security probably means protection from the media or others trying to get more information. For example, if you decide to have a meeting place for families at your school, it should be a place that is away from the media, comfortable for them to be in, that allows for the reception of news and information, and has food and water available. Families should be able to come and go without being swarmed by the media; in this situation, you have to think about the media both on campus and when and if family members travel to the hospital.

O. Postincident Evaluation and Training Based on Lessons Learned

As with any plans or procedures, they are never perfect and never one-size-fits-all solutions. It is always important to take time after an incident to examine what worked well and what didn't. There will always be lessons learned. Even if the process went well, there is usually at least one aspect that could be improved for a future situation. Everyone that was part of the response team should examine their contributions and/or their roles in the crisis and after it. It's common to have difficulty remembering everything days or even weeks later. It may be helpful to take notes or jot down comments on a daily basis. This will minimize the possibility of forgetting critical information and also create a journal for you to review and learn from. This information will also serve as a foundation for future training or planning and assist with redefining your emergency plan by considering lessons learned to improve the plan.

By no means is this information designed to make you a crisis counselor, psychologist, or social worker, owing to the amount of training required. This section is designed to raise your awareness about crises and the importance of having proper policies and procedures in place in order to respond to situations that go beyond day-to-day stresses. This information is intended to help you feel more comfortable about how and when to refer an individual on to the next level of care when needed. The well-being of the athletic trainer is dependent upon having good policies and procedures in place in the event that a crisis should occur. As with medical situations, emotional crises should be screened, triaged, and, when necessary, referred on to the next level of care with an appropriate professional. A general rule of good practice is: Whenever in doubt, consult with an appropriate professional or refer on to the next level of care.

WRAP-UP

A solid knowledge and understanding of the skills needed to help provide emotional support is key to responding to the mental health issues that will arise when an unthinkable, catastrophic event such as suicide, sudden death, or a travel accident occurs. These situations push the limits of emotional and physical health for you as well as your athletes, coaches, support staff, family, and friends. The athletic trainer is the primary health care provider who has the responsibility to triage the situation, must have a plan of action for referral, and be prepared with an emergency action plan in the event that the incident becomes a crisis situation. Although the goal of this chapter was to focus on the well-being of the athletic trainer, the principles applied are not unlike those that you would use to assist others. The athletic trainer must be able to recognize signs and symptoms of stress, both day to day and in a crisis situation. Following recognition, the athletic trainer must have a plan for both stress and crisis management. This chapter is not meant to provide the athletic trainer with a substitute for referral to a qualified mental health professional; rather, it is meant to give him or her an awareness of early psychological intervention skills until referral to a more qualified mental health professional can take place. The well-being of the athletic trainer is tied very closely to emergency preparedness. We

Scenarios

1. You are at preseason physicals and a freshman football player with a good sense of humor starts talking to you about his numerous injuries and states that you will probably get to know him well over the next 4 years. He comes to see you over the course of the season just to say hi. One day he comes in with another injured shoulder—a shoulder that has a history of injury. Consistent with your practice, you evaluate the injury, refer the athlete to the team physician—who recommends surgery—and then follow up with the athlete about the process. The athlete has the surgery and the rehabilitation process begins. Within 4 weeks after the surgery, you get a call in the middle of the night. You find out from one of the athlete's teammates that he was playing Russian roulette with a pistol in his dorm room and shot himself in the head.

   How could stress from recent medical events have contributed to the athlete's behavior and how might preincident education have addressed this situation?
   What postincident steps do you need to take in this situation?
   How should you deal with personal stress management in this situation?

2. It is September and the official basketball season has not yet started. According to NCAA guidelines, players are able to perform conditioning drills with a strength coach. The team is also "encouraged" to practice during open gym time to work on their skills. During open gym time, one of your players collapses on the court, never to get up again. He is later found to have experienced sudden death syndrome.

   What early psychological intervention skills should the athletic trainer employ in this situation?
   Could the athletic trainer have prepared himself for this situation? If so, how?

3. It is mid-February, and winter sports are in full swing at Obloy University. Basketball is a popular sport and the stands are packed at every home game. Obloy University is proud to have gained national recognition for its outstanding competitive cheer program. Because cheering is not recognized by the NCAA as an official sport, the athletic training squad is not required to provide health care to this team. On this particular day, at half-time of one of the biggest games of the year with rival Crowe University, the varsity cheer squad takes the floor. This squad is known for its outstanding stunts and the high degree of difficulty in its routines; today was no exception in that respect. What was different is that one of the stunts, the basket toss, went horribly wrong, and a team member fell to the floor, landing on her head. She did not move and no qualified health care provider was present at the scene. The athletic trainer was called to the scene after teammates tried to move the girl into an upright position. An ambulance was called, and the cheerleader was taken to the hospital. She was later diagnosed with a catastrophic spinal cord injury.

   What components of early psychological intervention would be most important to apply in this situation and why?
   The athletic trainer has been feeling guilty about these events—that he was not available at the time of the accident, when he might have prevented the catastrophic outcome. He has been unable to sleep, feels irritable, and is easily frustrated. Why is this happening and what would you recommend?

4. You are a certified athletic trainer and you have just accepted your first job at a local high school. Since this is your first year in a new job, you want to make a good impression; therefore, you put in overtime to make sure that you are taking care of as many athletes as you can. Two years later you are married. You are on top of the world. After several years, the late nights and weekends covering events and traveling with your teams start to take a toll on you, as demands for your time with family have increased, as well as demands by coaches to cover more and more events.

   What are some potential sources of stress facing you?
   What strategies can you employ to minimize the effects of these stressors?
   How will you know when the pressures of time have reached a critical point?

hope that the situations that have been described will never happen, but in the event that they do, having a solid knowledge base in when to seek help or refer to a mental health professional is important.

REFERENCES

1. Hendrix A, Acevedo E, Hebert E. An examination of stress and burnout in certified athletic trainers at division I-A universities. *J Athl Train.* 2000;35(2):139–144.
2. Dale J, Weinberg R. Burnout in sport: A review and critique. *Appl Sport Psychol.* 1990;2:67–83.
3. Perlman B, Hartman E. Burnout: Summary and future research. *Hum Relat.* 1982;35:283–305.
4. Smith R. Toward a cognitive–affective model of athletic burnout. *J Sport Psychol.* 1986;8:36–50.
5. Everly G, Mitchell J. *Critical Incident Stress Management (CISM): A new era and standard of care in crisis intervention.* Ellicott City, MD: Chevron; 1999.
6. Caplan G. *Principles of Prevention Psychiatry.* New York: Basic Books; 1964.
7. Mitchell J. *Critical Incident Stress Management (CISM): Group Crisis Intervention* (4th ed.). Ellicott City, MD: International Critical Incident Stress Foundation; 2006.
8. Mitchell J, Everly G. *The Basic Critical Incident Stress Management Course: Basic Group Crisis Intervention* (3rd ed.). Ellicott City, MD: International Critical Incident Stress Foundation; 2001.
9. Wilmore JH, Costill DL, Kenney WL. *Physiology of Sport and Exercise* (4th ed.). Champaign, IL: Human Kinetics; 2008.

10. Brummels K, Beach A. Role orientation of certified athletic trainers at institutions of higher education. *Athl Train Educ J.* 2008;1(Jan–Mar):5–12.

11. Everly G. *Assisting Individuals in Crisis* (4th ed.). Ellicott City, MD: International Critical Incident Stress Foundation; 2006.

12. American Red Cross (ARC). *Psychological First Aid: Helping People in Times of Stress. Instructors Manual.* Washington, DC: American Red Cross; 2006.

13. Mitchell J, Everly G. *Critical Incident Stress Debriefing: An Operations Manual for CISC, Defusing and Other Group Crisis Intervention Services* (3rd ed.). Ellicott City, MD: Chevron; 2001.

14. International Critical Incident Stress Foundation (ICISF). Critical Incident Stress Information Sheets, 2001. Retrieved July 30, 2008 from www.icisf.org/articles/Acrobat%20 Documents/TerrorismIncident/CISInfoSheet.pdf.

15. U.S. Department of Health and Human Services. *A Guide to Managing Stress in Crisis Response Professions.* DHHS Pub. No. SMA 4113. Rockville, MD: Center for Mental Health Services, Substance Abuse and Mental Health Services Administration; 2005.

16. Lerner MD, Volpe JS, Lindell B. *A Practical Guide For University Crisis Response.* Commack, NY: The American Academy of Experts in Traumatic Stress; 2004.

17. International Critical Incident Stress Foundation (ICISF). Early Psychological Intervention Points of Consensus Document, 2005. Retrieved July 30, 2008 from www.icisf.org/articles//NVOAD_commented.pdf.

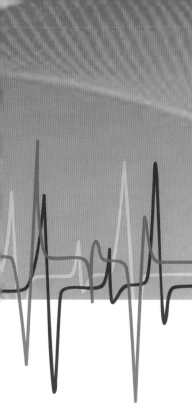

C H A P T E R 3

Legal Liability and Code of Ethics

CHAPTER OUTCOMES

1. Discuss actions an athletic trainer can take to limit legal liabilities in emergency situations.

2. Identify the legal rights and responsibilities of the athletic trainers and athletes during emergency situations.

3. Identify the standard of care as it relates to athletic trainer's job descriptions during emergency situations.

4. Identify and discuss the scope of practice of athletic trainers as it relates to emergency services.

5. Understand the "Good Samaritan" law and the provisions within the law that protect the rights of the athletic trainer.

6. Describe negligence and the main contributing factors that increase the chance of becoming negligent in emergency situations.

7. Identify and discuss the legal rights of the athlete in terms of confidentiality during emergency situations.

8. Identify and discuss how to obtain consent from an athlete for rendering emergency services.

9. Understand the importance of being compliant and following professional practice ethical standards.

NOMENCLATURE

Abandonment: stopping emergency services without the consent of the athlete or without making provisions for care by other qualified medical personnel

Commission: performing an act that results in harm

Expressed consent: consent given by the athlete to receive medical services

Implied consent: consent given by a legal guardian or parent for a infant or adolescent to receive medical services

Legal liability: when an athletic trainer who is legally responsible for services is liable for payment or damages

Omission: failure to do something one is trained to do and should do

Standard of care: degree of prudence and caution of the athletic trainer who is under a duty of care

Tort: civil wrongs recognized by courts of law as grounds for a lawsuit

BEFORE YOU BEGIN

1. What are some of the things an athletic trainer can do to decrease the likelihood of incurring legal liabilities when providing care for athletes?

2. Where does the athletic trainer find information about his or her standard of practice?

3. Does the athletic trainer have the legal right to refuse care for an athlete under his or her direct care?

4. Why is a code of ethics important for the athletic trainer?

Voices from the Field

Simply stated, a code of ethics identifies the principles one is obliged to follow. A professional code of ethics describes the essential values and guiding principles expected of all members of the profession. This all-encompassing code can be contentious, however. Some argue against creating a professional code of ethics because members of the profession may seek guidance from a personal moral code instead of a professional code. Others argue for the creation of a code of ethics because it clarifies the values of the profession for all affiliated individuals while also controlling for unethical practices within the profession. Whether or not the health care provider agrees with the creation of a code of ethics, he or she is still liable to the standard of care that is described by the profession's code. For the certified athletic trainer, this standard of care begins with the Board of Certification's Standards of Professional Practice.

The Standards of Professional Practice provide the framework from which the athletic trainer practices. It outlines the expected standard of care in athletic training by identifying the fundamental duties of the athletic trainer. It also guides the manner by which the athletic trainer satisfies these duties. Although the Standards of Professional Practice does not represent a policy and procedure manual, it does describe the general scope of practice for athletic training. Within this scope of practice is the duty to provide appropriate care to patients in an emergency situation. Failure to competently satisfy this duty can constitute negligence on the part of the athletic trainer. It can also violate a fundamental principle infused within the practice of athletic training. Whether the athletic trainer is guided more by personal or professional ethics, he or she is a health care professional and therefore is ethically compelled to respond to emergency situations.

Michael Hudson, PhD, ATC
Assistant Professor
Department of Sports Medicine and Athletic Training
Missouri State University

Athletic trainers, through their course work and clinical experiences, are taught to be prepared for emergency situations. Although they may have the knowledge ands skills to respond to these situations, another important skill comprises the knowledge that your services follow standards of practice to limit any type of **legal liability** that may occur. In this society, actions that are deemed immoral, unethical, or beyond the scope of practice can result in lawsuits and potentially cost you and your employers thousands of dollars and possibly your job. What can be done to limit your legal liability? The answer lies in the knowledge and understanding of what constitutes the actions that you can or cannot perform within your setting as an athletic trainer in responding to emergency situations and being ethical in rendering care to your athlete. This chapter focuses on your legal, moral, and ethical rights and the corresponding athlete's rights and responsibilities to ensure that in rendering services during an emergency situation, your focus and attention can be on your services, not on whether you may be held liable for your actions.

STANDARD OF CARE

Athletic trainers are required be certified in cardiopulmonary resuscitation (CPR) for Professional Athletic trainers, which encompasses CPR, automated external defibrillator (AED) training, and basic first aid. In addition, athletic trainers, through their curricula, are taught emergency rescues and transportation, splinting, and management of emergency injuries. Athletic trainers must demonstrate proficiency in these skills in caring for athletes. Because these skills are part of the athletic trainer's responsibilities, they are called the **standard of care** (Fig. 3.1). Only skills that reflect the training are included in the athletic trainer's standard of care. For example, if an athlete has a compound fracture of the humerus, the athletic trainer would properly splint the area and refer the athlete to medical personnel for follow-up care. Providing services that are not "standard" in this emergency situation may result in legal liability.

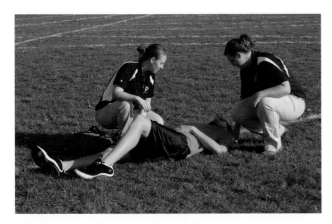

FIGURE 3.1   An athletic trainers working in the field.

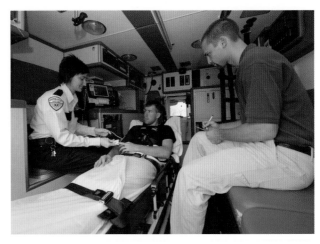

FIGURE 3.2   EMS performing their services.

SCOPE OF PRACTICE

Scope of practice implies providing medical services within the legal bounds of professional training and expertise to avoid harm. Providing care when not officially trained, knowledgeable, or illegally is "beyond" the individual's scope of practice and may lead to civil liability, especially if the injured athlete is harmed because of these actions. Each state has laws that govern the scope of practice for everyone from emergency medical technicians (EMTs) and nurses to physicians (Fig. 3.2). In athletic training, many practitioners' scope of practice is defined by state law, in addition to their scope of practice defined the role delineation study of the Board of Certification (BOC),[1] which delineates the knowledge and skills held by entry-level certified athletic trainers. All athletic trainers, regardless of their employment, must review their state laws for emergency services. To find the state laws, contact the athletic licensure or certification board or, if your state has no such board, contact the emergency services office or health and human services office.

These state laws or documents permit athletic trainers to provide care or services based upon their training and expertise. These laws also help protect injured athletes from receiving services from untrained individuals. In most cases, knowledge of essential emergency skills, such as lifesaving techniques for breathing, cardiac, and bleeding emergencies, can be performed by those trained CPR and first aid and can be rendered if these conditions become apparent. Starting an intravenous line in an emergency situation might be beyond the normal practices of an athletic trainer. Therefore, when rendering care in emergency situations, it is essential to know the extent and limitations of your professional responsibilities as defined by state law.

The Good Samaritan Law

When an athlete requires emergency aid, there may be uncertainty about who is legally qualified to provide such aid and about the potential legal implications of such treatment. Good Samaritan acts are "deeds in which aid is rendered to a person in need, when no fiduciary or legal obligation exists to provide such aid and no reward or remuneration from the aid is anticipated."[2] This law was established in 1959, initially to protect individuals such as doctors and nurses from civil liability when providing care in emergency situations where the athlete does not object to such treatment. These laws have since expanded and vary from state to state, so it's imperative that all athletic trainers know their state laws for rendering care in emergency situations. Although the Good Samaritan law does provide some protection to an individual rendering services, it does not protect against all legal actions for damages caused by the individual. In some states, the law may only protect those individuals who maintain a minimal level of first aid or CPR training certified by agencies such as the American Red Cross, American Heart Association, or National Safety Council. Therefore, when rendering emergency care, please follow these important rules:

1. If the injured athlete is conscious, ask him or her for consent before providing care.
2. Avoid unnecessary movement of the injured athlete if possible.
3. Call for emergency services.
4. Provide the care that a reasonable and prudent person with similar training would provide.
5. Provide care as you were trained. Do not render care outside your scope of practice.
6. If you start, provide the care until help arrives; do not abandon the athlete unless your own safety may be compromised or you become physically exhausted and cannot continue. Leaving the athlete in a condition that may allow him or her to become worse constitutes abandonment.

For example, suppose you are walking across campus and a faculty member collapses. Are you obligated to provide services? With your training and background in emergency situations, you may be qualified to assist (dependent upon your state's Good Samaritan law), and doing so may help save the life of the faculty member.

The above rules are meant to help you to avoid legal liability when you are providing care in an emergency situation. But does an individual have the right *not* to respond in an emergency situation? Depending upon state laws, you may not have to provide care unless you have a duty to act, meaning that your job requirement or responsibility requires you to act in a given situation. For example, if you are the parent or legal guardian of a child who needs emergency services, you are required to provide care. Failure to respond for the well-being of a child in an emergency situation will have legal implications in most states. If an emergency situation arises and you are working as an athletic trainer, you are required to render emergency services. This is called the **legal duty to act.** Whether you are being paid as an athletic trainer or volunteering, you are required to act when necessary to provide the standard of care defined by licensure or state statutes. In addition, once you begin rendering emergency services, you must continue to do so until help arrives. Stopping services before medical help arrives is called **abandonment,** which is defined as a stoppage of services without the consent of the injured person or without the provision of other qualified personnel to continue these services. For example, suppose, as the athletic trainer, you approach a football field and start providing care for an injured athlete when a bystander informs you that two other players are down at the other side of the field. You then leave the player without finishing your services or providing another qualified person to continue care. This would be an example of abandonment.

Patient's Right to Confidentiality

When emergency services are being performed, all information that may come to light should remain confidential. Information about the injured athlete's history and previous or current medical conditions should not be given out except to another qualified medical person who will also be providing care for the athlete. For example, if you are providing emergency services and another athletic trainer comes along to assist, some pertinent information as to the medical history or condition must be provided to ensure proper care; however, providing this information to a bystander is not appropriate. Discussing details with others at a later date is not warranted unless the athlete's name and medical history is protected or the athlete has given consent. If the athletic trainer gives out confidential information without consent, he or she may be found legally liable for **breach of confidentiality.**

Informed Consent

Informed consent means that the person being treated understands the risks or benefits of such treatment. It is meant

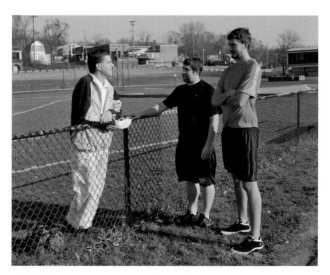

FIGURE 3.3   An athletic trainer discussing outcomes with athletes.

to allow athletes to make voluntary decisions or choices regarding their personal care, including possible results if care is not given (Fig. 3.3). Informed consent also protects the person from undue harm and ensures that the medical provider acts in a reasonable and prudent manner. In order for consent to be given by the injured athlete, the following conditions must be met: (a) the athlete must be competent to make such a decision; (b) the athlete must have been given all the necessary information to make such a decision, including the risks, benefits, and possible alternatives of treatment; and (c) the athlete must have the ability to understand the information given.[3] As a medical provider, before rendering services, you must make every possible effort to ensure that the athlete has understood the information given and has replied appropriately regarding the disposition of his or her situation. The athletic trainer should identify himself or herself to the athlete, stating his or her name and the type and level of training he or she possesses. Second, the athletic trainer should identify what has been observed (the type of medical emergency) and how he or she proposes to treat the athlete in this situation. The athletic trainer must identify the benefits of the treatment and the risks the athlete may face if treatment is not rendered. After this explanation, the athletic trainer must ask for understanding by the athlete; he or she cannot proceed unless the athlete consents to the treatment. When the injured athlete acknowledges that care should be given based upon the aforementioned criteria, he or she has provided **expressed consent.** Expressed consent can also be given by the athlete for only some medical services, such as the application of a splint but not transportation to a local medical facility.

Historically, informed consent was obtained by two different approaches, either the "professional practice" standard or the "reasonable person" standard.[4] The professional practice standard is geared to practices of physicians and other medical professionals who, based upon past practices, determine the kinds and amounts of information that may be disclosed to a patient.[5] Under the reasonable person standard, information given is in accordance with what a reasonable person would need and want to know, allowing the patient to be the agent of the decision-making process.[6] Patients, who are provided with all pertinent information may make a decision to accept or avoid medical treatment. Though not providing services may result in a potentially life-threatening condition for the patient, continuation of treatment of a competent person without consent may lead to legal liability.

As an athletic trainer, you must recognize that an athlete can refuse care; but in order to do so, you should follow some guidelines. First, the athlete must be an adult, 18 years of age or older, and not under the care of a legal guardian. The athlete should also be deemed competent; that is, able to comprehend and act in a reasonable manner. If an athlete refuses care and the athletic trainer suggests that care is needed, a thorough explanation of any or all consequences should be given to the athlete. Information should also be provided to the athlete who refuses care; that is, the athlete should be informed about signs and symptoms of the condition if it worsens and advised to seek medical referral if it does. It may be prudent for other medical personnel to intervene and explain the consequences of the athlete's condition and actions. However, the athlete may still refuse medical treatment. If all these procedures fail, it may be wise to leave the athlete with another competent adult if possible.

Minors pose a particular dilemma for emergency services. If a child or infant requires emergency medical services, consent from an adult or legal guardian must be obtained. The legal guardian may refuse treatment for their child. If this happens, and the athletic trainer feels that services are needed, he/she should provide a strong rationale for the necessity of care for the child's sake. If no guardian or parent is available in an emergency situation, it may automatically be assumed that consent has been given for medical personnel to render the appropriate services.

Implied Consent

Implied consent includes situations where the legal guardian or parent is not present for a minor, the athlete is unconscious, or the athlete has a life-threatening injury. In these situations, consent is "implied" and the athletic trainer can administer the appropriate care. The athletic trainer is protected because laws state that the parents or legal guardians would want emergency services rendered to their children and that injured persons of reasonable mind would want services.

Obtaining Consent

In the athletic training setting, consent prior to an emergency situation can be given in written form. Athletes participating in health care screening, such as preparticipation examinations or health history questionnaires, can be given a consent form that contains language for the sole purpose

of rendering care in case of an emergency or if the individual should become incapacitated. In creating informed consent documents, certain criteria should be met in order for the athlete to make the appropriate decisions. These criteria should include the types of treatments or procedures that might be offered, such as CPR/first aid, diagnostic tests, activation of medical emergency services, and transportation to a local hospital. Having the individual sign and date the consent will allow the athletic trainer to render emergency services in situations where consent cannot be given.

Negligence

If you provide care in an emergency situation outside your scope of practice or professional training or fail to provide any care at all in an emergency situation, you may be held liable for your actions. In law, negligence is a type of **tort** where an individual fails to render care as a reasonably prudent and careful person would have done under similar circumstances. For negligence to have occurred, the plaintiff must prove that the defendant met four conditions. These four conditions are duty to act, breach of that duty, causation, and damage.

The plaintiff must first establish that the athletic trainer (defendant) in fact had a legal responsibility to provide care. This is often defined by contract or job descriptions that determine the capacity and scope of practice for the athletic trainer. For example, Sam is employed as a certified athletic trainer to render athletic training services to his institution's ice hockey team. While Sam is covering a game, a player is struck in the throat with a puck. Sam has a duty to respond to the emergency situation as defined within the scope of practice of an athletic trainer.

Next, the plaintiff must prove that the defendant breached his or her duty to act. That is, did he or she exercise the same standard of care that another reasonable and prudent person with the same level of training and education would provide in a similar situation. Under this principle, an athletic trainer can be found negligent through an act of omission. **Omission** is the failure to act when there is a legal responsibility to act, while **commission** is acting incorrectly or beyond the scope of one's practice as compared with the actions of another reasonable and prudent person. For example, Sam determines that the player is not breathing and, rather than open the airway (as a reasonable and prudent person would do), Sam decides to perform a tracheotomy, which would be an act of commission.

In causation, the damages being claimed by the plaintiff are a direct result of the defendant's actions or inactions. In the situation given as an example, the player may be seeking recompense for medical expenses or speech therapy based upon the tracheotomy.

Last, did the defendant actually suffer physical, emotional, or financial harm as a result of Sam's services? This could be the case if, several weeks after the incident, it was determined that the ice hockey player lost his ability to speak because Sam placed the tracheotomy tube in the larynx rather than the trachea.

Simple physical acts, such as moving an athlete with a suspected spinal cord injury when there is no physical threat from the environment, providing services for which you have not been trained, or not providing care when you are obligated to do so (when you are working as an athletic trainer and encounter a person who has an life-threatening condition but you fail to provide services) can be classified as negligence.

If, however, one of the four points listed above cannot be proven, then negligence did not occur. For example, if an athletic trainer attempted to splint a severely painful, swollen, deformed leg using an unorthodox splinting technique (act of commission) but no harm or damage resulted, then negligence may not occur.

PROFESSIONAL ETHICS

As an athletic trainer working with various athletes, practicing and conducting yourself in ethical manner is paramount. The nature of professional ethics and what these mean for an athletic trainer should be part of every athletic training curriculum. Although many would argue that a discussion of professional ethics is not part of an emergency plan, the conduct and professionalism exercised in these instances reflects knowledge and pride in one's work. Professional ethics comprises the moral issues and responsibilities of an individual in his or her professional practice. Ethical standards are sets of guidelines, codes, or rules that guide an individual's professional behavior and protect the public served by that individual. They are meant to define what is acceptable behavior and to identify standards of practice. These codes of ethics are meant to help deter wrongdoing and usually have several components to guide professional organizations in developing their respective code of ethical practices.

> ### Breakout
>
> Links to Professional Organizations' Codes of Ethics
>
> National Athletic Trainers' Association: http://www.nata. org/codeofethics/code_of_ethics.pdf
>
> National Athletic Trainers' Association Board of Certification: http://www.bocatc.org/index.php?option=com_ content&task=view&id=51&Itemid=54
>
> National Strength and Conditioning Association (must log in as member): http://www.nsca-lift.org/
>
> American College of Sports Medicine: http://www.acsm. org/Content/NavigationMenu/MemberServices/Member Resources/CodeofEthics/Code_of_Ethics.htm
>
> American Physical Therapy Association: http://www. apta.org/AM/Template.cfm?Section=Ethics_and_Legal_ Issues1&Template=/TaggedPage/TaggedPageDisplay. cfm TPLID=48&ContentID=41162

Athletic trainers must know when and when not to apply certain services and how to conduct themselves in emergency situations. These actions reflect upon their overall professional training and responsibilities. The question of whether athletic trainers have a responsibility to act and whether they conduct themselves in legal and ethical manner is part of every emergency situation. Some codes of ethics are guided by state or federal laws, and individuals who breach these codes can often be held liable for their actions. Other codes of ethics are more "advisory" in nature and can result in actions ranging from warnings to dismissal from one's professional organization without criminal penalty. The code of ethics for athletic trainers may be found on the National Athletic Trainer's Association Web site. In addition, BOC, the athletic trainers' certification agency, also has a code of ethics. As a professional in an allied health field, it is imperative that you become cognizant of the codes of ethics affecting your practice and that you review these codes periodically.

WRAP-UP

> ### Breakout
>
> Common standards used for developing a code of ethics for a professional organization:
>
> 1. To promote honest and ethical conduct with services
> 2. To promote honest and ethical conduct when conflicts of interest arise
> 3. To be in compliance with all local, state and federal laws, rules, or regulations
> 4. To base professional conduct on scope of knowledge and training in the profession
> 5. To develop an internal means of reporting and investigating ethical code violations
> 6. To develop accountability for ethical violations

This chapter provides athletic trainers with legal and ethical considerations when rendering emergency care for injured athletes. The information presented should be a guide to ensure that emergency services follow standard scopes of practice and conform with state laws. It is the responsibility of the athletic trainer to become knowledgeable and aware of these laws prior to working with athletes. In addition, athletic trainers working with athletes should follow their professional organization's ethical standards and report those who violate such guidelines to the appropriate agency. By implementing the guidelines discussed in this chapter, the athletic trainer should feel confident that his

Scenarios

1. You are working as an athletic trainer at a swim meet. You notice some commotion in the stands and heard that a spectator has collapsed, needing CPR.

Do you help or do you ignore the situation and wait for EMS to arrive?

2. Working as an athletic trainer, you decided that a 14-year-old athlete with an ankle sprain and swelling should take an anti-inflammatory medication. Since you are busy, you tell the athlete just to grab the bottle and take some pills. The athlete, thinking that you meant take *all* the pills, and does so upon your request. Later, the athlete develops serious side effects that require medical intervention.

Are you, as the athletic trainer, liable for your actions?

3. You are about to graduate from a Commission on Accreditation of Athletic Training Education athletic training program and are looking for employment. You find a job in a neighboring state at a division 2 high school. You are sitting for the BOC examination about 3 weeks prior to your employment.

How do you find out if you will be qualified to work as an athletic trainer for said high school, and where can you find this information?

4. Prior to preseason practice, you conduct preparticipation physicals, orthopedic assessments, and health history documentation for your athletes. One aspect that just came to your attention is consent to treat.

What is needed for proper documentation and how should you obtain this information?

or her emergency services are legal and ethical and that the likelihood of legal liability is decreased.

REFERENCES

1. Board of Certification Role Delineation Study, 5th edition.
2. Daniels S. Ethical Issues in Emergency Medicine. *Emerg Med Clin North Am*. 1999;17(2):491–504.
3. Meisel A, Roth L. What we do and do not know about informed consent. *JAMA*. 1981;246:2473–2477.
4. Modern status of views as to general measure of physician's duty to inform patient of risks of proposed treatment. *Am Law Rep*. 3d,1978;88:1008.
5. Solomon RC. Ethical issues in medical malpractice. *Emerg Med Clin North Am*. 2006;24:733–747.
6. Physician's duty to inform of risks. *Am Law Rep*. 1986;88:1010–1025.

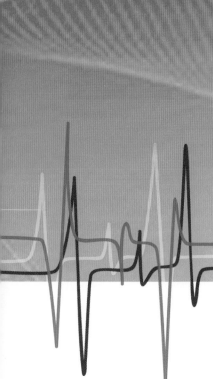

C H A P T E R · 4

Emergency Action Plans

CHAPTER OUTCOMES

1. Understand the rationale and importance of emergency action plans.

2. Be able to identify the major components of an emergency action plan.

3. Differentiate between the types of emergency action plans and their usage.

4. Understand that emergency action plans are venue- and sport-specific.

5. Be able to develop an emergency action plan based upon examples and components described in this chapter.

6. Understand the importance of emergency communication and appropriate ways to communicate with medical personnel.

7. Be able to identify and list responsibilities of all individuals associated with an emergency action plan.

8. Be able to describe where/how to locate necessary equipment, phones, stairs, and doors in emergency situations, using maps/drawings as part of an emergency action plan.

9. Identify means of conveyance used at athletic venues to transport athletes to various medical facilities.

10. Be able to outline, in bulleted form, highlights of an emergency action plan for use with visiting medical personnel or coaches/administrators.

11. Describe the need for information regarding blood-borne pathogens to be included in emergency action plans.

12. Discuss methods to properly implement/practice emergency action plans at each venue/site on a regular and basis.

NOMENCLATURE

Automated external defibrillator (AED): a portable electronic device that automatically diagnoses cardiac arrhythmias (ventricular fibrillation and ventricular tachycardia) and treats them with the application of an electrical charge to reestablish an effective rhythm

Emergency Medical Services (EMS): a service providing out-of-hospital acute/chronic care and

transport of patients with illnesses or injuries that are believed to constitute medical emergencies to medical facilities

First responder: the first medically trained person to arrive on scene of an injury or illness

Negligence: conduct that is culpable because it falls short of what a reasonable person would do to protect another individual from a foreseeable risk

Other potentially infectious materials (OPIMs): including semen, vaginal secretions, cerebrospinal fluid, synovial fluid, pleural fluid, amniotic fluid, or body fluid that is visibly contaminated with blood

Trauma: a body-altering physical injury

Venue: the location of a specific event

BEFORE YOU BEGIN

1. What are the main components of the emergency action plan (EAP)?

2. Who is responsible for developing the EAP at each venue?

3. Why is important to practice and rehearse the EAP?

4. What information must you provide to emergency medical services (EMS) when an emergency situation arises at your athletic venue?

5. What information should you include in an EAP for visiting personnel?

Voices from the Field

Athletic injuries can occur at any time and anywhere. How many times have you heard that line? As overused as that statement is, it holds very true. It is because of this statement that sports medicine teams and athletic departments have a duty to develop sound emergency plans that can be implemented when necessary and provide the appropriate standards of care to all sports participants. In formulating an emergency plan, it is a good idea to keep in mind that there are many components that must be identified. These include but are not limited to emergency numbers and communication, personnel roles and responsibilities, administrative policies and procedures, sudden injury/illness policy and procedures, serious/catastrophic injury policy and procedures, AED protocols, weather guidelines, blood-borne pathogen policy and procedures, and emergency action plans for each athletic venue. Creating a sound EAP is only half the battle. It is vital to routinely practice each and every possible scenario that involves implementing one or more of the elements of your EAP. This will allow you to step back and analyze what elements of the EAP are sound and what elements need some reconfiguring. The EAP should be routinely visited to ensure that all policies and procedures are up to date and that all personnel involved in athletics understand and can clearly identify their roles in an emergency situation. It also is a good idea to highly recommend that all coaches/personnel involved with athletics also be certified in first aid and cardiopulmonary resuscitation (CPR). It cannot be stressed enough that being prepared means being ready for any type of emergency. Whether you are revising an EAP or developing a new one, it is vital to make every effort to identify risks and provide appropriate responses, all the while keeping in mind that good judgment should prevail at the time of the emergency situation.

Scott Michel, MA, ATC
Head Athletic Trainer
Kalamazoo College
Kalamazoo, MI

This chapter discusses EAPs, which athletic trainers should follow when emergency situations arise; such plans also provide guidelines to prevent lawsuits or legal actions, often associated with **negligence** (see Chapter 3). As with all policies, an EAP must thoroughly cover medical/**trauma**-related events and how to respond in these situations. The EAP document provides succinct details and steps that must be followed in case an emergency should arise while working with athletes at any venue or occasion. In most cases, the EAP will cover situations not only with home events and practices but also events that take place while traveling or away from home. This includes tournaments, championship games, and other venues in which you may work from time to time.

The EAP is a written document that defines the actions that the athletic trainer and other medical personnel must follow if/when an emergency situation arises. All medical and athletic administration personnel who are involved in the care and administration of athletic events must be consulted and must work together closely in developing the EAP. Such personnel can include the athletic director, athletic trainer, physicians, police, and EMS in the community. The EAP is so important that the National Collegiate Athletic Association (NCAA)[1] and the National Federation of State High School Associations[2] recommend that each institution have one.

COMPONENTS OF AN EAP

According to the National Athletic Trainers' Association (NATA) position statement on emergency planning in athletics,[3] the EAP should, at a minimum, comprise those components that will give an organization a "blueprint" to follow in case of an athletic emergency. These components include qualifications of personnel, equipment that may be necessary, and communication and transportation guidelines. In addition, the EAP must be regularly rehearsed or practiced to let those involved become better acquainted with their specific tasks and responsibilities.

TYPES OF EAPs

According to Walsh,[4] EAPs can be classified into three distinct categories: standard injury protocol, weather-related emergency, and trauma/medical emergency in athletics. The standard injury protocol is an overall general action plan to address injuries or illnesses that require further attention or medical referral. This should include procedures to determine when to contact a physician (depending upon the extent of an injury), general instructions that athletes can take home to properly care for an injury, and information as to where the medical records of athletes are kept and how they are used for home and traveling events.

The weather-related action plan addresses severe weather emergencies, from tornadoes to extreme heat and humidity. Covered here are policies on how to suspend and resume physical activities based upon weather conditions (Fig. 4.1), who is in charge of assessing weather-related conditions, and who is to be notified in cases of extreme weather events. These protocols should address not only the athletes but also spectators at each athletic venue. Specific emergency action plans for athletes suffering from heat stress and how to provide appropriate care can be reviewed in the NATA position statements for exertional heat illness[5]; fluid replacement for athletes[6] can be included in the weather-related EAP.

Trauma/medical related emergency action plans should be the most specific in terms of management. Included

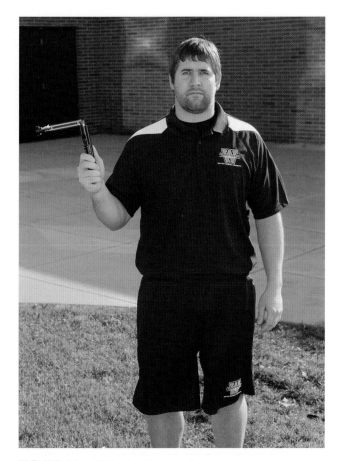

FIGURE 4.1   ATC using sling psychrometer.

in this EAP are protocols to follow in traumatic/medical emergencies for all athletic venues, home and away, and for all games, practices, or scrimmages. The NCAA provides guidelines in its *1998–1999 NCAA Sports Medicine Handbook* as to minimal requirements for athletic venues.[7] These include providing qualified persons who are trained in CPR/first aid, having on-site EMS, ensuring access to medical facilities, having appropriate emergency equipment and communication devices on hand, and having proper contact information readily accessible should emergency situations arise during athletic events.

DEVELOPING AN EMERGENCY ACTION PLAN

To develop an EAP, the primary medical personnel (e.g., athletic trainer, physician) must plan actions based upon their sport-specific venues. This means that the athletic trainer must list all practice and game sites, types of events covered, the personnel primarily working or available at these sites, access to gates or doors through which athletes may be transported, location of local hospital or medical facilities, emergency phone numbers, and other content (see the Breakout box on page 47). Once a list is created, a detailed plan for

Breakout

Example of an EAP for an Athletic Venue

A. Athletic Emergency—Certified Athletic Trainer (ATC) Present

   1. In the event of an emergency situation, the ATC will assume the role of **first responder** and activate EMS when necessary.

   2. Should a coach be sent to activate EMS, he or she should be prepared to provide the dispatcher with pertinent information regarding the student–athlete and then report back to the injury scene.

   3. In all situations where an ATC is present, necessary first aid and splinting supplies should be available.

B. Athletic Emergency–Athletic Training Student (ATS) Present

   1. In the event of an emergency situation, the ATS will assume the role of **first responder,** quickly assessing the situation and requesting assistance from the athletic training room or activating EMS.

   2. In this situation, a member of the coaching staff should assist the ATS by retrieving emergency supplies, calming the injured student–athlete, or clearing the immediate area.

   3. If the injured student–athlete should require transportation to a hospital, a member of the coaching staff should accompany the EMS staff in order to provide personal and insurance information to the hospital staff.

   4. When handling an emergency, it must be understood that an ATS is to act *only* as a first responder.

C. Only Coaches Present

   1. In the absence of an ATC or ATS, the coach should immediately assume the role of first responder. This involves a primary survey, basic life support, and activation of EMS. *At no time should a student–athlete assume the role of the first responder.*

   2. If the coach is providing basic life support, he or she must continue until EMS personnel arrive and take over.

   3. If the student–athlete requires transportation by EMS, a member of the coaching staff (person initially providing care for the student–athlete) must accompany the injured student–athlete to the emergency room. This is to make sure that the student–athlete's personal and insurance information is relayed to the appropriate personnel at the hospital.

   4. The supervising ATC for the team should be notified of the incident as soon as possible.

Activating EMS

A. Making the call

   1. The individual providing care for the injured student–athlete should *never* leave the injury site; instead, he or she should ask an ATS, coach, or manager to call.

   2. To activate EMS, use a cell or LAN-line telephone from the athletic training room (or easiest access) to dial campus police or EMS. The caller then should be prepared to give the following information:

   a. Name and title

   b. Name and age of student–athlete

   c. Injury that student–athlete has suffered

   d. Location of injured student–athlete

   e. Best place is to enter venue (venue directions, locations, entry spots, and maps are available in the appendices)

   3. Most importantly, *do not* hang up before the dispatcher does.

B. Once the call has been completed and before leaving, the caller should be instructed to report back to the injury site for any further instructions. Once returned, the caller should be sent to meet the EMS crew at the designated entrance site.

C. Insurance information on the injured student–athlete *must* be retrieved prior to arrival of the EMS crew. This information *must* be located in the medical kit.

Proper Notification and Follow-up

A. Once the injured student–athlete is en route to the hospital, a team physician must be notified of the situation immediately. Be prepared to report the mechanism of injury, injury sustained, management of the situation, and hospital to which the student–athlete was taken.

B. Ask the physician to call ahead to the hospital in an effort to contact the attending physician and expedite the registration process once the student–athlete has arrived.

C. Documentation

   1. Once the situation has been managed or following return to the athletic training room, the event should be documented *immediately*. This is to ensure that events and details are not forgotten.

   2. In addition, proper documentation and notification procedures must be completed as soon as possible.

Emergency Equipment and Transportation

A. Depending on the venue, emergency equipment will be on site and accessible for all teams competing. The equipment must be available at all scheduled practices and games.

B. The following emergency equipment should be available. (Availability will depend on the specific venue.)

   1. AED, Banyan kit, vacuum splints, leg immobilizers, SAM splints, crutches, and SportsChair.

C. Transportation to a local emergency room will be available by university vehicle (where applicable) or by ambulance service.

each venue can be developed. This plan can be duplicated for multiple venues if facilities or locations are similar. However, if differences exist, such as medical personnel, access to facility, and the like, the EAP must address these differences. In other words, each venue must have its own specific EAP. After the EAP is developed, it is recommended that it be reviewed by the organization's legal counsel and/or administrators before being officially posted and implemented.

Venue Communication and Personnel

In developing an EAP, the first step is to determine the location of telephones (land lines and cell phones) or other communication devices, such as two-way radios or walkie talkies (Fig. 4.2). The EAP should address not only who has access to these communication devices but also how to access outside numbers (if off campus) and specific phone numbers in that venue for emergency services.[4] These numbers should be posted or found next to phones at each site or in pocket cards for all medical personnel providing services. In addition, the EAP should include instructions pertaining to who will make phone calls requesting emergency services.

If the venue requires that an EAP be developed for weather-related emergencies, communication devices such as horns or whistles should be readily available and instructions as to when they are to be used and who will use them are required.[4] All parties involved in a given athletic venue must also know the meaning of signals given by these devices if the EAP is to functional properly in an emergency situation.

The personnel involved in emergency care at any athletic venue must be identifiable to visiting coaches, officials, athletic trainers, physicians, or other administrators prior to the event. In many instances, the person providing care is not the same person who summons assistance or is responsible for crowd control or clearing the scene. The EAP should be specific as to the roles of individuals at each venue. An action card can be created and distributed that lists those who will be available, their roles and responsibilities, and how to con-

tact them. This way, if an emergency situation arises, all visiting parties will have information at their disposal. Included on the card should be how to communicate properly with EMS or 911 services (see the Breakout box, above).

Emergency Equipment

One of the most important aspects of the EAP is knowing the types and locations of medical equipment. This includes spine boards, Epi-pens for allergic reactions, buoyancy devices for pool rescues, splints, **AEDs,** and other devices for sport-specific venues. Each piece of equipment should be in proper working order, functional, and readily available. All medical staff should be trained in the use of the equipment; they should practice and be tested in its use periodically to ensure competence (Fig. 4.3). For visiting medical personnel,

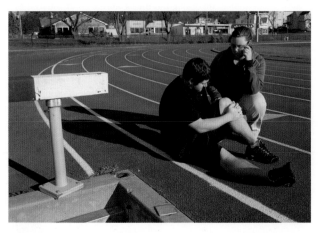

FIGURE 4.2 ATC using cell phone to call emergency services.

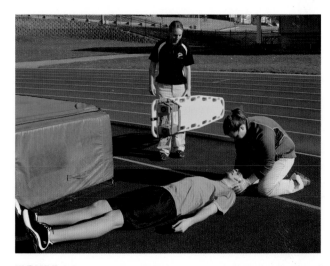

FIGURE 4.3 Situation in which an athlete will need to be placed on a spine board.

a listing of equipment should be provided, including its location. If the visitors are not properly trained in its use, they should be told how to summon help if necessary.

Blood-borne Pathogens

One often overlooked aspect of the EAP is exposure to blood-borne pathogens. Exposure to blood, bodily fluids, or **other potentially infectious materials** (OPIMs) can increase the risk of becoming infected. Exposure to such pathogens is common when caring for traumatically injured athletes, performing CPR, or in situations where towels may be soaked with blood. Similar risks are also involved in needle sticks associated with anaphylactic shock or when insulin injections may be required. Federal law states that a written exposure control plan (ECP) must be developed in facilities where risk may occur. The ECP should be included in the EAP, and the locations of all containers for devices exposed to OPIMs should be marked, making them easily accessible. For more specific information on blood-borne pathogens, see Chapter 7.

Transportation

During athletic events, emergency situations may arise that necessitate the transportation of an athlete to a medical facility. Usually, transportation involves activation of EMS. In many instances, however, EMS may not be available or appropriate. For each venue, the EAP should include protocols on how an athlete is to be transported to medical facilities. Although most EAPs provide instructions for emergency activation and personnel responsible for transportation to medical facilities, policies should also include multiple means of transportation in case more than one injured individual is involved.[4] For example, if a tornado caused injury during an athletic event and multiple athletes or spectators were injured, having a detailed plan for one vehicle as a mode of transportation may not suffice. In addition, it may also be reasonable to include driving directions to medical facilities for visiting personnel or individuals who are not familiar with the town/city/location of the athletic venue. The driving directions should include the names of the roads, distances traveled, and approximate times to reach the desired destination. It is advisable to provide alternate routes in places where traffic or construction could delay transport to medical care.

Schematic Maps

Often helpful in an EAP is a floor plan or hand-drawn map of the athletic venue.[4] A visual representation of the athletic venue can give medical personnel a better idea of where emergency equipment and services are located, enabling quicker access. Included in the maps should be the locations of doors, phones, emergency equipment (if not already present), ramps, elevators, steps, or other physical structures.

Locations of individuals who are assisting with the arrival of EMS or other medical personnel should be included in the venue map so as to facilitate their movement to and from the venue to the site of the injured athlete. The location of persons who are assisting is especially important for larger venues, such as stadiums or arenas, where there are multiple entrances and exits.

Flowcharts/Bulleted Points

Part of the EAP, usually near the end of the document, should contain flowcharts/bulleted points summarizing the steps involved for venue emergency situations. These

---

Breakout

EAP Instructions for Visiting Personnel

A. Nonemergency Injuries
  1. If an injury occurs that does not require the assistance of EMS, the visiting team's athletic trainer will perform an evaluation to determine participation status.

B. Emergency Injuries
  1. If a student–athlete or coach sustains an injury requiring immediate medical attention, it is the responsibility of the visiting team's athletic trainer to administrate emergency care until EMS arrives.
  2. The visiting team's athletic trainer, athletic training student, or coach will be responsible for activating EMS.
    a. Perform emergency CPR and first aid
    b. Instruct athletic training student, coach, or manager to call EMS.
    c. Provide the following information:
      Identify yourself and give general information
      Explain where you are located and direct EMS to your exact location.
      Offer any additional information and be the last to hang up.
    d. Coaching staff will head to the area specified in order to meet EMS.
  3. An AED is usually mounted on a wall near the athletic training room, and the AED box is wired to campus police. If EMS is needed, campus police should be contacted to activate EMS.
  4. An ATS or the visiting team's athletic trainer is responsible for providing the appropriate insurance information to the hospital.
  5. The visiting team's athletic trainer will assist EMS personnel.
  6. It is the responsibility of the visiting team's athletic trainer to contact the student–athlete's parent or guardian.
  7. Staff, coach, or visiting team's athletic trainer will accompany the student–athlete to the hospital.

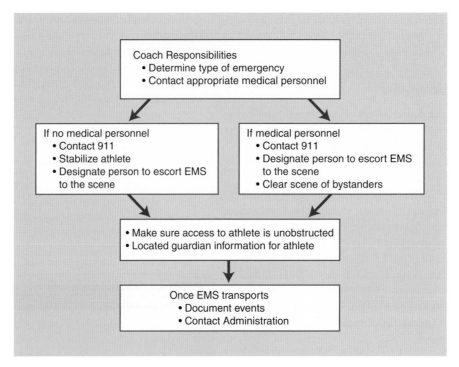

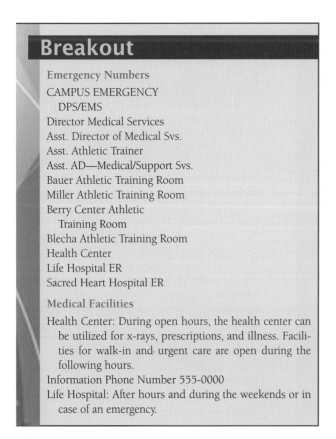

FIGURE 4.4   Example of an EAP flow chart for coaches.

elements should be general enough to provide crucial information in emergency situations. Although not as inclusive as the written EAP procedure, flowcharts and/or bulleted points are useful for visiting personnel, coaches, officials, or

administrators who need a quick overview of their responsibilities without reading a multiple-page document (Fig. 4.4). These sections can also serve as quick reviews for event staff, ATCs, and medical personnel to facilitate retention of procedures or protocols.

Breakout

Emergency Numbers

CAMPUS EMERGENCY
    DPS/EMS
Director Medical Services
Asst. Director of Medical Svs.
Asst. Athletic Trainer
Asst. AD—Medical/Support Svs.
Bauer Athletic Training Room
Miller Athletic Training Room
Berry Center Athletic
    Training Room
Blecha Athletic Training Room
Health Center
Life Hospital ER
Sacred Heart Hospital ER

Medical Facilities

Health Center: During open hours, the health center can be utilized for x-rays, prescriptions, and illness. Facilities for walk-in and urgent care are open during the following hours.

Information Phone Number 555-0000

Life Hospital: After hours and during the weekends or in case of an emergency.

EMERGENCY ACTION PLAN PRACTICE AND EDUCATION

Once the EAP is developed for all venues, it's time to practice activation of the EAP to determine feasibility. When a plan is developed on paper, it is prudent to act out a scenario that utilizes the protocols that have been developed so as to determine whether the written procedures can be accurately followed and implemented as planned. If the EAP is not thoroughly tested prior to implementation, actions thought to be trivial or commonsense may not work as devised or steps developed may be either too complicated or not beneficial in the emergency situation. After the initial practice, revisions can be made to ensure that the EAP is a functional document.

Once the EAP has been developed and determined to be feasible, it is important to educate all parties who will be involved in its implementation.[3] The education plan involves distribution of the EAP to all parties, reading and understanding the entire EAP, and reviewing individual roles. It may be pertinent to have inservices or structured meetings of all parties to review the components of the EAP, answer questions, and clarify roles and

Scenarios

1. Visiting athletic teams and athletic trainers report to your venue for a softball tournament. Your own team did not make the tournament playoffs and, because of additional clinical responsibilities, you will not be covering any part of the tournament. Your venue is off campus, approximately a mile, so all emergency equipment you feel may be required is brought on site each day by ATSs.

   Because you will not be present at the tournament, what should you do as the home athletic trainer to make sure all visiting parties are prepared for emergencies?

2. As a newly hired head athletic trainer at a small division II institution, you notice, upon beginning your employment, that the athletics department does not have an EAP for any venue or athletic site on or off campus. Knowing that emergencies will inevitably occur, one of your first tasks is to develop an EAP for each athletic facility at your institution.

   What are the specific components and tasks you should have in mind in order to develop an appropriate EAP?

3. An athlete required emergency services for an injury sustained during lacrosse. As the athletic trainer, you summoned EMS and provided care as specified in the EAP. However, some glitches occurred that hindered transportation during the emergency process (although these did not affect the care of the athlete).

   What should you do now that the emergency situation is over, and how should you correct the problem?

4. A visiting team comes to your volleyball venue for a game. The assistant athletic trainer approaches you prior to the start, asking how to proceed in case of an emergency.

   What information should you provide and how can you effectively supply/deliver that information?

responsibilities, especially for administrators or others who may be called into service who have minimal emergency training or experience.

Once the EAP has been found feasible, practicing it is recommended.[4] Practicing the EAP with all involved parties helps to refine skills and increase confidence in emergency situations. An EAP for each venue should be rehearsed and practiced, since the implementation may be different because of variations in emergency equipment, location of communication devices, personnel, etc. Most importantly, practice should be conducted not only prior to the sporting season or events but also during the entire season. Make sure that the EAP is reviewed by all parties associated with the event, including not only medical personnel (e.g., athletic trainer, physician, EMTs, etc.) but also event coordinators, coaches, officials, security, and even the sports information directors or public announcers. When all concerned know their roles and responsibilities prior to the event, you will be more comfortable knowing that if an emergency situation should arise, mishaps or errors may be avoided or kept to a minimum. In fact, arranging for an impromptu, unexpected scenario can be extremely beneficial for all parties.

ADDITIONAL DOCUMENTATION

In the event of an actual emergency situation, when care and management have been provided, a written summary of the event is recorded.[9] The written documentation should contain all pertinent information, such as how the event occurred, who provided care and their roles and responsibilities, and complications of the implementation of the EAP. Anderson[9] also recommends a debriefing of all parties involved to help determine difficulty or issues related to the EAP. The steps involved in the documentation of accounts after an emergency situation should be included in the EAP.

WRAP-UP

EAPs are integral parts of any athletic training venue. Considerable time and effort must be spent in developing an EAP that is venue-specific and can be implemented with little or no wasted time in any emergency situation. The criteria and examples presented in this chapter can serve as a starting point to gathering all the information needed; that is, the chapter can provide a template for the development of a properly working document. In addition to the development of an EAP, proper education of all parties involved and periodic practice with the EAP is required to ensure competence and confidence.

REFERENCES

1. Brown GT. NCAA group raising awareness on medical coverage. *NCAA News.* March 15, 1999:6–7.
2. Shultz SJ, Zinder SM, Valovich TC. *Sports Medicine Handbook.* Indianapolis, IN: National Federation of State High School Associations; 2001.
3. Andersen JC, Courson RW, Kleiner DM, McLoda TA. National Athletic Trainers' Association position statement: Emergency planning in athletics. *J Athl Train.* 2002;37(1): 99–104.
4. Walsh K. Thinking proactively: The emergency action plan. *Athl Ther Today.* 2001;6(5):57–62.

5. Binkley HM, Beckett J, Casa DJ, Kleiner DM, Plummer PE. National Athletic Trainers' Association Position Statement: Exertional heat illnesses. *J Athl Train.* 2002;37(3):329–343.

6. Casa DJ, Armstrong LE, Hillman SK, et al. National Athletic Trainers' Association Position Statement: Fluid replacement for athletes. *J Athl Train.* 2000;35(2):212–224.

7. Halpin T. *1999-2000 NCAA Sports Medicine Handbook (Serial),* 12th ed. Indianapolis, IN Natl Collegiate Athletic Assn;1999.

8. Davidson D, Eickhoff-Shemek JM. Is your emergency action plan complete? *ACSMs Health Fit J.* 2006;10(1):29–31.

9. Anderson B. Policies and philosophies related to risk management in the athletic setting. *Athl Ther Today.* 2006;11(1): 10–16.

10. American Red Cross. Emergency action plan. In: *Sport Safety Training: Injury Prevention and Care Handbook.* Yardley, PA: StayWell; 2005.

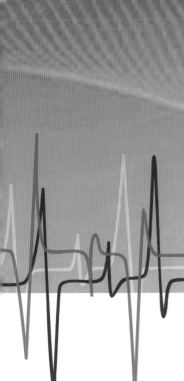

Human Body and Terms

CHAPTER OUTCOMES

1. Provide an overview of the structure and function of the systems comprised by the human body.

2. Describe anatomical positions and movements in relation to these positions.

3. Describe the planes and axes of motion of the body.

4. Describe specific body terms and regions necessary for understanding the relative position of athletes and for communicating athlete's positions to medical personnel.

5. Recognize and utilize the proper nomenclature and vocabulary when communicating with emergency personnel.

NOMENCLATURE

Aorta: the largest artery of the body

Aponeuroses: flat, broad tendons

Arterioles: small blood vessels, extending between arteries and capillaries

Atrium: top portion of the heart, divided into right and left sides

Axis: an imaginary line transecting the body or a body segment

Bicuspid valve: a valve controlling blood flow between the left atrium and left ventricle of the heart

Bronchi: passageways from the trachea to the lungs

Dermis: a layer of skin between the epidermis and subcutaneous layers

Diaphysis: the shaft of a bone

Electrolytes: ions of sodium, potassium, calcium, magnesium, chloride, hydrogen, phosphate, and hydrogen carbonate that help to regulate cellular function

Endosteum: the lining of the inner surface of the central medullary cavity of bone

Epidermis: the outermost layer of the skin

Epiphyseal plate: growth plate of bone

Epiphyses: bone ends

Esophagus: the passage through which food moves from the pharynx to the stomach

Fascia: soft tissue part of the connective tissue surrounding muscles, bones, nerves, and blood vessels

Lymphocyte: type of white blood cell

Organelles: subunits having specialized functions within a cell

Periosteum: outside surface of bone

Pharynx: the part of the throat that lies behind the mouth and nasal cavity, superior to the larynx

Planes: flat surfaces

Sebaceous glands: glands in the skin that secrete sebum (oily substances)

Subcutis: the deepest layer of the skin, under the dermis

NOMENCLATURE *(Continued)*

Trachea: the part of the throat that allows passage of air to and from the lungs

Tricuspid valve: a valve regulating the passage of blood between the right atrium and right ventricle of the heart

Venules: small blood vessels that carry deoxygenated blood from capillary beds to veins

BEFORE YOU BEGIN

1. How many body systems are there in the human body and what are their functions?

2. What are the most common anatomical descriptions used in athletic training?

3. What are the major types of joints found in the human body?

4. What are the structural components of muscle?

Voices from the Field

A thorough understanding of human anatomy is a necessary skill in becoming a highly effective emergency responder. As a certified athletic trainer with more than 30 years of experience, I have witnessed on numerous occasions emergency responses to a variety of injuries in athletic competitions. From broken bones to severe lacerations to emergency transport, the one thing that is critical in each situation is an understanding of the underlying anatomy. In an emergency situation, by being able to visualize and palpate the structures you are evaluating, you have a greater understanding of the possible injury or pathology in question. The use of visual recall or being able to see in your mind the anatomy you need to evaluate an injury makes it much easier to discern the actual structure(s) involved in an emergency situation and assists you in making a quicker and more accurate diagnosis of the problem. I highly encourage students to accentuate their anatomy learning any time they have an opportunity to get hands-on experience with a cadaver or in a surgical observation. Anatomy is a critical component of an emergency responder's education and should be continually reviewed throughout your career.

Brent Mangus, EdD
Dean, College of Education and Human Services
Texas A&M University—Commerce

An individual responding to a medical emergency must be able to communicate with other medical personnel using the appropriate medical terminology and must understand human anatomy in order to describe a patient's exact position or condition. Injuries or conditions that may look harmless can turn out to be medical emergencies. Therefore a thorough understanding of the systems of the human body and their functions, along with the medical terms associated with these, is essential. In this chapter, we discuss the basic anatomical and physiological components of the human body. The chapter is not intended to replace a course in human anatomy or physiology but rather to briefly remind the reader of basic structures and functions and to serve as an elementary foundation for the reader with limited experience.

ANATOMICAL DESCRIPTIONS

Before discussing human body systems, a review of anatomical terms is in order. These descriptions are divided into positional (location of the body as a whole) terms, directional (location of a body segment in relation to another) terms, and terms describing the body's planes.

Positional Descriptions

Anatomical position refers to an erect standing position, with arms to the sides and palms of the hands facing toward the front (Fig. 5.1). This position is considered the starting point for all movements of body segments, and any discussion about the specific location of an injury or direction of movement is referenced to this anatomical position. *Prone position* refers to the body lying face down on the stomach (Fig. 5.2). *Supine position* refers to the body lying face up on the back (Fig. 5.3). *Side-lying position* (lateral) refers to the body lying on either the right or left side with the knees slightly bent (Fig. 5.4).

Directional Descriptions (Fig. 5.1 and Fig. 5.5)

Anterior—front half of the body or toward the front as it relates to the anatomical position

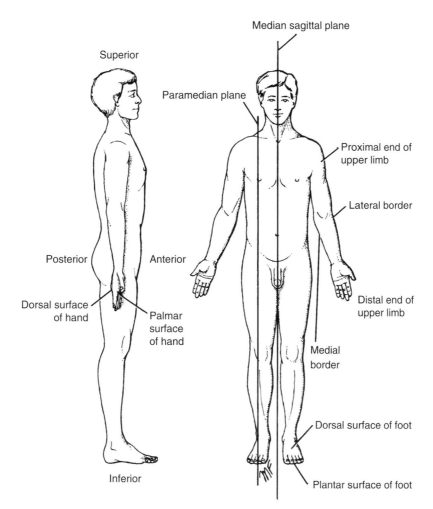

FIGURE 5.1 Anatomical terms used in relation to position. (From R. S. Snell. *Clinical Anatomy*, 7th ed. Philadelphia: Lippincott Williams & Wilkins; 2003.)

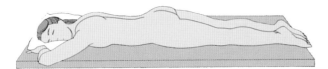

FIGURE 5.2 Prone position. (From J. Weber and J. Kelley. *Health Assessment in Nursing*, 2nd ed. Philadelphia: Lippincott Williams & Wilkins; 2003.)

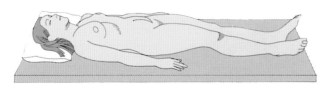

FIGURE 5.3 Supine position. (From J. Weber and J. Kelley. *Health Assessment in Nursing*, 2nd ed. Philadelphia: Lippincott Williams & Wilkins; 2003.)

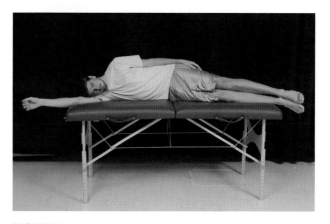

FIGURE 5.4 Side lying.

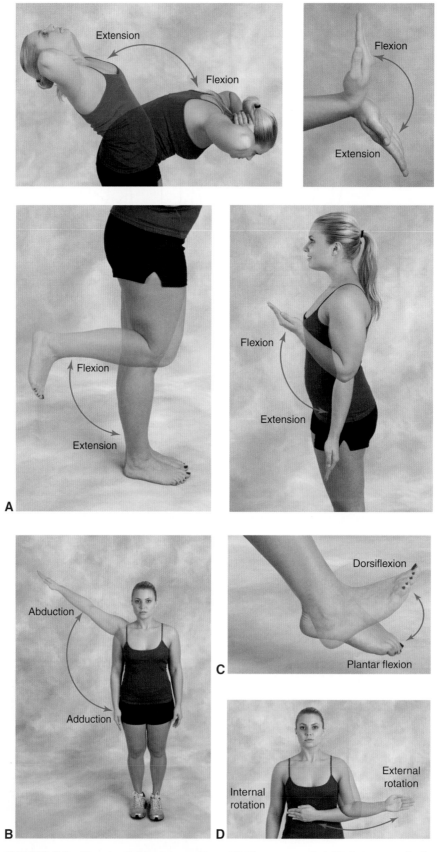

FIGURE 5.5 Directional descriptions. (From W. Thompson, ed. *ACSM's Resources for the Personal Trainer*, 3rd ed. Philadelphia: Lippincott Williams & Wilkins; 2010). *(continued)*

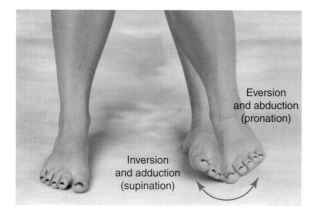

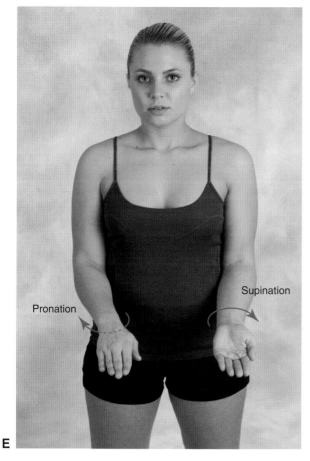

E

FIGURE 5.5   *(Continued)*

External—on the outside of the body

Flexion—decreasing a joint's angle (Fig. 5.5A)

Extension—increasing a joint's angle (Fig. 5.5A)

Elevation—gliding or moving a segment upward or toward the head

Depression—gliding or moving a segment downward or toward the ground

Abduction—movement away from the midline or trunk (Fig. 5.5B)

Adduction—movement toward the midline or trunk (Fig. 5.5B)

Dorsal—pertaining to the top

Volar—referring to the palm of the hand or bottom of the foot

Dorsiflexion—the upward movement of the ankle resulting in the foot/toes moving toward the body, decreasing the angle at the ankle (Fig. 5.5C)

Plantarflexion—the downward movement of the ankle resulting in the foot/toes moving toward the ground, increasing the angle at the ankle (Fig. 5.5C)

Inversion—movement turning inward, such as turning the outside of the foot inward to the body (Fig. 5.5D)

Eversion—movement of the sole of the foot away from the midline Fig. 5.5D

External rotation—rotation of a joint about its axis in the transverse plane away from the midline (Fig. 5.5D)

Internal rotation—rotation of a joint about its axis in the transverse plane toward the midline of the body (Fig. 5.5D)

Supination—rotation of the forearm placing the palm of the hand anteriorly or upward, or rotation of the foot such that the plantar surface is rotated upward (Fig. 5.5E)

Superficial—near the body's surface

Deep—beneath the surface, opposite of superficial

Pronation—rotation of the forearm moving the palm into a downward-facing position or the sole of the foot to face more laterally than when standing in the anatomical position (Fig. 5.5E)

Protraction—anterior movement of the arms at the shoulders in unison

Retraction—posterior movement of the arms at the shoulders in unison

Posterior—back half of the body or toward the back as it relates to the anatomical position

Superior—toward the head

Inferior—toward the feet

Medial—toward the middle or midline of the body

Lateral—away from the middle or midline of the body

Distal—away from a reference point or further from the trunk (e.g., the ankle is distal to the knee)

Proximal—toward a reference point or closer to the trunk (e.g., the knee is proximal to the ankle)

Internal—on the inside of the body

ANATOMICAL PLANES AND AXES

In the anatomical position, the body is divided into **planes** (flat surfaces), and movement about a plane is based upon its **axis** of rotation (Fig. 5.6). The body is divided into three planes that are perpendicular to each other; the sagittal plane, coronal/frontal plane, and transverse (horizontal) plane. Movements within these planes are dependent upon three axes: frontal, vertical (longitudinal), and horizontal (sagittal).

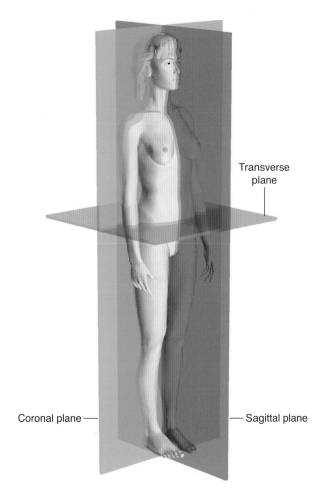

FIGURE 5.6 Anatomical planes. (LifeART image. Copyright © 2010 Lippincott Williams & Wilkins. All rights reserved.)

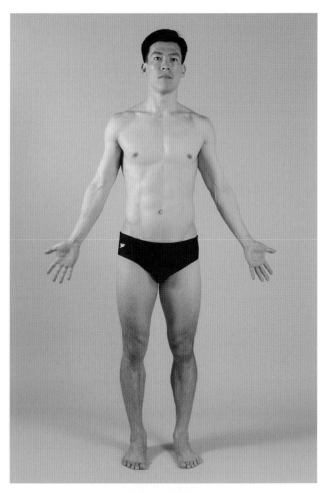

FIGURE 5.7 Body segments. (Courtesy of Anatomical Chart Co.)

The transverse (horizontal) plane divides the body into halves or top and bottom. The horizontal plane is the only plane that divides the body into equal top and bottom halves. Movement within this plane is based upon the vertical axis, which goes straight through the body from top to bottom; it is perpendicular to the transverse plane. These movements include rotation. The coronal (frontal) plane divides the body into anterior and posterior portions or front and back. The axis of rotation is a line perpendicular to the frontal plane; it extends from front to back. Movements that take place in the frontal plane with the sagittal axis are abduction and adduction. The sagittal plane divides the body into right and left sides. The frontal axis is a line running perpendicular to the sagittal plane; it allows movements such as flexion and extension.

BODY SEGMENTS

The body can be divided into various segments (Fig. 5.7). Extremities are the arms and legs. The spine is made up of the bones (vertebrae) on the posterior portion of the body,

making up the spinal column. The spinal column includes 5 cervical, 12 thoracic, 5 lumbar and 3 or 4 sacral vertebrae; the spinal cord runs within these. The thorax comprises the chest, upper back, and chest cavity (the space enclosed by the ribs, which contains the heart and lungs). The abdomen is the area below the thorax and above the genitals. Divided into four sections called quadrants (right upper, right lower, left upper and left lower), it is transected by an imaginary line across the umbilicus (belly button) and longitudinally down the center. Each of these four quadrants houses specific internal organs (Fig. 5.8). Finally, the pelvis, located immediately below the abdomen, encompasses the pelvic bones and pelvic cavity, which houses the reproductive organs, lower digestive tracts, and bladder.

BODY SYSTEMS

The body comprises major systems that are essential to life. These include the integumentary, musculoskeletal, circulatory, respiratory, gastrointestinal, lymphatic, endocrine, urinary, nervous, and reproductive systems. Each system is discussed briefly below, but their important anatomical characteristics are discussed in detail throughout this book wherever applicable.

Integumentary System

The integumentary system is comprised of the skin, hair, nails, and sweat and oil glands. The skin's primary functions are to protect the body from external pathogens or microorganisms, protect internal organs, help prevent the loss of fluids (dehydration), aid in the regulation of body temperature by loss of water (sweating) or retention of temperature (shivering and goose bumps), act as a barrier to external fluids, produce vitamin D from the sun, and act as a receptor for stimuli such as touch and pressure, temperature (heat and cold), and pain. The skin is the largest organ of the body; it's the thickness ranges from 1/32 to 1/8 in. or more.

The skin is made up of three layers: the **epidermis, dermis,** and **subcutis** (Fig. 5.9). The epidermis is the outer layer. It has several sublayers: the stratum corneum, stratum granulosum, stratum spinosum, and stratum basale. The primary function of the epidermis is to act as a barrier against foreign particles and liquids (dirt, chemicals, microorganisms, ultraviolet rays).

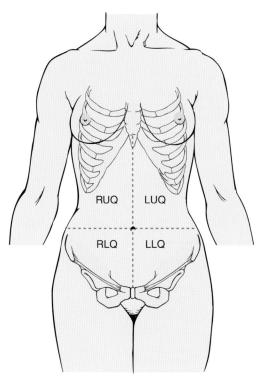

FIGURE 5.8 Abdominal quadrants. (Courtesy of Anatomical Chart Co.)

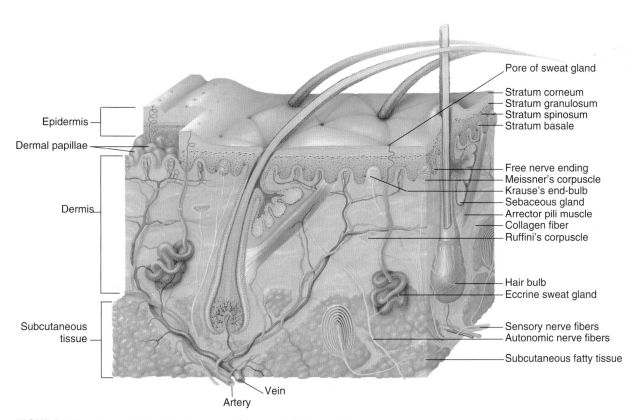

FIGURE 5.9 Layers of the skin. (Courtesy of Anatomical Chart Co.)

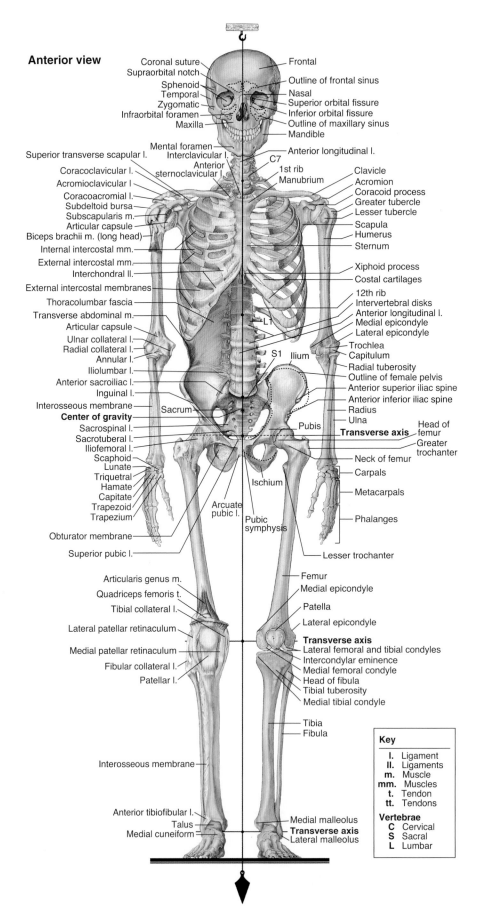

Anterior view

Coronal suture
Supraorbital notch
Sphenoid
Temporal
Zygomatic
Infraorbital foramen
Maxilla
Mental foramen
Interclavicular l.
Anterior sternoclavicular l.
Superior transverse scapular l.
Coracoclavicular l.
Acromioclavicular l
Coracoacromial l.
Subdeltoid bursa
Subscapularis m.
Articular capsule
Biceps brachii m. (long head)
Internal intercostal mm.
External intercostal mm.
Interchondral ll.
External intercostal membranes
Thoracolumbar fascia
Transverse abdominal m.
Articular capsule
Ulnar collateral l.
Radial collateral l.
Annular l.
Iliolumbar l.
Anterior sacroiliac l.
Inguinal l.
Interosseous membrane
Center of gravity
Sacrospinal l.
Sacrotuberal l.
Iliofemoral l.
Scaphoid
Lunate
Triquetral
Hamate
Capitate
Trapezoid
Trapezium
Obturator membrane
Superior pubic l.
Articularis genus m.
Quadriceps femoris t.
Tibial collateral l.
Lateral patellar retinaculum
Medial patellar retinaculum
Fibular collateral l.
Patellar l.
Interosseous membrane
Anterior tibiofibular l.
Talus
Medial cuneiform

Frontal
Outline of frontal sinus
Nasal
Superior orbital fissure
Inferior orbital fissure
Outline of maxillary sinus
Mandible
Anterior longitudinal l.
C7
1st rib
Manubrium
Clavicle
Acromion
Coracoid process
Greater tubercle
Lesser tubercle
Scapula
Humerus
Sternum
Xiphoid process
Costal cartilages
12th rib
Intervertebral disks
Anterior longitudinal l.
Medial epicondyle
Lateral epicondyle
Trochlea
Capitulum
Radial tuberosity
Outline of female pelvis
Anterior superior iliac spine
Anterior inferior iliac spine
Radius
Ulna
Head of femur
Transverse axis
Greater trochanter
Neck of femur
Carpals
Metacarpals
Phalanges
Lesser trochanter
Femur
Medial epicondyle
Patella
Lateral epicondyle
Transverse axis
Lateral femoral and tibial condyles
Intercondylar eminence
Medial femoral condyle
Head of fibula
Tibial tuberosity
Medial tibial condyle
Tibia
Fibula
Medial malleolus
Transverse axis
Lateral malleolus

L1
S1
Ilium
Sacrum
Pubis
Ischium
Arcuate pubic l.
Pubic symphysis

Key

l.	Ligament
ll.	Ligaments
m.	Muscle
mm.	Muscles
t.	Tendon
tt.	Tendons

Vertebrae
C Cervical
S Sacral
L Lumbar

FIGURE 5.10 Skeleton (anterior view). (Courtesy of Anatomical Chart Co.)

The dermis lies immediately beneath the epidermis. Blood vessels are located here, along with nerves, sweat glands, hair follicles, **sebaceous (sweat) glands,** and sensory nerves. The third and last layer is the subcutis, located beneath the dermis; it contains subcutaneous fat, which helps regulate body temperature and helps the skin to move independently of the tissues that lie beneath it (muscle and bone).

Musculoskeletal System

The musculoskeletal system comprises two separate but equally important systems: skeletal and muscular. The skeletal system includes 206 bones; more than 600 muscles make up the muscular system. Each system is discussed separately in this section, but they act congruently within the body, performing multiple functions.

Skeletal System

As stated above, the skeleton is made up of 206 bones that give the body its structural support (Fig. 5.10). The primary function of the skeletal system is to protect the internal organs from external forces, provide body shape and support, aid in mobility, produce red blood cells, and store calcium. The bones are classified according to shape: long, short, irregular, and flat. Long bones are primarily the femur, tibia, fibula, humerus, and ulna. Short bones include the carpals and tarsals. Irregular bones are the vertebrae and special areas of the skull. Finally, the ribs and scapulae are classified as flat bones.

A bone consists of an **epiphysis** at each end and a **diaphysis**, or bone shaft. Other components include an **epiphyseal plate** (growth plate), **periosteum** (outside surface), and **endosteum** (inner section). The epiphyseal plate (Fig. 5.11) is a cartilaginous structure that separates the epiphyses and allows the bone to grow. Upon maturation, the bones stop growing and these plates solidify, replacing the cartilaginous material with normal bone tissue. Damage to the growth plates during adolescence can disrupt the structure of the bone. Surrounding the entire outside of a bone is a thin layer of tissue called the periosteum. The ends of the epiphysis are covered by a specific cartilaginous structure called articular cartilage.

Joints of the Skeletal System

Bones that connect together form articular surfaces called joints. An articulation is where two or more bones meet. Most joints are classified as either immovable (skull bones), slightly movable (spinal column), or freely movable (knee and shoulder). Joints can be classified as diarthrodial or synarthrodial. Diarthrodial joints are special joints in which the bones are separated by a joint cavity; they are referred to as synovial joints. The synovial cavity is made up of (a) a synovial membrane lining the joints, which produces nutrients and fluid for lubrication, and (b) the articular capsule,

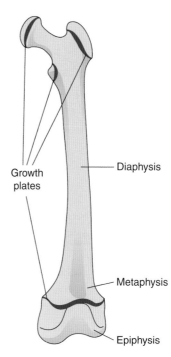

FIGURE 5.11 Epiphyseal plates. (From E. Rubin and J. L. Farber. *Pathology*, 3rd ed. Philadelphia: Lippincott Williams & Wilkins; 1999.)

which is an extension of the articular cartilage of the bone ends. Diarthrodial joints are usually divided into subcategories based upon their shape (Fig. 5.12), including:

> Ball and socket: such as the shoulder (humerus/scapula)—permits flexion, extension, adduction, abduction, medial and lateral rotation, and circumduction
>
> Hinge: such as the elbow (humerus/ulna)—permits flexion and extension
>
> Pivot: such as the neck (atlas/axis)—permits rotation
>
> Plane/gliding: such as carpal or tarsal bones—permit sliding or gliding
>
> Saddle: such as thumb area (trapezium/first metacarpal) permits flexion, extension, circumduction
>
> Condyloid: such as a knuckle (metacarpophalangeal)—permits flexion, extension, adduction, abduction, and circumduction

Synarthrodial joints do not have a synovial cavity and are fused together. They are subdivided into three categories: sutured, cartilaginous, and ligamentous. Sutured joints are sutured together (hence their name) and have no movement; examples include the bones connected in the skull (Fig. 5.13). Cartilaginous joints (Fig. 5.14) allow only slight movement; examples include the fibrocartilage spaces between the vertebrae in the spine. Ligamentous joints (Fig. 5.15) connect bones with ligaments and allow very limited motion or no motion at all. An example of this type

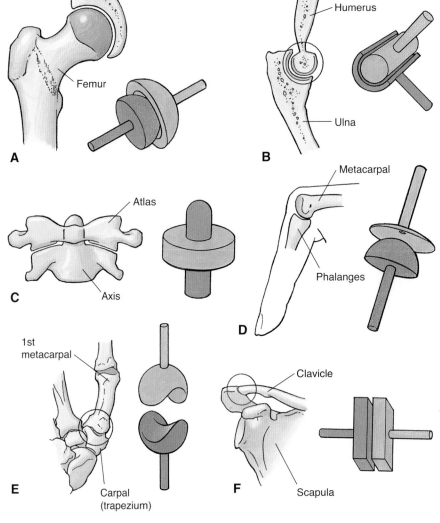

FIGURE 5.12 Types of synovial joints. **A.** Ball and socket. **B.** Hinge. **C.** Pivot. **D.** Ellipsoid or condyloid. **E.** Saddle. **F.** Gliding or planar. (From K. L. Moore and A.M.R. Agur. *Essential Clinical Anatomy*, 2nd ed. Baltimore: Lippincott Williams & Wilkins;.)

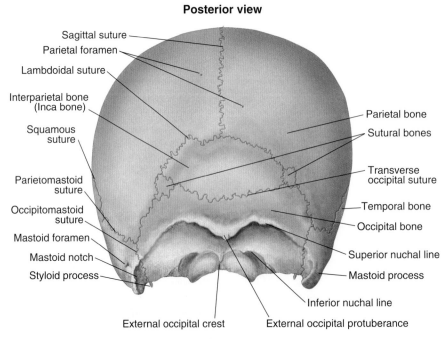

FIGURE 5.13 Examples of suture joints. (Courtesy of Anatomical Chart Co.)

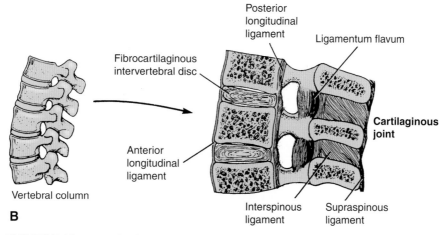

Posterior longitudinal ligament

Ligamentum flavum

Fibrocartilaginous intervertebral disc

Cartilaginous joint

Anterior longitudinal ligament

Interspinous ligament

Supraspinous ligament

Vertebral column

B

FIGURE 5.14   Example of a cartilaginous joint. (From R. S. Snell. *Clinical Anatomy by Regions*, 8th ed. Philadelphia: Lippincott Williams & Wilkins; 2008.)

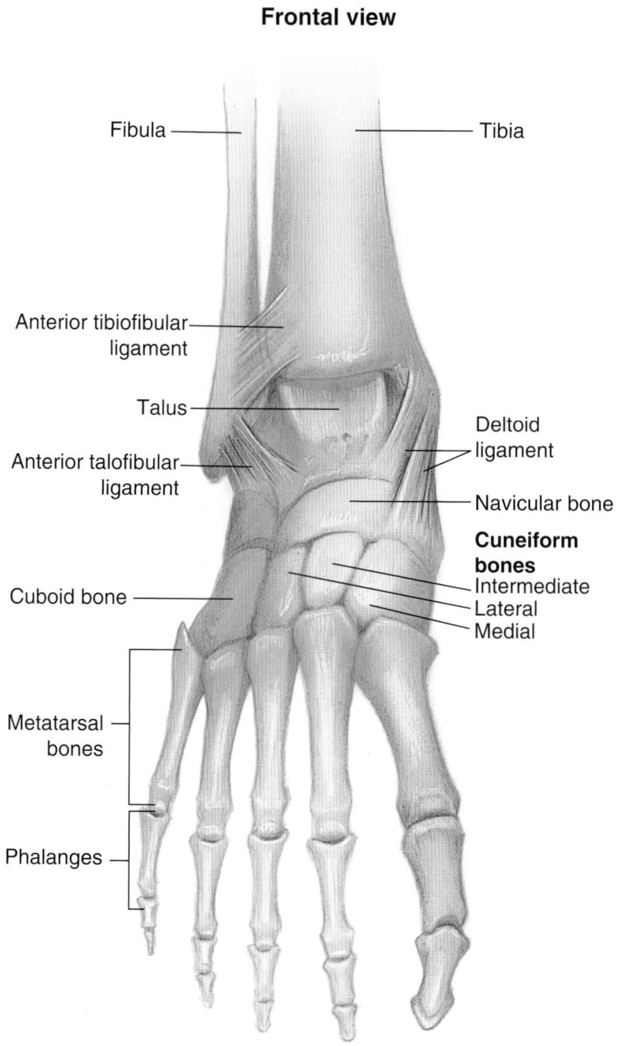

Frontal view

Fibula

Tibia

Anterior tibiofibular ligament

Talus

Deltoid ligament

Anterior talofibular ligament

Navicular bone

Cuneiform bones
Intermediate
Lateral
Medial

Cuboid bone

Metatarsal bones

Phalanges

FIGURE 5.15   Example of a ligamentous joint. (Courtesy of Anatomical Chart Co.)

of joint include the tibia and fibula or the ulna and radius, which are held together by ligaments. Ligaments are made up of strong, fibrous connective tissue that facilitates the movement and control of bones.

Muscular System

The muscular system constitutes approximately 40% of a person's total body weight[1] and has several main functions: force production for movement, posture, and breathing and the generation of heat (Fig. 5.16). Skeletal muscles usually connect to bone via tendons or **aponeuroses** and produce movement by contracting or relaxing. The muscular system is classified by voluntary action (skeletal muscles), involuntary action (smooth muscles found in the walls of certain organs, vessels, intestines), and cardiac movement (heart muscles).

Skeletal muscles have structural (connective) components (Fig. 5.17). These include connective tissue, which is an integral part of the muscle and muscle fibers. Muscles are separated from each other and held in position by a special connective tissue called **fascia**. The outermost layer of connective tissue surrounding or covering a muscle is called the epimysium. Muscle fibers in groups, called fasciculi, are surrounded by yet another type of connective tissue called the perimysium. The endomysium is loose connective tissue that surrounds each muscle fiber within a fascicle.

Individual skeletal muscles fibers include cellular proteins, **organelles,** and myofibrils. The myofibrils have specific components, called filaments, responsible for the contraction and relaxation of muscles. Thick filaments are called *myosin* and thin filaments are called *actin;* these give skeletal muscle its striated appearance because they are arranged in layers. When acted upon by a nerve cell (called a motor neuron),

Anterior view

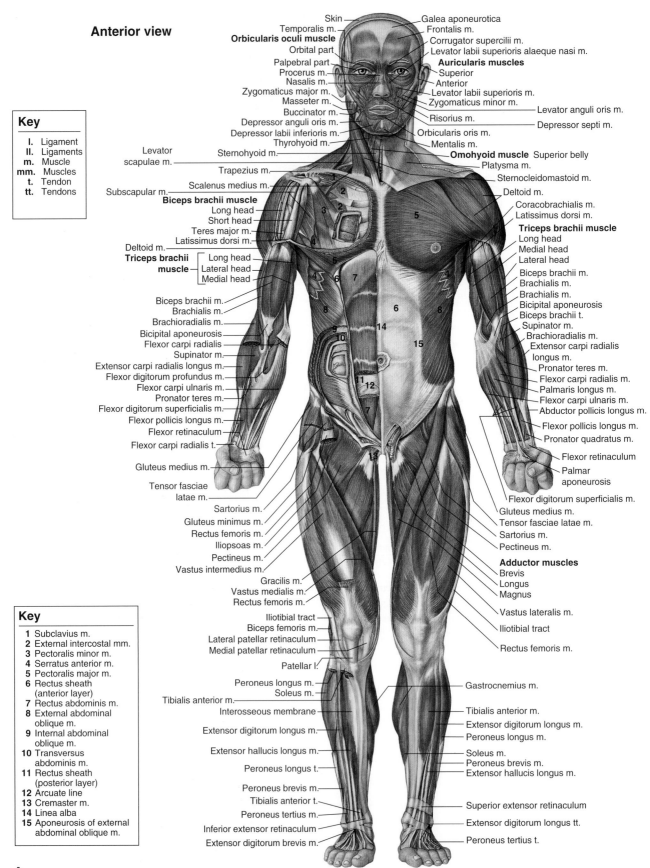

A

FIGURE 5.16 Skeletal muscles. **A.** Anterior view. *(continued)*

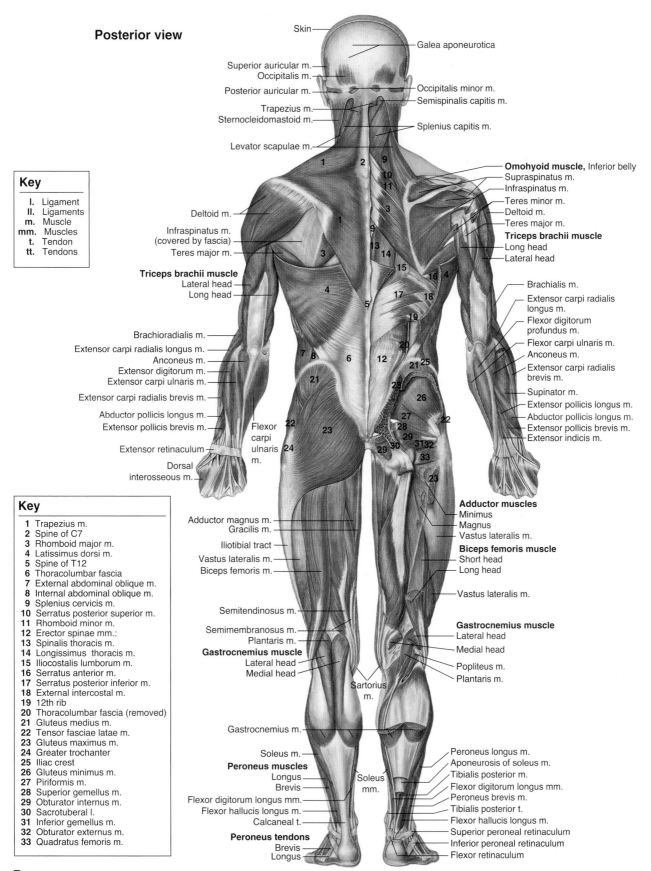

Posterior view

Skin
Galea aponeurotica
Superior auricular m.
Occipitalis m.
Posterior auricular m.
Occipitalis minor m.
Semispinalis capitis m.
Trapezius m.
Sternocleidomastoid m.
Splenius capitis m.
Levator scapulae m.

Omohyoid muscle, Inferior belly
Supraspinatus m.
Infraspinatus m.
Teres minor m.
Deltoid m.
Teres major m.
Triceps brachii muscle
Long head
Lateral head

Deltoid m.
Infraspinatus m.
(covered by fascia)
Teres major m.

Triceps brachii muscle
Lateral head
Long head

Brachialis m.
Extensor carpi radialis
longus m.
Flexor digitorum
profundus m.
Flexor carpi ulnaris m.
Anconeus m.
Extensor carpi radialis
brevis m.

Brachioradialis m.
Extensor carpi radialis longus m.
Anconeus m.
Extensor digitorum m.
Extensor carpi ulnaris m.
Extensor carpi radialis brevis m.

Supinator m.
Extensor pollicis longus m.
Abductor pollicis longus m.
Extensor pollicis brevis m.
Extensor indicis m.

Abductor pollicis longus m.
Extensor pollicis brevis m.
Extensor retinaculum
Flexor
carpi
ulnaris
m.
Dorsal
interosseous m.

Adductor muscles
Minimus
Magnus
Vastus lateralis m.
Biceps femoris muscle
Short head
Long head

Vastus lateralis m.

Adductor magnus m.
Gracilis m.
Iliotibial tract
Vastus lateralis m.
Biceps femoris m.

Semitendinosus m.
Semimembranosus m.
Plantaris m.
Gastrocnemius muscle
Lateral head
Medial head

Gastrocnemius muscle
Lateral head
Medial head
Popliteus m.
Plantaris m.

Sartorius
m.

Gastrocnemius m.
Soleus m.
Peroneus muscles
Longus
Brevis
Flexor digitorum longus mm.
Flexor hallucis longus m.
Calcaneal t.
Peroneus tendons
Brevis
Longus

Soleus
mm.

Peroneus longus m.
Aponeurosis of soleus m.
Tibialis posterior m.
Flexor digitorum longus mm.
Peroneus brevis m.
Tibialis posterior t.
Flexor hallucis longus m.
Superior peroneal retinaculum
Inferior peroneal retinaculum
Flexor retinaculum

Key
I. Ligament
II. Ligaments
m. Muscle
mm. Muscles
t. Tendon
tt. Tendons

Key
1 Trapezius m.
2 Spine of C7
3 Rhomboid major m.
4 Latissimus dorsi m.
5 Spine of T12
6 Thoracolumbar fascia
7 External abdominal oblique m.
8 Internal abdominal oblique m.
9 Splenius cervicis m.
10 Serratus posterior superior m.
11 Rhomboid minor m.
12 Erector spinae mm.:
13 Spinalis thoracis m.
14 Longissimus thoracis m.
15 Iliocostalis lumborum m.
16 Serratus anterior m.
17 Serratus posterior inferior m.
18 External intercostal m.
19 12th rib
20 Thoracolumbar fascia (removed)
21 Gluteus medius m.
22 Tensor fasciae latae m.
23 Gluteus maximus m.
24 Greater trochanter
25 Iliac crest
26 Gluteus minimus m.
27 Piriformis m.
28 Superior gemellus m.
29 Obturator internus m.
30 Sacrotuberal l.
31 Inferior gemellus m.
32 Obturator externus m.
33 Quadratus femoris m.

B

FIGURE 5.16 *(Continued)* **B.** Posterior view. (Courtesy of Anatomical Chart Co.)

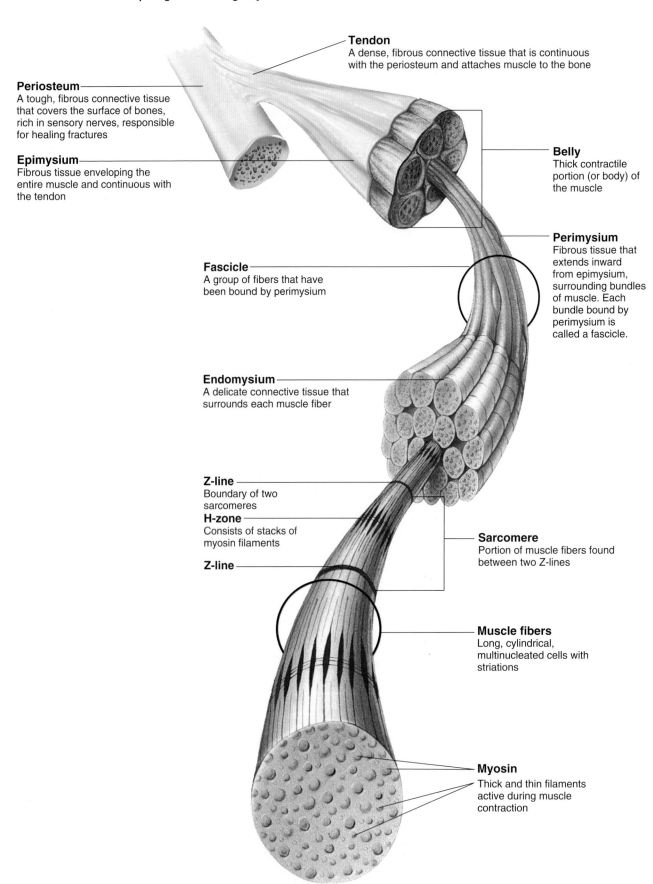

Tendon
A dense, fibrous connective tissue that is continuous with the periosteum and attaches muscle to the bone

Periosteum
A tough, fibrous connective tissue that covers the surface of bones, rich in sensory nerves, responsible for healing fractures

Epimysium
Fibrous tissue enveloping the entire muscle and continuous with the tendon

Belly
Thick contractile portion (or body) of the muscle

Perimysium
Fibrous tissue that extends inward from epimysium, surrounding bundles of muscle. Each bundle bound by perimysium is called a fascicle.

Fascicle
A group of fibers that have been bound by perimysium

Endomysium
A delicate connective tissue that surrounds each muscle fiber

Z-line
Boundary of two sarcomeres

H-zone
Consists of stacks of myosin filaments

Z-line

Sarcomere
Portion of muscle fibers found between two Z-lines

Muscle fibers
Long, cylindrical, multinucleated cells with striations

Myosin
Thick and thin filaments active during muscle contraction

FIGURE 5.17 Structural components of the muscle. (Courtesy of Anatomical Chart Co.)

the skeletal muscle begins a complex process involving contraction of the thick and thin filaments called the *sliding filament model*.

Circulatory System

The circulatory system comprises the heart and the vessels that carry both oxygenated and deoxygenated blood, nutrients, and waste products throughout the body. The heart is the part of the circulatory system responsible for pumping blood throughout the body. It has four chambers and is joined by right and left pulmonary arteries and veins as well as the **aorta** (Fig. 5.18). Deoxygenated blood flows to the heart from either the superior or inferior vena cava to the right **atrium.** The deoxygenated blood then flows past the **tricuspid valve** into the right ventricle, from which it is transported to the lungs via the right and left pulmonary arteries. After the blood is oxygenated in the lungs, it flows back to the heart via the right and left pulmonary veins into the left atrium and through the **bicuspid valve** into the left ventricle. From the left ventricle, oxygenated blood then is pumped out to the body through the aorta.

Blood travels through a mazelike network of vessels (Fig. 5.19). Oxygenated blood travels via arteries and **arterioles** to capillaries. Capillaries are special vessels that join the arterial and venous supply lines together in networks called capillary beds. It is here that oxygen-rich blood, nutrients, and other cellular materials are delivered to tissues. After cells take up these substances, the deoxygenated blood travels back to the heart via **venules** and veins to begin the cycle once more.

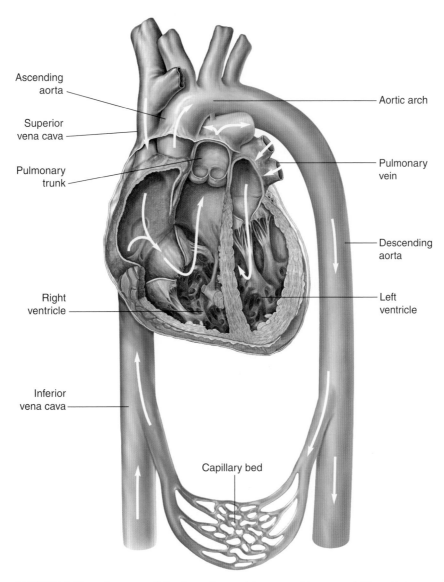

FIGURE 5.18   Schematic of blood circulation. (Courtesy of Anatomical Chart Co.)

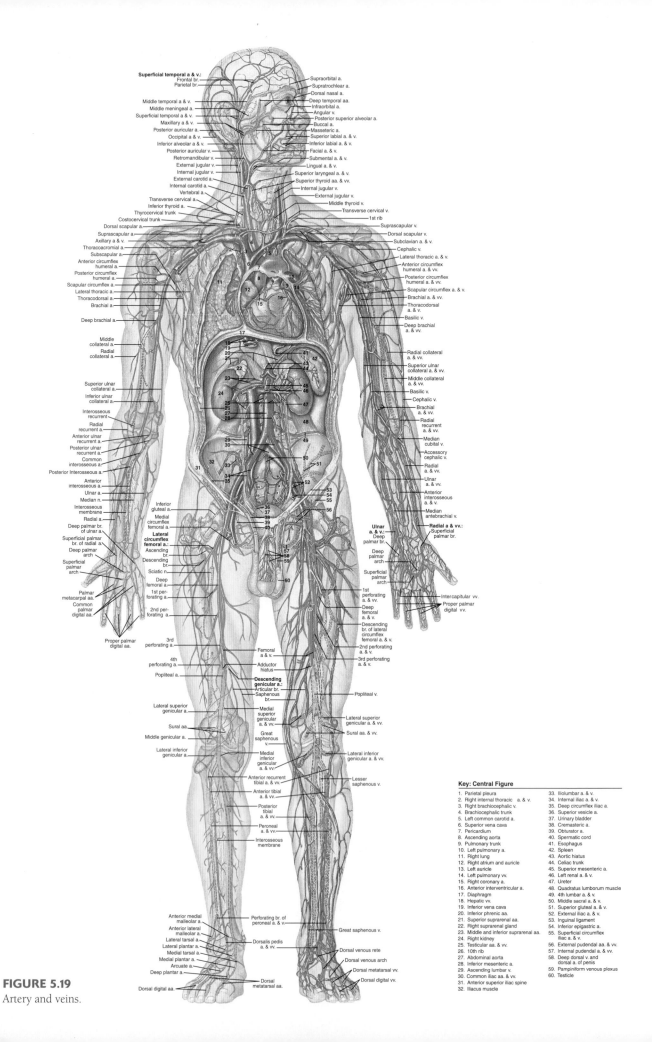

FIGURE 5.19
Artery and veins.

Key: Central Figure

1. Parietal pleura
2. Right internal thoracic a. & v.
3. Right brachiocephalic v.
4. Brachiocephalic trunk
5. Left common carotid a.
6. Superior vena cava
7. Pericardium
8. Ascending aorta
9. Pulmonary trunk
10. Left pulmonary a.
11. Right lung
12. Right atrium and auricle
13. Left auricle
14. Left pulmonary vv.
15. Right coronary v.
16. Anterior interventricular a.
17. Diaphragm
18. Hepatic vv.
19. Inferior vena cava
20. Inferior phrenic aa.
21. Superior suprarenal aa.
22. Right suprarenal gland
23. Middle and inferior suprarenal aa.
24. Right kidney
25. Testicular aa. & vv.
26. 10th rib
27. Abdominal aorta
28. Inferior mesenteric a.
29. Ascending lumbar v.
30. Common iliac aa. & vv.
31. Anterior superior iliac spine
32. Iliacus muscle

33. Iliolumbar a. & v.
34. Internal iliac a. & v.
35. Deep circumflex iliac a.
36. Superior vesicle a.
37. Urinary bladder
38. Cremasteric a.
39. Obturator a.
40. Spermatic cord
41. Esophagus
42. Spleen
43. Aortic hiatus
44. Celiac trunk
45. Superior mesenteric a.
46. Left renal a. & v.
47. Ureter
48. Quadratus lumborum muscle
49. 4th lumbar a. & v.
50. Middle sacral a. & v.
51. Superior gluteal a. & v.
52. External iliac a. & v.
53. Inguinal ligament
54. Inferior epigastric a.
55. Superficial circumflex iliac a. & v.
56. External pudendal aa. & vv.
57. Internal pudendal a. & vv.
58. Deep dorsal v. and dorsal a. of penis
59. Pampiniform venous plexus
60. Testicle

Lymphatic System

The lymphatic system contains vessels that connect to lymph nodes and various organs (e.g., the spleen). The lymphatic system is responsible for absorbing and transporting fat from the intestines, collecting plasma from the interstitial spaces, and transporting the plasma to the venous system. Most importantly, the lymphatic system defends the body against disease or foreign organisms and produces **lymphocytes** (white blood cells), which to fight infections.

Respiratory System

The respiratory system (Fig. 5.20) is comprised of the lungs and airways that facilitate the movement and absorption of oxygen. Air is inhaled through the nose or mouth into the **pharynx;** it then passes to the **trachea**. Air travels down the trachea into the right and left **bronchi,** which connect to the right and left lungs. The bronchi become narrower in the lungs, forming passageways called bronchioles, which eventually combine with more than 300 million tiny air sacs called alveoli. Within the small capillary vessels of the alveoli, oxygen and carbon dioxide are exchanged. Oxygenated blood travels to the heart via the pulmonary veins, as discussed previously in the discussion of the circulatory system.

The lungs are divided into right and left sides. The right lung has three lobes and the left lung has two. Each lung is covered by thins sacs called parietal pleura (outer layer) and a visceral pleura (inner layer); the space between these two layers is called the pleural cavity. Located directly underneath the lungs is a muscle called the diaphragm. When the diaphragm contracts, the thoracic cavity expands, drawing air into the lungs. When the diaphragm relaxes, the thoracic cavity becomes smaller and forces air to be expelled, carrying carbon dioxide and other elements out of the body. The process of inhalation and exhalation is called ventilation. Normally, the ventilatory rate is 12 to 20 breaths per minute in an adult, 15 to 30 in a child, and 25 to 50 in an infant.

Gastrointestinal System

The gastrointestinal system is comprised of organs and accessory organs to aid in the digestion of food and elimination of waste products (Fig. 5.21). Food and fluids consumed through the mouth flow down the **esophagus** to the stomach. After entering the stomach, the food is broken down into smaller particles by digestive enzymes. Organs such as the liver, pancreas, spleen, and gallbladder help break the food down into usable nutrients that are absorbed by the small intestine and filtered through the liver. Waste products or nutrients not used by the body continue to travel through the small intestine to the large intestine, from which they are eliminated via the anus.

Urinary System

The urinary system's primary functions are to filter wastes from the blood and eliminate them from the body (Fig. 5.22). It is also responsible for maintaining the body's fluid and **electrolyte** balance. The organs of the urinary system include the kidneys (right and left), located approximately at the T12 to L3 levels; ureters, which connect the kidneys to the bladder and carry urine; the bladder; and the urethra, which carries the urine from the bladder out of the body.

Nervous System

The nervous system is a broad arrangement of nerves and nerve fibers that function as the body's control center, regulating the body systems to communicate and work properly, and transmit impulses to coordinate movements (Fig. 5.23). The nervous system consists of two major structural components: the central nervous system (CNS) and the peripheral nervous system (PNS). The CNS contains the brain and spinal cord. The PNS has 31 pairs of spinal nerves that are attached to the **spinal cord** in nerve segments: 8 cervical, 12 thoracic, 5 lumbar, 5 sacral, and 1 at the coccygeal region, which carry information from the periphery back to the CNS. The PNS is divided into two divisions: afferent and efferent. The afferent division carries impulses to the CNS, while the efferent division carries impulses away from the CNS. The efferent division is also divided into two systems: the somatic nervous system, made up of sensory and motor neurons (which supply the skeletal muscles), and the autonomic nervous system, which innervates cardiac and smooth muscles as well as glands. The autonomic system has two divisions: sympathetic and parasympathetic. The sympathetic system is responsible for excitatory responses of the organs involved in emergency or stressful situations by increasing heart rate, blood pressure, and other functions. The parasympathetic system does the opposite, decreasing these functions and restoring blood flow and heart rate to normal levels.

Reproductive System

The reproductive system differs in men and in women. In men, the reproductive organs consist of testicles and penis (Fig. 5.24A). In women, they consist of the uterus, ovaries, and uterine tubes (which connect the ovaries to the uterus) as well as the vagina, labia, and clitoris (Fig. 5.24B). Men produce sperm in the testes and women produce eggs in the ovaries. Specific characteristics of each system are beyond the scope of this chapter.

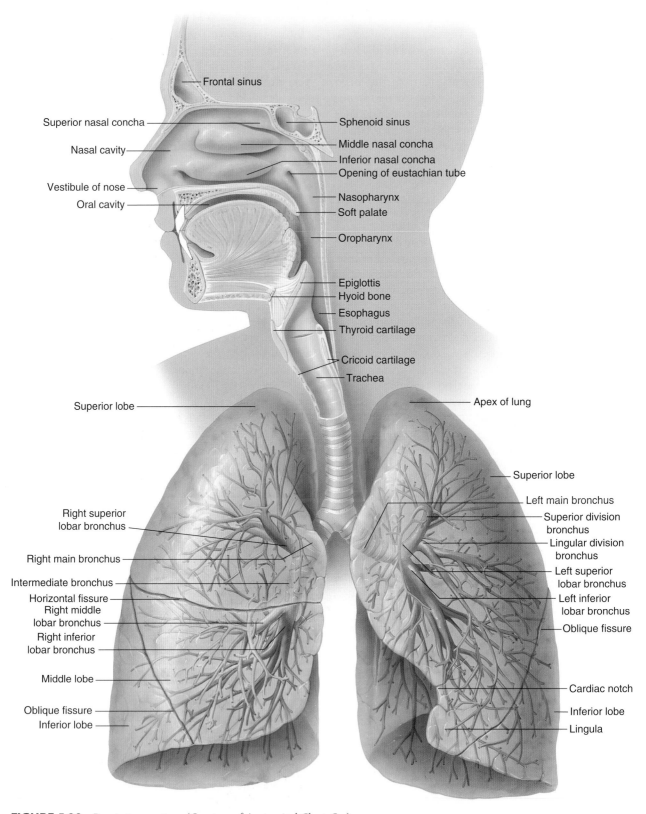

FIGURE 5.20   Respiratory system. (Courtesy of Anatomical Chart Co.)

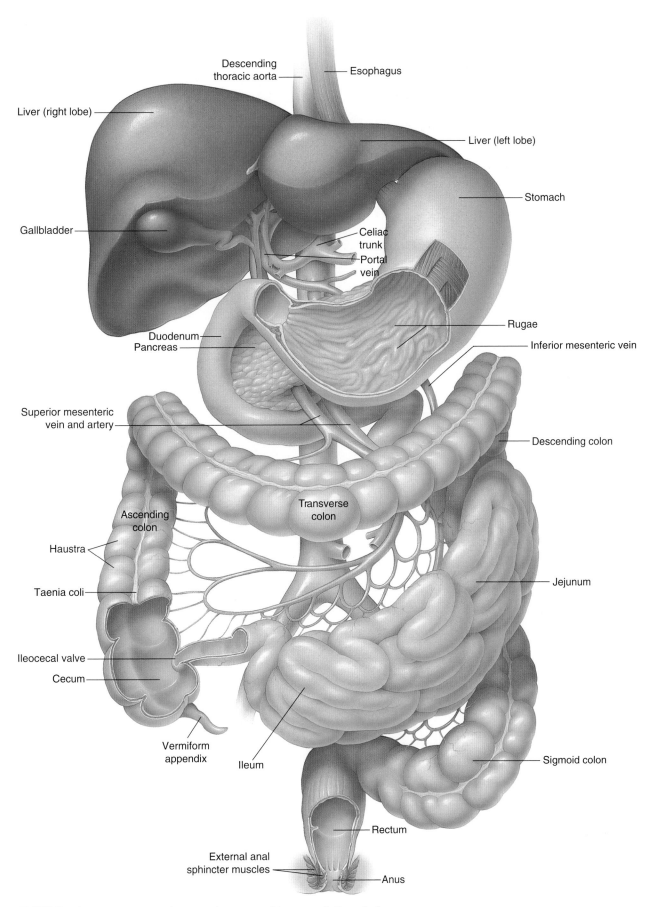

FIGURE 5.21   Gastrointestinal system. (Courtesy of Anatomical Chart Co.)

Anterior view

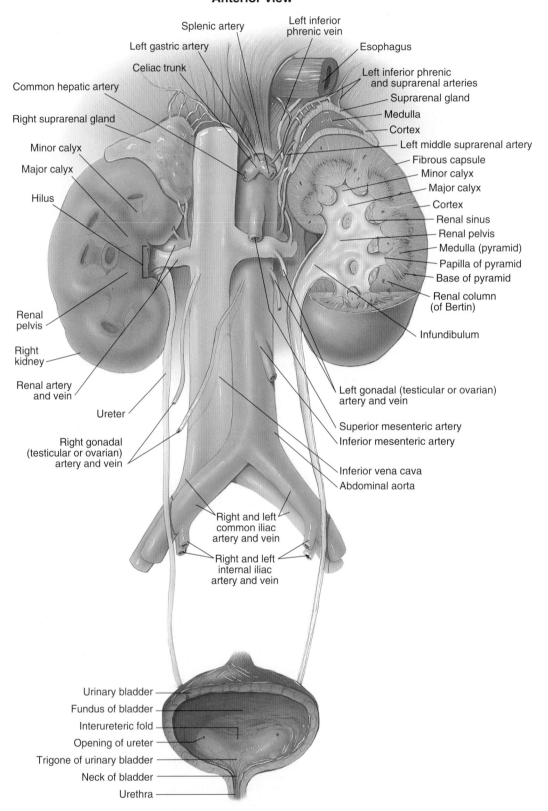

FIGURE 5.22   Urinary system. (Courtesy of Anatomical Chart Co.)

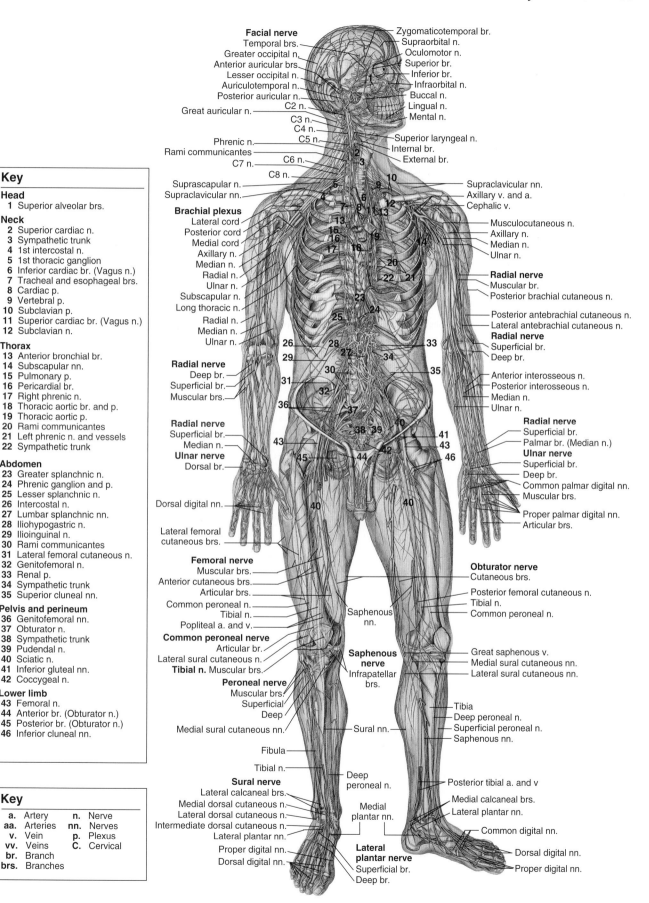

Key

Head
1 Superior alveolar brs.

Neck
2 Superior cardiac n.
3 Sympathetic trunk
4 1st intercostal n.
5 1st thoracic ganglion
6 Inferior cardiac br. (Vagus n.)
7 Tracheal and esophageal brs.
8 Cardiac n.
9 Vertebral p.
10 Subclavian p.
11 Superior cardiac br. (Vagus n.)
12 Subclavian n.

Thorax
13 Anterior bronchial br.
14 Subscapular nn.
15 Pulmonary p.
16 Pericardial br.
17 Right phrenic n.
18 Thoracic aortic br. and p.
19 Thoracic aortic p.
20 Rami communicantes
21 Left phrenic n. and vessels
22 Sympathetic trunk

Abdomen
23 Greater splanchnic n.
24 Phrenic ganglion and p.
25 Lesser splanchnic n.
26 Intercostal n.
27 Lumbar splanchnic nn.
28 Iliohypogastric n.
29 Ilioinguinal n.
30 Rami communicantes
31 Lateral femoral cutaneous n.
32 Genitofemoral n.
33 Renal p.
34 Sympathetic trunk
35 Superior cluneal nn.

Pelvis and perineum
36 Genitofemoral nn.
37 Obturator n.
38 Sympathetic trunk
39 Pudendal n.
40 Sciatic n.
41 Inferior gluteal nn.
42 Coccygeal n.

Lower limb
43 Femoral n.
44 Anterior br. (Obturator n.)
45 Posterior br. (Obturator n.)
46 Inferior cluneal nn.

Key

a.	Artery	n.	Nerve
aa.	Arteries	nn.	Nerves
v.	Vein	p.	Plexus
vv.	Veins	C.	Cervical
br.	Branch		
brs.	Branches		

FIGURE 5.23 Nervous system. (Courtesy of Anatomical Chart Co.)

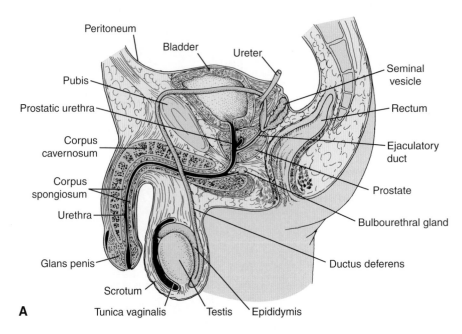

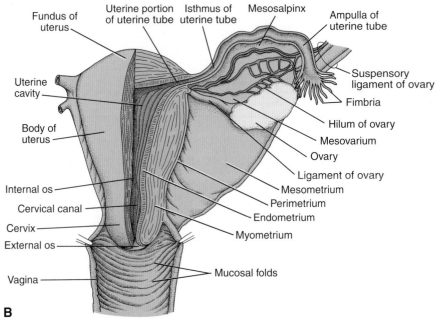

FIGURE 5.24   Reproductive systems. **A.** Male. **B.** Female.

WRAP-UP

Throughout this chapter, we discussed the various anatomical body parts and systems. Although not a complete and thorough review, the information provided should give the reader the rudimentary knowledge needed to understand how emergency trauma can affect or alter normal body systems or anatomy. More in-depth anatomical or physiological review can be obtain in various courses, workshops, seminars, or texts.

REFERENCE

1. Fox S. *Human Physiology*. New York: McGraw-Hill; 2002.

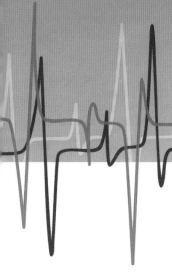

CHAPTER 6

Transportation and Ambulatory Techniques

CHAPTER OUTCOMES

1. Identify the proper mechanics for lifting and transporting an athlete.

2. Recognize when situations arise that require an athlete to be moved or transported.

3. Explain moves and transports to be done by one athletic trainer and by two or more athletic trainers.

4. Identify standard and fabricated equipment used to transport or move athletes.

5. Identify moves or drags using the athlete's torso or limbs.

6. Explain the various water rescues with or without emergency equipment.

7. Describe ambulatory aids and transport techniques for athletes with a lower extremity injury.

NOMENCLATURE

Ambulate: to walk, having only one foot leave the ground with each step

Axilla: armpit

Greater trochanter: the large eminence located approximately 1 cm lower than the head of the femur and a little to the side and back of the upper femur

Popliteal fossa: the space behind the knee joint

Power grip: also known as the supinated grip or underhand grip, palms facing up and knuckles facing down

Tandem: together, as in a group of persons working together, not necessarily in line

BEFORE YOU BEGIN

1. How would an athletic trainer ambulate an injured athlete off the field?

2. When should an injured athlete be moved off the field or away from the playing environment?

3. Should equipment lifts ever be used in the athletic training setting?

4. Should an athletic trainer be knowledgeable about removal techniques for athletes in water environments?

Voices from the Field

Safe and effective movement of an injured athlete requires training and technical skill development in a variety of situations to avoid aggravating the injury. The athletic trainer must be able to make quick decisions about the severity of the injury and condition of the athlete, whether there is an emergent need for removal from the environment, time until emergency medical transportation arrives, the equipment accessible for effective rescue and movement, and the number of people that are trained to assist. Once the decision to move an injured athlete takes place, the athletic trainer must choose which technique is going to be implemented to get the athlete to a safer location for further evaluation.

Knowing the different techniques available and the biomechanics of performing them is important for the protection of the athlete as well as the safety of the athletic trainer. The athletic trainer must be able to select the appropriate technique for the environmental condition (e.g., heat, cold, rain, snow), physical location (e.g., gym, field, pool), and the athlete's condition (e.g., conscious or unconscious, head or back injury, medi-

cal emergency). The athletic trainer needs to be competent in a variety of single athletic trainer moves to accommodate a variety of athlete sizes, situations, and conditions. In addition, the athletic trainer must know how to perform and instruct others in assisting with carries, lifts, and equipment rescues requiring more than one person to safeguard the athlete.

Communication is critical when transferring the athlete to the emergency medical services, hospital personnel, or other allied health professionals. Using appropriate medical terminology is essential to enhancing the credibility of the athletic trainer's assessment of the athlete's condition and expediting the care given to the injured athlete.

Helen M. Binkley, PhD, ATC, CSCS*D, NSCA-CPT*D
Associate Professor
Department of Health and Human Performance
Director, Undergraduate Athletic Training Program
Middle Tennessee State University
Murfreesboro, Tennessee

In most instances, the injuries or illnesses suffered by athletes are cared for on the sidelines or in athletic training, clinical, or physician rooms. The athletes themselves can usually ambulate to these areas with little or no support from medical personnel. However, there are instances where the athlete may suffer from a life-threatening situation, such as a fracture to an extremity where he or she cannot ambulate and needs assistance, where the terrain makes it difficult for the athlete to ambulate safely without assistance, or in rare instances when an athlete is located in a car or building and is in danger. Moving an athlete without the proper technique or knowledge may exacerbate an injury. Therefore, it is imperative that athletic trainers know the proper mechanics and types of ambulatory movements not only to transport an athlete safely but also to protect themselves from being hurt. In this chapter, we review equipment used by one person or by two or more people as well as other ambulatory aids that can be used to move and transport an athlete. Many of these techniques may never be used, but knowing the step-by-step procedures and when to use ambulatory movements may be useful when the need arises.

DECIDING TO MOVE AN INJURED ATHLETE

Before an athlete can be moved, the athletic trainer must decide how it can be done safely. First, can the athlete be moved by an athletic trainer without harm to either the athlete or the trainer? The size and strength of the athletic trainer and the size of the athlete will help to determine

whether equipment or more personnel are needed. A female gymnast who must be carried off the floor will pose less of a problem than a 300-lb lineman on a backboard. Another aspect to be kept in mind is the safety of the scene; in other words, must the athlete be moved in order to provide emergency care? If the answer is no, the athletic trainer should provide immediate care and call emergency medical services (EMS). If the answer is yes, the first step is to determine whether there are any potential spinal injuries, fractures, or life-threatening conditions. If it is determined that any of these conditions exist and the athlete must be moved, the appropriate measures for stabilization must be implemented and proper ambulatory methods used (these issues are discussed here and in Chapters 14 through 17). The method to move an athlete will depend upon the terrain and location, number of athletic trainers present (and their emergency training), their familiarity and experience with the lifts, and the type of injury suffered. The National Athletic Trainers' Association position statement is extremely useful in determining when to move an injured athlete (http://www.nata.org/statements/consensus/ NATAPreHospital.pdf). The decision-making process should take place based upon assessment of the scene and the condition of the athlete.

PROPER BODY MECHANICS IN LIFTING AN INJURED ATHLETE

When a decision has been made that an athlete must be moved to another location for follow-up or emergency

Breakout

Common Lifting and Moving Mechanics for the Athletic Trainer

1. When applicable, place your feet about a shoulder's width apart.
2. Bend at the knees, keeping your back straight as you bend down, similar to the bending squat position.
3. Use a power grip with the victim or equipment. The **power grip** has the palms facing up.
4. In lifting, use your legs to straighten up; (do not lift with the back), similar to the return motion during a squat.
5. Exhale as you stand.
6. Keep your head and chin up.
7. Keep the athlete or equipment close to your body to prevent reaching. It has been recommended that a athletic trainer should never reach more than 18 in.[2]
8. Lift slowly.
9. Do not twist or move in a jerky fashion.

services, proper body mechanics must be followed in order to limit the potential of injury to the athletic trainer. Using faulty body mechanics can lead to undue strain to the lower back, muscle strains in the arms and legs, or hernias. In most instances, ambulatory mechanics are the same whenever an athlete is being lifted or moved. These include proper foot and hand placements and breathing. The overall physical strength of the athletic trainer also plays a crucial role in lifting or moving an injured athlete. At no time should an athletic trainer risk his or her health to help another, especially since harm to the athletic trainer may limit emergency services provided. For these reasons, some of the two-person lifts and carries may not be appropriate, especially when there are other forms of equipment, such as spine boards or stretchers, available that can be used safely.

ONE-PERSON MOVES

It is critical to determine (a) the proper lifting or moving techniques and (b) when an injured athlete should be moved. You do not want to cause harm by moving the athlete unnecessarily; in some instances, however, there is no alternative to making a move. Before you do so, you must consider several factors, including the athlete's discomfort, extraneous conditions that may harm the athlete if he or she is not moved, your ability to move the athlete, and what equipment might be required. In most instances, the athletic trainer can **ambulate** the athlete with simple one-person moves (Table 6.1). These moves are classified by the positioning of the athlete/athletic trainer and are used for multiple purposes and multiple conditions. Each move is described in detail below, along with the proper mechanics of the move and the situations for which it is appropriate.

TABLE 6.1   One-Person Rescue Moves[1]

Type of Move	Indications
Shoulder drag	Spinal support, conscious/unconscious
Clothes drag	Spinal support, conscious/unconscious
Blanket drag	Spinal support, conscious/unconscious
Sheet drag	Moving short distance, no spinal injury, when victim has no shirt
Ankle drag	Moving short distance, no spinal injury
Piggyback carry	Conscious, lower extremity pathology, weight bearing is limited
Packstrap carry	Conscious/unconscious, when victim has no clothing to drag or equipment is not available to drag, moving over short distances, no spinal injury
Cradle carry	Child or light weight victim, conscious/unconscious, no spinal injury, carry over longer distance
Fireman's carry	Moving over rough terrain, no spinal or extremity fractures
Walking assist	Injury to one side of lower extremity

SKILL 6.1

Shoulder Drag

This move can be used if you suspect a spinal injury, the athlete is unconscious, and you are moving the athlete only a short distance.

1. Position yourself at the athlete's head (Fig. 6.1)
2. Kneel, placing one leg at a 90-degree angle, and rest on the knee of the opposite leg (Fig. 6.1).

3. Place your hands underneath the athlete's armpits (Fig. 6.1).
4. Cup your hands around the front of the athlete's shoulder with your fingers facing upward (Fig. 6.2).
5. Pull the athlete up slightly, resting the athlete's head against your chest for support (Fig. 6.2).
6. After supporting the athlete's head, slowly move backward, keeping your knees slightly bent, and pull the athlete to a safe place where care can be rendered (Fig. 6.3).

If you suspect a spinal injury, be careful not to flex the athlete's head too far forward.

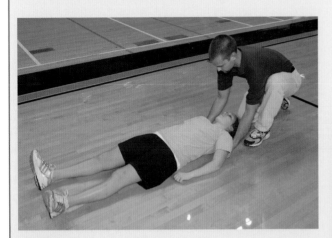

FIGURE 6.1

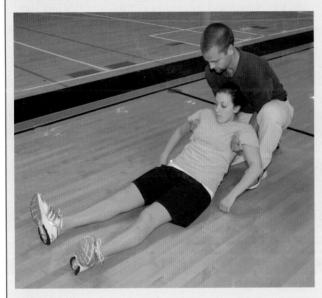

FIGURE 6.2

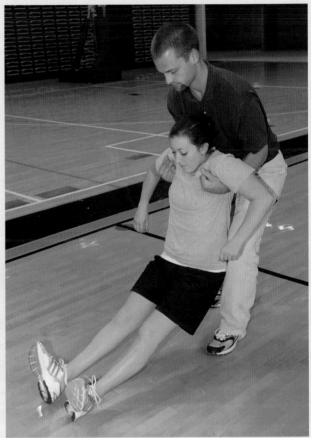

FIGURE 6.3

SKILL 6.2

Clothes Drag

This move is similar to the shoulder drag except that you move the athlete by his or her clothing at the shoulder/trapezius area.

1. Position yourself at the head of the athlete (Fig. 6.4).
2. Kneel, placing one leg at a 90-degree angle and resting on the knee of the opposite leg (Fig. 6.4).
3. Place your hands beside the athlete's neck and grab the clothing (shirt) at the shoulder/trapezius region (Fig. 6.4).
4. Pull the athlete up slightly, resting the athlete's head between your forearms (Fig. 6.5).
5. Keeping your leg and waist bent, slowly move backward to a safe place where care can be rendered (Fig. 6.6).

If you suspect a spinal injury, be careful not to flex the athlete's head too far forward.

The athlete's head should be cradled between your forearms.

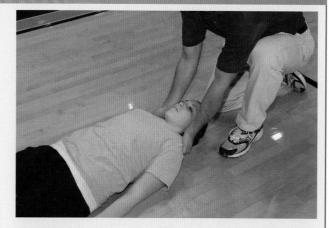

FIGURE 6.4

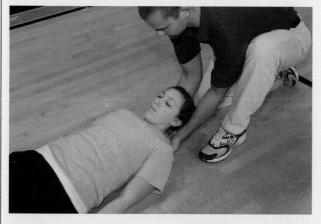

FIGURE 6.5

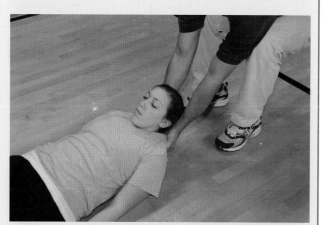

FIGURE 6.6

SKILL 6.3

Blanket Drag

The blanket drag is useful when an athlete must be moved a greater distance than with the shoulder or clothing drag. This method can also support the athlete's spine if you suspect a spinal injury. The only drawback is that you must have some type of blanket or sheet available to use for this purpose.

1. Place a blanket beside the athlete, with approximately 1 to 2 ft extending beyond his or her head and feet. If the blanket is not long enough to extend that far, make sure that the blanket extends beyond the head only (Fig. 6.7).
2. On the opposite side of the athlete, pull him or her toward you at the shoulders (Fig. 6.7).

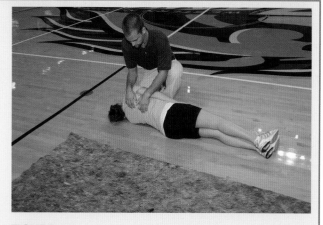

FIGURE 6.7

(Continued)

SKILL 6.3 *(Continued)*

Blanket Drag (Continued)

3. Grab the blanket and slide it as far as possible underneath the athlete; usually about half the body width can be covered (Fig. 6.8).
4. Repeat the procedure on the opposite side (Fig. 6.9). The blanket should extend 2 to 3 ft on either side.

5. Fold the blanket up at the athlete's feet. Fold in one side then the other, if possible tucking it in around the body (Fig. 6.10).
6. Grab the extended portion of the blanket at the athlete's head, pull tight, and then move the athlete (Fig. 6.11).

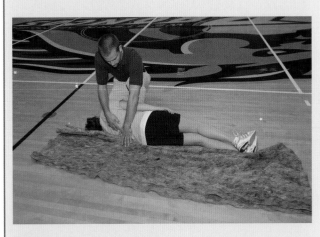

FIGURE 6.8

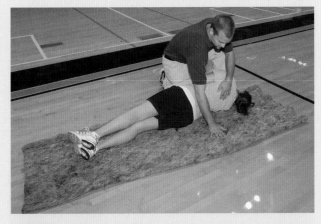

FIGURE 6.9

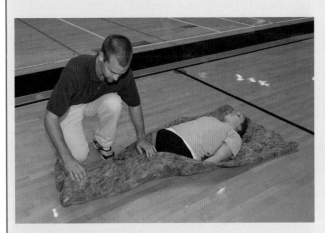

FIGURE 6.10

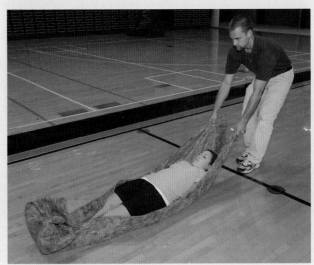

FIGURE 6.11

SKILL 6.4

Sheet Drag

The sheet drag is very similar to the shoulder and clothing drags except that a sheet or other material is wrapped around the torso and shoulders and the athlete is pulled backward. Again, this maneuver is best used when the athlete's clothing is not suitable for pulling, no spinal injury is suspected, and you are dragging for only a short distance.

1. Position yourself at the athlete's head (Fig. 6.12).
2. Roll or fold the sheet until it is only about 3 to 5 in. in diameter (Fig. 6.12).
3. Place the sheet across the athlete's chest just above the nipple and below the clavicle. Take both ends and fold them under the armpits, pulling the excess toward the athlete's head (Fig. 6.12).
4. Grab both ends of the sheet and twist it at the athlete's head to form a triangle (Fig. 6.13).
5. Pull up on the sheet, keeping your forearms and those of the athlete close together (Fig. 6.13).
6. Pull the athlete up slightly, resting the athlete's head between your forearms (Fig. 6.14).
7. Keeping your legs and waist bent, slowly move backward to a safe place where care can be rendered (Fig. 6.14). Be careful not to flex the athlete's head too far forward.

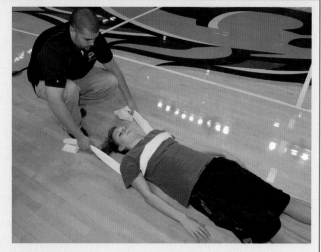

FIGURE 6.12

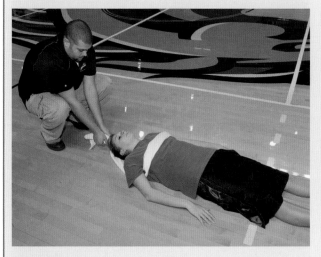

FIGURE 6.13

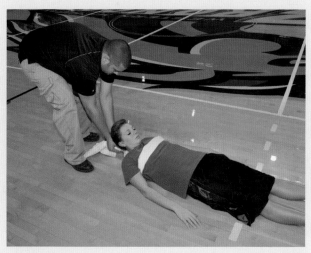

FIGURE 6.14

SKILL 6.5

Ankle Drag (Fig. 6.15)

If you do not suspect a spinal injury, the ankle drag is useful for moving the athlete a short distance over smooth terrain.

1. Arrange the athlete's arms over his or her head.
2. Place the athlete's legs and feet together.
3. Grab the athlete's ankle or lower leg area with both hands.
4. Keeping your knees and waist slightly bent, pull the athlete toward you as you walk backward.

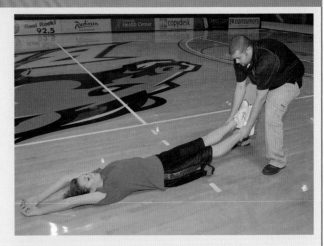

FIGURE 6.15

SKILL 6.6

Piggyback Carry

The piggyback carry is used when you have a fully conscious person, usually with a lower extremity injury, where full or partial weight bearing is limited and the distance to be traveled is relatively short. This carry requires significant effort on the athletic trainer's part, since the full weight of the athlete is placed upon the athletic trainer's back and shoulders. This carry is not recommended for athletes whose weight is significantly greater than that of the athletic trainer or those who are much taller than the athletic trainer. Good physical conditioning is also required of the athletic trainer who performs this maneuver.

1. Have the athlete face your back (Fig. 6.16).
2. Slightly bend your knees and waist (Fig. 6.16).
3. Have the athlete wrap his or her arms around your shoulders (Fig. 6.16).

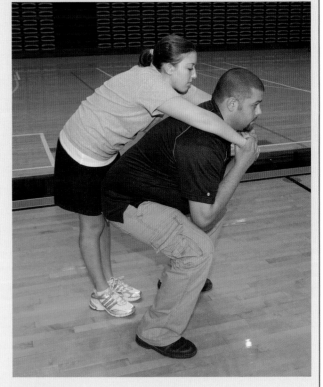

FIGURE 6.16

SKILL 6.6 *(Continued)*

Piggyback Carry *(Continued)*

4. Lift up using your knees (Fig. 6.17).
5. Reach back and grab the athlete's thighs so that his or her legs can rest on the your hips (Fig. 6.17).
6. Keeping your knees and waist slightly bent, pull the athlete toward you as you walk (Fig. 6.17).

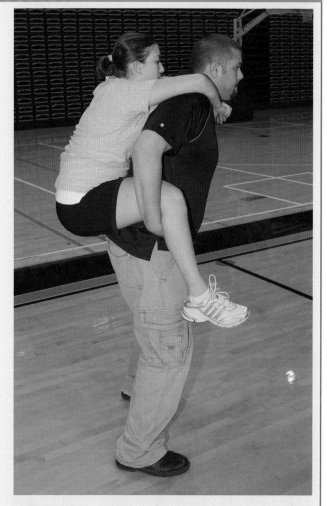

FIGURE 6.17

SKILL 6.7

Packstrap Carry

The packstrap carry is used to carry an unconscious or unresponsive person when a drag cannot be initiated because of inadequate clothing or lack of blankets or other essential equipment. As with the piggyback carry, the athletic trainer must have enough strength and conditioning to carry an athlete in this manner, because the athlete must be lifted off the ground. The packstrap carry should be used only for short distances.

1. The athlete should be face up on the ground with arms above his or her head.
2. Bend your knees and waist and grab the athlete's arms between the elbows and wrist joints.
3. Pull the athlete up to a sitting position.
4. Holding onto the athlete's arms, rotate your body to face away from the athlete (Fig. 6.18).

5. Place the athlete's arms over your shoulders (Fig. 6.18).
6. With your knees bent, slowly stand up without extending your back (Fig. 6.19).
7. Once the athlete is up, bend slightly forward at the waist to bring the athlete's feet off the ground (Fig. 6.19).

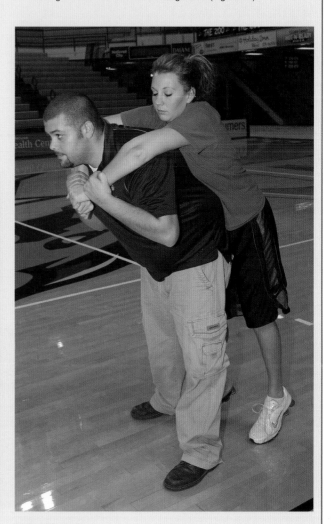

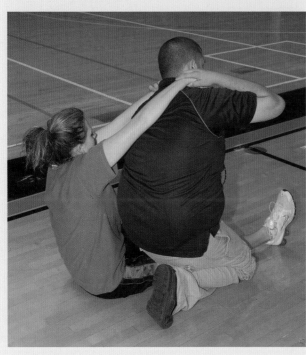

FIGURE 6.18

FIGURE 6.19

SKILL 6.8

Cradle Carry

The cradle carry is used to carry or move a child or lightweight athlete. The athlete can be either conscious or unconscious or unresponsive; he or she should not have any suspected spinal injuries. This carry can be used for longer distances if necessary. Again, the athletic trainer must have enough strength to perform this move.

1. Place the athlete on the ground in a supine position (Fig. 6.20).
2. Bend at the knees and waist, placing one of arm at the athlete's torso level and the other at his or her **popliteal fossa** area (Fig. 6.20).
3. Reach underneath these areas, hooking your hands to the opposite side of the athlete's body (Fig. 6.20).
4. With your knees bent, slowly stand up without extending your back (Fig. 6.21).

5. The athlete, if conscious, may then place his or her hands around your neck.

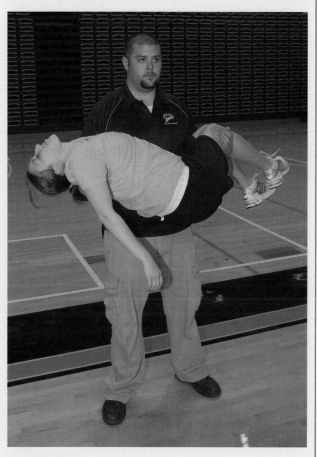

FIGURE 6.21

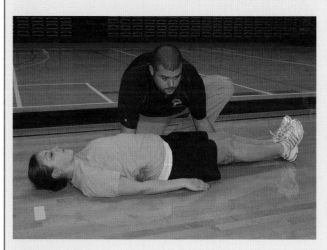

FIGURE 6.20

SKILL 6.9

Fireman's Carry

As a one-rescuer lift, the fireman's carry is complex and requires some physical strength to execute. The purpose of this carry is to move an athlete over irregular terrain, such as steps or rocks. The fireman's carry should not be used when you suspect a spinal injury or fractures to the extremities. This lift should not be attempted by anyone with low back pathology.

1. Place the athlete in the supine position (Fig. 6.22).
2. Place the athlete's heels several inches from his or her butt, with the knees bent and facing upward. The athlete's arms should be at the sides (Fig. 6.22).

3. Bend at the waist and knees and grab the dorsal side of the athlete's wrists (Fig. 6.22).
4. Place your feet on the athlete's toes (Fig. 6.22).
5. Leaning backward, pull the athlete's arms toward you (Fig. 6.23).
6. When the athlete is near the standing position, crouch toward the athlete, placing one of your knees at a 90-degree angle and the other leg behind your body (Fig. 6.23).

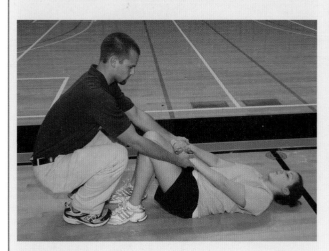

FIGURE 6.22

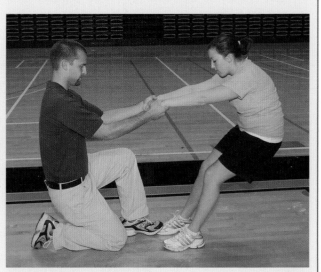

FIGURE 6.23

SKILL 6.9 *(Continued)*

Fireman's Carry *(Continued)*

7. Pull the athlete over one of your shoulders with one of the athlete's arms at the side of your head (Fig. 6.24).
8. While holding the athlete's arm at the side of your head, reach underneath the athlete and grab the athlete's leg adjacent to your head (Fig. 6.24).
9. Slowly rise up from the crouching position, maintaining contact with the athlete's arm and leg (Fig. 6.25).

10. Once fully erect, take the arm that you are holding and bring it to the hand holding the athlete's leg (Fig. 6.25).
11. With the hand holding the athlete's leg, grab the athlete's wrist and hold both together, freeing up your other arm (Fig. 6.25).

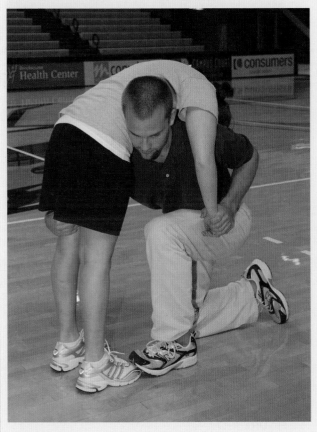

FIGURE 6.24

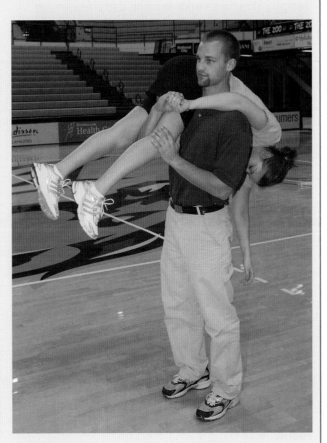

FIGURE 6.25

SKILL 6.10

Walking Assist

A walking assist is used to move an athlete who may have a lower extremity injury on one side only. The athletic trainer, in this case, acts like a crutch, supporting the athlete's body and injured extremity. This technique is often used to escort athletes who have suffered an ankle or knee injury off a playing field.

1. Place yourself at the side of the athlete's injured leg (Fig. 6.26).

2. Take the athlete's arm closest to you around your shoulder and grab it with your opposite hand (Fig. 6.26).
3. Place your arm that is closest to the athlete around his or her waist. You leg closest to the athlete will act like a crutch (Fig. 6.26).
4. In transporting, your "crutch" leg and the athlete's injured leg should move in **tandem** (Fig. 6.27).

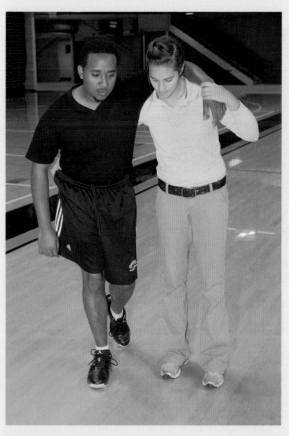

FIGURE 6.26

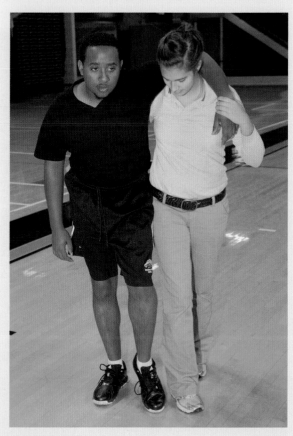

FIGURE 6.27

MOVES WITH TWO OR MORE ATHLETIC TRAINERS

Two-person moves are used when the athlete is either unconscious or unresponsive or has a fracture or injury, making it impossible for him or her to move without help. This type of move is generally used when the injured athlete is larger than the athletic trainer or the athletic trainer is not strong enough to support the athlete single-handedly. Two-person moves are also used when the athletic trainer feels more comfortable having assistance or there are two or more athletic trainers or medical personnel present, making transportation of an injured athlete easier for all involved (Table 6.2). When using two-person assistance techniques, each athletic trainer must communicate effectively to execute the lift; it is also important to use proper body mechanics to limit potential injuries associated with lifting/carrying an injured athlete.

Breakout

Communication Suggestions for Two or More Athletic Trainers[1]

1. Determine the lead athletic trainer.
2. The lead athletic trainer will be responsible for instructions to the second athletic trainer.
3. Determine the type of assist or carry that should be implemented based upon the athlete's condition.
4. The lead athletic trainer will instruct the secondary athletic trainer(s) as to the proper positions.
5. The lead athletic trainer should make sure that the athlete is properly stabilized and supported before proceeding.
6. When moving an injured athlete, the lead athletic trainer should establish a specific walking or moving cadence as appropriate.

TABLE 6.2	Two-or-More-Person Rescue Moves[1]
Type of Move	**Indications**
Two-handed carry	Moving short distances and over rough terrain, lifting athlete on elevated surface, lower extremity injury
Hammock carry	Conscious/unconscious athlete, no spinal injury
Two-person extremity lift	No spinal injuries, conscious/unconscious, must support weight of athlete
Two-person chair litter	Chair must be able to support the athlete's weight, athlete is conscious and can sit
Three-rescuer flat lift and carry	Conscious/unconscious athlete, no other equipment available, coordination of athletic trainers

SKILL 6.11

Two-Handed Seat Carry

This carry is good for moving an athlete a short distance, especially over unstable terrain, or in placing an athlete on a table or other elevated surface. This carry is often utilized when the athlete has a lower extremity injury and cannot support his or her weight.

1. Begin by determining who will be the lead athletic trainer.
2. The athletic trainers then place themselves on either side of the athlete, facing each other (Fig. 6.28).
3. The athlete is in a seated position with the athletic trainers standing with their knees bent and apart for stabilization (Fig. 6.28).

4. Each athletic trainer then places his or her arm closest to the back of the athlete around the athlete's back at the scapula level with the remaining hand placed on the other athletic trainer's shoulder (Fig. 6.28).
5. The athletic trainers then slide their arms under the athlete's thighs and interlock their hands (Fig. 6.28).
6. The athlete places his or her arms over the shoulders of the athletic trainers (Fig. 6.28).
7. The athletic trainers slowly stand up in tandem (Fig. 6.29).

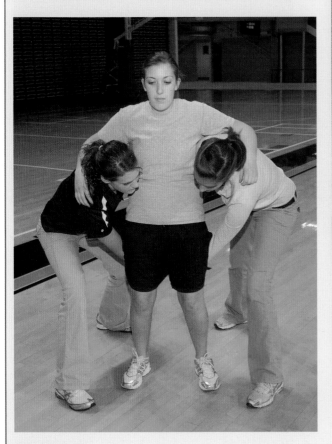

FIGURE 6.28

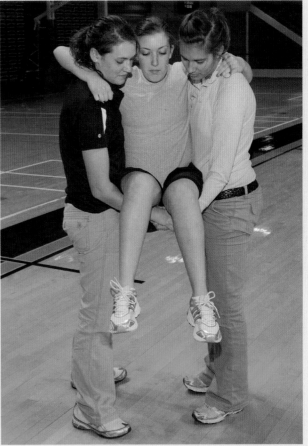

FIGURE 6.29

(Continued)

Two-Handed Seat Carry *(Continued)*

A variation of this technique is to have the two athletic trainers interlock their arms in the front and place their remaining arms on each other's shoulders to form a "seat." The athletic trainers then move behind the athlete, who leans back and "sits" in the cradle made by the athletic trainers' arms. The athlete then places his or her arms over the athletic trainers' shoulders.

Another variation can be performed by having the athletic trainers interlock their hands and arms together to create a "square seat":

1. The left hand of each athletic trainer grabs his or her right forearm, just below the wrist, to form a "T." This is called the supporting arm (Fig. 6.30).
2. The free hand of each athletic trainer then grabs onto the supporting arm of the other midway between the wrist and the elbow (Fig. 6.31). A square that acts like a seat has now been formed by the two athletic trainers.
3. The athletic trainers position themselves behind the athlete; in tandem, the athletic trainers bend at the waist and knees or kneel to position themselves closer to the ground (Fig. 6.31).
4. The athlete sits back on the "seat" and places his or her arms over the shoulders of the athletic trainers (Fig. 6.32).
5. The athletic trainers then slowly stand erect, supporting the athlete (Fig. 6.32).

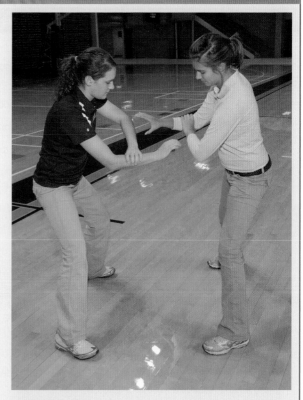

FIGURE 6.30

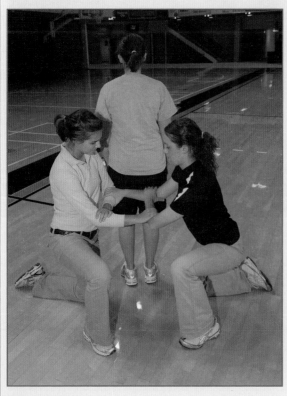

FIGURE 6.31

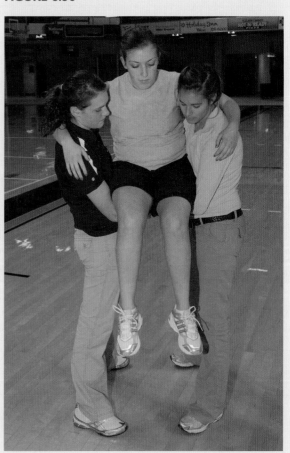

FIGURE 6.32

SKILL 6.12

Hammock Carry

The hammock carry is used when an athlete is unconscious or unresponsive and not suspected of having a spinal or severe extremity injury. This carry is performed by at least three persons but can accommodate up to six, depending on the size and weight of the athlete. The hammock carry with three athletic trainers is illustrated.

1. Place the athlete supine with arms folded across the waist (Fig. 6.33).

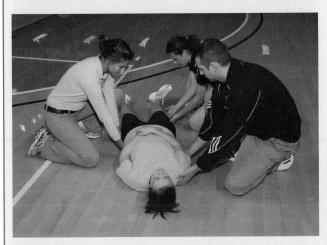

FIGURE 6.33

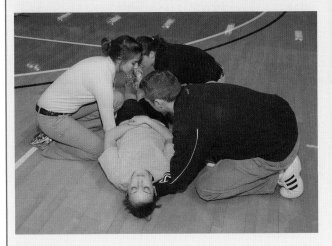

FIGURE 6.34

2. The lead athletic trainer determines where to position the other athletic trainers based on the athlete's size. In this scenario, one person will be at the athlete's shoulder level, one at the waist, and one at the knees. The athletic trainer at the waist should be on the side opposite the two other athletic trainers (Fig. 6.33).
3. All three athletic trainers kneel (Fig. 6.33).
4. The athletic trainers place their arms underneath the athlete, reaching to the other side (Fig. 6.34).
5. In unison, the athletic trainers slowly raise the athlete off the ground (Fig. 6.35).
6. Once the athlete is stabilized, the athletic trainers must transport him or her in a synchronous fashion, moving lengthwise to maintain good support (Fig. 6.35).

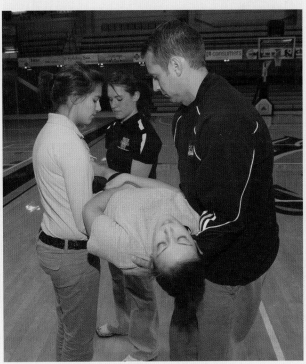

FIGURE 6.35

SKILL 6.13

Two-Person Extremity Lift

This lift can be utilized when there is no suspicion of spinal injuries. Used mainly when the athlete is unconscious or unresponsive, it may also serve for a conscious person who requires transportation to an appropriate setting. As with all lifts, the athletic trainers must be strong enough to support the athlete's weight without causing harm to themselves.

1. The athlete should be placed in a supine position (Fig. 6.36).
2. One athletic trainer is positioned at the athlete's head and the other at the feet (Fig. 6.36).
3. Kneeling, the athletic trainer at the head reaches under the athlete's shoulders and grabs the athlete's wrists, pulling the wrists toward his or her chest (Fig. 6.36).

4. The second athletic trainer, facing toward the athlete's feet, grasps underneath the knees of the athlete, reaching under to cup the popliteal fossa (Fig. 6.36).
5. In tandem, both athletic trainers stand, pulling the athlete off the ground (Fig. 6.37).

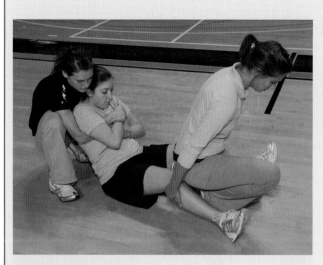

FIGURE 6.36

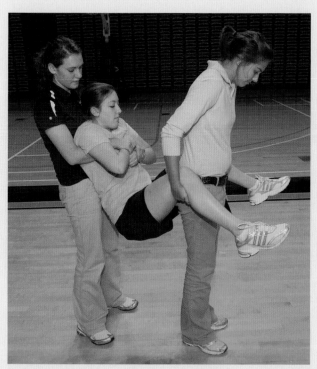

FIGURE 6.37

SKILL 6.14

Two-Person Chair Litter

This rescue utilizes a chair to lift the athlete for transport, and the chair must be strong enough to support the athlete's weight. The athlete should be conscious and should not have injuries that could be compromised in a sitting position. In emergency situations, this lift can be used for an unconscious athlete, but that is not recommended.

1. To begin, have the athlete sit in the chair (Fig. 6.38).
2. One athletic trainer stands behind the chair and the other kneels in front of it (Fig. 6.38).
3. The athletic trainer at the back grabs the sides of the chair while the athletic trainer in the front, facing forward, reaches back and grabs the chair's front legs (Fig. 6.38).

4. Raise the athlete in a controlled manner; the front athletic trainer must lift up while the athletic trainer at the rear slowly tilts the chair backward (Fig. 6.39).
5. When both athletic trainers are fully erect, the athlete should be slightly reclined, with his or her back supported by the back of the chair (Fig. 6.39).

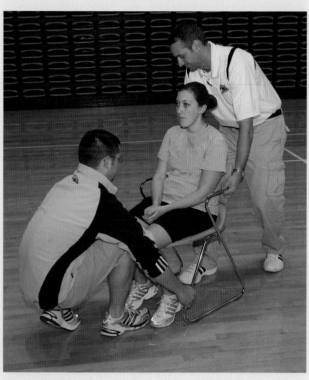

FIGURE 6.38

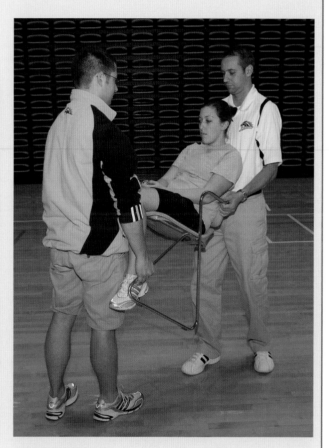

FIGURE 6.39

SKILL 6.15

Three-Person Flat Lift and Carry

This technique may be useful when no other equipment, such as a stretcher, chair, cot, or backboard, is available and there is no suspicion of spinal injuries. It is recommended with an injured, unresponsive athlete, either conscious or unconscious, who must be moved to a safer or more secure location. This technique requires coordination of moves and some skill, as the athletic trainers must move the athlete in unison. It is recommended that the athletic trainers have some previous experience or practice using this technique.

1. To begin, determine the extent of the injuries. Then all three athletic trainers place themselves at the side of the athlete with the least injury. It is recommended that the tallest of the athletic trainers be placed at the shoulders, with the other two at the waist and knees. In this fashion, when totally raised, the athlete is lying at a slight downward angle. If there are four athletic trainers, one is placed at the head, one at the chest, one at the waist, and one at the knees (Fig. 6.40).
2. With all the athletic trainers kneeling, the first athletic trainer reaches under the athlete's shoulder/neck region, the second reaches under the waist, and the third reaches under the knees, all grasping onto the athlete for good support (Fig. 6.40).
3. The athletic trainers place their knees at a 90-degree angle. In unison, the three athletic trainers lift the athlete and rest him or her on their knees (Fig. 6.41).

4. At this point, the three athletic trainers, in unison, rotate the athlete toward themselves, letting him or her rest on the inside of their elbow joints (Fig. 6.42).
5. Again in unison, the three athletic trainers stand erect, lifting the athlete as they do so (the athlete is facing them).
6. Once the athlete is off the ground and the athletic trainers are ready, they walk in a coordinated fashion as they transport the athlete to another setting.

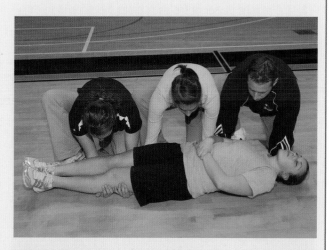

FIGURE 6.40

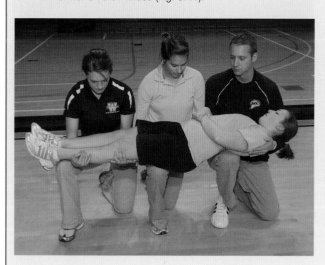

FIGURE 6.41

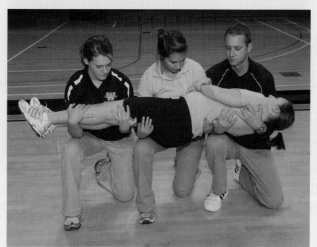

FIGURE 6.42

EQUIPMENT LIFTS

In addition to manual lifts, athletes can be transported or moved with equipment capable of holding and supporting them (Table 6.3). Each piece of equipment has a specific purpose and sometimes must be assembled before use. Therefore, it is imperative that the athletic trainer have a thorough understanding of how to assemble and use equipment specifically designed for athlete transport. Equipment lifts also require the assistance of two or more athletic trainers (preferably four to six) to properly stabilize the injured athlete and execute the move. The use of equipment lifts also requires adequate practice for all athletic trainers and good communication skills to ensure that all steps are being conducted properly and efficiently. In this section, we discuss and review the steps or techniques required to improvise or utilize the various types of equipment lifts.

When using equipment for lifting and moving injured athletes, it may be necessary to logroll the athlete and apply a cervical collar to stabilize the cervical spine. The logroll can be accomplished with as few as two athletic trainers, but three or four make the task easier; the latter is recommended to limit spinal movement and stabilize the athlete. The application of a cervical collar is addressed in Chapter 17, which discusses spinal injuries and backboarding procedures in emergency situations.

TABLE 6.3	Equipment Lifts
Equipment	**Indications**
Stretcher	No spinal injuries
Scoop stretcher	Spinal injuries
Blanket stretcher	No spinal or head injuries

SKILL 6.16

Performing a Logroll with Two or More Persons

1. The athletic trainer with the most experience should be designated as the leader or person in charge. The leader is placed at the athlete's head and holds the head with both hands, limiting motion (Fig. 6.43).
2. The other athletic trainers (two or more) are positioned at one side of the athlete, at the chest, pelvis, and knees (if only two athletic trainers, at the chest and pelvis) (Fig. 6.43).
3. The stretcher/backboard is placed at the other side of the athlete, as close to him or her as possible (Fig. 6.43).
4. The athletic trainer at the chest reaches across the athlete and grabs the upper arm and shoulder. The athletic trainer at the pelvis reaches across the athlete and grabs the lower back and pelvis (Fig. 6.44).
5. The athlete is logrolled when the leader makes the command, usually after a count of three, until the athlete is on his or her side (Fig. 6.44).
6. The stretcher/backboard is then pushed to where the athlete was just lying (Fig. 6.44).

7. The athlete is then rolled onto the stretcher/backboard after verbal command from the leader, usually after a count of three (Fig. 6.45).

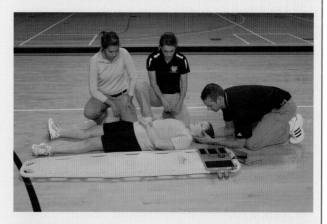

FIGURE 6.43

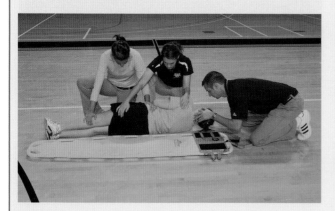

FIGURE 6.44

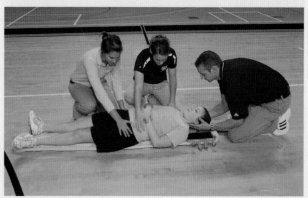

FIGURE 6.45

SKILL 6.17

Stretchers (Canvas or Vinyl) with Two Athletic Trainers

1. If no spinal injuries are suspected, the athlete is placed in the supine position.
2. The stretcher is unfolded and placed next to the athlete, on the side opposite the trainer.
3. A logroll is performed to place the athlete on the stretcher.
4. The athlete is placed into position on the stretcher by first sliding the shoulders on, then the waist, and then the legs.

Stretcher

One of the most commonly used pieces of equipment for transporting an injured athlete is the stretcher. Stretchers can be made of various materials—such as canvas or vinyl-coated nylon, with solid frames of wood or tubular frames—and most can support more than 300 pounds. A stretcher can also be improvised if a facility does not have one. For example, blankets can be used (this is discussed below as a specific technique), sheets (a combination of two sheets for extra support and strength) may be used, or clothing such as jackets or coats can be attached to long poles to create a stretcher (these types are not discussed in this chapter). Stretchers may be used to move athletes with or without spinal injuries.

SKILL 6.18

Scoop Stretcher

A scoop stretcher is similar in function to a regular stretcher except that it can be separated into halves to be placed on either side of the athlete. This method makes it easier to place the athlete onto the stretcher without logrolling, especially for athletes who may have spinal injuries. Usually two or more athletic trainers are required to use this technique, especially when lifting large athlete.

1. The athlete is placed in a supine position with the arms at the sides (Fig. 6.46).
2. The scoop stretcher is separated into halves, with one half placed on either side of the athlete (Fig. 6.46).
3. Half of the scoop stretcher is slid under the athlete to the midpoint of the body (Fig. 6.47).
4. The same is done with the other half.
5. Once the two halves are together, the scoop stretcher is fastened at the ends, where it was separated (Fig. 6.48).
6. Adjust the athlete (if needed) (Fig. 6.48).

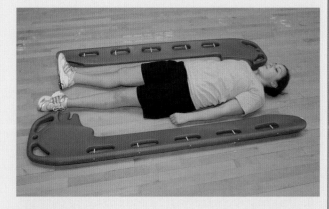

FIGURE 6.46

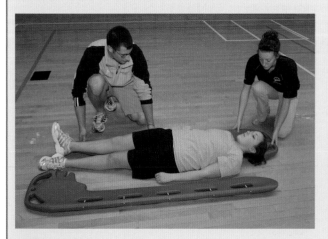

FIGURE 6.47

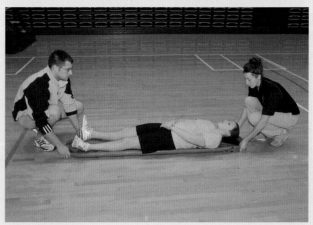

FIGURE 6.48

SKILL 6.19

Blanket Stretcher

A blanket stretcher can be improvised when you need to move an injured athlete over uneven terrain or obstacles or when you do not suspect a spinal injury or severe head injury. When using the blanket stretcher technique, it is imperative that the fabric of the blanket be free of holes and tears and strong enough to support the athlete. The blanket must also be considerably greater in length and width than the athlete in order to function properly as a stretcher. Use of this technique will require at least four athletic trainers to properly support and transport the athlete.

1. Place the athlete in a supine position, logrolling if necessary (Fig. 6.49).
2. Place the blanket on one side of the athlete, with the blanket extending beyond the athlete's head and feet (Fig. 6.49).
3. With three or four athletic trainers, logroll the athlete toward the position of the athletic trainers, until the athlete is on his or her side (Fig. 6.50).
4. The athletic trainers grab the blanket and slide approximately one third of it (in little folds or rolls) toward the athlete while each athletic trainer stabilizes the athlete with one arm (Fig. 6.50).
5. The athlete is logrolled onto the blanket, with the athletic trainers reaching underneath the athlete to pull out the blanket folds. If this is done correctly, approximately one third of the blanket should be on each side of the athlete. Make sure the blanket is evenly distributed on each side (Fig. 6.51).
6. With two athletic trainers on each side of the athlete, tightly roll the blanket toward the athlete (Fig. 6.51).
7. After creating the rolls, place an athletic trainer at the shoulder and knee area on each side of the athlete (Fig. 6.51).
8. Each athletic trainer should grab the blanket with his or her hands (shoulder width apart) at each respective site (Fig. 6.52).
9. The athletic trainers gently raise the athlete off the ground. With a blanket stretcher, the athlete will sink slightly as the fabric stretches with him or her (Fig. 6.52).

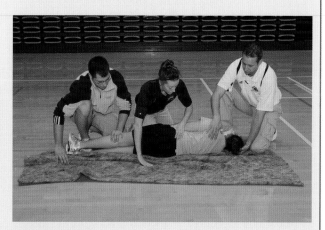

FIGURE 6.50

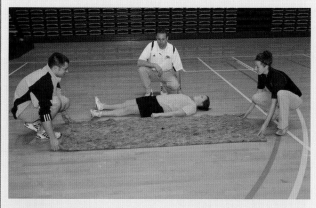

FIGURE 6.49

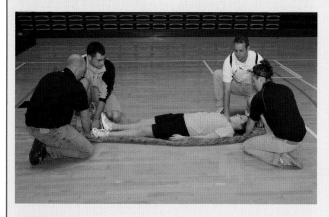

FIGURE 6.51

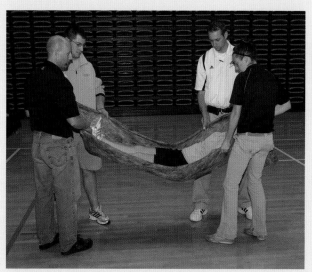

FIGURE 6.52

STRETCHER/BACKBOARD TRANSPORTATION

There are many types of stretchers that can be used to transport injured athletes safely to areas where care can be provided. However, one often overlooked aspect is the coordination and communication among athletic trainers when using a stretcher. Any athletic trainer who moves in a different direction may cause the athlete's support to become unbalanced, which can result in swaying or dropping of the athlete to the ground, potentially causing further harm. In order to transport an athlete safely, athletic trainers must practice the act of transportation, similar to practicing cardiopulmonary resuscitation or removing facemasks to gain access to airways. Practice securing an athlete to the stretcher with a manikin. Mistakes made in such practice can then be avoided when a real-life situation develops. Considerations for stretcher transportation are as follows:

1. Lift correctly, using your legs and not your back. Begin by having one leg at a 90-degree angle, with the sole of the foot on the ground. The other knee should be in contact with the ground, with the foot extending behind (Fig. 6.53).
2. Have the lead athletic trainer perform a "count" to ensure movement in unison. A count of "1, 2, 3, lift" will allow all athletic trainers to know when to initiate the movement.
3. Move the athlete in phases, first off the ground to the knee level and then to the waist level in two separate motions. Trying to lift to the waist may be difficult and cumbersome, depending on the type of equipment used (Fig. 6.54).
4. Make sure all athletic trainers are facing in the direction of movement. athletic trainers should all walk in

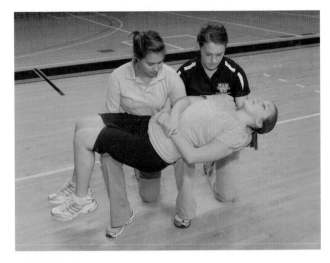

FIGURE 6.54

the same direction for ease of transportation, instead of some walking forward and some walking backward (Fig. 6.55).

Practice setting the athlete down on the ground in phases, from the waist to the knees and then to the ground, making sure that the athletic trainers bend at the knees instead of the waist.

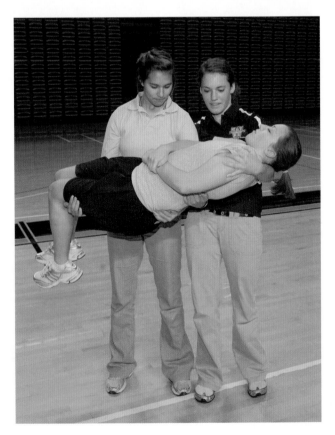

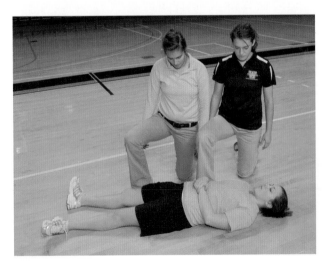

FIGURE 6.53

FIGURE 6.55

AMBULATION EQUIPMENT AND OTHER TRANSPORTATION TECHNIQUES

Although not an emergency transportation technique, the use of crutches or canes can be beneficial when moving an injured athlete. The use of crutches or canes is quite common when an athlete must be moved, must ambulate to a different area, or needs some support in everyday activities. Usually, the athlete has a lower extremity injury that impairs the use of one or both limbs and impedes locomotion. In emergency situations, an injured athlete may have a fracture, dislocation, or other pathology that can be treated at the scene. Once managed, the victim can be safely transported with a crutch or cane when other emergency equipment is not available or the use of drags or lifts is not appropriate. As with other transportation aids, the athletic trainers are responsible for implementing the correct fitting and ambulation techniques.

Crutches and canes can be made of wood, metal, or composites. Some are freely adjustable, while others are limited in possible adjustment. Whichever type you use, you should be familiar with the proper procedures to fit to the athlete. To fit a crutch properly, follow the procedures in Skill 6.20, below.

SKILL 6.20

Fitting a Crutch

1. Select a crutch of the appropriate size. Many crutches and canes come in various sizes depending on the height of the user. A crutch or cane that is too large or too small will not function properly.
2. If the athlete is standing, place the tip of the crutch about 6 in. in front and 2 in. to the side of the leg that is bearing weight (Fig. 6.56).

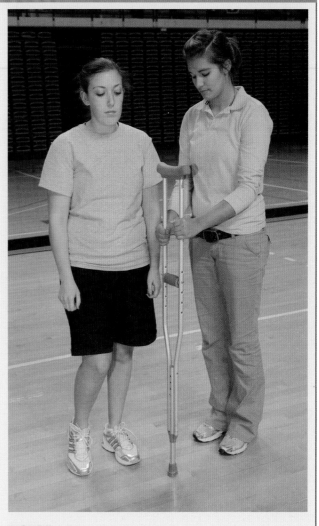

FIGURE 6.56

(Continued)

SKILL 6.20 *(Continued)*

Fitting a Crutch *(Continued)*

   a. If the athlete is lying on his or her back, measure the distance from one arm extended to a 90-degree bent arm on the other side at the elbow (Fig. 6.57).

3. The underarm brace should be approximately 1 in. below the **axilla.**

4. If adjustable, position the crutch at the appropriate height-adjustment markers based upon your measurements.

5. Have the athlete hold the crutch handle. Adjust it so that the athlete's arm is bent to approximately 30 degrees (Fig. 6.58).

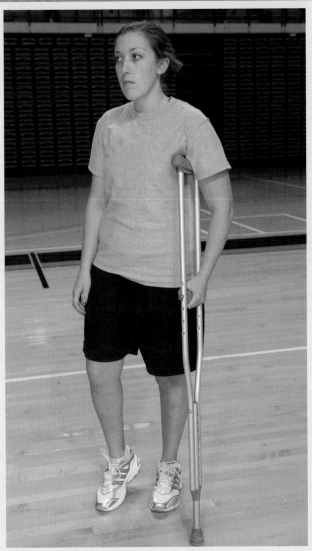

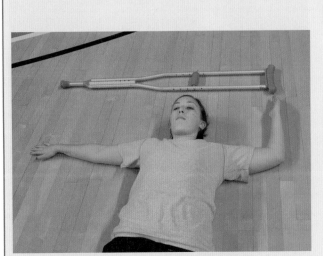

FIGURE 6.57

FIGURE 6.58

Cane Procedures

1. With the athlete standing or lying on his or her back, locate the **greater trochanter.**

2. Measure the distance from the ground to the superior aspect of the greater trochanter.

3. Select a cane that closely fits this measurement.

Crutch or Cane Ambulation

After fitting the injured athlete to the appropriate crutch or cane, the final step is to provide instruction in how to walk properly to limit further damage. There are two common methods for crutch ambulation—the tripod method and four-point method—and one common cane walking method.

SKILL 6.21

Tripod Method

1. After properly fitting the crutch, have the athlete stand with the crutches, placing his or her weight on the unaffected leg or, if both legs are injured, placing partial weight on both legs while using the crutches for support (Fig. 6.59).
2. Place the crutches about 12 to 18 in. in front of the body, slightly beside the center line of the feet (Fig. 6.59).
3. Have the athlete lean forward, moving the body with support of the arms between the crutches and placing the feet slightly in front of the tips of the crutches.
4. The athlete then swings the crutches about 12 to 18 in. in front of the center line of the feet and repeats the steps (Fig. 6.60).

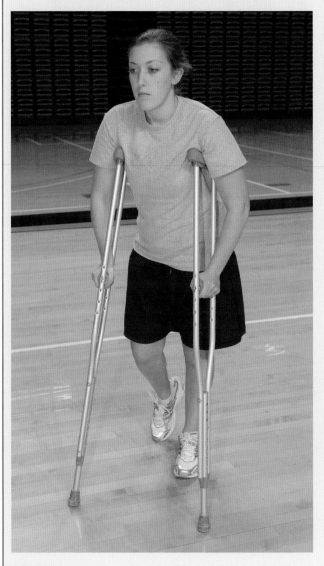

FIGURE 6.59

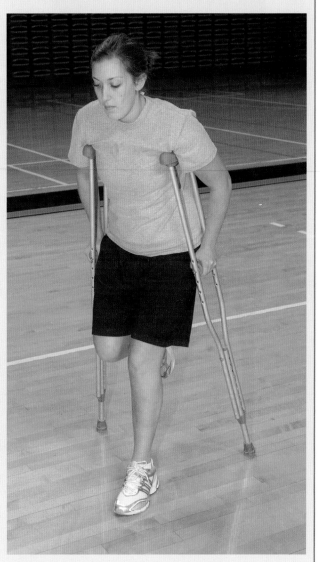

FIGURE 6.60

SKILL 6.22

Four-Point Method (Fig. 6.61)

1. Have the athlete stand on both feet, with weight supported on the crutches.
2. Begin by having the athlete move one crutch forward.
3. Have the athlete move the opposite foot forward.
4. Next, move the crutch that is on the same side as the forward foot slightly in front on the foot.
5. Have the athlete move the opposite foot forward, followed by the crutch.
6. Repeat.

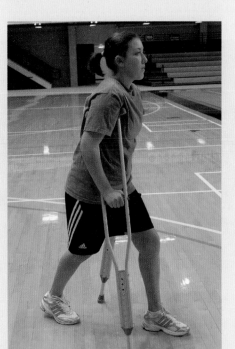

FIGURE 6.61A

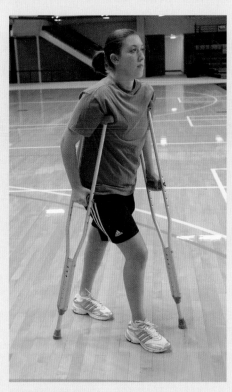

FIGURE 6.61B

SKILL 6.23

Moving Up Stairs

1. The athlete stands just below the first step with his or her weight on the crutches and the unaffected leg (Fig. 6.62).

2. The athlete places the uninjured leg on the first step (Fig. 6.63).
3. The athlete places his or her weight on the crutches.

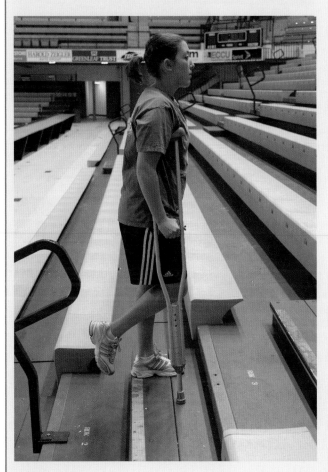

FIGURE 6.62

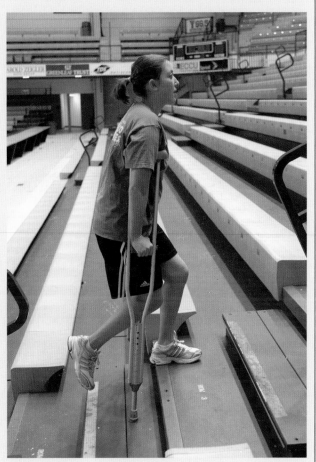

FIGURE 6.63

(Continued)

SKILL 6.23 *(Continued)*

Moving Up Stairs *(Continued)*

4. The athlete moves the injured leg and crutches onto the same step (Fig. 6.64).
5. Repeat.

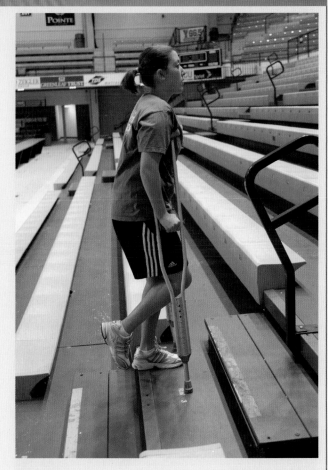

FIGURE 6.64

SKILL 6.24

Moving Down Stairs

1. The athlete stands at the top of the set of stairs (Fig. 6.65).

2. The athlete places his or her injured leg and both crutches on the first step (Fig. 6.66).

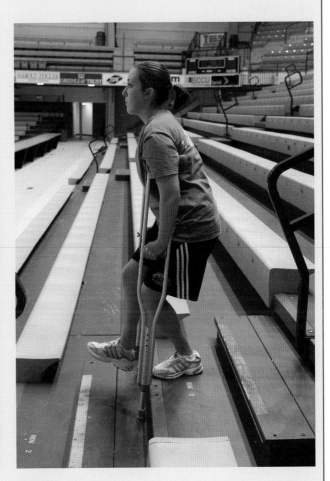

FIGURE 6.65   **FIGURE 6.66**

(Continued)

SKILL 6.24 *(Continued)*

Moving Down Stairs (Continued)

3. The athlete moves the uninjured leg down to same step (Fig. 6.67).

4. Repeat.

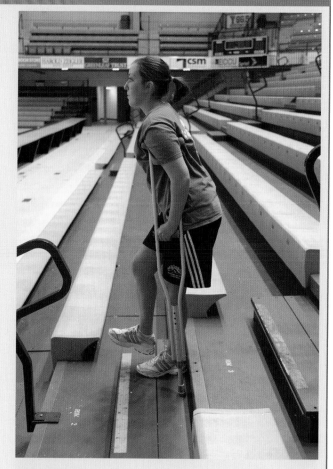

FIGURE 6.67

SKILL 6.25

Cane Walking (Fig. 6.68)

1. After proper measurement, place the cane at the side of the athlete's uninjured lower extremity.
2. To move, simultaneously move the cane and the athlete's injured leg forward.
3. Move the athlete's uninjured leg forward the same distance as the injured leg and cane.
4. Repeat.

This method can also be used with a single crutch.

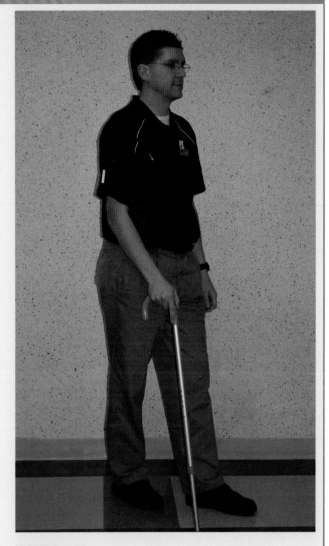

FIGURE 6.68

WATER RESCUES

Athletic trainers work with a variety of individuals and sports. One particular area that often goes unrecognized is the aquatic environment. Special considerations apply in emergency rescues for athletes participating in water sports. In this setting, mobilization and stabilization of an injured athlete is difficult. The athletic trainer must know the proper mechanics of aquatic rescue techniques to safely move an athlete out of a water environment when necessary, although a certified lifeguard is usually present during aquatic events. In many instances, lifeguards—excluding professional lifeguards working at beaches, water parks, or similar venues—have limited experience and skills. It may be more pertinent have an athletic trainer take charge of a spinal injury at a high school swimming and diving event than a certified teenaged lifeguard. In this section, we concentrate on techniques for moving and transporting a person from the water environment.

SKILL 6.26

Two-Person Front-and-Back Carry

The front-and-back carry is very similar to the two-person extremity lift.[2] However, this technique is used when removing the athlete from a body of water out of which the athletic trainers can walk. It should not be used when trying to pull an athlete out of the pool. It is used for an unconscious or unresponsive athlete with no suspected spinal injury or for an injured athlete who is having trouble getting out of the water without help. Special care should be taken when removing a large athlete, and attention should be given to the surface at the edge of the pool or the type of ground. Proper lifting mechanics are also important to decrease the chance of injury to the athletic trainers.

1. One athletic trainer is positioned at the head/shoulder region of the athlete and the other at the athlete's legs (Fig. 6.69).
2. The athletic trainer at the head reaches under the athlete's axilla and uses his or her right hand to grab the right wrist of the athlete. The same maneuver is performed on the athlete's opposite wrist (Fig. 6.69).
3. The athletic trainer then pulls both of the athlete's wrists/arms up and across the athlete's chest (Fig. 6.69).
4. The athletic trainer at the athlete's legs moves between his or her legs and faces in the same direction as the athletic trainers at the head. The athletic trainer, bending down, reaches around the outside of the athlete's legs and grabs under the popliteal fossa, hooking both hands in the popliteal fossa region (Fig. 6.70).

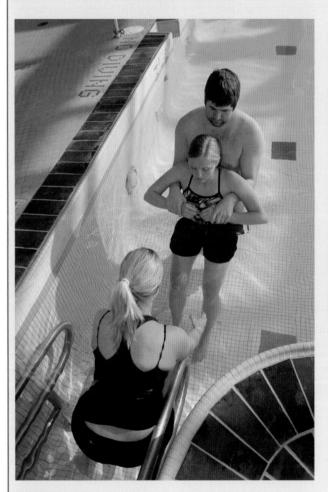

FIGURE 6.69

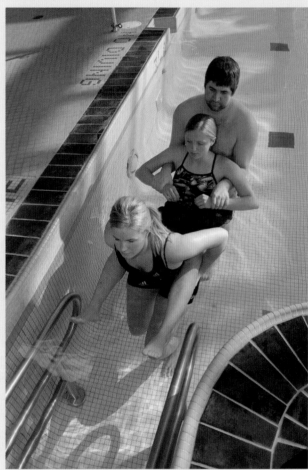

FIGURE 6.70

SKILL 6.26 *(Continued)*

Two-Person Front-and-Back Carry *(Continued)*

5. Once the athlete is secure, both athletic trainers lift the athlete up simultaneously and walk forward out of the water (Fig. 6.71).

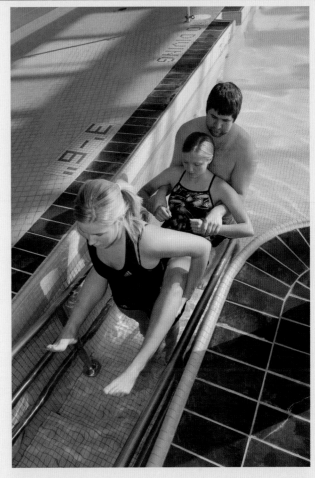

FIGURE 6.71

Anytime you suspect that a diving accident may involve a spinal injury or if you are dealing with an unconscious victim, proceed as though a spinal injury had occurred. Because of the water environment, stabilization is difficult, so you must stabilize the head and neck as best as you can. It is recommended by the American Red Cross[3] not to remove an injured athlete or one who may have a spinal injury from the water unless he or she has been properly secured to a backboard or other rigid support. Stabilizing the head/neck is recommended first; this is done by applying a head splint or cervical collar before placing the injured athlete on a backboard.

SKILL 6.27

Head Splint Technique[3]

1. If the athlete is prone, move the arms against the head.
2. Grab the athlete between the shoulder and elbow region. Note that the athletic trainer's left arm should grab the athlete's right arm and the athletic trainer's right arm should grab the athlete's left arm (Fig. 6.72).
3. Pull the athlete forward while holding onto the arms and, pressing the athlete's arms against his or her head, rotate the athlete onto his or her back (Fig. 6.73).
4. If the athlete is already in a supine position, grab each arm between the elbow and shoulder and bring them together over the athlete's head, squeezing the athlete's head between the arms (Fig. 6.74).
5. Move to the shallow part of the water if possible.

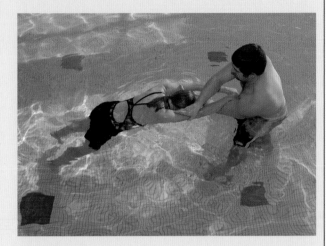

FIGURE 6.72

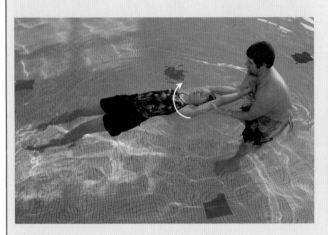

FIGURE 6.73

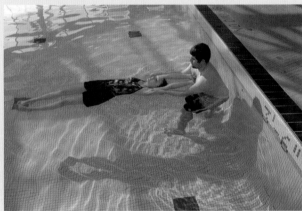

FIGURE 6.74

SKILL 6.28

Two-Person Backboard Removal from Water[2]

The two-person backboard removal technique is not intended for athletes who have suspected spinal injuries; rather, it is a means of helping to remove an athlete who cannot be walked out of a water environment or who has an injury that requires stabilization before removal from the water.

1. The first athletic trainer brings the athlete to the pool wall (Fig. 6.75).
2. A second athletic trainer will have a backboard with the straps removed at the wall (Fig. 6.75).
3. The second athletic trainer, with crossed hands, grabs the athlete's wrists and pulls the athlete slightly up out of the water (Fig. 6.75).
4. The primary athletic trainer then grabs the backboard and places it foot end down into the water next to the athlete (Fig. 6.76).
5. The second athletic trainer then rotates the athlete slowly 180 degrees onto the backboard (Fig. 6.76).
6. As the athlete is being rotated, the primary athletic trainer places the backboard between the athlete and the wall (Fig. 6.76).
7. The primary athletic trainer then exits the water and, standing side by side, the athletic trainers grab the athlete's closest wrist and the top of the backboard. If necessary, the athletic trainers can keep the backboard in place by using their legs (Fig. 6.77).
8. Simultaneously, both athletic trainers pull both the backboard and the athlete up and onto the pool deck or ground (Fig. 6.77).

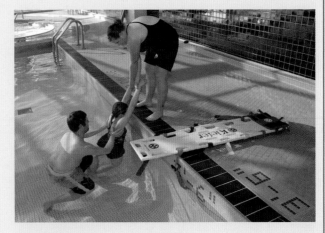

FIGURE 6.75

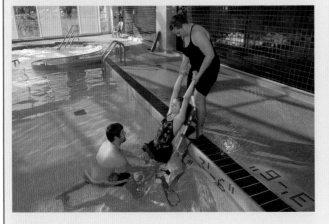

FIGURE 6.76

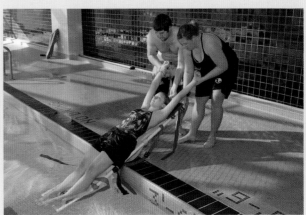

FIGURE 6.77

When an athlete sustains an injury to the spine or has a suspected spinal injury, removal from the pool with spinal stabilization is necessary. Backboarding an injured athlete in the water is extremely difficult and requires more than one athletic trainer. Practicing this technique is crucial to limiting spinal movement and building the athletic trainers' confidence. In describing this technique, we assume all of the injured athlete's major vital signs are intact.

SKILL 6.29

Backboarding an Injured Athlete

1. If athlete is prone, splint his or her head and neck, using the head splint technique, or gently rotate the athlete onto his or her back and continue stabilizing head and checking airway, breathing, and circulation (the ABCs).
2. If the athlete is in the supine position, use a head and chin support (Fig. 6.78).
   a. Place one forearm along the length of the athlete's spine, with one of your hands at the back of the lower head.

   b. Place the other forearm along the length of the breastbone, with one hand supporting the chin.
   c. Squeeze your arms together slightly.
3. Have another athletic trainer place a backboard underneath the athlete, starting at the athlete's legs and pulling it up and under the athlete lengthwise, to extend slightly past the athlete's head (Fig. 6.79).
4. Place the athlete's arms down to the sides and use the head splint technique.

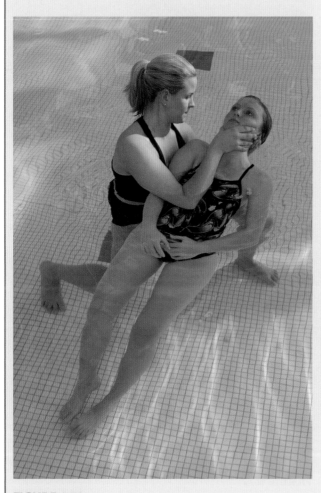

FIGURE 6.78

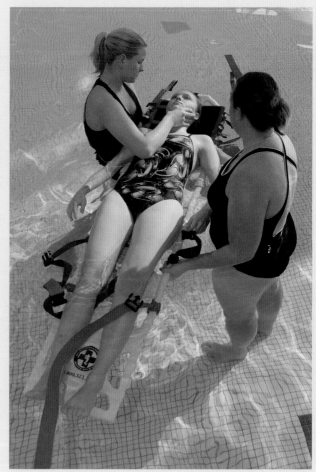

FIGURE 6.79

SKILL 6.29 *(Continued)*

Backboarding an Injured Athlete *(Continued)*

5. After the athlete's arms are at the sides, an athletic trainer places a rescue tube (flotation device) under the backboard at the athletes head/shoulder region, then grabs the head and stabilizes it so that the first athletic trainer can let go (Fig. 6.80).

6. The second athletic trainer or another athletic trainer then secures the athlete to the backboard with straps at the chest, waist, legs, and ankles.

7. Apply a head/neck support device (cervical collar).

8. Float the athlete to the side of the pool or edge of the water. The head of the backboard should be placed against the wall (Fig. 6.81).

9. Two or more athletic trainers pick up the athlete at the head of the backboard and pull the athlete up out of the water to the edge of the deck. If there are no extra athletic trainers, after placing the victim on the side of the deck, one athletic trainer exits the water and grabs the backboard at the head and pulls back. After the athlete is partially out of the water, the second athletic trainer exits the water and helps to pull the athlete the rest of the way onto the pool deck or ground (Fig. 6.82).

10. Once on land, two to four athletic trainers lift the athlete and transport him or her to appropriate medical facilities.

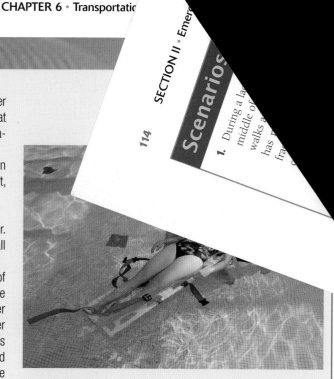

FIGURE 6.80

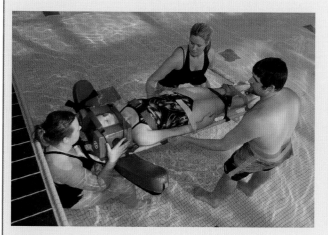

FIGURE 6.81

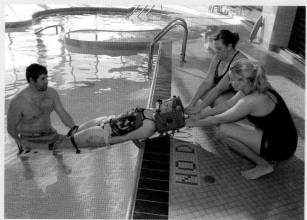

FIGURE 6.82

SECTION II • Emer

Scenarios

114

1. During a la
middle o
walks a
has
fra

...rosse game, you see two players collide in the ...the field. As you approach the scene, one player ...way slowly and seems to be shaken but apparently ...o serious injury. The other player obviously has a ...tured tibia. You splint and immobilize the fracture according to accepted standard practices. It is now time to transport the athlete off the field to meet an ambulance on the other side of the stadium.

Which transportation methods would be best suited for the athlete in this situation?

2. You are working as an athletic trainer during a cross-country meet. You are stationed in a heavily wooded area on a narrow trail. As the runners go by, they must transverse various obstacles on the trail. One runner falls, injuring her ankle. It is apparent that she cannot continue, and since you have limited supplies to effectively treat and manage the condi-tion, you decide that she must be transported to another location.

Which transportation method would be recommended to transport the athlete?

3. During a swimming event, a diver hits her head on the springboard and falls into the water. You dive in and pull her to the surface. She begins to breathe but you suspect a head or cervical neck injury.

Explain steps involved in placing a head splint before backboarding.

4. An athlete has recently been fitted with crutches at the sports medicine clinic. This is the athlete's first time on crutches.

Explain how the athlete would ambulate using the four-point walking method.

WRAP-UP

In this chapter, various lifts and moves were discussed, with step-by-step instructions to help ambulate or transport an injured athlete for proper follow-up or medical refer-ral. Many of these techniques are used only in unusual or extreme circumstances, but proper knowledge about them and proficiency in their use during emergency situations may be required at some time during the career of the athletic trainer. Although not all-inclusive, the techniques presented in this chapter should help the athletic trainer to develop a solid foundation in transportation techniques and can serve as a stepping stone to other techniques re-quired by athletic trainers or other medical personnel in emergency situations.

REFERENCES

1. Hafen BQ, Karren KJ, Frandsen KJ. *First Aid for Colleges and Universities,* 7th ed. Needhan Heights, MA: Allyn & Bacon; 1998.
2. Fundamentals of Emergency Care. In C. Richard Bebe and Deborah Funk, eds. *Lifting and Moving Patients.* Albany, NY: Delmar Thompson Learning; 2001.
3. American National Red Cross. *ARC Lifeguarding Manual,* 3rd ed. Yardley, PA: Banta Book Group; 2007.

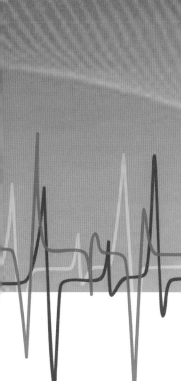

C H A P T E R · 7

Blood-Borne Pathogens

CHAPTER OUTCOMES

1. Define and describe blood-borne pathogens.
2. Describe what constitutes "other potentially infectious materials."
3. Explain how to minimize the risk of infection, such as hepatitis B and C and human immunodeficiency virus, associated with exposure to blood-borne pathogens.
4. Identify the signs and symptoms of infection due to common blood-borne pathogens.
5. Describe the ways in which an athletic trainer may be exposed to blood-borne pathogens and other infectious materials.
6. Develop an exposure control plan to be used in the athletic training setting.
7. Identify and describe universal precautions and body substance isolation procedures to limit exposure to blood-borne pathogens.
8. Describe the procedures or techniques required to minimize exposure to blood-borne pathogens in the athletic setting.
9. Describe personal protective equipment that can be used to limit exposure to blood-borne pathogens in the athletic setting.
10. Identify techniques of personal hygiene, specifically washing of hands, to limit exposure to blood-borne pathogens.
11. Identify and describe how to disinfect and decontaminant workplace environments to limit exposure to blood-borne pathogens.
12. Be able to describe and carry out the requirements for reporting an exposure to blood-borne pathogens.

NOMENCLATURE

Cirrhosis: scarring of the liver

Emesis: vomiting

Hepatitis B: a contagious liver disease caused by the hepatitis B virus (HBV)

Hepatitis C: a contagious liver disease caused by the hepatitis C virus (HCV)

Hepatocellular carcinoma: a carcinoma derived from parenchymal cells of the liver

Human immunodeficiency virus (HIV): a retrovirus that is the etiologic agent of acquired immunodeficiency syndrome (AIDS)

Microorganisms: organisms of microscopic or submicroscopic size

NOMENCLATURE *(Continued)*

Other potentially infectious materials (OPIMs): other bodily fluids or tissues that have been infected with pathogens, including (a) semen, vaginal secretions, cerebrospinal fluid, synovial fluid, pleural fluid, pericardial fluid, peritoneal fluid, amniotic fluid, saliva in dental procedures, any bodily fluid that is visibly contaminated with blood, and all bodily fluids in situations where it is difficult or impossible to differentiate between body fluids; (b) any unfixed tissue or organ (other than intact skin)

from a human or animal body (living or dead); (c) HIV-containing cell or tissue cultures, organ cultures, and HIV- or HBV-containing culture medium or other solutions; and (d) blood, organs, or other tissues from experimental animals infected with HIV or HBV

Parenteral: a route of administration that involves piercing the skin, such as an injection

Sputum: expectorated matter

BEFORE YOU BEGIN

1. What are examples of blood-borne pathogens?
2. What is hepatitis B and how is it contracted?
3. What are some examples of universal precautions?
4. What is the basic personal protective equipment needed to limit exposure to blood-borne pathogens?
5. How do you keep a work site clean and disinfected to limit risk of exposure to blood-borne pathogens?

Voices from the Field

The Certified Athletic Trainer (ATC) frequently encounters injuries and ailments with distinguishable signs and symptoms; based on those signs and symptoms, he or she determines the actions to be taken. However, the hazards of disease transmission through blood-borne pathogen contact are not always so easily recognizable. This should not negate or diminish the importance of taking precaution against exposure when providing care for an injured athlete.

It is imperative to the health and safety of both the ATC and the patient that the care giver take the "If I can't see it, it *can* hurt me" approach to applying universal precautions in any setting where care may be provided. It should be the responsibility of

the ATC, as the health care professional, to be both educated and prepared when dealing with blood-borne pathogen transmission. This awareness will not only protect you as the health care provider, but will also protect and reassure the patient. After all, the quality of care you provide is directly affected by the quality of your own health.

Heather Sjoquist MS, ATC, CSCS
Clinical Coordinator
Undergraduate Athletic Training Program
Western Michigan University
Kalamazoo, Michigan

Protecting athletic trainers against the health risks associated with exposure to blood and **other potentially infectious materials** (OPIMs) is the responsibility of the U.S. Department of Labor, specifically the Occupational Safety and Health Administration (OSHA). In 1992, OSHA enacted specific regulations to protect all workers at risk, not just athletic trainers, from potential exposure to blood-borne pathogens. Revised in 2001 to address the Needlestick Safety and Prevention Act,[1] these regulations outlined in the standards (29 Code of Federal Regulations [CFR] part 1910.1030) must be implemented by employers whose workers have been identified as facing a risk of occupational exposure to blood or OPIMs. An occupational exposure is defined as "reasonably anticipated skin, eye, mucous membrane, or **parenteral** contact with blood or OPIM that may result from the performance

of the employee's duties."[2] Standard 29 CFR 1910.1030 identifies how employers can minimize or eliminate occupational exposure through the use of (1) personal hygiene, (2) personal protective equipment (PPE), (3) engineering and work practice controls, and (4) training.[2]

BLOOD-BORNE PATHOGENS AND OPIMs

OSHA defines blood-borne pathogens as follows: any "pathogenic **microorganisms** that are present in human blood and can cause disease in humans. These pathogens include, but are not limited to, hepatitis B virus (HBV) and human immunodeficiency virus (HIV)."[2] Exposure to

Breakout

The following are the three categories of OPIMs as outlined by OSHA[2] (29 CFR 1910.1030[b]). As athletic trainers, we are greatest risk from the first category.

1. "The following human body fluids: semen, vaginal secretions, cerebrospinal fluid, synovial fluid, pleural fluid, pericardial fluid, peritoneal fluid, amniotic fluid, saliva in dental procedures, any body fluid that is visibly contaminated with blood, and all body fluids in situations where it is difficult or impossible to differentiate between body fluids";
2. "Any unfixed tissue or organ (other than intact skin) from a human (living or dead)"; and "HIV-containing cell or tissue cultures and organ cultures."
3. "HIV- or HBV-containing culture medium or other solutions; and blood, organs, or other tissues from experimental animals infected with HIV or HBV."

blood includes human blood, human blood components, and products made from human blood.[3] OPIMs include other bodily fluids or tissues that have been infected with pathogens, such as HBV and HIV.

Hepatitis B Virus

Hepatitis B is a contagious liver disease caused by the hepatitis B virus (HBV).[4] Acute hepatitis B can last several

weeks and occurs within the first 6 months after exposure to the virus. Chronic hepatitis B is a serious, possibly lifelong chronic condition that can result in long-term liver disease, liver cancer, and even death[4] (Fig. 7.1). Hepatitis B is transmitted through direct or indirect contact with infected blood and OPIMs.

Once infected, a person with acute hepatitis B may present with a variety of signs and symptoms, normally within 90 days after exposure. However, signs and symptoms can appear at any time between 6 weeks and 6 months after exposure.[4] Unlike other forms of hepatitis, hepatitis B can be prevented by a hepatitis B vaccine. As part of an employer's exposure-control plan, all employees with an occupational risk as defined by OSHA should be given "information on the hepatitis B vaccine, including information on its efficacy, safety, method of administration, the benefits of being vaccinated, and that the vaccine and vaccination will be offered free of charge."[2] The free vaccination must be provided at a reasonable time and place within 10 working days of initial assignment unless the employee offers proof of the vaccination or antibody testing reveals immunity. If an employee declines the vaccination, he or she must sign a declination form; however, the employee retains the right to accept the vaccination at a later date.[2]

Hepatitis C Virus

Hepatitis C, like hepatitis B, is a contagious liver disease caused by the hepatitis C virus (HCV).[5] Hepatitis C is the most common chronic blood-borne disease in the United States, with approximately 3.2 million individuals

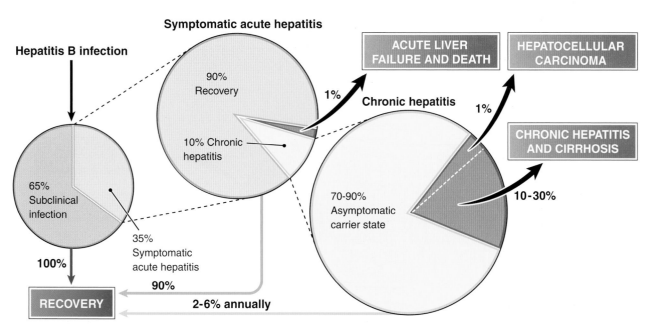

FIGURE 7.1 Outcomes of hepatitis B infection. (From McConnell TH. *The Nature Of Disease: Pathology for the Health Professions.* Philadelphia: Lippincott Williams & Wilkins; 2007.)

Signs & Symptoms

Common Blood-Borne Pathogens[4-6]

Hepatitis B

- Fatigue
- Loss of appetite
- Nausea
- Vomiting
- Abdominal pain
- Dark urine
- Clay-colored bowel movements
- Joint pain
- Jaundice (yellow color in the skin or the eyes)

Hepatitis C

- Fever
- Fatigue
- Dark urine
- Clay-colored stool
- Abdominal pain
- Loss of appetite
- Nausea

- Vomiting
- Joint pain
- Jaundice

Human Immunodeficiency Virus

The following are warning signs of advanced HIV infection:

- Rapid weight loss
- Dry cough
- Recurring fever or profuse night sweats
- Profound and unexplained fatigue
- Swollen lymph glands in the armpits, groin, or neck
- Diarrhea that lasts for more than a week
- White spots or unusual blemishes on the tongue, in the mouth, or in the throat
- Pneumonia
- Red, brown, pink, or purplish blotches on or under the skin or inside the mouth, nose, or eyelids
- Memory loss, depression, and other neurological disorders

chronically infected,[5] mostly likely as a result of the lack of a vaccine for HCV (Fig. 7.2). Individuals contracting hepatitis C are at risk for developing chronic HCV infection (75 to 85 individuals out of every 100), chronic liver disease (60 to 70 individuals out of every 100), **cirrhosis** (5 to 20 individuals out of every 100), liver cancer, or of dying (1 to 5 individuals out of every 100 die from liver cancer or cirrhosis).[5] HCV is transmitted through large or repeated percutaneous (through the skin) exposures to infected blood. In the health care setting, the greatest risk of HCV transmission is through needlesticks. Signs and symptoms of HCV are listed above.

Human Immunodeficiency Virus

The **human immunodeficiency virus (HIV)** is the virus responsible for causing acquired immunodeficiency syndrome (AIDS). Unlike other viruses, HIV attacks the immune system and destroys the white blood cells (T cells or CD4 cells) responsible for fighting infections. AIDS is the final stage of an HIV infection. Because of a weakened or depleted immune system, an infected individual is no longer to able to fight infections or other diseases. A person is said to have AIDS when he or she has one or more specific infections, certain cancers, or a very low T-cell count.[6]

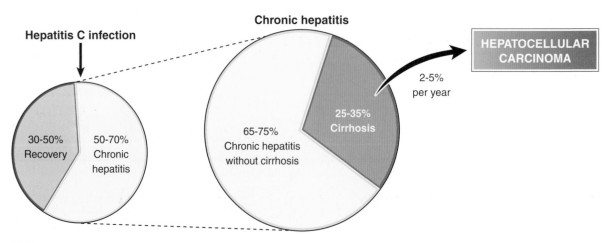

FIGURE 7.2 Out comes of hepatitis C infection. (From McConnell TH. *The Nature Of Disease: Pathology for the Health Professions.* Philadelphia: Lippincott Williams & Wilkins; 2007.)

Current Research

Risk of Exposure to HIV Infection as a Result of Occupational Exposure[3]

According to the Centers for Disease Control and Prevention (CDC), the risk of occupational exposure to HIV infections appears to be low. They report that

1. "The average risk of HIV infection after a needlestick or cut exposure to HIV-infected blood is 0.3% (i.e., three tenths of one percent, or about 1 in 300). Stated another way, 99.7% of needlestick/cut exposures do not lead to infection."
2. "The risk after exposure of the eye, nose, or mouth to HIV-infected blood is estimated to be, on average, 0.1% (1 in 1,000)," which is less than the average risk of needlestick or cut exposure."
3. "The risk after exposure of non-intact skin to HIV-infected blood is estimated to be less than 0.1%. A small amount of blood on intact skin probably poses no risk at all. There have been no documented cases of HIV transmission due to an exposure involving a small amount of blood on intact skin (a few drops of blood on skin for a short period of time)."

Identifying HIV, unlike hepatitis B or C, through signs and symptoms alone is difficult because it may take many years for the symptoms to manifest themselves. The only way to confirm the presence of HIV is to be tested for it.[6] According to the CDC, "one quarter of the HIV-infected persons in the United States do not know that they are infected." Many of these people may look and feel healthy, but they are still infected.[6]

Compared with HBV, which can survive outside the body for at least 7 days and still can be capable of causing a hepatitis B infection,[4] HIV is very fragile and cannot live for long outside the body.[6] Therefore, HIV is not transmitted via normal day-to-day activities (e.g., shaking hands, using a toilet seat, casual kissing). Found in blood and OPIMs, HIV is transmitted in several ways.[6] Although the risk of acquiring HIV in the health care setting is very small, one may become exposed to it in the following ways:

1. Sexual intercourse (anal, vaginal, or oral) with someone infected with HIV
2. Sharing needles and syringes with someone infected with HIV or through needlesticks in the health care setting (in the course of treating someone infected with HIV)
3. Being exposed (fetus or infant) to HIV before or during birth or through breast feeding
4. Exposure to infected blood

OCCUPATIONAL EXPOSURE TO BLOOD-BORNE PATHOGENS AND OTHER INFECTIOUS MATERIALS

For a blood-borne pathogen to infect an athletic trainer, the pathogenic agent must enter the host through one of four routes (Table 7.1):

1. Direct contact
2. Indirect contact
3. Vector-borne
4. Airborne

In the health care setting, including athletic training, direct and indirect contact are the two most common methods of disease transmission. These contacts include exposures through inadequate or inappropriate use of PPE (e.g., gloves) (Fig. 7.3) and from needlesticks or cuts from other sharp instruments (e.g., scalpels and razors).[3] However, the extent of the occupational exposure and risk of infection may vary and requires the following criteria be present[3,7]:

1. The pathogen involved (e.g., HBV, HIV)
2. The type of exposure (i.e., direct vs. indirect)/entry site
3. The amount of blood involved in the exposure (i.e., an adequate amount of pathogen must be present)
4. Susceptibility of a person to the pathogen

TABLE 7.1   Transmission of Blood-Borne Pathogens[3,7]

Method of Entry	Definition	Example
Direct	Infected blood or body fluids from one person enters another person's body at an entry site (skin, eye, mucous membrane, or parenteral).	An athlete is struck in the nose with a ball, there is no blood on the initial contact; however, as the athletic trainer is evaluating the nose, it begins to bleed, and the athletic trainer comes in contact with the blood.
Indirect	Individual touches an object that contains blood or bodily fluid from an infected person.	Soiled dressing and bandages, contaminated work surface and instruments.
Airborne	Individual inhales infected droplets that have become airborne.	Exposure to bacteria or virus through coughing and sneezing.
Vector	Infection transmitted by animals.	Exposure to infected animals such as dogs, raccoons, insects, and bats.

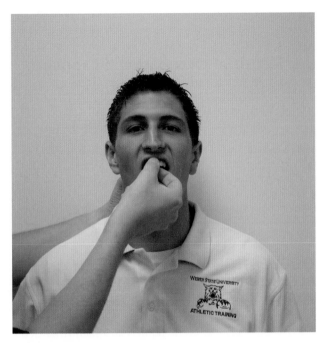

FIGURE 7.3 Exposure to blood-borne pathogens via direct exposure. Note the lack of use of personal protective equipment.

EXPOSURE CONTROL PLAN (ECP)

According to Standard 29 CFR 1910.1030(c)(1)(i), each employer having an employee(s) with occupational exposure "shall establish a written Exposure Control Plan designed to eliminate or minimize employee exposure."[2] This plan is, therefore, designed to limit occupational exposure to blood-borne pathogens and OPIMs by outlining the measures to be taken by the employer and employee to eliminate and/or minimize any chance of accidental exposure. An ECP must contain the following:

1. Exposure determination (identification of who is at risk based on job classification where exposure to blood or OPIMs occurs without regard to the use of PPE)
2. Schedule and methods of implementation of OSHA Standard 29 CFR 1910.1030
3. Procedure for the evaluation of circumstances surrounding exposure incidents as required by OSHA Standard 29 CFR 1910.1030 and recordkeeping

The employer is also responsible for ensuring that a copy of the ECP is accessible to employees at all times and that the ECP is "reviewed and updated at least annually and whenever necessary to reflect new or modified tasks and procedures which affect occupational exposure and to reflect new or revised employee positions with occupational exposure."[2] Finally, any employer with an established ECP is required to solicit input from any nonmanagerial employee who is at risk for occupational exposure and who provides direct patient care related to "the identification, evaluation, and selection of effective engineering and work practice controls."[2]

Methods of Compliance with OSHA Standards

OSHA standards identify several methods of compliance (as outlined in an ECP), including the use of universal precautions (UPs), which employers and employees must follow to eliminate and/or minimize any chance of accidental occupational exposure. These methods of compliance include (a) engineering and work practice controls, (b) PPE, and (c) equipment cleaning and disinfecting. Personal hygiene, while not specifically identified in the OSHA standard, is a component of UPs and body substance isolation (BSI); it is discussed below.

Universal Precautions and Body Substance Isolation

"Universal precautions shall be observed to prevent contact with blood or other potentially infectious materials."[2] Under this policy, all blood and certain body fluids (those identified as OPIMs) of all patients are considered potentially infectious for HIV, HBV, and other blood-borne pathogens[8] and now require the use of practice controls (i.e., gloves, gowns, aprons, masks, or protective eyewear) (Fig. 7.4) and

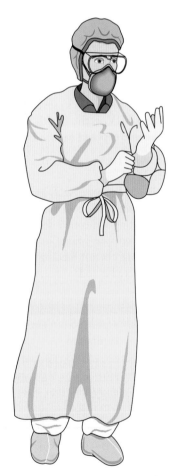

FIGURE 7.4 Man wearing body substance isolation (BSI) equipment. (LifeART image copyright ©2010 Lippincott Williams & Wilkins. All rights reserved.)

precautions to prevent injuries caused by needles, scalpels, and other sharp instruments. UPs do not cover or apply to items such as feces, nasal secretions, **sputum,** sweat, tears, urine, **emesis,** and saliva unless they contain visible blood.[8] BSI precautions take UPs one step further and suggest that precautions be taken for *all* moist body substances for all patients, regardless of their presumed infection status.[9] The of use of BSI has demonstrated a decrease in the transmission of secretions colonized with organisms (often resistant organisms),[10] thereby preventing the spread of infections.

Engineering and Work Practice Controls

Engineering and work practice controls are procedures/techniques used to eliminate or minimize employee (in the case of athletic training and athlete exposure as well) work site exposure to blood and OPIMs. Engineering practice controls are the use of medical devices designed to isolate or remove the risk of exposure to blood or OPIM hazards.[7,11] It includes the used of sharps disposal containers (Fig. 7.5), biohazard bags, otoscope speculums, thermometer covers,

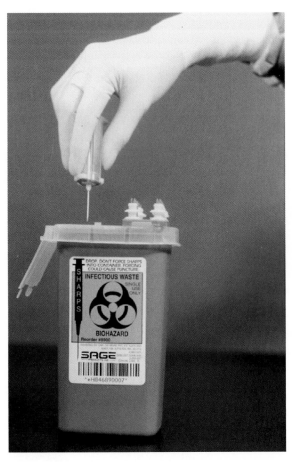

FIGURE 7.5 A type of sharps container. (McCall RE, Tankersley CM. *Phlebotomy Essentials,* 2nd ed. Philadelphia: Lippincott Williams & Wilkins; 1998. Courtesy of Sage Products, Inc., Crystal Lake, IL.)

self-sheathing needles, needleless systems, and PPE. Work practice controls are the behaviors performed by an athletic trainer (and athletes) to reduce the risk of exposure to blood or OPIM hazards.[7,11] Engineering and work practice controls should be examined, modified, and maintained on at least a yearly basis to ensure their effectiveness and a safe facility.

Breakout

The following are examples of work practice controls to reduce the risk of exposure to blood-borne pathogens or OPIMs in the health care setting[2,7,11]:

1. Proper and timely (immediately after removing gloves or PPE) hand washing using soap and water at a sink designated as utility or cleaning sink (i.e., do not use the same sink or hose used for filling water coolers). When a hand-washing facility is not available, the employer shall provide either an appropriate antiseptic hand cleanser in conjunction with clean cloth/paper towels or antiseptic towelettes.

2. Minimizing splashing and spraying of blood or bodily fluid while providing care and during equipment cleaning and disinfecting.

3. Proper cleaning and disinfecting of equipment (e.g., therapeutic rehabilitation and modality) and supplies (e.g., scissors, tweezers) following manufacturer's recommendations immediately after being soiled.

4. Proper disposal of all used supplies and equipment in properly labeled biohazard or sharps containers at the point of contact (i.e., bring the containers to the blood and bodily fluid rather than carrying the waste to the container in a different location). Contaminated needles and other contaminated sharps will not be bent, recapped, or removed. Do not overfill a sharps container.

5. Keep all food and drink away from areas where blood or bodily fluids may be present. This should apply to not only staff but to athletes as well.

6. No eating or drinking in areas where there is a risk of contamination.

7. Food and drink shall not be kept in refrigerators, freezers, shelves, cabinets, or on countertops or bench tops where blood, OPIMs, or urine may be stored.

8. Urine used for drug testing should be in a container that prevents leakage during collection, handling, processing, storage, transport, or shipping.

9. No smoking in areas where there is a risk of contamination.

10. Do not apply cosmetics, lip balm, or handle contact lenses in areas where there is a risk of contamination.

11. Do not touch or rub any mucous membranes (mouth, nose, eyes) while there is a risk of contamination.

12. Remove any nose, ear, and/or body piercings.

13. Do not reuse or allow sharing of items such as water bottles, mouth guards, towels, or self-adhesive electrodes where there is risk of contamination.

Personal Protective Equipment

According to the OSHA standards, "when there is occupational exposure, the employer shall provide, at no cost to the employee, appropriate personal protective equipment such as, but not limited to, gloves, gowns, laboratory coats, face shields or masks and eye protection, and mouthpieces, resuscitation bags, pocket masks, or other ventilation devices."[2] This PPE is considered "appropriate" according to the standard if it does not "permit blood or other potentially infectious materials to pass through to or reach the employee's work clothes, street clothes, undergarments, skin, eyes, mouth, or other mucous membranes under normal conditions of use and for the duration of time which the protective equipment will be used."[2] This means that items such as normal reading glasses and contact lenses are not considered PPE because protective goggles or glasses must have solid side shields. In athletic training, the most commonly used PPE would be gloves, breathing devices, and eyewear.

Gloves

Disposable gloves, made of either nitrile or vinyl (latex gloves may be utilized; however, some individuals are allergic or latex-sensitive so they are not recommended), are the first line of defense against blood and OPIMs. Gloves are required to be worn when dealing with any ill or injured athletes (particularly when there will be contact with blood, OPIMs,

mucous membranes, and nonintact skin) or when cleaning or handling any contaminated equipment or supplies.

Prior to donning gloves, be sure to cover any open wounds or sores and remove any jewelry that might pierce the gloves. After donning the gloves, inspect them for tears. If a glove tears or has been punctured while managing an athlete, it should be replaced as soon as feasible. As the name implies, disposable gloves are single-use medical devices and should not be washed or decontaminated for reuse (Skill 7.1).[2]

Barrier Devices

Barriers such as a resuscitation masks, face shields, and bag-valve-mask (Chapter 11) devices are designed to limit exposure to blood and blood-containing saliva, respiratory secretions, and vomitus. Devices such as resuscitation masks and face shields are further intended to be used by a single athletic trainer and should not be shared between athletic trainers. These devices are intended for one-time use on a specific athlete and should be properly disposed of once they have been utilized.

Personal Hygiene

Personal hygiene, including frequent simple hand washing, is believed to help in reducing the transmission of infectious pathogens[12,13] and health care–associated infections.[14] There are several ways of ensuring personal hand hygiene, including (a) handing washing, (b) antiseptic hand wash, (c) alcohol-based hand rub, and (d) surgical hand hygiene/antisepsis (Table 7.2).

SKILL 7.1

Removing Disposable Gloves

1. Pinch one glove at the wrist, being sure to touch only the glove's outer surface. If necessary, place any contaminated waste to be removed in the gloved hand (Fig. 7.6).

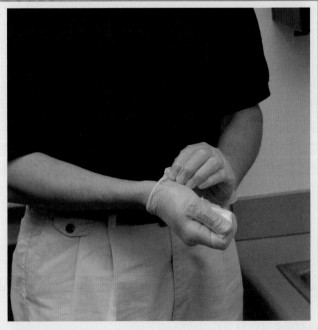

FIGURE 7.6

SKILL 7.1 *(Continued)*

Removing Disposable Gloves *(Continued)*

2. Grasp the clean inner surface of the other gloved hand, being careful to avoid touching any contaminated surfaces (Fig. 7.7).
3. Pull the glove toward the fingertips, completing removal so that it is inside out. Be sure to dispose of the used gloves in a biohazard container (Fig. 7.8).

4. Wash hands thoroughly (Skill 7.2).

Note: Extra disposable gloves should always be conveniently available and gloves should always be changed between patients.

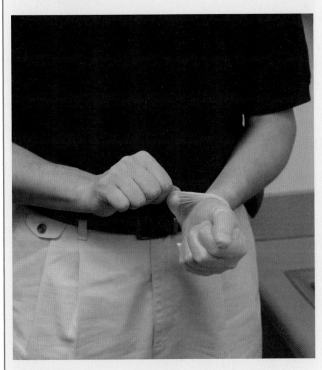

FIGURE 7.7

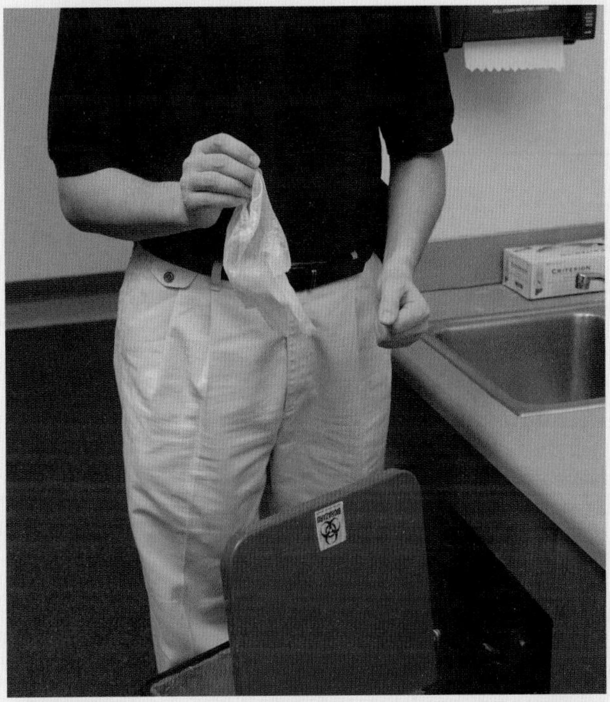

FIGURE 7.8

Hand washing, which is defined as washing hands with soap and water, is indicated before patient contact and donning gloves and after contact with any intact skin, contact with body fluids or excretions, nonintact skin or wound dressings, and removal of disposable gloves.[14]

Hand washing has also been recommended before and after using a rest room, using ordinary soap (i.e., non antimicrobial) and water or antimicrobial soap and water.[14] To wash hands properly, follow the skill steps outlined in Skill 7.2.

TABLE 7.2   CDC Definitions of Hand Hygiene*

Term	Definition
Hand washing	"... washing hands with plain soap and water. Hand washing with soap and water remains a sensible strategy for hand hygiene in non–health care settings and is recommended by CDC and other experts."
Antiseptic hand wash	"... washing hands with water and soap or other detergents containing an antiseptic agent."
Alcohol-based hand rub	"... alcohol-containing preparation applied to the hands to reduce the number of viable microorganisms."
Surgical hand hygiene/ antisepsis	"... antiseptic hand wash or antiseptic hand rub performed preoperatively by surgical personnel to eliminate transient and reduce resident hand flora. Antiseptic detergent preparations often have persistent antimicrobial activity."

*The Centers for Disease Control and Prevention in their *Guideline for Hand Hygiene in Health-Care Settings* have identified several different terms related to the proper management of hand hygiene. The term "hand hygiene" refers to the act of hand washing, antiseptic hand wash, alcohol-based hand rub, or surgical hand hygiene/antisepsis.[14]

SKILL 7.2

Hand Washing[14]

1. Remove all jewelry and wet hands with water (Fig. 7.9).
2. Apply the amount of soap recommended by the manufacturer. Rub hands together for at least 15 seconds, cleaning and covering all surfaces of the hands and fingers (Fig. 7.10).
3. Rinse hands thoroughly with water (Fig. 7.11).
4. Dry hands thoroughly with a disposable paper towel.
5. Turn off the water faucet using the disposable paper towel (Fig. 7.12).

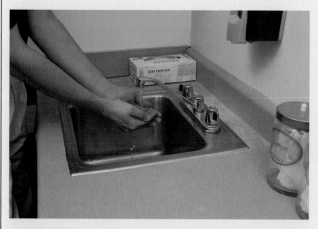

FIGURE 7.9

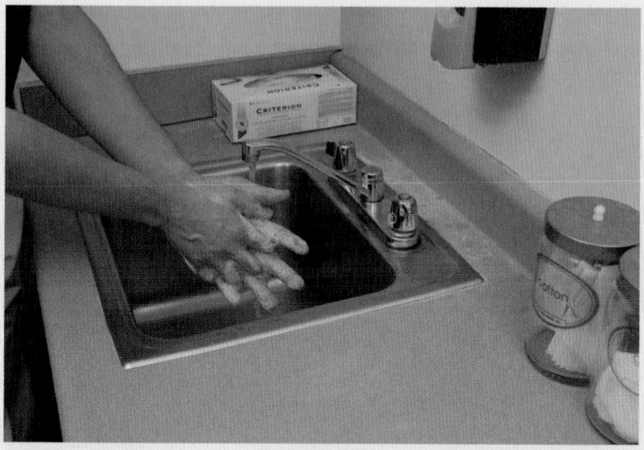

FIGURE 7.10

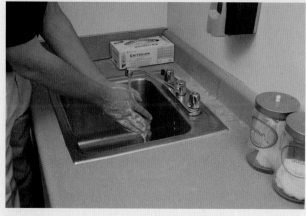

FIGURE 7.11

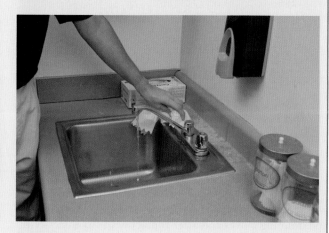

FIGURE 7.12

When soap and water are unavailable, the use of a waterless antiseptic hand cleaner (alcohol-based) is an appropriate method of hand hygiene, assuming that the hands are not visibly dirty.[14] In fact, in one study, the use of an alcohol-based hand rub was faster and more convenient; it improved the health care worker's hand hygiene compliance and microbial colonization did not change. The alcohol-based rub demonstrated increased efficacy in removing pathogens already present on the health care worker's hands.[15] Studies examining alcohol-based hand rubs have also demonstrated significantly less skin dryness and irritation compared with hand washing with liquid detergents.[12,14] When decontaminating hands with an alcohol-based rub, place the correct volume (according to

the manufacturer's directions) on the palm of one hand. Rub both hands together, making sure that all surfaces of the hands and fingers are covered, until the hands are free of the product.[14]

Equipment Cleaning and Disinfecting

The OSHA standards state: "Employers shall ensure that the work site is maintained in a clean and sanitary condition. The employer shall determine and implement an appropriate written schedule for cleaning and method of decontamination based upon the location within the facility, type of surface to be cleaned, type of soil present, and tasks or procedures being performed in the area."[2] Specific procedures and protocols, while defined by the employer's ECP, must be followed out on a daily basis by the facility employees. This may include the cleaning of items such as tables, floors, medical apparatuses (autoclaving tweezers, scissors, etc.), and rehabilitation tools, and appropriate disposal and handling of laundry. Remember that all soiled or contaminated items should be handled using PPE and precautions; decontamination using commercial cleaning solutions should follow the manufacturer's recommendations; and any contaminated material should be disposed of in the appropriate receptacles (Fig. 7.13).

Spill Cleanup

Cleaning and decontamination of spills of blood or bodily fluid should be prompt and done observing UPs or BSIs by trained individuals. When a spill occurs, the first and probably most important step is to contain the spill. Continue cleaning the spill by following the steps in Skill 7.3.

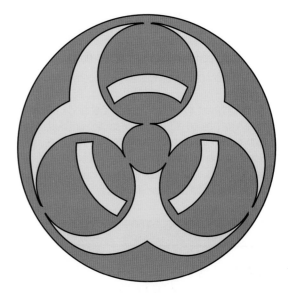

FIGURE 7.13 Biohazard symbol. (LifeART image copyright ©2010 Lippincott Williams & Wilkins. All rights reserved.)

SKILL 7.3

Cleaning and Decontaminating a Blood-Borne Pathogen Spill

1. Begin cleaning the spill by donning disposable gloves, at a minimum. If there is potential for splashing to occur, consider protective eyewear, gown, and mask (Fig. 7.14).

2. Soak up blood or bodily fluid using any absorbent material such as paper towels, cloth towels (rags), or commercially designed hazardous material containment kits. Any large sharp objects should be removed using tongs or two pieces of cardboard and should be disposed of properly (Fig. 7.15).

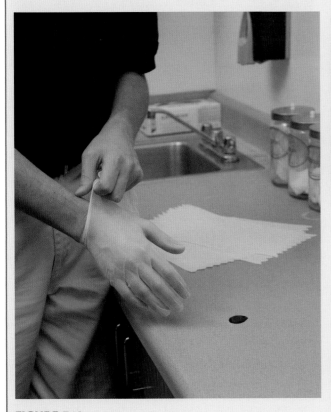

FIGURE 7.14

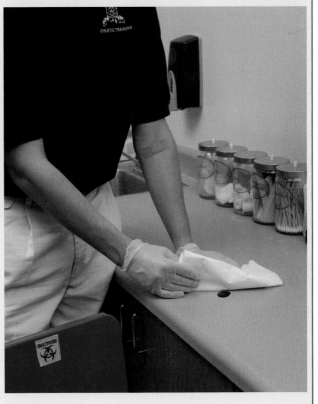

FIGURE 7.15

(Continued)

SKILL 7.3 *(Continued)*

Cleaning and Decontaminating a Blood-Borne Pathogen Spill (Continued)

3. Place the contaminated waste in a properly marked biohazard container.
4. Thoroughly wet the surface using either a 1½ c liquid chlorine bleach to 1 gallon of fresh water solution or Environmental Protection Agency–approved disinfectant for 10 minutes (Fig. 7.16).
5. Soak up the solution using an absorbent material such as paper towels, cloth towels (rags), or commercially designed hazardous material containment kits.

6. Place the contaminated waste in a properly marked biohazard container (Fig. 7.17).
7. Let the area air dry. Dispose of any PPEs in a properly marked biohazard container.
8. Wash hands (refer to Skill 7.2).

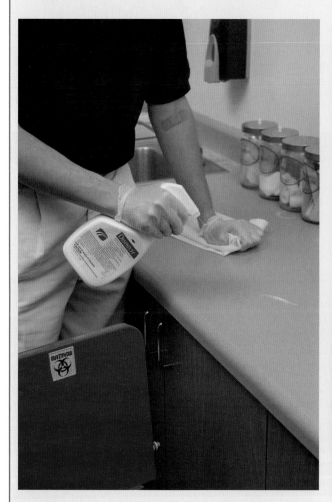

FIGURE 7.16

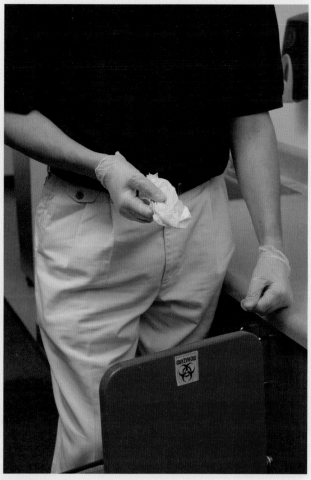

FIGURE 7.17

EXPOSURE INCIDENT

An exposure incident occurs when an individual experiences a "specific eye, mouth, other mucous membrane, nonintact skin, or parenteral contact with blood or other potentially infectious materials that results from the performance of an employee's duties,"[2] often as a result of a needlestick, sharps injury, or improper/faulty PPE usage.

When and if this occurs, follow these steps listed below immediately.[2,11,16,17]

1. Remain calm; stop what you were doing and wash needlestick, sharps wound, and any remnants of blood or OPIMs with soap and water.
2. Flush splashes of blood or OPIMs reaching the nose, mouth, or skin with tap water.

3. Flush splashes of blood or OPIMs to the eyes with clean water, saline, or sterile irrigation solution from the inside out.

4. Immediately report the incident to your department supervisor responsible for managing exposure incidents. Prompt reporting is essential, as postexposure treatment may be necessary and should be started as soon as possible.

5. Immediately seek medical treatment from a licensed health care provider following the recommended guidelines established by the facility's ECP. This medical care should be provided free of charge. Medical treatment may include postexposure prophylactic medication and counseling, which includes recommendations for avoiding transmission and prevention of HIV. All medical treatments prescribed will follow appropriate current U.S. Public Health Service recommendations.

6. Within 15 days, you will receive a copy of the physician's written opinion of your medical evaluation. The report will identify whether a HBV vaccination was recommended and whether or not the employee received the HBV vaccination as well as being informed of any medical conditions resulting from exposure to blood that require further evaluation or treatment.

Prompt reporting of an exposure incident is also important for several other reasons.[17] It helps to avoid the spread of blood-borne infection between other workers and family and friends. Reporting an exposure allows for testing of the blood of the source individual to determine HBV and HIV infectivity if the status is unknown and permission is granted for the testing. In some cases state or local law may prohibit the disclosure of the source individual. As the exposed employee, you have the right to be informed of any tests results regarding the source individual.

As part of the postexposure control plan, the exposure should be noted in an employee's medical records, which remain confidential and are unavailable to the employer without written permission. Furthermore, all records must be maintained for the duration of the employee's service plus 30 years, in accordance with 29 CFR 1910.1020 of the OSHA Standards.

WRAP-UP

This chapter outlines multiple means and methods for preventing exposure to blood-borne pathogens in the athletic training setting. The tables and figures give step-by-step details of some of the most important barrier controls, including the fitting and removal of gloves and disinfection of the workplace environment. Disease states, including hepatitis and AIDS, are reviewed to inform the athletic trainer about what can occur if workers are not properly protected or vaccinated. Finally, and most important, this chapter provides information about developing work site protocols and how to inform and contact appropriate medical personnel if an athletic trainer should come into contact with blood-borne pathogens in an unsafe manner. By reviewing and following all of the aforementioned procedures and processes, the athletic trainer should be confident that he or she will be protected and that their work site will be safe from potential hazards due to blood-borne pathogens.

Scenarios

1. An athlete reports to the athletic training room for a wound he sustained in practice. The wound appears to be a large abrasion over his lower back. The athletic training student (ATS) does a very thorough job cleaning the wound appropriately. However, after cleaning the wound, the ATS just pulls off his gloves and disposes them in the garbage.

   How should the ATS have removed the gloves and what type of container should the gloves have been placed in for correct blood-borne pathogen disposal?

2. An athletic trainer has been hired at a local high school to provide athletic training services. The high school had never previously had an athletic trainer and the athletic director asks that the athletic training facility have all the proper equipment and supplies necessary. One thing that you notice is missing is a posting of the OSHA guidelines for blood-borne pathogen engineering controls.

   What should the athletic trainer request for the facility in order to follow OSHA guidelines?

3. During a softball game, an athlete sustains a blow to the nose, resulting in profuse bleeding. The athletic trainer, wearing gloves, controls the bleeding.

   According to this chapter, what are the routes of transmission entries of which the athletic trainer must be aware and how should the athletic trainer be prepared to control these transmission methods?

4. Approximately 6 months earlier, an ATS came in contact with a person who had an open wound. Evidently, controls for preventing the transmission of blood-borne pathogens were not followed precisely owing to lack of knowledge. The ATS, after learning of blood-borne pathogen controls in a class, suspects that she may be infected with a pathogen.

   Which pathogen is the mostly likely to be contracted via this method and what are the signs and symptoms that should be monitored?

REFERENCES

1. Needlestick Safety and Prevention Act; 2000. http://frwebgate. access.gpo.gov/cgi-bin/getdoc.cgi?dbname=106_cong_public_laws&docid=f:publ430.106.

2. Occupational Safety and Health Administration. Bloodborne pathogens.–1910.1030. Occupational Safety and Health Administration. http://www.osha.gov/pls/oshaweb/owadisp.show_document?p_table=STANDARDS&p_id=10051. Accessed August 26, 2009.

3. Centers for Disease Control and Prevention, Diseases NCfI, eds. *Exposure to Blood: What Healthcare Personnel Need to Know.* Centers for Disease Control and Prevention. Atlanta, GA; 2003.

4. Centers for Disease Control and Prevention. *Hepatitis B.* Centers for Disease Control and Prevention. http://www.cdc.gov/hepatitis/HepatitisB.htm. Accessed August 20, 2009.

5. Centers for Disease Control and Prevention. *Hepatitis C.* Centers for Disease Control and Prevention. http://www.cdc.gov/hepatitis/HCV/HCVfaq.htm#section2. Accessed August 20, 2009.

6. Centers for Disease Control and Prevention. *HIV/AIDS.* http://www.cdc.gov/hiv/topics/basic/index.htm#hiv. Accessed August 20, 2009.

7. American Red Cross. *Bloodborne Pathogen Training: Preventing Disease Transmission.* Yardley, PA: Staywell; 2003.

8. Centers for Disease Control and Prevention. *Universal Precautions for Prevention of Transmission of HIV and other Bloodborne Infections.* Centers for Disease Control and Prevention. http://www.cdc.gov/ncidod/dhqp/bp_universal_precautions.html. Accessed August 20, 2009.

9. Gardner JS. Guideline for isolation precautions in hospitals. The Hospital Infection Control Practices Advisory Committee. *Infect Control Hosp Epidemiol.* 1996;17(1):53–80.

10. Lynch P, Cummings MJ, Roberts PL, et al. Implementing and evaluating a system of generic infection precautions: Body substance isolation. *Am J Infect Control.* 1990;18:1–12.

11. Mitus MC. *Bloodborne Pathogens.* Wild Iris Medical Education, LLC. http://www.nursingceu.com/courses/248/index_nceu.html. Accessed August 20, 2009.

12. Kampf G, Kramer A. Epidemiologic background of hand hygiene and evaluation of the most important agents for scrubs and rubs. *Clin Microbiol Rev.* 2004;17(4):863–893.

13. Ejemot RI, Ehiri JE, Meremikwu MM, et al. Hand washing for preventing diarrhoea. *Cochrane Database Syst Rev.* 2008;23(1):CD004265.

14. Centers for Disease Control and Prevention. Guideline for hand hygiene in health-care settings: Recommendations of the Healthcare Infection Control Practices Advisory Committee and the HICPAC/SHEA/APIC/IDSA Hand Hygiene Task Force. *MMWR Morb Mortal Wkly Rep.* 2002;51(RR-16):1–45.

15. Mody L, McNeil SA, Sun R, et al. Introduction of a waterless alcohol-based hand rub in a long-term-care facility. *Infect Control Hosp Epidemiol.* 2003;24(3):157–159.

16. American Red Cross. *CPR/AED for the Professional Rescuer Participant's Manual.* Yardley, PA: Staywell; 2006.

17. Occupational Safety and Health Administration. *Reporting Exposure Incidents.* U.S. Department of Labor. www.osha.gov/OshDoc/data_BloodborneFacts/bbfact04.pdf. Accessed August 20, 2009.

C H A P T E R · 8

Primary, Secondary, and Ongoing Assessment

CHAPTER OUTCOMES

1. Discuss and identify potentially harmful surroundings in approaching the scene of an injured athlete.

2. Identify signs of potential hazards at an emergency scene.

3. Understand how to appropriately manage an emergency scene to prevent or limit further injury to the athlete and the athletic trainer.

4. Identify how to survey the scene to determine what additional resources may be needed to care for an injured athlete.

5. Identify the proper use of a motorized vehicle to block traffic and secure the scene to prevent or minimize further harm to the athlete or athletic trainer.

6. Identify and utilize various illumination and sound devices to warn others that a potential hazard is nearby as well as to ensure the safety of the athletic trainer, all injured athletes, and any bystanders.

7. Identify the appropriate use of flares in emergency situations.

8. Examine the scene visually to determine the extent of injuries or emergency conditions.

9. Check the mental status of the injured athlete during the initial assessment.

10. Check airway, breathing, and circulation (the ABCs) in a thorough but quick manner in an injured responsive or unresponsive athlete.

11. Determine which conditions warrant high-priority intervention and/or referral to a medical facility.

12. Differentiate between a trauma victim and a medical patient in an emergency situation.

13. Understand the secondary assessments for conscious and unconscious victims of trauma and medical conditions.

14. Recite and conduct the OPQRST (onset, provocation, quality, radiation/region/relief, severity, time) and SAMPLE (signs and symptoms, allergies, medications, past medical history, last oral intake, events) secondary assessment procedures for the athlete requiring medical attention.

15. Understand the appropriate communication procedures with other medical personnel about emergency situations and scenes.

16. Understand the importance of conducting an ongoing assessment for an athlete requiring intervention for a medical condition or trauma.

17. Recognize that although an athlete's vital signs may be stable, they can deteriorate rapidly, leading to a medical emergency.

18. Identify the parameters used for the ongoing assessment with regard to the ABCs.

19. Identify the parameters used for the ongoing assessment as they pertain to an athlete's medical history and physical findings.

NOMENCLATURE

Battle sign: discoloration behind the ears, indicative of skull fracture

Cerebrospinal fluid (CSF): a clear fluid surrounding the brain and spinal cord

Chief complaint: a patient's primary symptom

Flail chest: an injury to the chest in which the ribs break off from the rib cage

Hyphema: a blood collection in the anterior chamber of the eye

Jugular vein distention: bulging of the jugular veins of the neck

Sucking chest wound: sound of air flowing through a puncture of the lung cavity

Raccoon eyes: discoloration around the eyes as a result of skull fracture or trauma to the brain

Rhinorrhea: discharge of fluid from the nose

Unobstructed: readily accessible

Vomitus: contents from the stomach; if red or coffee-grounds color, may indicate internal bleeding

BEFORE YOU BEGIN

1. What are some of the ways in which a motorized cart can be used to ensure safety at the scene of an emergency?

2. What are the steps an athletic trainer must take when conducting the primary assessment of an injured athlete?

3. What are some illumination devices that can be used at a medical emergency/trauma scene?

4. What are the major steps in a secondary assessment?

5. What does acronym SAMPLE mean?

6. What are some things that should be checked in the ongoing assessment?

7. How often should you reassess an injured athlete?

8. Name some conditions that can develop slowly and become life-threatening, necessitating further ongoing assessment.

9. Why should the athletic trainer conduct more than one medical history of the injury?

Voices from the Field

As Certified Athletic Trainers (ATCs), we come across injury after injury on a daily basis. We are first on the scene for on-the-field injuries and, many times, the first medical professionals to evaluate the patient in the clinical setting. As we grow in our profession and gain more knowledge and experience, we at times become overconfident with our evaluations and may jump to conclusions without properly assessing the entire individual. The ATC should never allow injury assessment to become monotonous.

When assessing injuries and illnesses, ATCs must hone a combination of traits and use many different tools that set them aside from other health care professionals. The art of blending the traits of speed (both physically and mentally), diligence, and having an eye for detail will allow the professional to provide

optimal care. Enhancing these traits and utilizing the resources in an ATC's well-rounded arsenal, whether that includes using a John Deere Gator or not, can help aid and protect the patient.

Athletic injuries do not become routine on their own; we allow ourselves to get in a rut. We must challenge ourselves to improve our use of a systematic approach to assess injuries. If we use this approach, we will always ensure proper triage and referral for our patients without missing the minutest detail.

Andrew T. Doyle, MA, ATC, LAT, CSCS
Assistant Athletic Trainer
Indiana Wesleyan University
Marion, Indiana

In an emergency situation, the initial and secondary examinations of an injured athlete are vital to determine the appropriate treatment plan; however, there is a critical third step, the ongoing assessment that is sometimes forgotten. This process of checking and re-checking the patient for any changes in physical or mental state is one that, as an ATC, you may already be performing in some cases, especially those cases deemed life threatening. However, it is important to make this part of all trauma conditions in order to ensure you are providing the best and highest quality care. It is important for ATCs to know the proper guidelines to follow in these emergency situations

because ATCs are in most cases at the center of the sports emergency care team and, therefore, must be proficient in the skills needed for sports emergency care. Also, ATCs must be knowledgeable about how to perform the ongoing assessment and the importance of this process in providing proper care for an athlete in these emergency situations.

Jessica Groth, MA, ATC, CSCS
Athletic Trainer
Select Medical Corporation
Clearwater, FL

In athletic training, the ATC is often called upon to manage an emergency at a scene that may be dangerous (as when a cross-country runner collapses on a road shared by vehicular traffic). Although care of the athlete is of immediate concern, it is also vitally important to survey the scene and arrange appropriate barriers, so that care can be provided safely. One of the first priorities in any emergency situation is to secure and maintain a safe environment and apply safety precautions that will limit harm to both the athletic trainer and the athlete. Once the scene is safe, the athletic trainer must conduct an initial assessment to determine the extent of the athlete's injuries and the next steps needed. After the initial assessment, a more thorough secondary assessment is conducted to look for injuries that are not life-threatening. In this chapter, we discuss ways to ensure safety at any emergency scene. This is followed by descriptions of the initial and secondary assessments required for appropriate treatment for the injured athlete.

THE SCENE

Approaching the Scene

One of the first preventative measures for the safety and well-being of the athletic trainer in any emergency situation is to know the surroundings before rendering care; this is sometimes referred to as a "size-up." It can be accomplished by surveying the scene and identifying potential hazards. The size-up involves looking at the "big picture"— the entire area or scene. For example, an athletic trainer may be working at a football game when a player sustains an injury on the field. Making sure that the play has ended, knowing where the remaining players are located, and being aware of the field conditions (slippery surfaces as a result of weather, watering, etc.) are all necessary. Rushing out to the downed player without taking the necessary precautions could cause the athletic trainer to take a fall or be hit by another football player, leading to personal injury and thus interfering with or delaying care and management of the injured athlete.

If an injured athlete is located in a secluded area or other part of an athletic venue, away from sight, it is the responsibility of the athletic trainer to know the terrain and potential hazards of that area. This can be accomplished by exploring the area ahead of time or by direct communication with facility managers, athletic directors, coaches, players, and so forth. Knowing about the scene and potential hazards or environmental conditions, the athletic trainer can avoid mistakes. For example, it would be a mistake to take a motorized cart across a field only to find boggy conditions, holes, traffic, power lines, or other hazards that would limit access to the injured player with that transportation method. In addition, it is also prudent to know how to transport an athlete out of an area that is not readily accessible. By

---

Breakout

Signs of Potential Hazards

1. Try to determine whether the injury is traumatic (fractured bone, sprained ligament) or medical (seizure, hypoglycemia) in nature and if the cause of the injury was associated with the environment you will be entering.
2. Look for smoke or fire.
3. Determine if there is heavy automobile or other vehicular traffic.
4. Determine if there are objects (small holes, uneven terrain, sharp edges, glass) that may impede your response time and ability to provide care.
5. Identify potentially hazardous materials or gases (e.g., chlorine fumes from a swimming pool).
6. Look for bleeding or blood near the athlete and determine the probable cause.
7. Identify animals (dogs, wild game, etc.) that may thwart care.
8. Examine the scene for downed electrical wires. If any are seen, treat them as a fully energized wires and keep clear of them.
9. Look for unpredictable interference, such as unruly persons (threatening words, fighting, suspicion of alcohol or drug use).

---

knowing what to expect and identifying conditions that could cause injury to himself or herself, the athletic trainer should be able to adjust to the situation, ensure safety, and provide the care that is needed. Some situations may place the athletic trainer in a hostile environment (visiting game or scrimmage), where the fans may throw debris and place the athletic trainer and injured athlete at risk. Finally, by knowing the scene, the athletic trainer can determine what type of equipment may be needed to properly care for the athlete.

Managing the Scene

After noting all the potential hazards or conditions that may make the scene dangerous, the athletic trainer must manage and control the scene. In terms of priority, athletic trainers who arrive at the scene of an emergency must always protect themselves, protect the public at the scene (if applicable), and then protect the downed or injured athlete from harm or hazards. If it is determined that proceeding into the scene is unsafe or risky, the athletic trainer has the right not to provide care. However, it must be determined that personal harm could result from entry into an unsafe scene. The athletic trainer has the legal responsibility to provide care and must do so if the scene is safe; in such a situation, the athletic trainer cannot decide simply not to act (refer to Chapter 3 for a discussion of legal liability).

Resources at the Scene

The athletic trainer must also determine the nature or causes of the condition or illness of the injured athlete. This task is completed at the same time as the scene is sized up. This process begins by determining the athlete's level of consciousness, the possible mechanism of injury and scope of damage, and the type of care needed. Based upon this information, the athletic trainer can make a rational decision about the resources available to handle the situation. If an athlete is unconscious, other trained medical personnel may be needed to secure the athlete on a backboard or perform cardiopulmonary resuscitation (CPR). If the athlete is unable to support his or her body weight, another athletic trainer or medical personnel may be required to move the athlete to the athletic training room or other location for medical services. Additional personnel may also be required if there is severe bleeding or more medical supplies are needed. Having determined the extent of the injury, the athletic trainer can summon the additional assistance and supplies necessary without leaving the injured person.

SCENE SAFETY

Using Motorized Vehicles as Barriers

In situations where an athletic event takes place on roadways used by motorized vehicles, the athletic trainer must be cognizant that passing traffic can pose a danger. For self-protection, the athletic trainer can follow some simple rules/steps to minimize risk in these situations. When these are carried out appropriately, the safety of all parties (athletic trainer, injured athlete, bystanders) is ensured. First, if the care of an injured athlete requires the use of a motorized vehicle (e.g., car, cart), that vehicle can be used as a barrier to protect the athlete and athletic trainer. Park the vehicle far enough away from the injured athlete to leave sufficient space for access and treatment while also letting the vehicle serve as a protective barrier. For example, if the injured athlete is located along the side of a road (having fallen during a cross-country meet while running along a road used by vehicular traffic), place your vehicle (in this situation a cart) approximately 50 ft in front to shield both the athletic trainer and the injured athlete. If the traffic on the road is moving at higher speeds, place the barrier up to 30 yds away in order to allow enough time for ongoing traffic to view the cart and avoid the area.

Illumination and Sound Devices

In situations where visibility may be poor (because of fog, minimal light during sunrise and sunset, and nighttime activities), it may be necessary to use illumination. Flashlights, flares, and lights from a motorized vehicle (hazard lights) are examples of illumination equipment that may be required. Flashlights can be used by the athletic trainer or bystanders, coaches, etc. to help illuminate the site or used as warning lights for oncoming traffic. The light can be a continuous beam, but turning it on and off at 1- to 2-second intervals will be more effective in gaining attention. Road flares, which are typically found in car emergency kits, are also used as warning devices to alert others to a nearby hazard. It is recommended to place one flare about 120 ft from the scene when traffic is in a rural area (local town and street traffic speeds, up to 30 mph). Traffic speeds above 50 mph should have the flare placed 200 ft or more from the scene. If enough flares are available, the athletic trainer should place them 50 ft apart when walking back toward the scene (but remember, never turn your back on oncoming traffic). To light a flare, follow the steps shown in Skill 8.1.

In addition to using an illumination device, it may also be prudent to use some type of sound device, such as a small portable air horn that you can blast intermittently in situations of poor visibility. These short blasts should catch the attention of others nearby and warn them of a problem in the area. For example, an athletic trainer may be on the scene, attending to a rower who has sustained a non-life-threatening injury on a river edge in foggy conditions, where visibility is limited to several feet. Here it would be useful to have a bystander, another teammate, or another athletic trainer

---

SKILL 8.1

Lighting a Flare

1. Locate and wear protective gloves. Thicker gloves, such as garden gloves or gloves that are flame-resistant, are good choices.
2. Preferably, the athletic trainer should be wearing a long-sleeved shirt or jacket to protect his or her arms from stray sparks.
3. Wear protective goggles or safety glasses.
4. Remove the striker from the top or head of the flare.
5. Grab the flare in midshaft or at least 6 in. from the top.
6. Using the striker, strike the head (the flare's igniter) in a direction away from your body. It may take several strikes before ignition occurs.
7. If applicable, place the flare on the ground at the proper location in the flare stand (which may come with certain flares) or stick it into the ground with a ground spike.

blast an air horn once every minute or less. This sound could serve as a warning to others who may be on the river, such as boats or other rowers, to proceed with caution.

INITIAL ASSESSMENT

Whenever an athlete is injured and the scene is determined to be safe, it is imperative that an initial assessment be conducted (Algorithm 8.1). In order to render the appropriate care, the initial assessment must be made within the first 15 seconds of arrival on the scene. The purpose of the initial assessment is to determine life-threatening conditions or problems; it is often divided into several parts or segments in a systematic manner. These steps are to (a) obtain a quick overview of the injury, (b) determine the athlete's mental status, and (c) assess the athlete's airway, breathing, and circulation (the ABCs). By following these steps, the athletic trainer can make all necessary and correct interventions for care as required. Each one of these steps is examined more closely in the following sections of this chapter.

Overview of the Injury

Usually, by examining the athlete as you approach the scene (after determining the scene's safety), you can quickly determine what may have happened and all the necessary

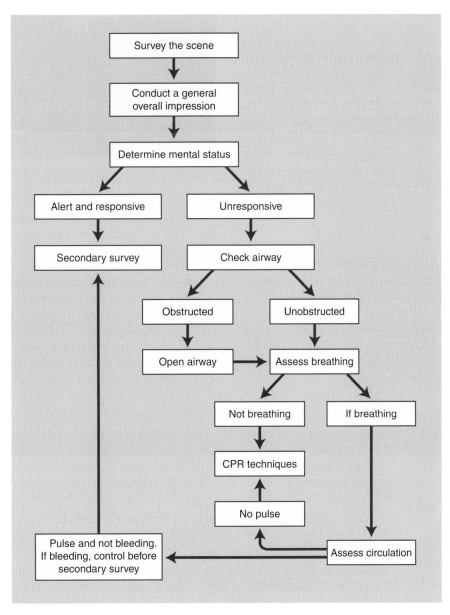

ALGORITHM 8.1   Initial assessment steps.

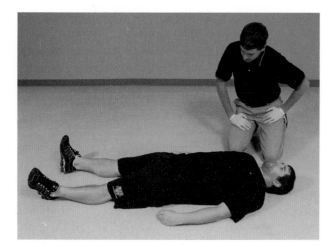

FIGURE 8.1 Examination of the athlete.

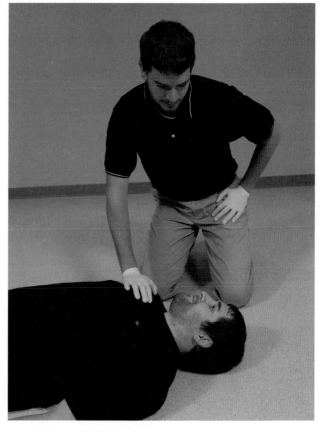

FIGURE 8.2 Checking the mental status of the athlete.

actions that may be necessary to provide proper care. Look for signs or clues of what may have caused the injury, such as an object (e.g., baseball, hurdle) or another player who may be able to provide clues as to the mechanism of the injury or the scope of the damage (Fig. 8.1). Examine the body position, the location of the extremities, and the head and neck for obvious signs of deformity. Pay close attention to the environmental conditions (e.g., extremely cold or hot, wet, or rainy) or other factors, such as noxious gases, that may cause you to alter your treatment or even location when providing care.

Mental Status

The next step is to determine the athlete's mental status. Begin by talking to the athlete to find out what happened (Fig. 8.2). On the basis of the athlete's responses, the athletic trainer can determine the athlete's level of consciousness: whether he or she is fully alert, somewhat groggy, or more or less unresponsive. This can be accomplished by remembering the acronym AVPU (alert, verbal response, painful response, and unresponsive) (Table 8.1).

If the athlete does respond, assess mental status by establishing orientation, as to a person, place, and time. A response from the athlete will indicate a degree of alertness, but he or she may have some cognitive dysfunction (e.g., a concussion), being disoriented as to who or where he or she is. When the athlete's mental status is depressed or diminished, expect a potentially life-threatening injury—which could include shock, spinal cord damage, or brain injury—and be prepared to initiate the appropriate action. If you suspect any type of spinal or neck injury during the assessment, manual stabilization of the head and neck must be

TABLE 8.1 AVPU	
Alert	The athlete is awake (eyes are open) and responds sensibly to questions (aware of his or her surroundings and condition). Ask questions about time, place, and person to assess this. If all replies appear to be normal, the athlete is said to be "alert and orientated times three," or A/O×3.
Verbal response	Athlete may respond only when prompted, sometimes by the athletic trainer's loud or yelling voice. This sign is indicative of depressed mental status. The athlete often closes his or her eyes and is not aware of the surroundings.
Painful response	Athlete responds only to a painful stimulus, such as pressing on the sternum with a knuckle or pinching a finger or toe. Begin with a tap on the shoulder before progressing to more noxious stimuli.
Unresponsive	Athlete does not respond to verbal or painful stimuli.

Current Research

The AVPU method has been effective in assessing the mental status of poisoned patients, has been less useful with alcohol-intoxicated individuals.[1] However, the AVPU may not be the best scale to use for critically ill neurosurgical patients compared with other mental status assessments.[2]

conducted (see Chapter 17). When following AVPU, please note the response you get within each level. This information will be useful when the athlete is referred for medical attention.

Airway, Breathing, Circulation

Airway, breathing, and circulation (the ABCs) are usually assessed concurrently while assessing the injury and mental status. If the athlete is talking and alert, all the necessary vital information to determine the ABCs is apparent. If, on the other hand, the athlete is unresponsive, a more thorough assessment of the ABCs is required. First, determine whether the athlete's airway may be blocked. Look for signs of struggling as the athlete tries to breathe or for drooling from the mouth, which can be a sign of an airway obstruction. The use of head-tilt, chin-lift, jaw-thrust maneuvers, as discussed in Chapter 10, should be followed. If a blocked airway is interfering with the athlete's breathing, one of these maneuvers should allow air to pass freely.

Perform the "look, listen, and feel" technique to determine whether the patient is breathing (Fig. 8.3).[3] Look

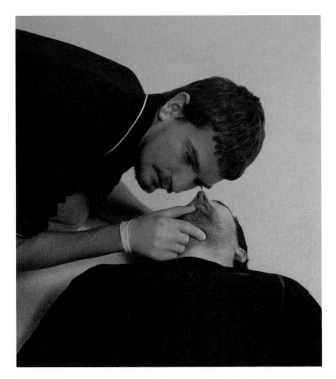

FIGURE 8.3   Performing the "look, listen, feel."

for the chest to rise. Athletes who may have a **flail chest** will have paradoxical rib movement, with the flail section moving backward during inspiration and forward during expiration. Listen for breathing by placing your ear close to the athlete's mouth and nose or placing a stethoscope just below the clavicles on each side. Abnormal sounds, as in a **sucking chest wound,** will impede airflow into the lungs. Finally, feel for the chest to rise and for deformity of the chest by placing your hands on the chest wall. If the athlete is breathing, assess the quality of the breaths and their rate. Supplemental oxygen may be required if breaths are fewer than 8 or greater than 24 per minute (see Chapter 11, on breathing devices). If the athlete is not breathing, rescue breathing should be initiated (see Chapter 10).

After determining the condition of the airway and breathing, the third step is to assess the circulation. This can be accomplished by first checking the carotid artery at the neck, followed by checking for a pulse at the radial artery (Fig. 8.4A), femoral artery (Fig. 8.4B), and tibial artery (Fig. 8.4C). Check the pulse at each location (if necessary) for approximately 5 to 10 seconds. Look for warm, pink skin (skin color and temperature); then check the nail beds and lips for color, especially for people with dark skin. After determining the pulse, look for signs of external bleeding. One common method to determine the presence of blood underneath the athlete is to swipe your hands beneath both sides and look for blood on your hands. If the athlete is breathing and there is significant external bleeding, implement the necessary steps to control the loss of blood.

It is also imperative that baseline vital signs be assessed (i.e., heart rate, respiratory rate, and blood pressure). Once these baseline signs have been determined, assess pupil reaction, skin temperature, and capillary refill for fingers and toes. All this information should be documented and reassessed periodically to assess the condition of the athlete over time. While assessing the vital signs, note any abnormal signs that may require emergency transportation, such as abnormal heartbeats, pupils that become nonreactive over time, difficulty breathing, or a breathing rate that increases or decreases over time.

After the major vital signs have been assessed, the next step, before continuing with a secondary assessment, is to determine the priority of the injured athlete. If the athlete is deemed sufficiently stable for a secondary assessment, proceed; if the athlete requires immediate transport or the condition is of high priority, activate

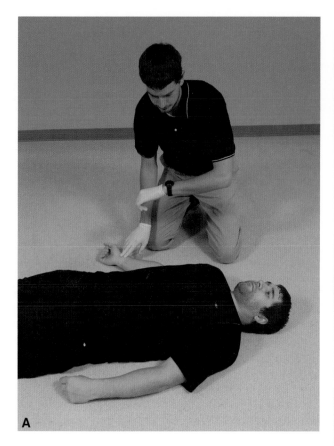

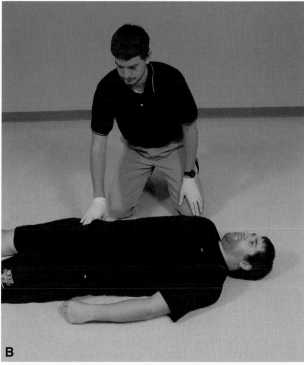

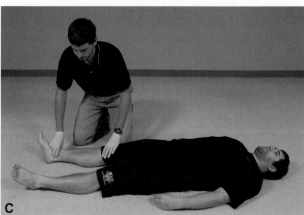

FIGURE 8.4   Performing artery palpation: **A.** Radial. **B.** Femoral. **C.** Tibial.

emergency medical services (EMS) for transport to the nearest medical facility. By following these initial steps of the primary survey, the athletic trainer can make the important judgment of what type of care will be appropriate.

The steps outlined above can be implemented rather quickly in an emergency situation; the subsequent actions of the athletic trainer will then determine the athlete's outcome. Only practice and due diligence can mentally and physically prepare the athletic trainer for these situations.

SECONDARY ASSESSMENT

In any emergency situation, the primary responsibility of the athletic trainer is to determine the extent of the injury and, if a medical emergency exists, to initiate the actions necessary to sustain life. However, in most cases an injury is either not life-threatening or not immediately life-threatening, but it has the potential to become life-threatening if not properly cared for. In these instances, after the initial assessment has been conducted and it has

Breakout

Conditions that are of High Priority

1. Shock
2. Childbirth
3. Unresponsiveness
4. Breathing difficulty
5. Uncontrolled bleeding
6. Extreme pain anywhere in the body
7. Chest pain

been determined that the athlete is not in serious danger, a more thorough assessment must take place to determine the extent and specific type(s) of injury. This assessment is called the secondary assessment and focuses on the physical examination of the athlete.

Secondary Assessment Communication and Basic Procedures

The procedures of the physical examination are intimate in nature, focusing on touching and assessing the body. As with any physical assessment, it is important to obtain the athlete's consent for these procedures. Never touch the athlete without consent unless he or she is unconscious or unresponsive. If the athlete declines your medical services, document that you offered to assist and that medical services were declined. By doing so, you have documentation that can be used to support your case if legal actions should be pursued because of subsequent damage due to the injury. In order to obtain the athlete's consent and trust, follow the basic rules of engagement. These rules will not only make the athlete feel more relaxed but can also provide the athletic trainer with initial navigational steps to be followed when conducting the physical examination.

Breakout

Basic Guidelines to Follow During the
Physical Examination

1. Be cognizant of the athlete's injury or injuries and apprehension.
2. Conduct yourself in a professional and polite manner. Maintain eye contact when necessary and answer all the athlete's questions as truthfully as possible.
3. Introduce yourself to the athlete and give your qualifications (if applicable). Ask for permission to conduct the physical assessment and explain the medical need for such an assessment.
4. Be courteous to the athlete, using his or her first name if appropriate. If the athlete is older, use an appropriate title, such as Mr. Barnes or Ms. Cheatham. In fact, ask how the athlete would like to be addressed.
5. Explain the processes that you are following while conducting the physical assessment. When performing special tests, explain what they are used for and why they are needed. This will help to ensure that the athlete is comfortable with your actions and will allow you to make appropriate decisions regarding his or her care.
6. Respect the athlete's privacy. Do not undress the athlete without consent and do so only when necessary. If there is a need to undress, provide some type of drape or barrier between the athlete and bystanders. When you have finished this assessment, cover the body to limit exposure.

The secondary assessment often falls into two distinct categories: assessment for trauma and assessment for a medical condition. A secondary assessment for trauma focuses on identifying trauma/injuries that were not apparent after the initial assessment but that could be serious. For an athlete with a medical condition, the secondary assessment examines illnesses or conditions that are brought forward by a medical issue, such as a disease. In either case, the secondary assessment is important to identify trauma or medical issues that need management and have the potential to be life-threatening.

Secondary Assessment for the Athlete Who Has Suffered Trauma (Rapid Secondary Assessment)

For the athlete who has been a victim of trauma, a rapid secondary assessment should be conducted once potential life-threatening injuries have been ruled out. The rapid secondary assessment is a very quick scan of the body, looking for serious conditions/injuries that may have been missed or not identified in the initial assessment (see Fig. 8.1 and Algorithm 8.2). During this secondary assessment, use the acronym DCAP-BTLS (deformity, contusion, abrasion, puncture–burn, tenderness, laceration, swelling) as a guide (Table 8.2). These steps will allow you to proceed through a secondary evaluation in a systematic manner, thus ensuring a thorough examination.

Begin with the head/neck and look for signs associated with the acronym DCAP-BTLS (Fig. 8.5). Next, use your fingers to quickly scan the hair/scalp, feeling for deformities and looking for blood. Check the face in the same manner, including the jaw. Examine the mouth and nose for bleeding, fluids, or foreign objects. Proceeding to the neck, examine the trachea for deformity and the jugular veins for **jugular vein distention.** Palpate the posterior neck from the base of the skull to the shoulder, looking for deformity, tenderness, and/or blood. If a neck fracture or head injury is suspected, apply a rigid cervical immobilization device and be prepared for spinal immobilization (see Chapter 17).

Once the head and neck have been examined, proceed to the chest and abdomen (Fig. 8.6). It may be necessary to loosen or remove clothing to properly assess for injuries to the chest area. If you must do so, remove clothing only to assess one section at a time and cover that section before proceeding to another. While examining the chest, look for the chest to rise and fall slightly during respiration. Notice the ease or difficulty of the breaths. Listen for breath sounds (Skill 8.2) and feel for movement. A flail chest will show paradoxical motion, and air will escape from a sucking chest wound while the athlete is breathing. Next, palpate the chest wall, anteriorly and laterally, feeling for crepitus, deformities, and tenderness. After examining the chest, proceed down the chest wall to the abdominal region between the pelvis and diaphragm. Using the umbilicus as a reference guide, divide the abdomen into four quadrants: upper, lower, left, and

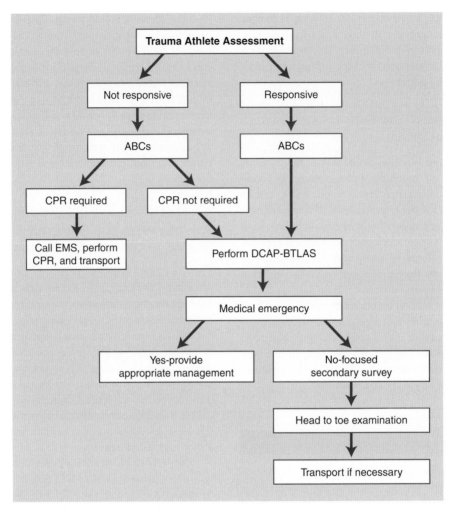

ALGORITHM 8.2   Secondary assessment of the athlete with trauma.

TABLE 8.2	**DCAP-BTLS**
Deformity	Look for any type of deformity to the body, including the extremities, torso, and head/neck.
Contusion	Examine the entire body for signs of bruising or contusions as a result of trauma. Discoloration of the tissues and pooling of blood may be noticeable.
Abrasion	Damage to or removal of the outer layer of the skin due to rubbing or friction. Not an immediate priority but can lead to infection if not properly treated.
Puncture	Penetration of the skin and/or soft tissue by a sharp object. Puncture wounds can be superficial or deep. If there is a deep puncture wound, refer to a medical facility.
Burn	Skin/soft tissue damage due to extreme heat. Burns are classified according to severity, from first to third degree. The higher the number, the more severe the burn or the more delicate the areas of the body burned.
Tenderness	Sensitivity of the skin to palpation, which causes some degree of pain. During examination, look for signs such as facial expressions, verbal expressions, or guarding of the area by the athlete.
Laceration	A deep cut through the skin that most likely would call for sutures or Steri-Strips to approximate the edges. Lacerations (if deep or long) can cause severe damage to the underlying tissues and should be referred to a medical facility for physician care.
Swelling	Increased size of the area/body part compared with the contralateral side as a result of an injury. May be warm to the touch and red.

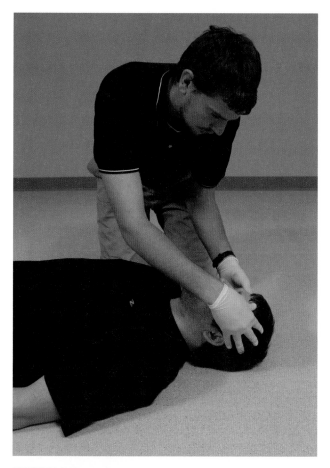

FIGURE 8.5   Performing DCAP-BLTS.

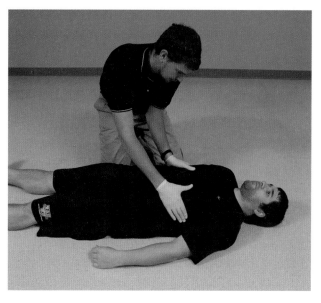

FIGURE 8.6   Scanning the chest and abdomen.

right. Visually inspect the area for discoloration and bleeding; then gently palpate the quadrants. The abdomen should be relatively soft and nondistended. Feel for guarding of the abdomen and notice tenderness and rebound tenderness. The pelvis can also be examined during the abdominal examination. Examine the pelvis in the same manner as the chest, dividing it into left and right and looking for deformity and discoloration and palpating for physical signs of injury.

SKILL 8.2

Assessing Breath Sounds (Fig. 8.7)

1. Place a stethoscope against the bare skin, not over clothing.
2. Listen for breath sounds that are equal between the right and left lungs.

Listen at these sites: apex of the midclavicle on the left and right sides, base of both clavicles, and the axillae. Abnormal sounds should be noted and the athlete referred for medical intervention.

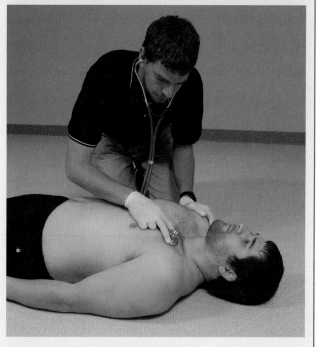

FIGURE 8.7   Examining breath sounds.

After the abdomen, chest, and pelvis have been scanned, proceed to the extremities (Fig. 8.8). Start on one side of the body (either left or right) and examine the left arm, then the right, and follow the same procedures for the lower extremity. Look for deformities, contusions, abrasions, lacerations, and tenderness. Palpate starting at the most proximal end (at the shoulder for the upper extremity and inguinal area for the lower extremity). Locate the radial and pedal arteries to check for a pulse in each extremity. Check for sensation equally within the upper and lower extremities and examine for movement of the fingers and toes. To help remember extremity testing, use the acronym PMS (pulse, movement, and sensation).

Secondary Assessment for a Trauma Patient (Focused Secondary Assessment)

The initial assessment followed by a rapid secondary assessment is used to identify life-threatening injuries, bleeding, and obvious fractures. These two assessments should take only a few minutes to complete. A more focused secondary assessment is then warranted to identify specific injuries in athletes who are either unconscious or whose level of consciousness is compromised. The focused secondary assessment is used to identify injuries that may not have been severe or that may have been overlooked in the rapid assessment. Most often, a focused secondary assessment is conducted while the athlete is transported to the hospital, but it can also be performed on the sidelines or in the athletic training room if the athlete is able to get there either alone or with help. Like the rapid assessment, the focused assessment is a head-to-toe examination, in which the athletic trainer can follow the DCAP-BTLS steps. However, unlike the rapid secondary assessment, the focused secondary assessment is more thorough and detailed; only the differences are discussed in this section.

Secondary Assessment Focused on the Head, Face, and Neck

Begin at the head and proceed down the body in the same way as in the rapid secondary assessment. While at the head, make sure that the entire skull, from the occiput to the temporal and frontal bones, is palpated. Again, palpate for deformity and look for blood. If necessary, use a penlight to examine the scalp for small lacerations (Fig. 8.9). After inspecting the head, proceed to the face and the ears. While inspecting the ears, look for fluid or drainage. Clear fluid, called **cerebrospinal fluid** (CSF), may indicate brain damage or skull fracture (see Chapter 17 for more information on head injuries). If

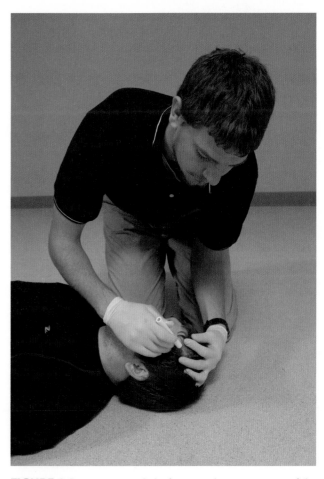

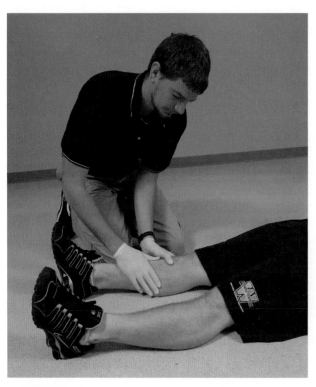

FIGURE 8.8 Secondary assessment of extremity.

FIGURE 8.9 Using a penlight for secondary assessment of the head.

you suspect CSF, do not attempt to stop the drainage but apply gauze to absorb the fluid. Stopping the drainage may increase the pressure within the skull and cause more brain damage. Look behind the ears for a discoloration called **Battle sign,** indicating a skull fracture (Chapter 17). Next, examine the eyes for discolorations called **raccoon eyes** and check for **hyphema.** Examine each pupil for shape, size, tracking, and reaction to light. If the pupils appear unequal or do not respond to light, the athlete may have a skull fracture or brain damage. If an object is impaled, treat according to the procedures in Chapter 14. Foreign substances that can be brushed away should be removed; however, if there is an object in the eye that is not impaled, leave it to medical personnel to remove. Inspect the nose for deformity, bleeding, and drainage **(rhinorrhea).** Examine the outside and inside the mouth. If lacerations are found on the outside of the mouth, control the bleeding to help prevent the blood from draining into the throat. Objects in the mouth can dislodge or fall into the airway, causing difficulty breathing and leading to a medical emergency. If loose objects, such as teeth, are found in the mouth, remove them and send them along with the athlete to the proper medical personnel. Inspect the teeth and look for bleeding. Finally, inspect the neck for tracheal deformity, discoloration, or other signs of injury.

Chest and Abdomen-Focused Secondary Assessment

Continuing down the body, the focused examination of the chest and abdominal area is very similar to the rapid secondary assessment, but with more detail. Examine chest expansion and depression during respirations closely by looking, feeling, and listening. A more thorough examination of the axillae and flanks may be needed, along with overall inspection of the entire chest wall/ribs for fractures and discomfort. Pay particular attention to the sternum for fractures/deformities; this is seldom examined in the rapid assessment. If no obvious deformities are noted, each side of the rib cage should be palpated with firm compression of the ribs to help rule out fractures. Finally, palpate the entire length of the clavicle, examining for deformities, discomfort, dislocations, and possible fractures.

The abdomen is examined very much as in the rapid secondary assessment. The priority is to look for abdominal distention and signs of internal pathologies. Asking the athlete about abdominal pain or mechanisms may help to diagnose the injury. Pay close attention to the patterns of referred pain involving the abdominal organs, as described in Chapter 16. Other signs include loss of bladder control, which may be indicative of spinal pathology. If urine stains are found, it may be prudent to use a spine board or immobilize the spine, as discussed in Chapter 17. While examining the pelvic region for urinary incontinence, perform pelvic distraction and compression tests to rule out fractures or discomfort.

Extremity-Focused Secondary Assessment

A visual inspection of both the upper and lower extremities with the focused assessment is very similar to the quick inspection during the rapid secondary assessment discussed previously. Each arm and leg should be examined independently, starting at the proximal ends and working distally. The athletic trainer should focus on small cuts, abrasions, or other superficial wounds along with discoloration and swelling or size differences between the extremities. Working down the extremity, palpate for signs of tenderness, crepitus, or deformities. Take note to the presence of any physical signs and compare with the opposite extremity. If a fracture is suspected, immobilize the body part according to the guidelines in Chapter 16.

During palpation, assess for movement bilaterally and skin sensation throughout the whole extremity. Have the athlete move his or her fingers and squeeze your hand (Fig. 8.10). Have the athlete raise his or her toes upward and then push downward against slight resistance from your hand. Pressure should be equal bilaterally with these movements. Assess the pulses at the wrist (radial) or the feet (pedal) and compare bilaterally.

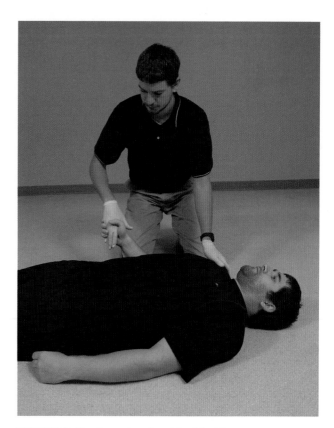

FIGURE 8.10   Squeezing the athlete's hands.

Secondary Assessment for an Athlete with a Medical Condition

In the preceding section, the assessment was conducted on an athlete suffering from a traumatic event. Athletes may also suffer from nontraumatic medical events, such as hypoglycemia or epilepsy. The secondary survey for these individuals is similar to that in the case of trauma, but instead of focusing on traumatic injuries, the secondary survey for a medical event focuses on the illness or medical condition necessitating the emergency care and response (Algorithm 8.3). In addition, the secondary assessment in such a case will also differ slightly depending on whether the athlete is conscious or unconscious. Regardless of the athlete's responsiveness, detailed information must be obtained in order to provide proper care. Before initiating the secondary assessment of an athlete with a medical condition, it is prudent to first survey the scene, conduct an initial assessment, and then proceed to the examination.

Assessment of a Conscious Athlete

In most circumstances, the athlete will be responsive and a detailed history can be obtained to help determine the nature of the medical condition and its causes. During the history, pay close attention to the responses and condition of the athlete before deciding on the appropriate medical referral (either immediately, after the secondary assessment, or not at all). When asking about the **chief complaint,** the athletic trainer may use the OPQRST acronym to guide the questions and help specify the problem[4] (Table 8.3). In addition to OPQRST, the athletic trainer must detail the examination further by obtaining a SAMPLE history (Table 8.4). Both of these examination methods will allow the athletic trainer to be sure the majority of possible conditions have been covered for a full medical history. In fact, these methods can also be used for nonemergency responses to athletes with injuries or illnesses in the athletic training setting.

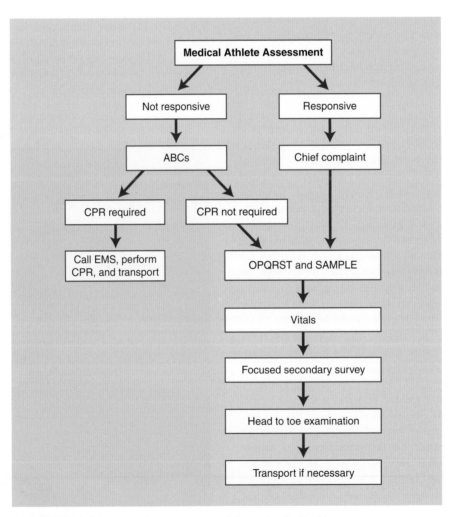

ALGORITHM 8.3   Secondary assessment of the medically ill athlete.

TABLE 8.3   OPQRST History Procedures

Acronym	Significance	What Questions to Ask
O—Onset	Determines when the athlete began having symptoms.	What happened? When did you first notice your symptoms?
P—Provocation	Determines what factors may have caused the problem/condition.	Please describe what you were doing when you first noticed your symptoms. Are there any actions that increase or decrease your current symptoms?
Q—Quality	Determines the characteristics and quality of the symptoms the athlete is experiencing.	Please describe your symptoms.
R—Radiation/ region/relief	Determines whether the symptoms experienced by the athlete are felt elsewhere, where they may be located, and what makes the athlete feel better.	Do you have any symptoms elsewhere from your chief complain? Do your symptoms appear to be moving up or down related body parts? Where exactly are your symptoms? What makes your symptoms feel better?
S—Severity	Determines how severe the illness is—useful to know when describing the symptoms.	Please rate your pain on a scale from 1 to 10, with 10 being the most severe pain.
T—Time	Determines the time when the illness or condition occurred and for how long the athlete has been experiencing the symptoms.	Do you remember when your symptoms began?

TABLE 8.4   SAMPLE History Procedures

Acronym	Significance	What Questions to Ask
S—Signs and symptoms	Determines what the athlete feels and provides the athletic trainer with clues as to the extent and type of condition/illness.	Can you describe your chief complaint? What makes it feel better/worse? What body part is affected?
A—Allergies	Determines if there are medications or environmental factors that may have caused the illness/condition.	Are you taking any medications? Have you been bitten by anything? Are you allergic to anything?
M—Medications	Determines whether the athlete is currently taking prescribed medications or if medications were used that may have caused the condition. It is also important to survey the scene and look for medications in the vicinity. If medications are found, record the type/dose taken or obtain a sample for further analysis if necessary.	Are you taking any medications? Did you swallow or contact something?
P—Past medical history	Determines what conditions or illnesses the athlete may have had in the past that may be related to current symptoms.	What medical conditions have you had in the past? Could any of these be related to what you have now? Who is your regular physician?
L—Last oral intake	Determines what medications or other substances the athlete may have ingested.	Have you taken anything by mouth recently? When was the last time you ate or drank?
E—Events	Determines all events and actions leading up to the athlete's current condition and symptoms.	What were you doing when you experienced your symptoms? How long were you doing this?

Assessment of an Unconscious Athlete

Assessment of the unconscious medical patient is very similar to that of the unconscious trauma patient. However, a detailed history may not be obtainable; therefore, the course of action is to conduct a rapid secondary assessment, check vital signs, perform a SAMPLE examination, and then transport the patient to a medical facility. While the rapid secondary assessment is being conducted, it is imperative that the athletic trainer look for a medical alert bracelet on the athlete, either at the wrist or around the neck. Usually, athletes with medical illnesses or conditions wear such a bracelet to ensure proper treatment in the event of an emergency during which they may become unresponsive or unconscious. If, during the examination, as with all physical examinations, the athletic trainer discovers a condition that needs immediate attention, provide the appropriate care before proceeding on to the next part of the head-to-toe evaluation.

TABLE 8.5	Time Line for Ongoing Assessment
Time Interval for Assessment	**Athlete's Condition**
Every 15 minutes	Alert and responsive
	Normal vitals
	No apparent serious injury or medical condition
Every 5 minutes	Altered mental status
	Difficulty with ABCs
	Uncontrolled bleeding or severe blood loss
	Serious physical trauma or medical condition

REPEATING THE INITIAL ASSESSMENT

After the initial evaluation to determine life-threatening injuries and the secondary assessment to examine and identify other signs of trauma or conditions that warrant immediate medical attention (as addressed in Chapter 8), a third process called the "ongoing assessment" ensures the athlete's stability while treatment is rendered or while the athlete is transported to a medical facility. The ongoing assessment is a seldom-considered part of the management plan of an athlete in the athletic training setting, but there are many circumstances in which a stable athlete can become unstable over time (e.g., hypoglycemia, compound fractures, head injuries). As with the initial and secondary assessments, the information gathered in the ongoing assessment should be documented and may be used by other medical personnel if the athlete suddenly becomes unstable.[5] In addition, the ongoing assessment should always be repeated periodically, especially in the case of life-threatening conditions.

Rarely does an athlete fully recover from trauma or medical illness in an emergency situation when en route to a medical facility, although stabilization can sometimes be achieved (see Fig. 1.15). On the other hand, an athlete can deteriorate rapidly over the course of an evaluation, even with the appropriate interventions; therefore, the athletic trainer must be prepared to manage an athlete in these circumstances and must know how to monitor him or her and identify possible changes in condition. It is often recommended that the ongoing assessment be repeated about every 5 minutes for a high-priority or unstable athlete (Table 8.5) and every 10 to 15 minutes for a stable or low-priority athlete.[6] If time permits, more frequent reassessment of the athlete is acceptable and encouraged. As with

the secondary assessment procedures, the athletic trainer should communicate to the athlete in a courteous manner, maintain eye contact where appropriate, and do what is possible to reassure the athlete and thus to decrease his or her anxiety. In this chapter, we focus on how to properly perform an ongoing assessment for athletes waiting to be transported, in the process of transportation to the medical facility, or being managed on site for a long period of time.

The ongoing assessment is essentially a repetition of the initial rapid assessment, where the ABCs are determined (Algorithm 8.4). This also includes baseline vital signs and the reexamination of areas that may have been considered speculative, such as fracture sites, head injuries, and bleeding or additional trauma or changes in the athlete's condition. In addition, if emergency devices were employed, such as splints or neck collars, they should also be reexamined to make sure that circulation and stability are maintained.

Mental Status

The first aspect to reexamine is the athlete's mental status (Fig. 8.2). As with the initial rapid assessment, the acronym AVPU should be used to reassess the athlete and determine whether any changes have occurred since the initiation of management. Head injuries and bleeding within the skull may take time to cause symptoms. Also, in exertional heat illness, a reduction in core temperature will improve mental status. Reexamining the mental status may alert the athletic trainer to changes in symptoms that were not apparent during the initial and secondary assessments. If the athlete's metal status is altered, provide the appropriate care as needed, based upon the symptoms, and arrange for immediate transport of the athlete if this is not already in process.

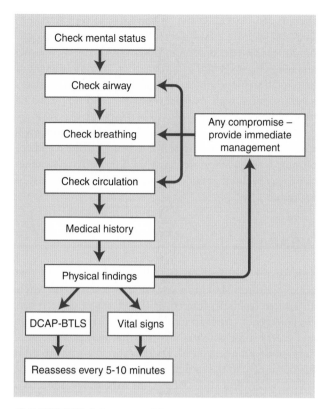

ALGORITHM 8.4   Steps of the ongoing assessment.

Airway

After checking the athlete's mental status, examine the airway to make sure it is still open and **unobstructed** (see Chapter 10 for equipment removal procedures). An athlete who is unconscious and breathing without effort during the initial assessment can develop an obstruction and may quickly do so (e.g., when the tongue falls back into the throat or from **vomitus** in the airway). Removal of foreign matter (blood, secretions, and vomitus) using a finger sweep or adjunct breathing device (or suction if trained to do so; see Chapter 11) and head-tilt/jaw-thrust procedures to open the airway may be needed based on the mechanism of injury/nature of illness. If an oropharyngeal or nasopharyngeal airway was inserted, check its placement to make sure that it is still functioning correctly and determine whether it is still needed. If the athlete is being artificially ventilated with a bag-valve-mask device or resuscitation mask, make sure that there is no resistance and that the chest is rising and falling adequately.

Breathing

After confirming that the airway is open, the athletic trainer should look, listen, and feel for adequate breathing. This means noting the presence of breaths as well as their rate and depth; unusual sounds should also be noted, preferably with a stethoscope (see Chapter 10 for use of the stetho-

scope) (Fig. 8.7). Changes in the breathing pattern—such as poor quality and rate (increase or decrease)—can indicate a pathology or condition not directly observed in the initial assessment. Actions to correct abnormal breathing, such as the use of artificial ventilation with supplemental oxygen, must be readjusted and/or readministered with immediate transportation to the medical facility (see Chapter 10 on breathing emergencies).

Circulation

After examining breathing, checking the circulation is the next step. Reexamine areas where bleeding was found in the initial or secondary assessments to determine whether the bleeding has been controlled, slowed, or stopped. If the bandages used to control bleeding are soaked, add additional layers to the area without removing the old bandages. If you notice bleeding that was overlooked initially, control the bleeding with the appropriate techniques (see Chapter 14). Also reexamine the body carefully for signs of internal bleeding, such as discoloration in the abdominal and flank areas of the body; this may be indicative of an internal injury that was initially noted.

Check the rate and quality of the pulse at the wrist and foot and check capillary refill at the fingers and toes (Fig. 8.4). An increase in pulse rate with poor quality may suggest continued bleeding, most notably internal bleeding if there are no observable signs. A decrease in pulse rate and improvement in the overall condition of an athlete whose pulse was initially high is suggestive of improved breathing and circulation. Notice the temperature and overall color of the skin compared with the initial and secondary assessment documentation. Skin that becomes cool and clammy indicates shock; warm and discolored skin may indicate swelling and internal injuries. Changes in the circulation and uncontrolled bleeding are a high priority; in such cases, transportation will be required. Skin color and temperature that return to normal indicate improvement.

ONGOING ASSESSMENT: HISTORY AND PHYSICAL EXAMINATION

Medical History

After completing reexamination of the vital signs, the athletic trainer should ask again about the injury/illness and repeat a physical assessment, such as SAMPLE. Occasionally, when the athletic trainer questions an athlete about an injury or medical condition, the athlete may not be able to provide all details or may forget some of the details; also, his or her physical condition or symptoms may change during the assessment. When completing the secondary assessment, the athletic trainer should repeat the history questions again to confirm earlier findings or to make sure that all subsequent changes have been reported by the athlete. Many times, the shock of the trauma or medical condition or the unfamiliarity of the site will confuse the athlete or prevent him or her from thinking clearly. A review of the medical history will also allow the athletic trainer to ensure that the treatment or management procedures are correct. In those cases where the athlete's circumstances have changed, it may be necessary to revise the management procedures or decision to transport.

Physical Exam

After conducting another medical history, the athletic trainer should perform another physical examination over the entire body of the athlete, using the DCAP-BTLS procedures, and compare these findings with the initial findings of the secondary assessment.[7] This procedure should take only a few minutes, but changes in the physical findings may occur because signs of injury or medical pathologies can develop over time. Again, changes should be documented, managed if necessary, and any new information assessed to determine priority and transportation to a medical facility.

INTERVENTIONS

After reexamination of the ABCs, physical exam, and medical history, determine whether the planned interventions remain appropriate. Ensure adequate delivery of adjunct breathing devices, bleeding control, cardiac management, spinal and joint immobilization, and management of hyperthermia. To determine the effectiveness of your interventions, ask yourself questions such as: Has there been an improvement or deterioration in vital signs? Is the chest rising and falling as it should? Has there been an improvement or deterioration in the athlete's mental status? Has the athlete's color improved with artificial ventilation and supplemental oxygen?

If improvements are not noted, the athletic trainer will have to reconsider the interventions being provided and determine whether they are being used properly or whether there may be another underlying injury/illness that must be addressed.

WRAP-UP

This chapter focused on the steps and procedures that athletic trainers should follow on arrival at a scene where an athlete has been injured or is suffering from a medical emergency. Always approach the scene with caution and survey it for potential hazards that may pose a risk of harm to everyone involved. Try to secure the scene to limit further injury to the athlete and to safeguard the athletic trainer when providing care. If the athlete has suffered a traumatic injury, perform a rapid initial assessment, followed by a more focused secondary assessment to discover potential injuries/conditions, life-threatening or not. If the athlete has a medical issue, follow the same procedures with a more focused examination of his or her medical history and conditions that might have caused the event. By following the practices outlined in this chapter, the athletic trainer can implement the appropriate steps and techniques to examine and treat an athlete involved in an emergency situation.

Scenarios

1. As an athletic trainer, you are working a high school wrestling meet on a Saturday. You have been fairly busy caring for bloody noses, bruises, and a dislocated finger. However, one wrestler suddenly collapses against a wall. His brother, Tom, who is on the same team, summons you to the area. Tom states that his brother had not eaten all day because he wanted to be sure to make his weight class. You are also told that the wrestler is a diabetic.

   Based upon what you have learned, what should be your course of action?

2. As the athletic trainer, you are summoned for immediate care for a downed cross-country runner a mile away. You take your motorized cart across the field to where you've been told she is lying. As you approach, you notice several people flagging you down. Upon arrival, you notice the runner flat on her back with other runners dashing by as the meet continues.

   What is your first course of action?

3. An athlete has suffered a head injury while playing volleyball. You have just finished your rapid initial assessment and all secondary assessments. The athlete has been securely attached to a spine board for transportation to the hospital. As you wait for emergency medical services to arrive, another person notices that the athlete's lips have a bluish tint. It is then apparent that the athlete has stopped breathing and rescue breathing is successfully initiated.

   What should the athletic trainer have done in this situation?

4. While an athlete is being transported, you notice that his level of consciousness has changed. However, during the initial assessment, the athletic trainer who was providing care did not record any information on the athlete's loss of consciousness.

   What should have been done to control this situation?

REFERENCES

1. Kelly CA, Upex A, Bateman DN. Comparison of consciousness level assessment in the poisoned patient using the alert/verbal/painful/unresponsive scale and the Glasgow coma scale. *Ann Emerg Med.* 2004;44:108–113.

2. McNarry AF, Goldhill DR. Simple bedside assessment of level of consciousness: Comparison of two simple assessment scales with the Glasgow coma scale. *Anaesthesia.* 2004;59:34–37.

3. Perkins G, Walker G, Christensen K, et al. Teaching recognition of agonal breathing improves accuracy of diagnosing cardiac arrest. *Resuscitation.* 2006;70(3):423–437.

4. Beevers G, Lip G, O'Brien E. ABC of hypertension: Blood pressure measurement. *Br Med J.* 2007;322:981–985.

5. Flegel MJ. *Sport First Aid: A Coach's Guide to Preventing and Responding to Injuries,* 3rd ed. Champaign, IL: Human Kinetics; 2004.

6. Beebe R, Funk D. *Fundamentals of Emergency Care.* Albany, NY: Delmar Thomas Learning; 2001.

7. Limmer D, O'Keefe MF. *Emergency Care,* 10th ed. Upper Saddle River, NJ: Prentice Hall; 2005.

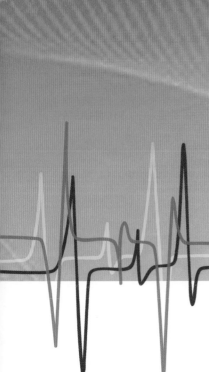

CHAPTER 9

Assessment of Vital Signs

CHAPTER OUTCOMES

1. Describe the vital signs commonly assessed by athletic trainers during prehospital emergency care of an ill or injured athlete.

2. Identify and describe the methods to obtain commonly used vital signs in athletic training, including (a) pulse rate; (b) respiration rate; (c) blood pressure (palpation and auscultation); (d) skin temperature, condition, and color; (e) capillary refill; and (f) pupils.

3. Demonstrate the ability to obtain and document commonly used vital signs in athletic training, including (a) pulse rate; (b) respiration rate; (c) blood pressure (palpation and auscultation); (d) skin temperature, condition, and color; (e) capillary refill; and (f) pupils.

4. Recognize and describe normal and abnormal vital sign values when assessing the following: (a) pulse rate; (b) respiration rate; (c) blood pressure (palpation and auscultation); (d) skin temperature, condition, and color; (e) capillary refill; and (f) pupils.

NOMENCLATURE

Agonal breathing: irregular gasping or shallow breathing, a common sign of the early stages of cardiac arrest, suggesting that death is imminent

Anisocoria: a condition in which the two pupils are not of equal size

Apnea: cessation of breathing—a life-threatening condition if left untreated

Apneustic breathing: abnormal respiratory pattern consisting of a pause at full inspiration

Arteriolosclerosis: often referred to as "hardening of the arteries"—occurs when plaque accumulates along the arterial wall, resulting in a loss of elasticity of the affected artery

Atherosclerosis: a condition where fatty substances, cholesterol, cellular waste, calcium, and other substances collect along the inner lining of an artery, resulting in a narrowing of the vessel

Atrial fibrillation: rapid, irregular twitching of the heart's muscular wall, causing the ventricles to respond irregularly

Baseline vital signs: initial set of objective measurements of pulse, respiration, blood pressure, skin, and pupils as a means of assessing general health and cardiorespiratory function

Biot breathing sign: irregular breathing pattern, with a continually varying rate and depth of breathing

Bradycardia: slowness of the heartbeat, usually at less than 60 beats per minute

Bradypnea: abnormally slow respiration, at less 10 breaths per minute; commonly occurs before apnea

Cheyne–Stokes respiration: breathing pattern with a gradual increase in depth and sometimes in rate to a maximum, followed by a decrease resulting in apnea; cycles ordinarily are 30 seconds to 2 minutes in duration, with 5 to 30 seconds of apnea

Cyanosis: dark bluish or purplish coloration of the skin, nail beds, lips, or mucous membranes due to deficient oxygenation of the blood

Dyspnea: shortness of breath, a subjective difficulty or distress in breathing, usually associated with disease of the heart or lungs; occurs normally during intense physical exertion or at high altitude

Diabetic ketoacidosis: state of inadequate insulin levels resulting in increased blood sugar levels and accumulation of organic acids and ketones in the blood

Diaphoretic: relating to or causing perspiration

Eccrine gland: coiled tubular sweat gland (other than apocrine glands) located in the skin on almost all parts of the body

Hypertension stage 1: high blood pressure; generally established guidelines are values of 140 to 159 mm Hg systolic and 90 to 99 mm Hg diastolic blood pressure

Hypertension stage 2: high blood pressure; generally established guidelines are values of 160 mm Hg and above systolic and 100 mm Hg and above diastolic blood pressure

Hypotension: subnormal arterial blood pressure

Hypothermia: body temperature significantly below 98.6°F (37°C)

Interstitial fluid: fluid in spaces between the tissue cells, constituting about 16% of the weight of the body; closely similar in composition to lymph

Jaundice: yellowish staining of the integument, sclera, and deeper tissues and the excretions with bile pigments, which are increased in the plasma

Kussmaul respiration: deep, rapid respiration as the body attempts to lower the acid levels that occur in diabetic ketoacidosis

Pulse: palpable, rhythmic expansion of an artery, produced by the increased volume of blood forced into the vessel by the contraction of the heart

Pulse points: areas of the body where major arteries are located close to the skin's surface and lie directly over a bone, allowing for easy palpation of the pressure wave caused by the contraction of the heart

Respiration: fundamental process of life wherein oxygen oxidizes molecules of organic fuel, thus generating energy as well as by-products such as carbon dioxide and water

Respiration rate: frequency of breathing, recorded as the number of breaths per minute

Sympathetic nervous system: the branch of the autonomic nervous system that promotes heightened awareness, increased consumption of nutrients, and other changes associated with the "fight-or-flight" reaction, including increased heart rate and respiration, cold and pale skin, dilated pupils, and raised blood pressure

Tachycardia: Rapid beating of the heart, conventionally applied to rates of more than 100 per minute

Tachypnea: rapid breathing, greater than normal values for an age group

Thready pulse: a weak, fine pulse, feeling like a small cord or thread under the fingers

Ventilation: replacement of air or other gas in a space by fresh air or gas

Wheezing: whistling, squeaking, musical, or puffing sound, seen in individuals suffering from asthma or bronchiolitis, made by air passing through the space between the cavity of the mouth and the pharynx, epiglottis, or narrowed tracheobronchial airways during exhalation

BEFORE YOU BEGIN

1. What are baseline vital signs? Why are they so important to an athletic trainer during an emergency?

2. What is the difference between pulse rate, strength, and rhythm? Where are the pulse points in a conscious adult and child?

3. What is the difference between respiratory rate, rhythm, and effort? Describe how to assess respiratory rate in an ill or injured athlete.

4. Identify and discuss the four categories of respiratory effort.

5. What does "skin CTC" stand for? What are the differences between these categories?

6. An athlete whose blood is poorly oxygenated will present with what sort of skin color? Why?

7. What does skin turgor indicate? Describe how this assessment is performed.

8. Discuss and demonstrate how to assess pupil shape and size, equality, and reactivity.

9. Define blood pressure. What is the difference between systolic and diastolic blood pressure?

10. Discuss the difference between blood pressure assessment via palpation and auscultation.

Voices from the Field

The athletic trainer of a team is responsible not only for the athletes but also the staff. The accurate assessment of vital signs in any emergency is imperative. A prehospital evaluation requires the athletic trainer to be able to examine breathing, pulse, pupils, and blood pressure. This will determine any further actions by the athletic trainer.

Fortunately, the taking of vital signs is not a daily occurrence; but for that reason it requires periodic refreshing of all procedures. This can be set up on a schedule, so that everyone will have an idea as to when it will occur.

Being able to measure vital signs at any time is important when one is traveling with a team. This past Summer League, I was awakened at 3:00 A.M. by a staff member saying his heart was racing. I took his pulse, which was 160 bpm, and checked his blood pressure, which was normal. I also questioned him and found out that he had been awakened at 1:00 A.M. by an urgent phone call.

After calming him down I rechecked his pulse, and it had slowed to 84 bpm. He was seen by our team physician and told he needed to be defibrillated to settle his pulse back to normal. This was done successfully, and he was told it was caused by a number of factors.

I have also been asked, at our preseason physicals, to recheck a player's blood pressure after a high reading was detected by our physician. This was done and reported daily until either it returned to a normal range or the player was removed from practice for further testing.

I always hope I won't have to take any vital signs, but I am always prepared to do so.

Gary Briggs, LAT, ATC, PES, CES, IMT
Head Athletic Trainer
Utah Jazz
Salt Lake City, Utah

In Chapter 8 we discussed the steps involved in the primary and secondary assessments of an ill or injured athlete. As you may remember, the primary assessment included (a) forming a general impression, (b) assessing the level of consciousness, (c) assessing the airway, (d) assessing breathing, and (e) assessing circulation. The secondary assessment included a physical examination (head to toe, or focused) and SAMPLE history. The type of athlete managed and the nature of the condition determined whether the physical examination or SAMPLE came first (Fig. 9.1). However, a quick but thorough evaluation of **baseline vital signs** such as pulse, respiration, and blood pressure is also a necessary component of the secondary assessment as well as the ongoing assessment. During the secondary assessment, vital signs are used to further establish the condition of the athlete and, after the necessary medical interventions have been implemented, to determine whether this condition is improving or deteriorating. This chapter describes in detail a variety of normal and abnormal baseline vital signs commonly utilized by athletic trainers when responding to an emergency. The techniques described in this chapter are commonly used by athletic trainers not only during emergencies but also in everyday practice. However, in situations where an athletic trainer does not utilize these skills on a regular basis, we strongly recommend reviewing and practicing these skills in order to maintain clinical competence.

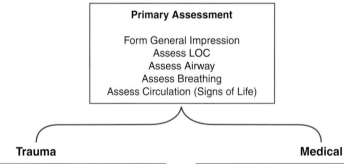

FIGURE 9.1   Review of primary and secondary assessment procedures. LOC, level of care; MOI, mechanism of injury.

VITAL SIGNS

Vital signs are indicators of the body's most basic physiological functions (e.g., breathing and heartbeat); their measurement by athletic trainers as well as many other health care professionals helps to determine the relative stability of these functions during an emergency. Because vital signs can reflect changes in the respiratory, circulatory, or neurological systems, they are often used to evaluate an individual's general condition, identify any potential threats to life that may compromise the delivery of oxygen to the brain and other vital organs, and determine whether the interventions provided during an emergency were effective. The four main vital signs routinely monitored by athletic trainers and health care professionals include (a) pulse rate, (b) respiration rate, (c) blood pressure, and (d) skin color, temperature, and condition. However, vital signs such as capillary refill (in children) and pupillary reflex/reaction are also indicators of the status of the respiratory, circulatory, and neurological systems.

It should be noted that normative vital sign values can and do change with a person's age, fitness level, level of anxiety, and medical condition. In fact, in some well-trained athletes, what would be considered abnormal in the general population is actually normal. For example, a resting pulse rate of 80 to 90 beats per minute in an endurance athlete might be considered abnormal because many well-conditioned endurance athletes have a resting pulse rate between 40 and 60 beats per minute.[1] This is why it is critical to review the preparticipation physical examinations prior to an athletic event in order to identify the normal rate in such an individual.[2]

Baseline Vital Signs

The first vital signs recorded during the secondary assessment are called the baseline vital signs. Baseline vital signs establish the athlete's normative values for the current situation and offer a starting point for the athletic trainer to determine whether there has been any compromise to the body's physiological functions. By comparing normative vital sign data against those of the athlete during an emergency, the athletic trainer can determine significant problems involving the cardiovascular or respiratory systems and provide appropriate care to minimize the risk of further injury. Baseline vital signs should be assessed as soon as possible on the uninjured side, but *not* before providing care for life-threatening situations. Be sure to document the findings either on paper or on the athletic trainer's gloved hand in order to avoid the loss of data.

Quantitative Versus Qualitative Vital Signs

Vital signs provide quantitative and/or qualitative data. Quantitative data provides objective measurements of the athlete's condition by measuring the number of times (i.e., rate) an athlete breathes or his or her heart beats; this data can then be compared with normal ranges for the person's age and medical condition, as discussed later in this chapter. Qualitative data assess the rhythm and strength of these biological functions (e.g., the strength of the pulse). For example, when assessing the pulse, the rate (number of times the heart beats) may be 136 beats per minute, with an irregular rhythm and poor strength (i.e., a **thready pulse**), suggesting that the athlete may be in shock.

Ongoing Assessment of Vital Signs

Vital signs will have to be reevaluated periodically in order to determine whether an intervention or medication is having the desired effect. Pulse, respiration, and blood pressure as well as skin color, temperature, and condition are reassessed during the ongoing assessment and are compared with the documented baseline vital signs assessed during the secondary assessment. Stable athletes should be reassessed approximately every 15 minutes, whereas an unstable athlete should be reassessed approximately every 5 minutes to make sure that his or her condition has not worsened.

PULSE

The **pulse** is defined as the "palpable rhythmic expansion of an artery, produced by the increased volume of blood thrown into the vessel by the contraction of the heart,"[3] reflecting the rate, rhythm, and strength of the heart's contractions. Restated, the heart is a pulsating pump that pushes blood intermittently into the arterial system in order to provide blood and oxygen to the rest of the body.[4] Assessment of the pulse rate requires the identification of **pulse points** or areas where the major arteries are very close to the skin's surface and lie directly over a bone. These pulse points allow for easier palpation of the pressure wave created by the beating heart (Fig. 9.2). The following section discusses and demonstrates how to properly assess this vital sign.

Locating the Pulse

Radial Pulse

The athlete's age and whether he or she is responsive or unresponsive will determine where an athletic trainer should locate the pulse. In an individual over 1 year of age (child or adult) who is responsive (i.e., has a pulse and is conscious), the radial artery at the wrist will be the point of contact. To locate the pulse, place your index and middle fingers perpendicular to the distal end of the anterior forearm on the radial or thumb side of the wrist (Fig. 9.3). Gently press down on the artery located between the flexor carpi radialis and brachioradialis tendon, looking for an intermittent pulse wave or pulsation. Note the rate, rhythm, and quality of the pulse. Be sure you are not using your thumb because the thumb has its own pulse. Also do not press too hard because this will cause the artery to collapse.

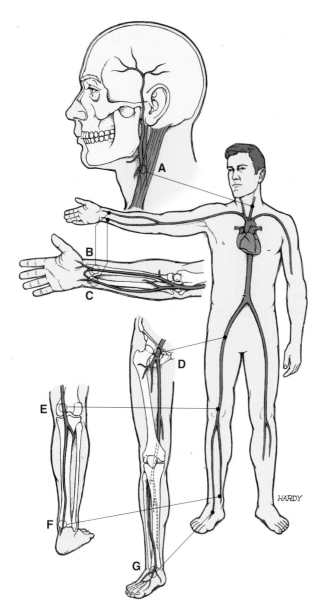

FIGURE 9.2   Pulse points in the human body. A = Carotid, B = Radial, C = Ulnar, D = Femoral, E = Popliteal, F = Posterior tibial, G = Dorsalis pedis.

Carotid Pulse

In an individual over 1 year of age (child or adult) who is unresponsive (unconscious), use the carotid artery located between the trachea and the sternocleidomastoid muscle as the pulse point. To locate the carotid pulse, kneel perpendicular to the athlete and place your index and middle fingers on the midline of the throat at approximately the thyroid cartilage (Adam's apple). Gently slide your fingers downward until they rest in the groove between the trachea and sternocleidomastoid (Fig. 9.4). Although the pulse can be located on either side of the neck, we recommend locating it on the side from which you are evaluating. Also, because the carotid artery is a central artery and is fed directly from the

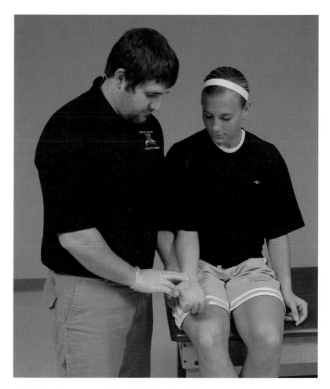

FIGURE 9.3   Locating the radial pulse in a conscious adult or child.

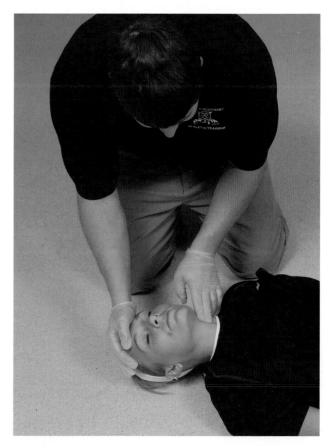

FIGURE 9.4   Locating the carotid pulse in an unconscious adult or child.

TABLE 9.1	Measuring the Pulse Rate	
Technique	**Formula**	**Pulse Rate Example**
15 seconds	Beats × 4	15 beats × 4 = 60 beats/min
30 seconds	Beats × 2	30 beats × 2 = 60 beats/min
60 seconds	Beats × 1	60 beats × 1 = 60 beats/min

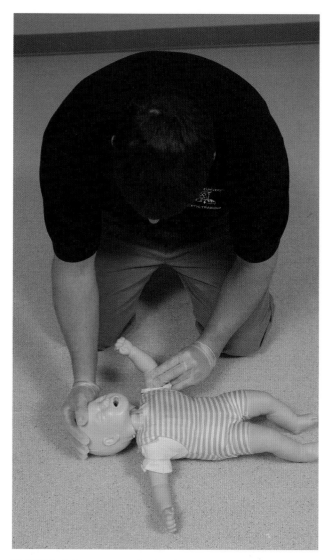

FIGURE 9.5 Locating the brachial pulse in an unconscious infant.

Brachial Pulse

In individuals under 1 year of age, the radial and carotid arteries are difficult to locate; therefore, the brachial artery is used to assess the pulse. To locate the brachial pulse, place the infant supine and rotate the arm to a 90-degree position to expose the inner arm; then place your index and middle fingers perpendicular to the midshaft of the upper arm. Gently compress two fingers (index and middle) between the triceps and short head of the biceps and coracobrachialis (Fig. 9.5), compressing the artery against the humerus.

Assessing the Pulse

Pulse Rate

Once the appropriate pulse point has been located, it will be necessary to determine the pulse rate, or the number of times the heart beats per minute (recorded as beats/min or bpm). Several techniques exist to determine pulse rate, and all require either a digital watch or an analog watch with a second hand. These techniques include recording the number of beats for 15, 30, or 60 seconds. At the end of the counting interval, multiply the number of heartbeats recorded by the factors found in Table 9.1. In situations where the rhythm or quality of the pulse is poor, where it is difficult to locate, or the athlete is **hypothermic,** assessing the pulse for 30 to 45 seconds is recommended.[5,6]

Normal Pulse Rates   In adults, the normal pulse rate is between 60 and 100 beats per minute. In children, the normal rate is between 70 and 130; in infants, it is between 140 and 160. Individuals who participate in regular vigorous or strenuous physical activity will normally present with markedly lower pulse rates as a result of morphological, functional, and electrophysiological changes in cardiac structure and function

aorta, it may provide more information relative to the status of the cardiovascular system than a peripheral (i.e., radial or brachial) pulse. Finally, remember that the carotid artery supplies the brain with oxygenated blood, so applying too much pressure for too long or to both arteries simultaneously can reduce blood flow to the brain, potentially resulting in serious harm to the athlete.

Current Research

Only Time Will Tell Which Method Best Assesses Pulse Rate

Research suggests that use of the 30-second count is more accurate in predicting 1-minute resting radial pulse rates in adults, as opposed to 15-, 30-, and 60-second counts.[4,7] Hwu et al.[4] further suggest that a 15- or 30-second count could be used to predict the 1-minute resting pulse when the pulse rate is counted from 1. However, Hollerbach and Sneed[7] suggest that in those with a pulse rate above 100 beats per minute, the 15-second counting interval should not be used.

TABLE 9.2	Normal Pulse Rates for Different Age Groups
Age (years)	Range (beats/min)
Birth to 1	140 to 160
1 to 3	80 to 130
3 to 5	80 to 120
6 to 12	70 to 110
13 to 18	55 to 105
19 to 40	60 to 100
41 to 60	70 to 100
>60	Dependent on health status

due to training.[8,9] Individuals with this condition, known as the athletic heart syndrome, may present with **bradycardia** and pulse rates ranging from 35 to 50 beats per minute. Additionally, medications such as beta blockers affect the **sympathetic nervous system,** acting to decrease vital signs such as pulse rate and blood pressure. Other factors affecting pulse rate include (a) degree of exercise just completed, (b) medical condition, (c) blood loss, (d) stress, (e) body temperature, and (f) fear and anxiety. Normative values for pulse rate by age group may be found in Table 9.2.[6]

Abnormal Pulse Rates   In an adult, a rapid heartbeat—that is, a rate above 100 beats per minute—is referred to as **tachycardia**. It can result in the inadequate delivery of blood to various parts of the body because the heart's chambers cannot fill adequately between contractions. However, in an athletic environment, it is expected that athletes will have a heart rate greater than 100 beats per minute if they are engaged in athletic competition; this should not be confused with the condition of a tachycardic patient who has been sitting in a chair for an expended period of time; such a situation would constitute a possible medical emergency. Tachycardia can be caused by hypoperfusion (shock), bleeding, heat illness, dehydration, fever, pain, and anxiety and must be documented (e.g., "pulse is 100, rapid, and thready") and will often require advanced medical care.

Bradycardia, on the other hand, is defined as slowness of the heartbeat, usually a rate less than 60 beats per minute in adults and 100 beats per minute in infants. It can be caused by issues such as heart disease and medications and can result in fatigue, weakness, dizziness, light-headedness, or fainting due to inadequate perfusion of the brain.

Pulse Quality

Once the pulse rate has been established, it will be necessary to determine and document the quality of the heartbeat, including its rhythm and strength. Both rhythm and strength are assessed by maintaining the index and middle fingers over the same pulse point used to determine pulse rate.

Rhythm   Pulse rhythm examines the evenness of an individual's pulse. A pulse can be either regular or irregular (Fig. 9.6). A regular pulse (normal) can be rapid or slow; however, the interval between each contraction of the heart's ventricle remains constant. In an irregular pulse, the beats are unsteady and/or uneven. The athlete may experience missed beats or extra beats, or the interval between beats may be irregular and unpredictable. Any individual presenting with an irregular pulse and signs and symptoms of a cardiovascular disorder requires referral to more advanced medical care as quickly as possible. An irregular pulse may be due to a condition known as **atrial fibrillation** (AF), which involves rapid, irregular twitching of the heart's muscular wall, causing the ventricles to respond irregularly. It is a major risk factor for stroke.

Strength   Pulse strength examines the force of the pulse as the blood is forced into the artery by the heartbeat. A normal pulse will be regular or strong. Otherwise, the individual may present with a pulse that is either bounding, weak (thready), or absent (Table 9.3).

When strength and rhythm are paired, the athletic trainer may recognize a pulse that is:

1. Rapid and strong, resulting from early stages of shock, overexertion, fright, anxiety, heat illness, diabetic emergency (hyperglycemia), or fever
2. Rapid and weak, resulting from internal bleeding, later stages of shock, heat illness, diabetic emergency (hypoglycemia), or a failing circulatory system

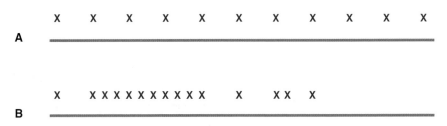

FIGURE 9.6   Regular versus irregular pulse rhythm. **A** demonstrates the heart beating at regular intervals, indicated by the X. **B** demonstrates the heart beating at irregular intervals, also indicated by the X.

TABLE 9.3   Abnormal Pulse Strength

Pulse Observation	Identification	Cause
Bounding	A strong, forceful pulse due to large amounts of blood being pumped with each heartbeat.	Heavy exercise, pregnancy, fever, high anxiety, fluid overload (e.g., congestive heart failure)
Weak	A pulse that is difficult to detect owing to decreased amounts of blood flowing through the arteries.	Bleeding, shock, heat illness, diabetic emergency, failing circulatory system
Absent	No pulse detected.	Blocked or injured artery, low blood pressure, lack of heart electrical signal (cardiac arrest)

3. Slow and strong, resulting from a stroke, skull fracture, or brain trauma
4. No pulse, normally suggesting cardiac arrest (Chapter 12)

RESPIRATION

Respiration is a fundamental process of life, whereby oxygen is used to oxidize organic fuel molecules, providing a source of energy as well as producing by-products such as carbon dioxide and water. The respiratory system (i.e., the lungs) is responsible for ensuring an adequate exchange between oxygen and carbon dioxide, a waste product from the red blood cells, through the process of **ventilation** (i.e., breathing). The movement of oxygen and carbon dioxide into and out of the lungs consists of the actions of inhalation and exhalation (Fig. 9.7). Inhalation is an active process that draws in oxygen (causing the chest to rise); it depends upon the action of the muscular system under the direct control of the nervous system. Exhalation is a passive process (causing the chest to fall), which blows off the carbon dioxide exchanged at the alveoli. Together, one rise and one fall of the chest equals one breath. The frequency of breathing, recorded as the number of breaths per minute, is called the **respiration rate.**

The following section discusses and demonstrates how to properly assess the vital sign respiration.

Assessing Respirations

Assessment of an individual's respiratory status requires evaluation of the respiration rate and the quality of the breaths. However, the general status of the respiratory system (whether the athlete is breathing at all) is first evaluated as part of the primary assessment. This includes observation of the chest in order to answer the follow questions:

1. Does the chest rise and fall, evenly or unevenly?
2. Do you feel or hear an exchange of air through the nose and mouth, noting any obstructions?

3. Do you hear breath sounds when you are auscultating each lung with a stethoscope?

Respiration Rate

Respiration rate is the frequency or the number of times a person breathes (one cycle of inspiration and expiration) in 1 minute. As when assessing pulse rate, the athletic trainer will have to count the number of breath cycles for 30 seconds and then multiply this by 2 to determine the number of breaths per minute. This too requires the use

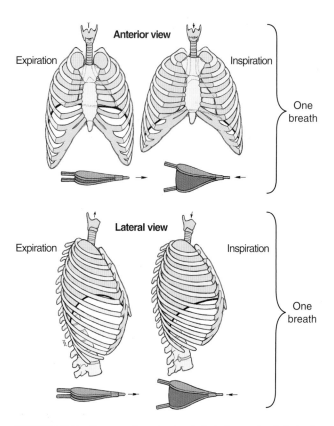

FIGURE 9.7   Process of respiration (inhalation and exhalation). Respiration at expiration: volume is low so pressure is high, causing air to leave lungs to equalize pressure. Respiration at inspiration: volume is high so pressure is low, causing air to enter lungs to equalize pressure.

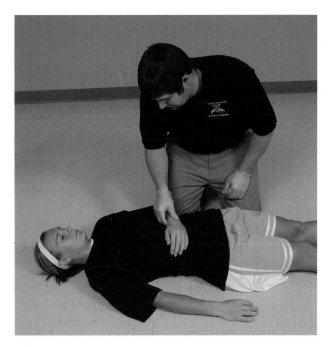

FIGURE 9.8   Assessing respiration rate in an athlete. Count the number of breath cycles at the same point in the cycle, normally at the peak of inspiration.

TABLE 9.4	Normal Respiratory Rates for Different Age Groups
Age (years)	**Range (breaths/min)**
Birth to 1	25 to 50
1 to 3	20 to 30
3 to 5	20 to 30
6 to 12	20 to 30
13 to 18	12 to 20
19 to 40	12 to 20
41 to 60	16 to 20
>60	Dependent on health status

of a digital or analog watch with a second hand. Document the findings immediately to avoid forgetting them at later time.

In a responsive adult or child, continue to palpate the radial pulse and relocate his or her arm up to the lower rib cage, near the xiphoid process (Fig. 9.8). In this position, count the number of breaths at the same point in the breath cycle, normally at the peak of inspiration (rise in the chest and belly). This position works well because you can feel each breath cycle and the individual will typically remain unaware of what is occurring. Be sure not to allow the athlete to speak while assessing respiration rate; verbal communication will interfere with the assessment and often leads to an undercount because breathing ceases during communication. In addition, if the athlete becomes consciously aware of what you are doing, it will lead him or her to override the normal breathing pattern, resulting in breaths that are now slower and/or deeper.

In an unresponsive adult, child, or an infant, the same procedure can be utilized after the pulse is assessed at the appropriate location. An alternative method is to simply count the breaths by watching the rise and fall of the chest; however, in some situations, as in the presence of protective equipment or when the athlete is breathing rapidly, it is very easy to lose count of the breaths. Once this occurs you will either have to restart the count, delaying care, or you will be using inaccurate data to determine the interventions required to manage the situation.

Normal Respiration Rates

In an adult, the normal respiration rate ranges from 12 to 20 breaths per minute. In a child, the normal rate is between 20 and 30; it is between 25 and 50 in an infant. Normative values for respiration rate by age group may be found in Table 9.4.[6]

Factors affecting respiration rate include (a) age, (b) size, (c) physical conditioning, (d) degree of exercise recently completed, (e) history of illness and medical conditions, (f) rise in body temperature, and (g) fear and anxiety. In an emergency situation, fear and anxiety, in particular, will often increase the respiration rate. Similarly, exercise and the higher body temperature accompanying it can increase the respiration rate; however, an athlete should recover to a near normal value within 5 or 10 minutes. Failure to return to a normal value within that time should be documented and treated accordingly.

Abnormal Respiration Rates

An adult with a respiration rate below 8 to 10 or above 20 to 24 breaths per minute or a child whose rate is below 20 breaths per minute is breathing inadequately and requires assisted ventilations and high-flow supplemental oxygen to avoid becoming critically ill. An adult presenting with rapid breathing, normally greater than 20 breaths per minute, and shallow breathing, may be experiencing **tachypnea.** This may be caused by respiratory and cardiac disease (e.g., asthma, chronic obstructive pulmonary disease, pneumonia or other lung infections), pain, and anxiety. **Bradypnea,** on the other hand, is abnormal slowness of respiration, normally less than 10 breaths per minute, and commonly occurs before **apnea.** It is caused by conditions such as **diabetic ketoacidosis,** central nervous system depression (caused by increased intracranial pressure), and respiratory failure. Apnea is the cessation of breathing; this is obviously a life-threatening situation if left untreated (Chapter 10).

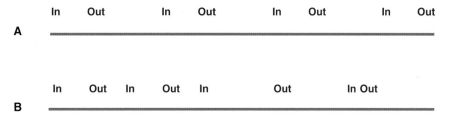

FIGURE 9.9 Regular versus irregular respiration rhythm. **A** demonstrates regular inhalation (in) and exhalation (out) intervals. **B** demonstrates the respiration at irregular intervals.

Quality

The quality of respiration can be assessed while determining the rate and, as in the case of the pulse, quality depends on the associated rhythm and effort.

Rhythm

The rhythm of respiration is examined much like that of the pulse; it can be either regular or irregular (Fig. 9.9). A regular respiratory rhythm will present with equal intervals between inhalation and exhalation. In a responsive athlete, however, rhythm will be affected by such things as speech, movement, and anxiety and may therefore not be entirely reliable. In an unresponsive athlete, respiratory rhythm should be regular. If an unresponsive or responsive individual presents with an irregular respiratory rhythm or a breathing cycle that is unsteady and/or uneven (Table 9.5), this must be documented (e.g., "respirations are 18, irregular, and shallow") and will often require advanced medical care.

Effort

Respiratory effort is broken down into four categories and documented as either (a) normal, (b) shallow, (c) labored, or (d) noisy.

Normal Breathing   An athlete who can speak and carry on a conversation without pausing and presents with normal or average equal movements of the chest without the use of accessory muscles (e.g., the sternocleidomastoid and scalenes) is considered to have normal breathing. The challenge lies in determining what constitutes "normal." Observations of the athlete's breathing during the waking hours and when at rest normally define what constitutes normal.

When an athlete cannot speak without taking an additional breath or an expanded pause, he or she may be experiencing difficulty breathing, or **dyspnea;** this will alter his or her normal respiratory efforts.

Shallow Breathing   An athlete with shallow respirations will present with decreased expansion of the chest or

TABLE 9.5 Irregular Breathing Patterns		
Breathing Pattern	**Signs and Symptoms**	**Implications**
Agonal breathing	Irregular gasping or shallow breathing—a common sign of the early stages of cardiac arrest, suggesting that death is imminent.	The body's last attempts to save itself. A primal reflex seen as an athlete dies. Do not confuse the gasping noise for breathing.
Apneustic breathing	Abnormal respiratory pattern consisting of a pause at full inspiration.	Lesion at the level of the medulla oblongata.
Biot breathing sign	Completely irregular breathing pattern, with continually varying rate and depth of breathing.	Lesions in the respiratory centers in the brainstem; increased intracranial pressure.
Cheyne–Stokes respiration	Pattern of breathing with a gradual increase in depth and sometimes in rate to a maximum, followed by a decrease resulting in apnea; the cycles are ordinarily 30 seconds to 2 minutes in duration, with 5 to 30 seconds of apnea.	Severe head trauma resulting in brainstem lesions and increased intracranial pressure. Also seen in congestive heart failure, cerebrovascular disease, altitude sickness, and spinal cord–injured athletes.
Kussmaul respiration	Deep, rapid respiration as the body attempts to lower the acid levels that arise in diabetic ketoacidosis.	Characteristic of diabetes or other causes of acidosis or crush syndrome.

Adapted from references 3, 10, and 11.

abdominal wall, thus limiting the exchange of gases with each breath. There are many different causes of shallow breathing, including but not limited to (a) respiratory diseases (e.g., asthma, bronchitis, pulmonary edema, pneumonia), (b) poisoning, (c) shock, (d) heat illness, and (e) heart failure.

Labored Breathing   An athlete with labored breathing constitutes a medical emergency. Causes of labored breathing include but are not limited to (a) airway obstruction, (b) heart attack, (c) chest trauma, (d) lung disease, and (e) diabetic emergency. Such a individual will present with[6]:

- Increased breathing effort (the individual works harder to breathe in and out)
- Use of accessory muscles, nasal flaring (widening of the nares), and retractions (supraclavicular and intercostal in children and infants)
- Noisy breathing

An athlete with labored breathing may attempt to find a position that allows for the greatest exchange of gases. The tripod position and sniffing position (Fig. 9.10) are commonly used to improve respiratory mechanics. The tripod position is said to allow for recruitment of all of the muscles of respiration so as to maximize gas exchange during upper and lower airway obstruction and in the presence of respiratory distress. In one study, however, respiratory function was no different in the tripod position as compared with the sitting and supine positions.[12] In children, the sniffing position (with nasal flaring) is used to open the upper airway by flexing the cervical spine toward the chest and extending the head in order to align the oropharynx (mouth), larynx, and trachea.

Noisy Breathing   Noisy breathing can be assessed with or without a stethoscope (auscultation), depending upon the severity of the condition. To determine normal breath sounds via auscultation, place the bell of the stethoscope along the midclavicular and midaxillary line. These areas allow for assessment of vesicular breath sounds, which can normally be heard over the entire lung surface. A soft, low-pitched blowing or rustling sound during all of inspiration and about a third of the way through expiration indicates normal vesicular breath sounds. When the respiratory system is compromised, abnormal sounds such as snoring, wheezing, gurgling, crowing, grunting, or a stridor may be heard upon

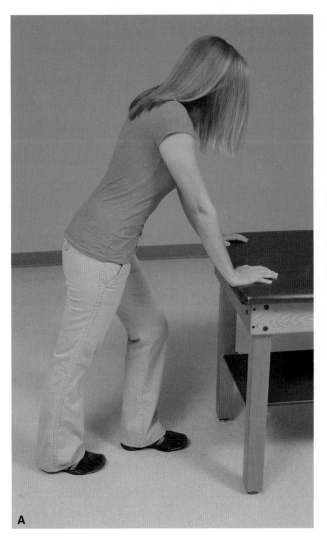

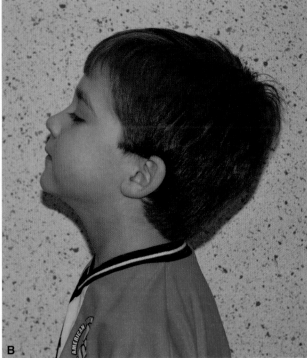

FIGURE 9.10 (A) Tripod position using either single or double arms for support. (B) Sniffing position may lean slightly forward with the head and nose tilted forward and upward as though they are sniffing something in the air.

TABLE 9.6   Abnormal Breath Sounds Indicating Respiratory Compromise

Sounds	Presentation	Conditions/Treatments
Crowing	Harsh sound produced when inhaling.	Blockage of the upper airway; requires prompt transport by EMS.
Grunting	"Uh" sound normally heard during exhalation.	Difficulty breathing; consider placing in tripod position to assist respirations.
Gurgling	Coarse sound heard over large cavities or over a trachea nearly filled with secretions.	Fluid in the airway; may require the use of suction to clear.
Snoring	Rough, rattling inspiratory noise created by an upper airway obstruction, such as the tongue falling back in the throat of an unconscious individual.	Blocked airway, requires opening of airway.
Stridor	High-pitched, noisy respiration, like the blowing of the wind; a sign of respiratory obstruction, especially in the trachea or larynx or with croup in a child.	Foreign-body obstruction, swelling.
Wheezing	Whistling, squeaking, musical, or puffing sound made by air passing through the space between the cavity of the mouth and the pharynx, epiglottis, or narrowed tracheobronchial airways during exhalation (heard during inhalation as well).	Constriction of airway or partial airway obstruction due to inflammation, swelling, or spasm of smooth muscle, as seen in asthma, bronchiolitis, or anaphylaxis. In case of asthma or anaphylaxis, use of prescribed medications such as a metered-dose inhaler or EpiPen will be required while waiting for EMS.
Absent	No exchange of air.	Respiratory arrest.

Abnormal breath sounds occur when air passes through a passage that has become narrowed due to swelling, moisture, or inflammation (i.e., of the membranes lining the chest cavity and lungs).[3,6,13–16] They are heard best with a stethoscope during auscultation. EMS, emergency medical services.

auscultation (Table 9.6). Remember: as with labored breathing, abnormal breaths, if left untreated, can lead to serious consequences and will often require advanced medical care.

When assessing an athlete wearing protective equipment, it will often be necessary to cut the straps securing the pads. If you are unable to gain immediate access, do not delay immediate care. Assessment of respiration rate, rhythm, and noisy breathing without a stethoscope should provide ample information to provide care.

SKIN

Assessment of skin color, temperature, and condition (CTC) provides valuable information regarding the status of the athlete's peripheral circulation, perfusion, and body temperature. This is because the skin, in particular the dermis, contains many blood vessels that help to perfuse tissues and organs adequately. The skin and blood vessels also work in conjunction to help to regulate body temperature through the dilation or constriction of the superficial blood vessels. And, although the skin can survive for hours without blood flow, alterations in CTC may be suggestive of potential failure in peripheral circulation as a result of an injury or illness. The following section discusses and demonstrates how to properly assess skin CTC.

Skin Color

Skin color is determined by the amount of blood circulating through the blood vessels, oxygen levels, and the type of pigmentation (amount of melanin) in the skin. In adults, skin color is normally assessed by observing (possibly with a penlight when applicable) anatomical structures such as the nail beds, inner lower eyelid (conjunctiva), sclera (white of the eye), mucous membrane inside the mouth (inner cheek), and plantar surfaces (soles) of the feet, particularly in dark-skinned individuals.[6] This is because these areas have less skin pigmentation, so changes in skin color are more easily seen. In infants and children, the plantar surfaces of the feet and volar surfaces of the hands should be assessed.[6] Alterations in skin color are also seen more easily here because the blood vessels are very superficial and any compromise in the peripheral circulation can quickly be identified at these sites.

When the circulatory system is functioning properly and the blood is saturated with oxygen, the combination of red blood cells and skin pigment will cause the skin to appear pinkish. Hemorrhaging, vasoconstriction or vasodilatation, inadequate breathing, inadequate heart function, as well as other conditions will cause the skin's color to change, indicating compromise to the circulatory system (Table 9.7).

Breakout

Auscultation of the Lungs

Auscultation of the lungs requires the use of the stethoscope. The diaphragm or disk at the end of stethoscope should be used because lungs sounds are naturally high-pitched and the diaphragm is designed to assess these sounds.

With the athlete supine, place the diaphragm just below the clavicles, halfway between the sternum and acromion (Fig. 9.11A). If the athlete is conscious, instruct him or her to breathe deeply through an open mouth. If the individual is unconscious, listen for at least one full breath. Note the presence or absence of each breath as well as the quality of each breath. Repeat on the other side and compare bilaterally.

Now place the diaphragm over the person's lateral rib cage, halfway between the axilla and the 12th rib (Fig. 9.11B). Instruct a conscious athlete to breathe deeply through an open mouth. If the individual is unconscious, listen for at least one full breath. Note the presence or absence of each breath as well as its quality. Repeat on the other side and compare bilaterally.

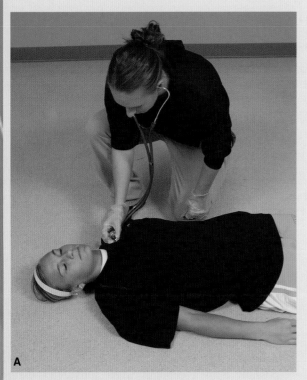 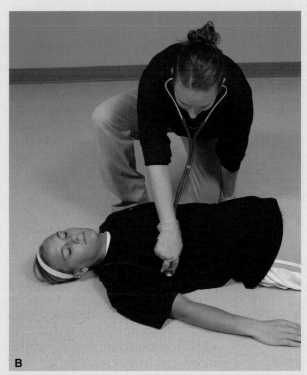

A   B

FIGURE 9.11 **(A)** Assessment of normal breath sounds over midclavicular area. Stethoscope is placed at the second intercostal space just below the clavicle. Assess bilaterally to compare sounds. May also be used to assess for the presence or absence of air movement during inspiration and expiration. **(B)** Assessing normal breath sounds over midaxillary area. Stethoscope is placed between the fourth and fifth intercostal space, just below the axillary. Assess bilaterally to compare sounds. May also be used to assess for the presence or absence of air movement during inspiration and expiration.

Skin Temperature

The skin serves multiple functions, and the regulation of skin temperature is one of these. During periods of increased heat production—either through normal metabolic activities or as the result of illness, exposure to extreme heat, or intense exercise—vasodilatation of superficial blood vessels will allow large amounts of blood to reach the skin's surface. This allows the heat to be released to the environment through the process of sweating and eventually cooled through evaporation of the sweat. When subjected to cold, the same blood vessels will vasoconstrict to retain body heat in and around the vital organs. In some cases certain diseases, lifestyle choices, and medications will limit or restrict blood flow to peripheral tissues.

Skin temperature is assessed by feeling the individual's skin with the back of a hand or wrist on the forehead (Fig. 9.12) or, in a child, on the calf or forearm. However, it may be necessary to assess other areas of the body such as the

TABLE 9.7 Assessment of Skin Color

Skin Color	Causes	Conditions
Pale, white, ashen, or gray	Poor peripheral circulation	Decreased blood flow caused by a variety of factors such as blood loss, shock, decreased blood pressure, emotional distress, exposure to cold.
Blue	Deficient oxygenation of the blood	Commonly referred to as **cyanosis.** Can results in central or peripheral cyanosis. Central (whole body) cyanosis = inadequate breathing (i.e., airway, ventilation, respiration) or heart function. Peripheral (extremities) cyanosis = constriction of peripheral arterioles.
Flushed or red	Vessels engorged with blood, inability to dissipate heat	High blood pressure, fever, heat exposure, thermal burns, and emotional distress.
Yellow	Staining of the skin, sclerae, and deeper tissues (due to liver disease or dysfunction) and accumulation of bilirubin	Often referred to as **jaundice.** Seen in newborns and in adults as a result of chronic liver disease.

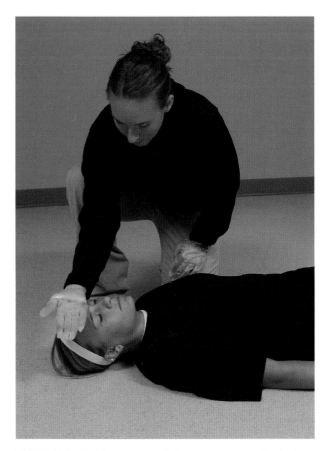

FIGURE 9.12 Assessment of skin temperature. If blood or bodily fluid is present, do not remove the glove.

neck, abdomen, or extremities, depending on the emergency and whether or not an athlete is wearing protective equipment. The skin should normally feel warm. Abnormal skin temperatures include[6]:

1. Cool skin
2. Cold skin
3. Hot skin

Cool skin is suggestive of the early stages of shock, mild hypothermia, or inadequate circulation. Cold skin is suggestive of exposure to cold, including the development of hypothermia and/or frostbite and profound shock. Hot skin is suggestive of fever, exposure to heat, and sunburn. Note that the only definitive method of assessing body temperature—particularly as it relates to core temperature, which is the "gold standard" used in the assessment of hypothermia and hyperthermia—is by the use of a rectal thermometer (Chapter 18). Isolated hot spots may indicate a localized infection, whereas "goose pimples" may suggest the chills, a communicable disease, exposure to cold, and/or fear.

Skin Condition

Skin condition or wetness of the skin can be assessed simultaneously with skin temperature. The skin should normally be dry, but as peripheral blood flow changes, so does skin temperature. Abnormal skin conditions include:

1. Clammy skin
2. Moist skin
3. Wet skin

Skin that is clammy is often described as being moist, cool, and pale due to a reduction in blood flow to the superficial blood vessels. Clammy skin—particularly around the palms, forehead, and soles—is caused by the release of moisture (sweat) from **eccrine glands** after a comfortable body temperature is exceeded or as a sympathetic response to stress. Clammy skin is often suggestive of shock (of varying types), heat exhaustion, cardiac distress, pain, and anxiety. However, clammy skin is unlikely to be seen in infants, particularly when they are in shock, because of their immature eccrine glands and their inability to sweat. **Diaphoretic** or wet, moist skin occurs because of vasodilatation of the superficial blood vessels in an attempt to regulate body temperature, particularly during strenuous exercise or again through the activation of the eccrine glands. Moist or wet skin is often suggestive of strenuous exercise, exposure to heat, or fever; it will require the athletic trainer to examine the mechanism of injury/nature of illness to determine the severity of the moist or wet skin arising from participation in athletics.

When skin color and condition are paired, several combinations may occur. The four most common include:

1. Cool, moist skin, which occurs because of shock, heart attack, or anxiety
2. Cold, dry skin, which occurs after exposure to cold or because of a diabetic emergency
3. Hot, dry skin, which occurs because of exposure to heat or in the presence of fever or a spinal injury
4. Hot, moist skin, which occurs because of exposure to heat or in the presence of fever or a diabetic emergency

When documenting the skin's vital signs, remember to include all three measures of skin appearance (CTC). For example, you might document the findings as follows: "Skin: blue, cold, and dry."

Skin Turgor

Skin turgor assesses the degree of fluid loss or dehydration (usually moderate to severe dehydration) by determining the elasticity of the dermal layer of skin. Decreased skin turgor or inelasticity occurs when fluid in the spaces between the tissue cells **(interstitial fluid)** is forced into circulation; this can happen when there is a loss of fluid volume due to excessive vomiting, diarrhea, increased urination (caused by diuretics or alcohol), malnutrition, or in reaction to corticosteroids.

Assessment of skin turgor requires you to pinch and lift the skin of the forehead, sternum, dorsal surface of the hand, or abdomen (in a child) to create a tenting effect (Fig. 9.13) for several seconds. If normal skin turgor is present—that is, the skin is adequately hydrated—it should immediately snap back to its normal resting position. If the skin remains tented (Fig. 9.14) or holds it position for an extended time (up to 30 seconds) and returns to its normal position slowly, decreased skin turgor is present. The longer the skin remains elevated, the greater the fluid loss. The athlete's skin CTC will also generally be flushed, warm, and moist.

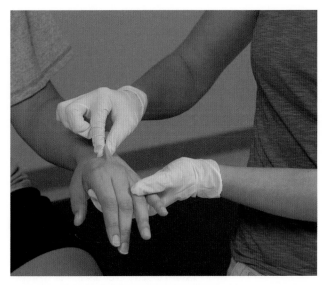

FIGURE 9.13 Assessment of skin turgor.

Capillary Refill

Capillary refill time (CRT) is a measure of peripheral circulation and tissue perfusion and is associated with adequate cardiac output and peripheral vascular resistance.[17] Typically assessed in individuals younger than 6, CRT can also be evaluated in adults if necessary. Pressure is applied to the athlete's nail bed (Fig. 9.15) with the thumb until the nail bed has become blanched (turned white). Blanching occurs as the blood is forced from the capillaries in the nail bed. Once this has occurred, the pressure is immediately released and the amount of time it takes for the nail bed to return to its normal pink color is recorded. Normal capillary refill should be prompt and color to the nail bed should return in less than 2 seconds. If the color takes more than 2 seconds to return, the peripheral circulation may be compromised. Condi-

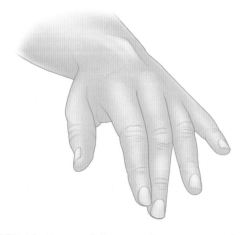

FIGURE 9.14 Decreased skin tugor. Skin remaining in the tented position for up to 30 seconds and slowly returns to its normal position suggests a dehydrated state.

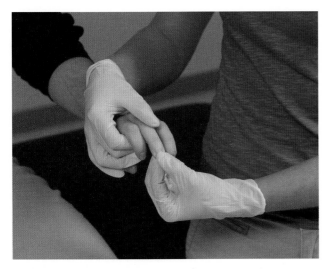

FIGURE 9.15   Assessment of capillary refill time. When assessing adults the index or middle finger (elevated at or above heart level) is a commonly accepted site.[21] Top of the hand, hypothenar eminence, or foot are also possible sites.

tions such as dehydration and shock are likely causes of delayed capillary refill. When documenting capillary refill, identify whether CRT was greater or less than 2 (i.e., "CRT <2" or "CRT >2").

PUPILS

By changing its size, the pupil or the spherical black center of the eye determines the amount of light entering the eyes. When the pupils are exposed to a bright environment or a penlight is directed into the eye, the pupil will constrict to limit the amount of light that is allowed to enter (Fig. 9.16). This helps to minimize damage to the eye's structures. In a dim environment or when the penlight is taken away, the pupil dilates to allow more light to enter. This allows a person to see even in low-lit environments. The pupil's reactivity and responses to changes in light are used to assess the function of the brainstem (i.e., cranial nerves), including adequate perfusion and condition (e.g., trauma). The following section discusses and demonstrates

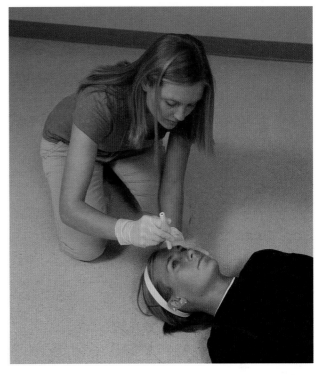

FIGURE 9.16   Use of a penlight to assess the status of the pupils.

how properly to assess pupil shape, size, equality, and reactivity.

Shape and Size

Upon initial assessment, normal pupils should be of the same shape and size. That is, the pupils should be neither large nor small, rotated neither upward nor downward, but rather sitting midline, with the pupils themselves somewhere between large and small. Be sure to note this before using a penlight to actually assess equality and reactivity. Carefully observe for conditions such as **anisocoria** or teardrop pupil (normal pupils should be round and not oblong). A teardrop-shaped pupil may indicate a globe rupture (Fig. 9.17). Anisocoria occurs when the pupils are not of equal size (Fig. 9.18). It may be congenital (in physiological anisocoria, asymmetry is less than 2 mm in diameter)[19] or due to trauma of the head or face (e.g.,

Current Research

Delayed Capillary Refill Alone Is Not a Significant Vital Sign

Delayed capillary refill times without the presence of other associated changes in heart rate, respiratory rate, and level of consciousness may be an unreliable vital sign, particularly in pediatric patients. Factors such as age, sex, temperature, lighting, preexisting medical conditions, medication, hypothermia, and the presence of a simple fractures will affect CRT.[17] For example, in one study, CRT time was less than 2 seconds in children and male adults when the environmental temperature was 71°F. However, CRT increased in female adults (to more than 3 seconds) and in older adults (above age 62).[18] Therefore, CRT without concomitant observations and/or other signs and symptoms of trauma or illness should not be considered significant.

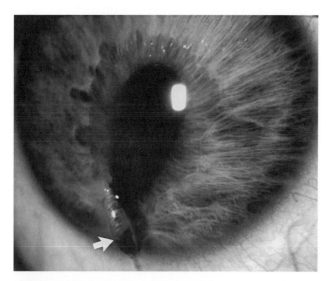

FIGURE 9.17 Elliptical tear drop pupil. This is considered a serious eye condition and is often the result of a corneal laceration (full-thickness) or ruptured globe.

TABLE 9.8	Classification of Pupillary Reaction Speed[11,15,37,38]
Classification	**Presentation**
Normal (Brisk)	Bilateral, prompt pupillary constriction in response to the penlight. This is a normal finding.
Sluggish	Unilateral or bilateral, sluggish or abnormally slow pupillary constriction in response to the penlight.
Nonreactive	Pupils fail to constrict in response to light or dilate when the penlight is moved away.
Fixed	Pupils that are unresponsive to all stimuli and maintain a stationary position.

oculomotor nerve palsy, damaged iris), illness, or medication. Because anisocoria occurs in about 20% of the population[20] be sure to document any congenital difference in the size of an athlete's pupils during the preparticipation physical examination. This will help to alleviate any concerns of potential head trauma when an athlete sustains a blow to head because unequal pupillary size is sign of head trauma and stroke.

If both pupils are dilated at the initial assessment, it may be difficult to observe any of the iris's pigmentation. Dilation of both pupils is suggestive of depressed brain function, trauma to the oculomotor nerve, fright, blood loss, drug use (e.g., stimulants and hallucinogens), and the application of eye drops specifically designed to dilate the pupils. Constriction of both pupils is suggestive of drugs (e.g., narcotics), disease, and the application of eye drops designed to constrict the pupils.

Equality and Reactivity

Pupil equality and reactivity is determined by shining a penlight into the pupils and observing the pupillary reaction to this light relative to size equality (symmetry vs. asymmetry) and reaction speed. Normally the reaction to light should produce equal pupillary changes; reaction speed is based on four classifications, as shown in Table 9.8.

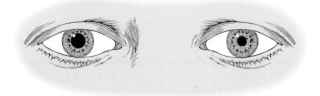

FIGURE 9.18 Anisocoria. Physiologic anisocoria, which is not a medical emergency, occurs when pupil asymmetry is 1–2 mm between pupils with preserved light responses and no other symptoms.

The assessment of pupillary reaction begins by examining the pupils' *direct light reflex*. Begin by having the individual look at a distant object with both eyes open. Shine the penlight into the pupil for 1 to 5 seconds. Repeat with the opposite eye. Normally both pupils should constrict in the presence of the bright light. Next, assess the *consensual light reflex*. With both eyelids open, shine the penlight into the right eye while watching the left pupil. A normal finding is brisk constriction of both pupils. If a penlight is not available the eye to be tested can be covered and the pupil observed when the eye is exposed to light.

A variety of circumstances and medical conditions (e.g., glaucoma, drug use, degenerative disease of the central nervous system, and diabetic neuropathy) can cause abnormal reaction of the pupils. For example, a stroke, head trauma (pressure on the oculomotor cranial nerve), eye injury (trauma to iris, eye lesion), and an artificial eye will cause the pupils to be of unequal size. Trauma to the optic nerve will result in constriction of the opposite eye (consensual reflex) and dilatation of the pupil being assessed with the penlight (direct reflex) (Fig. 9.19).[24] If the affected pupil presents as fixed and dilated in response to either a direct or consensual light reflex, then trauma to the oculomotor nerve should be suspected,[24] often as result of intracranial bleeding. A sluggish pupillary response may suggest increased intracranial pressure (swelling or bleeding).[25] Bilateral or unilateral pupils that are midsized, in midposition, and nonreactive are suggestive of trauma to the midbrain, which results in severe swelling or bleeding.[19,21,25] Bilaterally fixed, dilated, nonreactive pupils suggest either massive intracranial swelling and bleeding, profound hypoxia, or brain death.[21] It should also be noted that certain medications will affect pupillary equality and reactivity. Depressants (e.g., opioids and alcohol) cause pupillary constriction, whereas stimulants (e.g., cocaine, amphetamines) cause dilatation.

Assessment of the pupils in an athlete wearing a face or eye shield may be more difficult. Current cervical spine

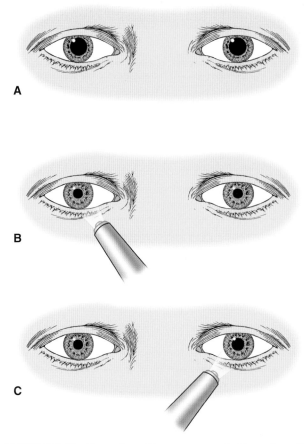

FIGURE 9.19 Normal pupillary response. **A.** Normal pupils. **B.** Normal consensual light reflex where both pupils constrict. **C.** Trauma to the optic nerve results in constriction of the opposite eye (consensual reflex) and dilation in the pupil being assessed with the penlight (direct reflex). (From Bickley, LS and Szilagyi, P. *Bates' Guide to Physical Examination and History Taking*, 8th Ed. Philadelphia: Lippincott Williams & Wilkins 2003.)

management protocols call for the removal of the facemask in a football player with suspected cervical trauma. In other sports, these guidelines are less clear. Assess the pupils when it is safe to do so and you have access.

When documenting eye vital signs in athletes with normal pupil size, equality, and reactivity, many health care professionals use the acronym PEARRL (see the Highlight, below). If an abnormality is noted during the assessment, it will be necessary to document the findings and to relay this information to emergency medical services or other medical personnel. For example, "Pupils are unequal and round; right pupil is sluggish and smaller in size; left pupil is brisk and regular in size."

BLOOD PRESSURE

Blood pressure is defined as the "the pressure or tension of the blood within the systemic arteries, maintained by the contraction of the left ventricle, the resistance of the arterioles and capillaries, the elasticity of the arterial walls, as well as the viscosity and volume of the blood."[3] Restated, blood pressure measures the amount of force exerted by blood, as it travels throughout the body, against the blood vessel walls each time the heart contracts. The pressure created when the heart contracts, pushing blood into the arteries, is known as the *systolic blood pressure*. It is the pressure the heart must overcome to efficiently move blood throughout the body's arterial system. *Diastolic blood pressure* is the pressure remaining in the arteries when then left ventricle relaxes and is allowed to refill. Without the ability to maintain adequate blood pressure (i.e., a pressure that is not too high or too low), the athlete will experience poor circulation and inadequate perfusion of the vital organs. Blood pressure should be measured in every individual 3 years of age or older. The following section

---

Highlight

PEARRL is a mnemonic used to document normal pupillary findings:

P = Pupils
E = Equal
A = And
R = Round
R = Regular
L = React to light

Another mnemonic seen in the literature is PERRLA (Pupils Equal, Round, Reactive to Light, and Accommodation). However, this mnemonic, much like PEARRL, may fail to adequately describe the pupillomotor function. Spector suggests that although PERRLA is a convenient tool used by many, it also gives only an "incomplete description of pupillomotor function. It specifically omits important clinical data such as the actual size and shape of each pupil, the speed and extent of pupillary constriction, and the results of determining an afferent pupillary defect."[26] Levin,[27] in a letter in the *Annals of Internal Medicine*, also suggests that the use of "PERRLA is not only incorrect and inexact—it is also, more seriously, incomplete." Levin suggests that accommodation (pupillary constriction when the eye is focused on a near object) is not tested with PERRLA. He suggests moving away from the use of ambiguous abbreviations when documenting clinical findings. However, unlike Spector, Levin does recommend the use of PERRL-RAPD (Pupils Equal, Round, Reactive to Light—Relative Afferent Pupillary Defect). For further information, we recommend reviewing Levin's clinical observation letter in the *Annals of Internal Medicine*.

TABLE 9.9	Components and Features of a Sphygmomanometer[19]
Component	**Design and Function**
Cuff	Inelastic cloth that encircles the arm and encloses the inflatable rubber bladder and secured with Velcro to the adjoining surfaces. Most are labeled to provide the athletic trainer with visual reference points to ensure proper placement of the bladder over the artery.
Bladder	May be sewn into the cuff or removable, the inflatable bladder applies pressure to the artery when air is forced into the device through the ball-pump cutting off blood flow.
Ball Pump	Attached to the inflatable bladder, the ball-pump uses a turn-valve allows air to enter the cuff when closed. When the turn-valve is open air is allowed to escape from the bladder at a controlled rate.
Pressure Gauge	Designed to measure the pressure that exists in the artery under the bladder, records pressure in millimeters of mercury (mm Hg).

discusses and demonstrates how to properly assess the vital sign blood pressure.

MEASURING BLOOD PRESSURE

Equipment to Measure Blood Pressure

To measure blood pressure accurately, you will need both a sphygmomanometer and a stethoscope.

Sphygmomanometer

A sphygmomanometer, or blood pressure cuff as it is commonly called, is designed to apply pressure to the artery when assessing blood pressure. Blood pressure cuffs come in a variety of sizes (e.g., adult, pediatric, and thigh) and is fastened to either the upper arm, approximately 1 in. above the crease at the elbow (antecubital crease), or around the thigh, depending on the circumstance. The sphygmomanometer consists of four components, including the (a) cuff, (b) bladder, (c) ball-pump, and (d) pressure gauge (manometer) (Fig. 9.20 and Table 9.9). Three types of cuffs are available: (a) mercury, (b) aneroid, and (c) automatic (digital).

Mercury Sphygmomanometer   A mercury sphygmomanometer is commonly used in hospitals and physicians' offices; it is considered the gold standard for blood pressure measurements. These instruments are durable, easy to read, do not require readjustment, and may include an attached stethoscope. However, they are bulkier than other devices and, because the mercury is toxic, should not be stored in athletic training bags because the mercury could spill.

Aneroid Sphygmomanometer   An aneroid sphygmomanometer is the measurement device most commonly used by athletic trainers. These are fairly inexpensive, light in weight, and much more portable and safe than the mercury type. The pressure gauge is attached to the cuff via tubing and can be removed and read from any position. Like mercury sphygmomanometers, some models have an attached stethoscope and a D-ring cuff for easy one-handed application. They are not as delicate as mercury units; however, they can become unreliable and inaccurate when bumped, dropped, or jostled. Because of this, they should be checked yearly against a mercury sphygmomanometer by attaching the aneroid gauge to the mercury gauge.[29] When inconsistencies are noted, you have two choices: return to the manufacturer for repair or purchase a new sphygmomanometer.

Automatic Sphygmomanometer   An automatic (digital) sphygmomanometer is a self-contained unit that electronically measures the athlete's blood pressure. They are easy to use and are secured using a D-ring cuff (Fig. 9.21), may minimize human error, and allow for assessment of other vital signs during analysis. In fact, some units have a built-in pulse-rate measurement that is displayed in conjunc-

Current Research

Improper Calibration of Aneroid Sphygmomanometers Leads to Improper Classification of Hypertension

Rouse and Marshall[30] found that, in the primary care setting, mercury, aneroid, and automatic sphygmomanometers were rarely if ever calibrated. Calibration errors of the 1,462 mercury and aneroid sphygmomanometers tested ranged from equal to or less than 30 mm Hg to equal to or greater than 30 mm Hg, with 80% of sphygmomanometers demonstrating an error between -2.0 to $+1.9$ mm Hg. The authors suggest that these errors increase the risk of improper classification of patients as hypertensive.

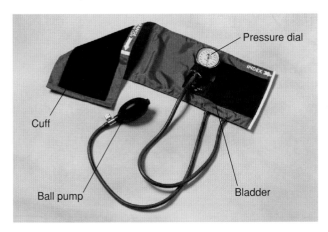

FIGURE 9.20 Aneroid sphygmomanometer and blood pressure cuff. (From Thompson WR, editor. *ACSM's Resources for the Personal Trainer*, 3rd edition. Baltimore: Lippincott Williams & Wilkins; 2010:279.)

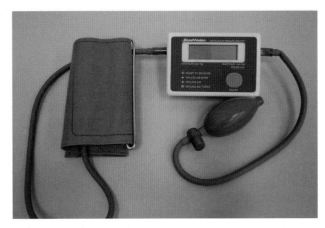

FIGURE 9.21 D-ring cuff automatic sphygmomanometer. A D-ring cuff is specifically designed to allow a user to self-administer the unit.

tion with the blood pressure. These units, though are bulky, require batteries (which could die during an emergency) and are very fragile and sensitive to being bumped or jostled. They are more appropriate for the athletic training room or clinical setting to monitor changes in blood pressure rather than being used on the field or court during an emergency. To secure the blood pressure cuff correctly around the athlete's upper arm, follow the instructions in Skill 9.1.

SKILL 9.1

Securing a Blood Pressure Cuff

1. Select a cuff of the appropriate size (i.e., infant, child, adult, large adult, or thigh cuff) based on the size of the individual (Fig. 9.22). A blood pressure cuff that is too narrow can result in overestimation of blood pressure, whereas one that is too wide can result in an underestimation of blood pressure.[31]

2. Place the arm, either left or right, palm up in a supported, horizontal position at the level of the heart if possible. Note that errors in the measurement of systolic and diastolic pressure can be as great as 10 mm Hg if the athlete's arm is allowed to drop below the heart (overestimation) or is elevated above the heart (underestimation).[28] If both arms are injured, blood pressure can be assessed with a thigh cuff if available; otherwise continue assessing other vital signs and providing the appropriate interventions.

3. Place the blood pressure cuff so that the inflatable bladder is centered directly over the brachial artery (at the antecubital fossa on the medial side of the upper arm). This is accomplished by following the arrows stamped onto most blood pressure cuffs.

4. Make sure that the index line fits within the range lines inside the cuff. If the index line does not fall within the range lines, move to a size larger or smaller depending on where the index line falls. In obese or muscular athletes, an adult large (thigh) cuff will probably have to be used to ensure proper bladder inflation.

5. Wrap the cuff snugly around the upper arm so that the bottom of the cuff is approximately 1 in. above the elbow crease. Be sure that the tubes entering the bladder and the pressure gauge are not tangled up in the cuff (Fig. 9.23).

6. Secure the Velcro, but be sure not to overtighten the cuff.

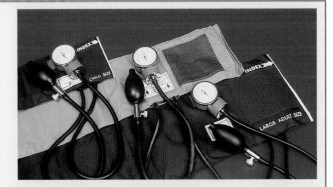

FIGURE 9.22 (From Carol R. Taylor, Carol Lillis, RN, et al. *Fundamentals of Nursing: The Art and Science of Nursing Care*, Sixth Edition. Philadelphia: Lippincott Williams & Wilkins, 2008.)

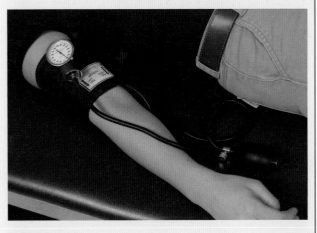

FIGURE 9.23

Determining Blood Pressure via Palpation

Blood pressure via palpation is designed to quickly evaluate systolic blood pressure and does not require the use of a stethoscope. It is not as accurate as blood pressure recorded via auscultation, but it is often used when the environment is very noisy, during transport, or in individuals whose auscultatory endpoints are difficult to hear (e.g., in cases of shock). To determine blood pressure via palpation, begin care by following the directions in Skill 9.2.

Determining Blood Pressure via Auscultation

Blood pressure via auscultation requires a properly fitted cuff and a stethoscope. To determine blood pressure via auscultation, begin care by following the directions in Skill 9.3.

SKILL 9.2

Determining Blood Pressure via Palpation

1. Secure an appropriately sized blood pressure cuff.
2. Using your nondominant hand, identify the radial pulse and do not remove your hand until the assessment is complete (Fig. 9.24).
3. Using your dominant hand (thumb and index finger) to close the turn valve on the ball-pump (Fig. 9.24).
4. Begin inflating the cuff by squeezing the ball-pump until the radial pulse under your fingertips disappears. Continue to inflate the blood pressure cuff until the pressure gauge is 20 to 30 mm Hg above the point of the lost radial pulse.
5. Deflate the cuff slowly by opening the turn valve (counterclockwise) slowly to allow air to escape from the bladder at a rate of approximately 2 to 3 mm Hg per second. If the valve is opened too quickly, you will be unable to get an accurate reading. If the valve is opened too slowly, circulation to the athlete's arm will be restricted and the he or she will report heaviness and tingling distal to the cuff.
6. Continue to deflate the cuff until you feel the radial pulse return. Once the pulse returns, note the reading on the pressure gauge. This is the point of the estimated systolic pressure.
7. Fully open the turn valve to remove any remaining air from the bladder.
8. Document the time of determination and the results as systolic blood pressure over palpation ("120/P" or "120 by palpation").

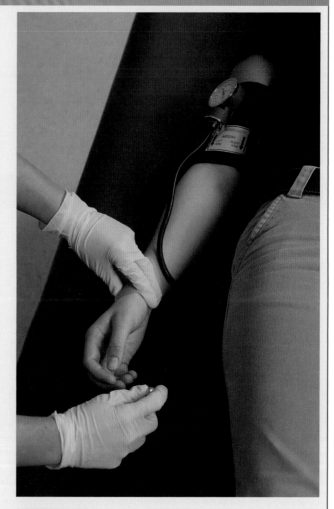

FIGURE 9.24

SKILL 9.3

Determining Blood Pressure via Auscultation

1. Secure an appropriately sized blood pressure cuff.
2. Place the earpieces of the stethoscope in your ears, ensuring they are positioned forward in the ear canal (Fig. 9.25). Improper placement of the earpieces is a common reason for difficulty in assessing blood pressure.
3. Palpate the brachial artery.
4. Using your nondominant hand, place the diaphragm of the stethoscope directly over the brachial artery (Fig. 9.26). Be sure not to place the stethoscope underneath the cuff because this will result in an inaccurate reading.
5. Using your dominate hand (thumb and index finger), close the turn valve on the ball-pump.
6. Begin inflating the cuff by squeezing the ball-pump. Continue to inflate 20 to 30 mm Hg above the loss of the pulse sound (brachial artery) or at the point of the lost radial pulse found during blood pressure via palpation.
7. Deflate the cuff by opening the turn valve slowly to allow air to escape from the bladder at a rate of approximately 2 to 3 mm Hg per second.
8. While deflating, watch the pressure gauge while listening for the start of a tapping or clicking sound as the blood begins to flow again. The first sound heard is the systolic pressure and indicates the passage of the first pulse wave along the artery below the cuff.
9. Continue to deflate the cuff until you no longer hear any of the tapping or clicking sounds. The point at which you no longer hear any sound is referred to as the fifth Korotkoff phase (or sound).
10. Once the systolic and diastolic pressures have been identified, fully open the turn valve to remove any remaining air from the bladder.
11. Document the time of determination and the results as systolic blood pressure over diastolic blood pressure (e.g., "120/80"). Also document the athlete's position (i.e., lying, semirecumbent, sitting).
12. If you believe your reading was inaccurate either wait 1 minute between readings or place the cuff on the other arm. If the inaccuracy was due to inability to hear the blood pressure sounds, check the stethoscope's position for loose connections and proper placement and check for kinks in the tubing. If the second attempt is again unsatisfactory, terminate the procedure and document the problem.

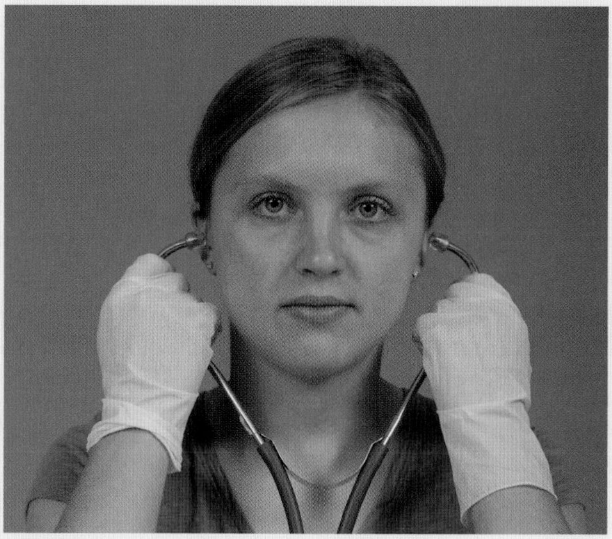

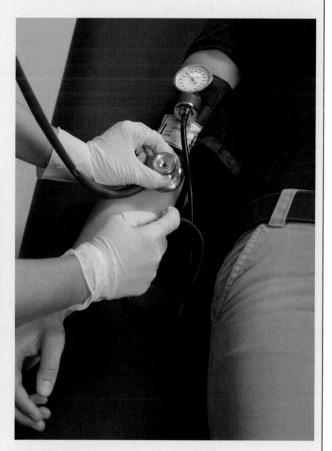

FIGURE 9.25

FIGURE 9.26

Highlight

Korotkoff Sounds

Korotkoff sounds are sounds you hear while assessing blood pressure by auscultation. They are named after Nikolai Sergeyevich Korotkoff, a Russian doctor and scientist who, in 1905, reported on a new auscultatory method of assessing arterial pressure. His work described five sounds or phases (four originally, the fifth was demonstrated later),[32] which are due to vibrations and pressure changes within the arterial walls as blood flows through them.[33]

Korotkoff found that as the pressure of the inflated cuff fell, the first sound heard (a clear-cut snapping or tapping tone, lasting from about 10 to 15 mm Hg) indicated that the first pulse wave was passing through the artery and that the pressure gauge reading where the first sound appeared corresponded to the systolic pressure.[34] This is now known as Korotkoff phase 1 (or sound 1). Korotkoff phase 2 consists of a murmur-like sound lasting from approximately 14 to 20 mm Hg. Thereafter the tapping tone returns and becomes louder and sharper with phase 3.[33,35] Then the tapping tone is replaced by a dull, muffled sound—phase 4.[33,35] Finally, Korotkoff phase 5 represents the complete disappearance of the sounds as blood begins flowing through the artery again, which Korotkoff found corresponded to the diastolic pressure.[34]

Even today, the auscultatory method of assessing arterial pressure developed by Korotkoff is one of the few medical techniques to survive relatively unchanged. Systolic blood pressure is still the point at which the first Korotkoff sound is heard, and the disappearance of the Korotkoff sound (onset of phase 5) defines the diastolic blood pressure.[36]

Blood Pressure Ranges

Generally, normal ranges for blood pressure vary between age groups, with normal adult pressure being equal to or less than 120 mm Hg systolic and equal to or less than 80 mm Hg diastolic[36] (Table 9.10). Blood pressure measurements can also vary from one measurement to another[28] owing to changes in respirations, emotion, temperature, and pain; they can also vary between athletic trainers (or the persons taking the measurements). Blood pressure measurements are also influenced by age (children vs. elderly), race, and health status (e.g., obesity and arrhythmias).[36] Thus the first blood pressure reading may not be reliable, requiring subsequent measurements over time to determine the person's actual status. In fact, when there is a drop in circulation due to loss of blood, loss of vascular tone and arterial constriction to maintain pressure, and failing cardiac function (output), the body immediately begins to compensate by increasing the pulse rate and causing vasoconstriction of the peripheral blood vessels in order to maintain adequate perfusion of the vital organs. Baseline vital signs will demonstrate a near-normal blood pressure; however, respiration and pulse rate will be increased, and skin CTC will be cool, clammy, and pale.

As the circulatory system begins to deteriorate and can no longer compensate for the reduced circulation of blood, the blood pressure will also begin to fall below its normative ranges. This is referred to as **hypotension.** Hypotension without any associated signs or symptoms should be of little concern to an athletic trainer; it is common among athletes because of the same morphological and functional changes in cardiac structure and function seen with a lowered pulse rate. However, when hypotension is accompanied by trauma or illness (such as anaphylaxis), arterial bleeding (internal or external), and the later stages of shock, it becomes life threatening.

TABLE 9.10 Normal Blood Pressure Rates for Different Age Groups

Age (years)	Range*
Birth–1	Systolic blood pressure increases from 70 mm Hg at birth to 90 mm Hg at one year. Normal diastolic is 50 mm Hg.
1–3	Normal systolic blood pressure is between 70 to 100 mm Hg. Normal diastolic is below 80 mm Hg.
3–5	Normal systolic blood pressure is 80 to 110 mm Hg. Normal diastolic is below 80 mm Hg.
6–12	Normal systolic blood pressure is between 80 to 119 mm Hg. Normal diastolic is below 80 mm Hg.
13–18	Normal systolic blood pressure is between 80 and 119 mm Hg. Normal diastolic is 80–81 mm Hg.
19–40	Optimal blood pressure is <120/80.
41–60	Optimal blood pressure is <120/80.
>60	Dependent on health status, but optimal blood pressure is <120/80.

*In children and adolescents, normal BP is defined BP < 90th percentile for age, height, and gender while hypertension is defined as elevated BP that persists on repeated measurement at the 95th percentile or greater for age, height, and gender.[6,20,39]

Hypertension is the opposite of hypotension; it occurs when the blood pressure is higher than normal, as the arteries become narrower owing to the accumulation of fatty deposits **(atherosclerosis);** they gradually lose their elasticity and become hardened **(arteriolosclerosis).** Hypertension (Table 9.11) can occur in children or adults, but it is more commonly seen in individuals over the age of 55 with a family history of hypertension, obesity, smoking, heavy drinking, diabetes mellitus, or kidney disease; it is also seen in women over 35 years of age who have a history of oral contraceptive

TABLE 9.11	Classification of Hypertension in Adults[20]		
Blood Pressure Classification		**Systolic BP**	**Diastolic BP**
Prehypertension		120–139	80–89
Stage 1 hypertension		140–159	90–99
Stage 2 hypertension		>160	>100

Breakout

Cushing's Triad[19,38,39]

In the case of head trauma with intracranial bleeding that results in excessive pressure on the brainstem (medulla), the athlete will present with:

1. Hypertension (systolic blood pressure rises)
2. Bradycardia
3. Slow, irregular respirations

These changes are the late signs of head trauma; they are known as Cushing's triad and occur because of markedly increased intracranial pressure. The increased blood pressure leads to continued abnormal perfusion of the brain, causing it to swell, whereas the changes

in heart rate occur due to increased pressure on the vagus nerve, located near the brainstem. The vagus nerve (the parasympathetic nerve that innervates the heart) then prompts an increased release of acetylcholine, resulting in bradycardia. Vomiting and decorticate or decerebrate posturing (Fig. 9.27) may also indicate increased intracranial pressure.

It should be noted that the changes in vital signs associated with Cushing's triad are the opposite of those seen in an athlete in shock. When an athlete is in shock, he or she will present with the opposite signs:

1. Hypotension
2. Rapid, weak pulse
3. Rapid, shallow breathing

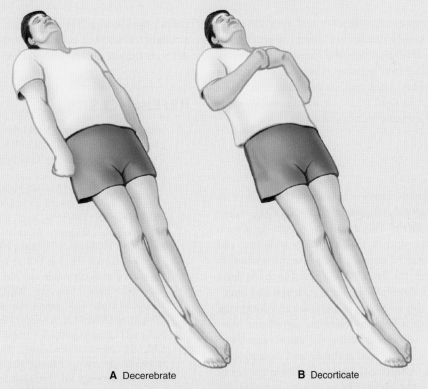

A Decerebrate   **B** Decorticate

FIGURE 9.27 Body Posturing. **A.** Decerebrate rigidity is characterized by extension in all four extremities. **B.** Decorticate rigidity is characterized by extension of the legs and flexion of the elbows, wrists, and fingers. Both conditions indicate a severe brain injury. (From Anderson MK, et al. *Foundations of Athletic Training: Prevention, Assessment, and Management,* 4th ed. Baltimore: Lippincott, Williams & Wilkins; 2009.)

Scenarios

1. During a high school football game, the starting wide receiver was tackled by three opposing players. Once the pile cleared, the wide receiver remained on the ground supporting his right arm. You are covering the event and immediately respond to the athlete. Upon arrival, you quickly determine that the athlete' skin is pale, cool, and clammy.

   What other types of vital signs should be assessed as part of the baseline examination after the primary assessment has been completed?
   Would capillary refill be an appropriate vital sign to assess?
   If all of the vital signs were within the normal range, would delayed capillary refill be a concern?

2. While covering a cross-country meet you are summoned to the 1-mile marker for an athlete in distress. As you approach the scene, your general impression reveals a 16-year-old female who appears to be having difficulty breathing.

   Which vital sign would be the most important to assess based on the general impression alone?
   Describe how to assess this vital sign quantitatively.
   What would be considered normal?
   If the athlete reported a history of asthma, what type of noisy breathing would you expect?

3. A 19-year-old tennis player begins to complain of shortness of breath during a tennis match. You are summoned onto the court to assess her condition. Her respiration rate is 21 and labored; pulse is 102, rapid, and bounding. You notice unequal movement of the chest wall.

   Describe assessment for the presence or absence of air within the lung.
   What are the signs of labored breathing?
   What are the clinical implications of the athlete's blue skin color?
   Discuss the difference between tachycardia and bradycardia.

4. You are treating a 52-year-old man who had recently undergone a total knee arthroplasty. While he is performing passive range of motion exercises, he begins to complain of nausea, chest pain, and light-headedness. You immediately stop what you are doing and give him a glass of water. Two minutes later, he begins to complain of increased chest pain. You immediately call 911 and begin to assess his condition. Pulse rate is 112, rapid, and thready; respirations rate is 20 and labored, skin is cool, clammy, and pale.

   What other baseline vital signs would you look for?
   Describe how to properly perform assessment of these vital signs.
   If you were assessing an athlete in a noisy stadium, describe an alternative method to assess the same vital signs.

use.[36] The blood pressure classification and coexisting diseases (diabetes or kidney disease) will often determine the type of medical intervention required (lifestyle changes vs. drug therapy). High blood pressure is seen in medical illnesses such as a heart attack and stroke, idiopathic nosebleeds, trauma such as head injury, or with exertion, emotional distress, and extreme excitement.

WRAP-UP

The proper and prompt assessment of the vital signs of an athlete is a fundamental component of both the secondary and ongoing assessments. Without data on vital signs such as pulse, respiration, skin (CTC), pupillary response, and blood pressure, it may be impossible to determine whether and to what degree the body's biological functions have been compromised. Baseline vital signs gathered and documented as part of the secondary assessment and compared against normative data help to determine significant trauma and medical conditions affecting the cardiovascular or respiratory systems. Vital signs gathered and documented during the ongoing assessment allow an athletic trainer to determine whether the interventions provided during the emergency were appropriate. The techniques described in this chapter are commonly used by athletic trainers not only in emergency situations but also in some cases of everyday clinical practice. However, in situations where an athletic trainer does not utilize these skills on a regular basis, we strongly recommend periodic practice of these skills in order to maintain clinical competence.

REFERENCES

1. Swank A. Adaptations to aerobic endurance training programs. In: Bacechle TR, Earle RW, eds. *Essentials of Strength Training and Conditioning.* Champaign, IL: Human Kinetics; 2008:121–140.
2. Carek PJ, Mainous AG. A thorough yet efficient exam identifies most problems in school athletes. *J Fam Pract.* 2003;52(2):127–134.
3. Stedman TL. *Stedman's Medical Dictionary.* Philadelphia: Lippincott Williams & Wilkins; 2001.
4. Hwu Y-J, Coates VE, Lin F-Y. A study of the effectiveness of different measuring times and counting methods of human radial pulse rates. *J Clin Nurs.* 2000;9(1):146–152.
5. American Heart Association. Part 4: Adult basic life support. *Circulation.* 2005;112(24 Suppl):IV-19–IV-34.
6. National Highway Traffic Safety Administration. In: NHTSA-EM, ed. *National Emergency Medical Services Education Standards: Emergency Medical Responder Instructional Guidelines.* Department of Transportation; 2009, http://www.safercar.gov/staticfiles/DOT/NHTSA/ems/811077b.pdf. Accessed May 15, 2010.
7. Hollerbach AD, Sneed NV. Accuracy of radial pulse assessment by length of counting interval. *Heart Lung.* 1990;19(3):258–264.

8. Puffer JC. The athletic heart syndrome. *Phys Sportsmed.* 2002; 30(7):41.

9. O'Connor FG, Kugler JP, Oriscello RG. Sudden death in young athletes: Screening for the needle in a haystack. *Am Fam Physician.* 1998;58(15):1760–1761.

10. Starkey C, Ryan J. *Evaluation of Orthopedic and Athletic Injuries,* 2nd ed. Philadelphia: FA Davis; 2002.

11. Frisbie JH, Sharma GVRK. Cheyne–Stokes respiration, periodic circulation, and pulsus alternans in spinal cord injury patients. *Spinal Cord.* 2005;43(6):385–388.

12. Bhatt SP, Guleria R, Luqman-Arafath TK, et al. Effect of tripod position on objective parameters of respiratory function in stable chronic obstructive pulmonary disease. *Chest.* 2007;132(4):610b.

13. Assessing breath sounds. *Nursing.* 1983;13(8):68.

14. Visich MA. Knowing what you hear: A guide to assessing breath and heart sounds. *Nursing.* 1981;11(11):64–79.

15. Anderson M, Parr GP, Hall S. Injury assessment. In: *Foundations of Athletic Training: Prevention, Assessment, and Management,* 4th ed. Lippincott, Williams and Wilkins, 2008: 86–128.

16. Owen A. Respiratory assessment revisited. *Nursing.* 1998;28(4): 48–49.

17. Bumke K, Maconochie I. Paediatric capillary refill times. *Trauma.* 2001;3(4):212–220.

18. Schriger D, Baraff L. Defining normal capillary refill: Variation with age, sex and temperature. *Ann Emerg Med.* 1988; 17:932–935.

19. Merck Research Laboratories. *The Merck Manual of Diagnosis and Therapy.* http://www.merck.com/mmpe/index.html. Accessed September 4, 2009.

20. Eggenberger ER. Anisocoria. *eMedicine.* 2009. http://emedicine.medscape.com/article/1158571-overview. Accessed June 5, 2010.

21. Darovic G. Assessing pupillary responses. *Nursing.* 1997;27(2):49.

22. Fairley D, Pearce A. Assessment of consciousness: Part one. *Nursing Times.* 2006;102(4):26–27.

23. Anness E, Tirone K. Evaluating the neurologic status of unconscious patients. *Am Nurs Today.* 2009;4(4):8–10.

24. Magee DJ. *Orthopedic Physical Assessment.* 5th ed. Philadelphia: Saunders; 2007.

25. Adoni A, McNett M. The pupillary response in traumatic brain injury: A guide for trauma nurses. *J Trauma Nurs* 2007; 14(4):191–196.

26. Spector R. The pupils. In: Walker HK, Dallas WD, Hurst JW, eds. *Clinical Methods: The History, Physical, and Laboratory Examinations,* 3rd ed. Burlington, MA: Butterworth-Heinemann; 1990.

27. Levin LA. The perils of PERRLA. *Ann Intern Med.* 2007; 146:615–616.

28. Beevers G, Lip G, O'Brien E. ABC of hypertension: Blood pressure measurement. *Br Med J.* 2005;322:981–985.

29. Yeats M. The maintenance of an aneroid sphygmomanometer (Electronic version) In: *Update in Anaesthesia.* 1993, http://www.nda.ox.ac.uk/wfsa/html/u03/u03_018.htm. Accessed March 13.

30. Rouse A, Marshall T. The extent and implications of sphygmomanometer calibration error in primary care. *J Hum Hypertens.* 2001;15:587–591.

31. Cuppett M, Walsh KM. Medical evaluation techniques and equipment. In: Cuppett M, Walsh KM, eds. *General Medical Conditions in the Athlete.* St. Louis: Elsevier; 2005:13–31.

32. Kircheva PD, Krivoshiev S. A centenary of auscultatory blood pressure measurement: A tribute to Nikolai Korotkoff. *Kidney Blood Press Res.* 2005;28:259–263.

33. Rudy SF. Take a reading on your blood pressure techniques. *Nursing.* 1986;16(8):46–49.

34. Shevchenko YL, Tsitlik JE. 90th Anniversary of the development by Nikolai S. Korotkoff of the auscultatory method of measuring blood pressure. *Circulation.* 1996;94(2): 116–118.

35. Allen J, Gehkre T, O'Sullivan JJ, King ST, Murray A. Characterization of the Korotkoff sounds using joint time—frequency analysis. *Physiol Meas.* 2004;25:107–117.

36. National Institutes of Health, U.S. Department of Health and Human Services. *Prevention, Detection, Evaluation, and Treatment of High Blood Pressure.* Washington, DC: National Heart Lung and Blood Institute; 2003.

37. National High Blood Pressure Education Program Working Group on High Blood Pressure in Children and A. The fourth report on the diagnosis, evaluation, and treatment of high blood pressure in children and adolescents. *Pediatrics.* 2004;114(2):555–576.

38. Ayling J. Managing head injuries. *Emerg Med Serv.* 2002; 31(8):42.

39. Schultz SJ, Houglum PA, Perrin DA. *Examination of Musculoskeletal Injuries,* 2nd ed. Champaign, IL: Human Kinetics; 2005.

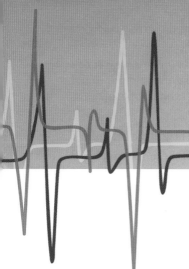

CHAPTER · 10

Recognition and Management of Breathing Emergencies

CHAPTER OUTCOMES

1. Identify and describe the major structures of the respiratory system and how these structures affect the breathing process.

2. Identify and describe the difference between adequate and inadequate breathing.

3. Define respiratory distress and describe how it develops.

4. Identify and describe the signs and symptoms of respiratory distress.

5. Identify and describe specific conditions associated with respiratory distress.

6. Define respiratory arrest and describe how it develops.

7. Identify and describe the signs and symptoms of respiratory arrest.

8. Demonstrate proper care for an athlete suffering from respiratory distress or arrest, including properly opening the airway using a head-tilt/chin-lift and jaw-thrust maneuver.

9. Identify special considerations for managing an athlete in respiratory arrest.

10. Demonstrate how to care for an athlete with a special consideration, including mouth-to-mouth, mouth-to-nose, and mouth-to-stoma resuscitation, the management of athletic equipment, and dealing with cervical spine injuries.

11. Define foreign-body airway obstruction and describe the difference between partial and complete airway obstructions.

12. Describe how foreign-body airway obstructions develop.

13. Identify and describe the signs and symptoms of partial and complete foreign-body airway obstructions.

14. Demonstrate how to clear partial and complete foreign-body airway obstructions in a responsive adult, child, and infant.

15. Demonstrate how to clear a foreign-body airway obstruction in an unresponsive adult, child, and infant.

NOMENCLATURE

Aspirate: fluid or foreign body that has been inhaled into the airway, such as vomit

Bronchitis: acute or chronic inflammation of the mucous membrane of the bronchial tubes

Cephalad: toward the head

Cricoid cartilage: lowermost region of the laryngeal cartilage, distal to the cricoid cartilage at the beginning of the trachea

Crowing: harsh sound produced during inhalation

Dyspnea: shortness of breath, a subjective difficulty or distress in breathing, usually associated with disease of the heart or lungs; occurs normally during intense physical exertion or at high altitude

Epiglottis: leaf-shaped plate of elastic cartilage, covered with mucous membrane, at the root of the tongue; serves as a diverter valve over the superior aperture of the larynx during the act of swallowing; stands erect when liquids are being swallowed but is passively bent over the opening of the trachea when solid foods are being swallowed

Epiglottitis: inflammation of the epiglottis, possibly caused by a respiratory obstruction, especially in children; frequently due to infection

Foreign-body airway obstruction: anything introduced into the airway and that restricts the passage of air

Grunting: "uh" sound normally heard during exhalation

Gurgling: coarse sound heard over large cavities or over a trachea nearly filled with secretions

Hypothermic: body temperature significantly below 98.6°F (37°C)

Influenza: an acute infectious respiratory disease, caused by an influenza virus

Nasopharynx: upper section of the airway behind the nasal cavity

Oropharynx: lower section of the airway below the oral cavity

Paradoxical breathing: deflation of a lung or of a portion of a lung during the phase of inspiration and the inflation of the lung during the phase of expiration

Patent: open or exposed

Pharynx: throat—the joint opening of the gullet and windpipe

Pneumonia: inflammation of the lungs primarily due to infection by bacteria or viruses; occasionally due to inhalation of chemicals or trauma to the chest wall

Respiratory arrest: cessation of breathing

Respiratory distress: first sign of a life-threatening condition, demonstrated by abnormal breathing (increased effort and frequency of breathing), abnormal skin appearance, and other symptoms

Sinusitis: inflammation of the lining membrane of a sinus, especially of one of the paranasal sinuses

Snoring: rough, rattling inspiratory noise created by an upper airway obstruction, such as the tongue falling back into the throat of an unconscious individual

Stoma: an artificial opening between two cavities or canals or between a body space and the surface of the body

Stridor: high-pitched, noisy respiration, like the blowing of the wind; a sign of respiratory obstruction, especially in the trachea or larynx or in a child with croup

Ventilation: replacement of air or gas in a space by fresh air or gas

BEFORE YOU BEGIN

1. What is the difference between inhalation and exhalation? Why are these processes so important?

2. Describe the difference between adequate and inadequate breathing. What are some signs of inadequate breathing? How do you assess the differences in breathing?

3. What is the difference between respiratory distress and respiratory arrest? What are some of the likely causes of these conditions?

4. What are the signs and symptoms an athlete in respiratory distress may display?

5. Describe the appropriate steps to take when caring for an adult, child, or infant suffering from respiratory distress.

6. Describe the appropriate steps to take when caring for an adult suffering from respiratory arrest.

7. What is the Sellick maneuver? When should this procedure be performed and by whom?

8. What type of emergency equipment should an athletic trainer carry to properly manage an athlete suffering a respiratory emergency?

9. What are two primary causes of an airway obstruction?

10. Describe the appropriate steps to take when caring for an adult or child who is conscious with a complete airway obstruction.

Voices from the Field

An easy lesson is that you get better from practicing. Sport is the epitome of "practice makes perfect," and athletic trainers have a front-row seat. Athletic trainers rarely treat acute respiratory emergencies, but when they do occur, it is vital that you be prepared to do your best in the emergency situation. Practicing your skills, drilling with case scenarios, and role playing are all a means to improve skills that are vital when dealing with any emergency situation. In any emergency care situation, the athletic trainer should establish and maintain an open airway. Various procedures and devices are available to assist in this fundamental step. Athletic trainers should become familiar with these devices and their use. Each year, our staff devotes one day to practicing emergency skills, including airway management, cardiopulmonary resuscitation (CPR) recertification, and responses to other life-threatening injuries.

John R. Bowman, MEd, ATC
Assistant Athletic Director for Sports Medicine
Ohio University
Athens, Ohio

An athlete suffering from acute trauma or illness that impairs the function of the airway or lungs is at risk for a breathing emergency. The two types of breathing emergencies athletic trainers must be able to recognize and manage are **respiratory distress** and **respiratory arrest.** Caused by a variety of traumas (e.g., obstructed airway, lung injury) and/or illnesses (e.g., allergic reaction, asthma, poisoning), respiratory emergencies lead to inadequate breathing and eventually cessation of breathing, decreasing or limiting the delivery of oxygen to body cells and vital organs. Without oxygen, these vital organs, especially the brain, begin to suffer damage within minutes and eventually death occurs if the condition is left untreated. This chapter identifies and describes how to manage individuals of all ages (infant, child, and adult) suffering from respiratory distress and arrest as well as airway obstructions. The techniques described in this chapter, like all clinical skills, require review and practice to maintain clinical competence. The skills presented should be reviewed annually or semiannually by an athletic trainer along with the emergency action plan (EAP), facility policies, and other emergency procedures. Remember too that, according to the Board of Certification, all certified athletic trainers must maintain and demonstrate proof of a valid emergency cardiovascular care—that is, CPR certification.[1]

Before we begin, let us first answer the question "Why discuss respiratory distress and arrest techniques for infants and children in a book designed for athletic trainers?" First, not all athletes treated by athletic trainers are over the age of 12. Organized youth sports are a popular form of recreational activity, with many youths participating in sports like tackle football (ages 5 to 15)[2,3] and soccer (ages 4 to 19).[4,5] In fact, the U.S. Youth Soccer and American Youth Soccer Associations boast more than 3.2 million and 650,000 players (ages 5 to 19), respectively.[4,5] And just like adult athletes, children do get hurt. In one study of youth football injuries (grades 4 to 8), the overall injury rate was 17.8 injuries per 1,000 athlete exposures.[6] Of those injuries, 58.6% did not require restriction from participation but did require assessment or first aid provided by a certified athletic trainer.[6]

The second reason for discussing respiratory distress and arrest techniques for infants and children is simple: social responsibility. As allied health care providers, we have an obligation to assist others when they are ill or injured, regardless of whether they are engaged in athletics or sitting on the sidelines. Whether or not you choose to study the information pertaining to infants and children is up to you and your classroom instructor. However, we leave you with this scenario to think about. You are covering a Pop Warner

Highlight

National Safe Kids Campaign Sport Injury Rates

In 2002, the following number of children ages 5 to 14 were treated in hospital emergency rooms for sports-related injuries:

- 207,400 children were treated for basketball-related injuries.
- 187,800 children were treated for football-related injuries.
- 116,900 children were treated for baseball- or softball-related injuries. (Baseball also had the highest fatality rate of all sports for children aged 5 to 14.)
- 76,200 children were treated for soccer-related injuries.
- 21,200 children were treated for gymnastics-related injuries.

Data from National Safe Kids Campaign.[7]

football game one Saturday morning; everything is going great until Timmy's little brother starts choking on some cookies. You turn to the commotion in the stands and realize that the baby is not breathing. None of the bystanders in the stands are taking charge of the situation; however, because young children and infants do not participate in sports and you do not know how to treat them, you continue to stand on the sidelines. How would you sleep that night?

RESPIRATORY SYSTEM

The respiratory system's main purpose is to supply the body with oxygen and remove carbon dioxide, a waste product from cellular metabolism, through the process of **ventilation.** Any trauma or illness involving the nose, mouth, throat, or lungs predisposes an athlete to a respiratory emergency. Therefore, the athletic trainer must have a thorough understanding of the anatomy and function of the respiratory system. The following section reviews its anatomy and physiology.

Anatomy

Our discussion of the respiratory system begins with the mouth and nose. This is the beginning of the airway or the path taken by air on its way to the lungs. Air enters the respiratory system through the **oropharynx** (mouth) and **nasopharynx** (nose) (Fig. 10.1). Air passing through the oropharynx first encounters the lips and teeth, which are securely embedded in the upper and lower jawbones. The mandible forms the lower

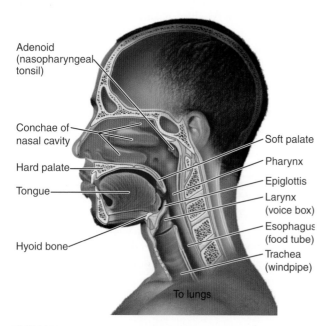

Adenoid (nasopharyngeal tonsil)

Conchae of nasal cavity

Hard palate

Tongue

Hyoid bone

Soft palate

Pharynx

Epiglottis

Larynx (voice box)

Esophagus (food tube)

Trachea (windpipe)

To lungs

FIGURE 10.1 Throat region, lateral cross-sectional view. (From Anderson MK, Parr GP, Hall SJ. *Foundations of Athletic Training: Prevention Assessment, and Management,* 4th ed. Baltimore: Lippincott Williams & Wilkins; 2009.)

jawbone and is the point of attachment for the tongue, a skeletal muscle covered by a mucous membrane and attached to the floor of the oral cavity by the lingual frenulum. When the airway of an unconscious athlete becomes blocked, the tongue is most often responsible. The upper jawbone or maxilla supports the roof of the mouth and separates the oropharynx from the nasopharynx. Most breathing occurs through the nasopharynx, which has two external openings, the nares (nostrils). Air passing the through the nostrils into the nasal passage is warmed and humidified; the nostrils trap foreign particles before the air moves down the pharynx and into the lungs.

The inhaled air then passes through the **pharynx** to the **epiglottis,** the point at which the oropharynx and nasopharynx meet. A leaf-shaped structure, the epiglottis is responsible for preventing the passage of food and fluid down the trachea during swallowing and air into the stomach during breathing. The epiglottis is the uppermost portion of the lower airway and is the opening of the sound-producing portion of the throat. Air continues to move past the larynx (voice box), vocal cords, and **cricoid cartilage.** The larynx is the most superficial structure and prominent feature of the throat and is covered superiorly by the thyroid cartilage (Adam's apple) and inferiorly by the cricoid cartilage. Because the larynx is relatively unprotected, it is vulnerable to injury during athletic events, particularly with a severe blow to the anterior throat.[8] Fortunately, these injuries are uncommon[9,10] and represent less than 1% of all blunt trauma.[11]

The inhaled air continues down the trachea toward the lungs (Fig. 10.2). The trachea is a membranous, semiflexible tube covered by a series of cartilaginous rings anteriorly to protect it from trauma. At the level of the lungs, the trachea divides into the right and left bronchi, which enter the right and left lungs, respectively. The right and left bronchi further divide into three and two segmental bronchi, serving the lobes of the right and left lungs.

Once inside the lung, the bronchi progressively become smaller and smaller, forming bronchioles. These bronchioles get smaller as well, eventually ending as alveoli, the terminal branches of the bronchioles. The alveoli are tiny, thin-walled sacs within the lungs where oxygen and carbon dioxide are exchanged; this is occasionally referred to as the "point of vital exchange" (Fig. 10.2).

The walls of the alveoli contain tiny vessels known as pulmonary capillaries, which carry the carbon dioxide from the body to the lungs and the oxygen from the lungs to the body (Fig. 10.3). The exchange of gases between the capillaries and alveolar sacs occurs through the process of passive diffusion, whereby molecules move from an area of high concentration to one of low concentration. That is, oxygen in the alveolar sacs moves into the bloodstream because there are more oxygen molecules in the sacs than in the bloodstream. The reverse occurs for the movement of carbon dioxide. The movement of oxygen and carbon dioxide molecules between the alveolar sacs is facilitated by the movement of the diaphragm and accessory muscles. The diaphragm, below the lungs, is a muscular structure responsible for the physiological

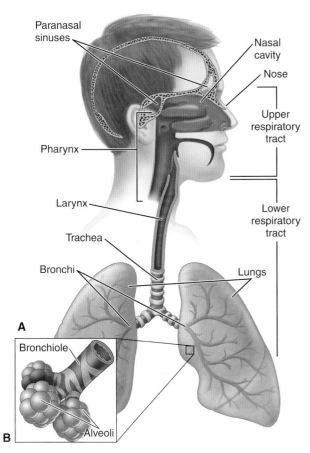

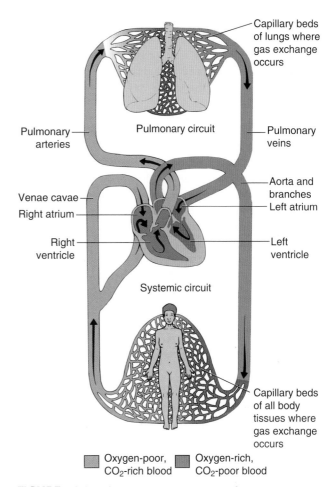

FIGURE 10.2 The respiratory system. **A.** The trachea, bronchi, and lungs. **B.** Oxygen and carbon dioxide are exchanged at the alveolar sacs, the terminal ends of the bronchial tree. (From Anderson MK, Parr GP, Hall SJ. *Foundations of Athletic Training: Prevention Assessment, and Management,* 4th ed. Baltimore: Lippincott Williams & Wilkins; 2009.)

FIGURE 10.3 The respiratory system works in conjunction with the cardiovascular system to allow for the exchange of oxygen and carbon dioxide within the body.

processes of inhalation and exhalation. It separates the chest cavity from the abdominal cavity.

Physiology

Breathing consists of two actions: inhalation and exhalation.

Inhalation

Inhalation is the act of bringing air into the lungs; it is an active process. This active process of breathing depends upon the action of the muscular system and is under the control of the nervous system. When the diaphragm, which is controlled by the phrenic nerve, contracts, it is drawn downward, increasing the volume of the chest cavity. At the same time, the external intercostal muscles of the chest cavity move the ribs upward and outward, causing the chest cavity and lungs to expand, thus increasing the volume (see Fig. 9.7). This increase in volume lowers the air pressure in the alveoli to below atmospheric pressure. And because air flows from a region of higher pressure to a region of lower pressure, the air now rushes in through the upper respiratory tract to the

alveoli. This is referred to as negative-pressure breathing, because the air rushing into the lungs through the nasopharynx and oropharynx attempts to equalize the pressure inside the lungs relative to the pressure of the outside atmosphere.

Air drawn into the lungs is moved to the alveoli. The small alveolar sacs are clumped together like clusters of grapes on a grapevine. The oxygen from the inspired air is transferred to the capillaries passing by the alveolar sacs to the bloodstream, where it is transported from the lungs to the heart. From the heart, the now-oxygenated blood is pumped to the rest of the body (Fig. 10.3). At the same time, deoxygenated blood is picked up from the cells and returned to the heart. It is then sent back to the lungs, where the carbon dioxide moves from the bloodstream to the alveolar sacs for removal during exhalation.

Exhalation

Exhalation is the opposite of inhalation. It is the process of blowing off carbon dioxide exchanged at the alveolar sacs. Exhalation, unlike inhalation, is a passive process. The diaphragm and internal intercostal muscles now relax, causing the diaphragm to return to its original position while the chest cavity moves down and inward. This movement compresses the chest cavity and lungs, generating a positive pressure within the chest cavity and forcing the air (including carbon dioxide) out of the lungs.

ADEQUATE AND INADEQUATE BREATHING

We are acutely aware that breathing is a prerequisite for life and completely under control of the brain. As we have learned, breathing involves a balance between inhalation and exhalation. When oxygen and carbon dioxide are properly exchanged, one can say that an athlete is breathing adequately. Adequate breathing, therefore, is breathing that can sustain life.[12] Inadequate breathing, on the other hand, is a condition that, if left untreated, cannot sustain life. This can occur when an individual breathes too slowly or weakly, often because of trauma or illness affecting the respiratory system or the central nervous system. This section examines the difference between adequate and inadequate breathing.

Adequate Breathing

To assess whether an individual is breathing adequately, we only need to remember three simple words learned in Chapter 8: "look, listen, and feel." Once an airway has been established, the athletic trainer should be looking for the chest to rise and fall equally, listening for an exchange of air and for abnormal breath sounds (Table 10.1) and also feeling for an exchange of air.[13] Adequate breathing can also be assessed by comparing the findings of the rate, rhythm, and quality of the breathing to the range of values considered normal (Chapter 9). Furthermore, an athlete who is breathing adequately will normally be able to speak without gasping for air; he or she will also present with normal skin color and mental status. However, an athlete demonstrating adequate breathing one minute can, with little to no warning, quickly begin to demonstrate signs of inadequate breathing, so always remain prepared and observant.

Inadequate Breathing

Inadequate breathing is a condition in which the current breathing pattern cannot sustain life. Athletes who are breathing inadequately may experience alterations in breathing rate, rhythm, and quality.[13] If the athletic trainer fails to recognize inadequate breathing in an athlete, the risk of respiratory arrest increases significantly. For this reason, it is essential to assess and document the athlete's breathing status immediately during the initial on-field assessment. Furthermore, the athletic trainer should continue to look for changes in breathing status during the ongoing assessment in order to minimize the development of inadequate breathing. The signs of inadequate breathing include changes in respiratory rate, rhythm, and quality as well as other signs and symptoms, as listed in Table 10.2.

TABLE 10.1	Abnormal Breath Sounds Indicating a Compromised Respiratory System	
Sounds	**Presentation**	**Conditions/Treatments**
Crowing	Harsh sound produced when inhaling.	Blockage of the upper airway; requires prompt transport by EMS.
Grunting	"Uh" sound normally heard during exhalation.	Difficulty breathing; consider placing athlete in tripod position to assist respirations.
Gurgling	Coarse sound heard over large cavities or over trachea nearly filled with secretions.	Fluid in the airway; may require the use of suction to clear airway.
Snoring	Rough, rattling inspiratory noise created by an upper airway obstruction such as the tongue falling back into the throat of an unconscious individual.	Blocked airway, requires opening of airway.
Stridor	High-pitched, noisy respiration, like the blowing of the wind; a sign of respiratory obstruction, especially in the trachea or larynx or with croup in a child.	Foreign-body obstruction, swelling.
Wheezing	Whistling, squeaking, musical, or puffing sound made by air passing through the space between the cavity of the mouth and the pharynx, epiglottis, or narrowed tracheobronchial airways during exhalation (heard during inhalation as well).	Constriction of airway or partial airway obstruction due to inflammation, swelling, or spasm of smooth muscle as seen in asthma, bronchiolitis, or anaphylaxis. In case of asthma or anaphylaxis, use of prescribed medications such as a metered dose inhaler or EpiPen will be required while waiting for EMS.
Absent	No exchange of air.	Respiratory arrest.

Abnormal breath sounds occur when air passes through a passage that has become narrowed by swelling, moisture, or an inflammation of the membranes lining the chest cavity and lungs.[19,53–57] These sounds are heard best with a stethoscope during auscultation. EMS, emergency medical services.

TABLE 10.2   Indications of Inadequate Breathing[19,55,58,59]

Rate*	Respiration above or below normal baseline for vital signs	Adult <8 or >24 breaths per minute
		Pediatric <20 or >60 breaths per minute, depending on situation and age
Rhythm†	Irregular breathing patterns	Agonal breathing: irregular gasping or shallow breathing, which is a common sign of the early stages of cardiac arrest and suggests that death is imminent. Do not confuse the gasping noise for breathing.
		Apneustic breathing: abnormal respiratory pattern consisting of a pause at full inspiration
		Biot's breathing sign: completely irregular breathing pattern, with continually varying rate and depth of breathing; seen with increased intracranial pressure
		Cheyne–Stokes respiration: pattern of breathing with gradual increase in depth and sometimes in rate to a maximum, followed by a decrease resulting in apnea; cycles 30 seconds to 2 minutes in duration, with 5 to 30 seconds of apnea
		Kussmaul respiration: deep, rapid respiration as the body attempts to lower high acid levels due to diabetic ketoacidosis
Quality	Breath sounds	Absent or decreased upon auscultation (midaxillary and midclavicle for adults and midaxillary for pediatric athletes)
	Chest expansion	Unequal or inadequate
Paradoxical breathing	Tidal volume	Inadequate or shallow
	Effort	Labored or normal‡: use of accessory muscles (muscles other than the diaphragm or intercostals muscles) to assist breathing (commonly seen in pediatric athletes) as well as nasal flaring and retractions above the clavicles, between the ribs, and below the rib cage
Other	Altered mental status	
	Skin pale or blue (cyanotic§); cool and clammy	
	Abnormal breath sounds (Table 10.1)	
	Inability to speak a full sentence	
	Excessive coughing	
	Athlete assumes tripod position (sitting upright or leaning forward with a hand on the table or chair to support the upper body)	
	Barrel chest in older athletes with known chronic lung disease	

*If the athlete is responsive with signs of inadequate breathing, consider assisted ventilations using a bag-valve-mask device.
†In the case of athletics, irregular breathing may indicate head trauma and the athlete will normally be unresponsive.
‡If the athlete is using only the diaphragm to breathe, suspect spinal cord trauma to the nerves supplying the intercostals muscles.
§Tongue, nail beds, and inside of the lips and conjunctiva.

BREATHING DIFFICULTY

Respiratory Distress

An athlete suffering **dyspnea** should or shortness of breath as a result of trauma (e.g., blow to the chest) or illness (e.g., anaphylaxis) may be experiencing respiratory distress, some-times referred to as difficulty breathing. Breathing difficulties in the general population occur more frequently and for many more reasons than what is generally seen in the athletic population. Causes of breathing difficulty in the general population include but are not limited to an obstructed airway, medical illness, electrocution, shock, drowning, heart disease or heart attack, injury to the chest or lungs, allergic

TABLE 10.3 Possible Causes of Breathing Difficulty in the Athletic Population

Location	Mechanism of Injury/ Nature of Illness	Injury*
Facial trauma	Blunt trauma	Nasal fracture
		Deviated septum
		Foreign-body airway obstruction (tongue, dislocated teeth, bleeding from soft tissue injuries)
	Penetrating trauma	Cheek-embedded object with excessive soft tissue bleeding
Throat trauma	Blunt trauma	Hyoid fracture
		Thyroid fracture
		Cricoid cartilage fracture
		Laryngeal trauma
	Soft tissue	Throat laceration
Chest trauma	Blunt trauma	Pulmonary contusion
		Pneumothorax
		Hemothorax
		Hemopneumothorax
		Flail chest
		Rib fracture/contusion
		Sternal fracture
	Penetrating trauma	Sucking chest wound
Medical	Acute conditions	Exercise-induced asthma
		Bronchospasm
		Hyperventilation
		Anaphylaxis
		Prolonged seizures
		Upper and lower respiratory infections (e.g., **bronchitis, pneumonia, influenza, sinusitis, epiglottitis**)
	Chronic conditions	Chronic obstructive pulmonary disease
		Pleural effusion
		Pulmonary embolism

*The injuries and illnesses identified in this list are not all-inclusive; any trauma/illness altering an athlete's ability to breathe adequately requires immediate attention.

reactions, drugs, and poisonings.[12,14–18] Possible causes of breathing difficulty in the athletic population are listed in Table 10.3. Remember that the symptoms experienced by an athlete in respiratory distress are subjective and may not accurately reflect the extent of his or her condition. Fear, anxiety, and uncertainty all may cause an individual to overreact to a situation, particularly if it is exacerbated or influenced by the overreaction of the coach, teammates, and/or parents. In fact, an athlete experiencing a breathing difficulty may display signs of either adequate or inadequate breathing, depending on his or her reaction to the situation. Therefore, the athletic trainer must complete a thorough on-field or on-court primary assessment to determine the severity of the breathing emergency. The findings of the primary assessment will then determine the required interventions, including immediate assisted positive-pressure ventilations.

Signs and Symptoms of Breathing Difficulty

The signs and symptoms of breathing difficulty may be exacerbated by the athlete's age and medical history. For example, compared with a high school or college athlete, an older athlete with a history of lung disease may present with signs and symptoms more quickly and with little ability to compensate. These changes are often the result of the aging process. As an athlete ages, physiological changes such as loss of muscle tone and flexibility of the chest wall and stiffness of the alveolar sacs affect the ability to exchange carbon dioxide and oxygen. Pediatric athletes, on the other hand, have tongues that are proportionally larger than those of adults in relation to the amount of free space in the oropharynx (increased risk of airway obstruction), an underdeveloped and flexible trachea (increased risk of narrowing or occlusion), and underdeveloped chest wall muscles, often requiring the use of the

Signs & Symptoms

General Signs and Symptoms of Breathing Difficulty

- Shortness of breath (i.e., inability to speak a full sentence)
- Restlessness, combativeness, and/or altered mental status due to hypoxia
- Dizziness or disorientation, also due to hypoxia
- Increased pulse rate
- Changes in breathing rate, either increased or decreased
- Pale, cyanotic, or flushed skin, particularly the skin or nails of the fingers and toes. In a pediatric athlete, look for pale skin, as cyanosis is a late finding in children.
- Cool, moist skin due to the loss of blood flow to the distal extremities
- Noisy breathing, particularly grunting, wheezing, and stridor in pediatric athletes
- Coughing
- Using accessory muscles in the effort of breathing
- Flaring nostrils in an attempt to increase the size of the airway
- Retractions of the skin above the sternum and between the ribs
- Poor peripheral perfusion, delayed capillary refill greater than 2 seconds, particularly in pediatric athletes
- Tripod position (see Fig. 9.10)

abdominal muscles to assist in the breathing process. When experiencing breathing difficulty, a pediatric athlete may suffer from a see-saw breathing pattern, a combination and alternation between abdominal and diaphragmatic breathing. Pediatric athletes will also present with nasal flaring in order to increase the size of the airway; they may also make use of accessory muscles, such as those of the neck and abdomen, to assist in ventilation. Cyanosis in the pediatric athlete is a late sign of difficulty breathing; retractions of the skin above the sternum and between the ribs are easier to visualize in a child than in an adult athlete. The general signs and symptoms of breathing difficulty, regardless of age, are outlined in the Signs and Symptoms box above.[19]

Respiratory Arrest

An athlete suffering from respiratory distress or inadequate breathing who has not received the appropriate level of intervention may fall victim to a condition referred to as respiratory arrest. Respiratory arrest, or respiratory failure, is a condition seen in an athlete who is unconscious and not breathing at all during the primary or ongoing assessment. The causes of respiratory distress or difficulty breathing are also the same conditions seen in an athlete suffering from respiratory arrest; however, the athlete has now progressed to the point where breathing has ceased. As a result, the

athlete is unable to properly exchange oxygen and carbon dioxide between the lungs and body cells. Eventually, he or she will begin to suffer brain damage as a result of the lack of adequate oxygen perfusion to the brain cells, with brain damage occurring in as little as 4 to 6 minutes.[20] This is followed by cardiac arrest, as the heart also begins to suffer from the lack of oxygen.

EMERGENCY MEDICAL CARE FOR BREATHING EMERGENCIES

Respiratory Distress

The signs and symptoms of respiratory distress are typically obvious and require immediate attention. Delaying appropriate interventions and advanced medical care increases the athlete's risk of respiratory arrest. Regardless of the causes of respiratory distress, the athletic trainer should begin care by:

1. Initiating the facility's EAP.
2. Completing a primary assessment to determine any compromise in the athlete's ABCs (airway, breathing, and circulation, including external bleeding) by opening and adequately maintaining the airway.
3. Summoning advanced medical personnel if necessary, as in the case of rapid breathing and any underlying injuries and/or illness that may be contributing to the breathing emergency. If the athlete appears to be suffering from a breathing emergency caused by anxiety or fear and you believe that you will be able to manage the situation appropriately, delay summoning advanced care.
4. Place the individual in a position of comfort in order to assist breathing. Many athletes who experience respiratory distress find sitting or standing in the tripod position (see Fig. 9.10) to be more comfortable than being supine because breathing may be easier in this position. Consider limiting the number of bystanders (e.g., coaches, teammates) in order to reduce the athlete's anxiety and fear.
5. Complete a SAMPLE history, focusing on the questions using the mnemonic OPQRST, as defined below.[21]
   - **O**nset, when did the problem start?
   - **P**rovocation, what makes the symptoms better or worse?
   - **Q**uality, what does it feel like? Can you describe the pain and/or symptoms?
   - **R**adiation, where do you feel it?
   - **S**everity, how bad is it on a scale from 0 to 10?
   - **T**ime, how have the symptoms changed over time?
   If the athlete is unable to provide any answers because of problems speaking, consider interviewing bystanders, such as the coach, teammates, or referees if appropriate.
6. Complete a focused physical exam.
   - Assess for dismissed or absent breath sounds by auscultation. Assess for unequal and/or inadequate chest

expansion, inadequate or shallow tidal volume, and effortful breathing (i.e., use of accessory muscle, nasal flaring, etc.).

7. Assist the athlete with medications such as a prescribed metered-dose inhaler or EpiPen. Be sure to consult your individual state practice acts, facility's policies and procedures, and/or standing medical orders to determine how and when these medications should be administered. The proper uses of these medications is discussed further on.

8. Assist the athlete with the use of supplemental oxygen if appropriate and if you are trained to do so. The proper use of supplemental oxygen is discussed in Chapter 11.

9. Assist the athlete in trying to control his or her breathing. In the case of asthma or anxiety, ask the athlete to exhale slowly through pursed lips to help maintain pressure in the airway, thus preventing the airway from collapsing and making inhalation easier. Pursed-lips breathing is accomplished by keeping the lips half closed and breathing forcefully against them. An individual who is hyperventilating should close his or her mouth and block one nostril in order to slow down his or her breathing rate.

10. Perform an ongoing assessment, watching for changes in the airway, level of consciousness, and vital signs, particularly in situations where medication has been administered.

If at any time the athlete's respiration rate is below 8 or above 24 breaths per minute (in an adult) or the airway is threatened, immediate action[23] such as the administration of supplemental oxygen and/or positive-pressure ventilation using a bag-valve-mask (BVM) device (Chapter 11) may be

Breakout

Using a Stethoscope through Clothing

The proper method of auscultation is to place the stethoscope directly on the athlete's bare chest. Many health care providers, including doctors and pulmonologists, violate this basic principle. Although exposing the chest is always recommended in a respiratory emergency, it may not always be practical to do so; therefore, the athletic trainer will have to auscultate through clothing. A recent study designed to evaluate the sensitivity of two common stethoscopes found that the effect of one or two layers of indoor clothing (T-shirt and flannel material) on lung sounds can be negated by increasing the pressure on the stethoscope head as it makes contact with the athlete's clothing. However, the authors remind us that auscultation through clothing still remains problematic owing to the inability to inspect the chest and because of the risk of acoustic artifacts caused by clothing.[22]

warranted. If the athlete becomes unconscious, reassess his or her condition and provide appropriate care based on the current signs and symptoms.

Respiratory Arrest

An athlete in respiratory arrest during the primary assessment will demonstrate no signs of breathing but will have a pulse. In addition, the athletic trainer may detect the condition commonly referred to as agonal breathing. This is

Current Research

Assessing Normal versus Abnormal Breathing

It is vitally important that the athletic trainer be able to accurately assess the breathing and circulation status of a collapsed athlete in order for the most appropriate interventions to be implemented. However, discriminating between "normal" and "abnormal" may be difficult for a variety of reasons, including an inadequate level of training, insufficient previous experience with actual situations, and unusual environmental circumstances. Perkins et al.[24] examined the ability of medical students to discriminate between simulated normal and abnormal breathing patterns and to select the correct treatment. In their study, 48 medical students (none of whom had previous experience performing CPR on a patient) were shown six 10-second video clips of simulated breathing, including (a) normal, (b) abnormal (i.e., shallow, rapid, agonal/obstructed, agonal/unobstructed airways), and (c) absent breathing. It was found that the medical students, who had been trained in basic life support, were unable to reliably differentiate normal breathing from abnormal breathing as shown on the video clips. In actual practice, their decisions would have resulted in numerous inappropriate, potentially harmful actions or omissions. According to the researchers, the students' diagnostic accuracy for recognizing normal breathing and knowing when it was appropriate to perform rescue breathing was only marginally better than chance (72% and 61%, respectively). The positive predictive value of the decision to perform rescue breathing (which is the number of times the athletic trainer correctly reports that rescue breathing is required compared with the total number of times it was reported as being required) was also disappointingly low, at 67%.[24] The researchers did note a major limitation of the study—that is, the use of video clips rather than live patients. They pointed out, however, that the expert group had 100% agreement as to the breathing type and indicated the appropriate treatment for their patients.

This study serves as a reminder that although we may believe we have learned a skill, what we see and how we respond may be very different when we are confronted with a real-life situation. In fact, the actions we select may actually be contraindicated. This is why continued practice and review of even the most elementary skills is necessary on a yearly, semiannual, or quarterly basis.

an irregular gasping or shallow breathing that is not to be confused with normal breathing.[20] In fact, agonal breathing commonly marks the early stages of cardiac arrest and suggests that death is imminent. It is often mistaken by lay responders as a sign of life, leading them to withhold CPR.[24,25] If, during the primary assessment, the athletic trainer does determine that the athlete has a pulse but is not breathing or demonstrating movement, the athletic trainer should immediately begin rescue breathing.

Rescue Breathing

Rescue breathing or artificial ventilation is a technique used by athletic trainers to move air containing oxygen into the athlete's lungs. Because the heart is still beating, rescue breathing ensures that the athlete in respiratory arrest will continue to receive at least a portion of the oxygen required to perfuse vital tissues. A healthy adult demonstrating adequate breathing will breathe 12 to 20 times per minute. With each inspired breath at sea level, he or she is drawing in 21% oxygen, 78% nitrogen, and 1.4% carbon dioxide and other gases. However, only a small portion of the inspired oxygen is utilized by the body; the remainder is exhaled with each breath. In fact, with each exhalation, an athlete will blow off 16% to 17% oxygen, which is more than enough to sustain life and perfuse the vital tissues. When rescue breathing is used in conjunction with other adjunct respiratory devices, the athletic trainer may be able to deliver up to 90% or more oxygen with each artificial breath (Chapter 11). Rescue breathing, therefore, helps to maintain adequate tissue perfusion by delivering oxygen until the individual begins breathing independently or until more advanced medical personnel arrive on the scene.

Rescue Breathing in Adults and Children   To perform rescue breathing, begin by carefully following the directions in Skill 10.1 or referring to Algorithm 10.1 for an emergency action decisional algorithm.

When performing rescue breathing, consider your body position. By remaining close to the athlete and avoiding excessive bobbing up and down in between breaths, you will help to limit the development of fatigue and ensure adequate ventilations.

Rescue Breathing in Infants   Depending upon the facility where he or she is employed, the athletic trainer may at some point be called upon to perform rescue breathing in an infant. If this should be your experience, follow the same steps identified in Skill 10.1 with the exception of the following:

- Airway
  - Open the airway using a head-tilt/chin-lift maneuver by tilting the head to a neutral position (Fig. 10.4).
- Rescue breaths
  - Secure a resuscitation mask or BVM device of the appropriate size over the infant's face. If no barrier device is used, it will be necessary to place your mouth over the infant's mouth and nose.
  - Deliver each breath over 1 second with enough volume to ensure that the chest clearly rises. Remember, infant lungs are much smaller than those of an adult or child and will require significantly less tidal volume.
- Circulation
  - While maintaining the airway, identify the brachial artery (Fig. 10.5).

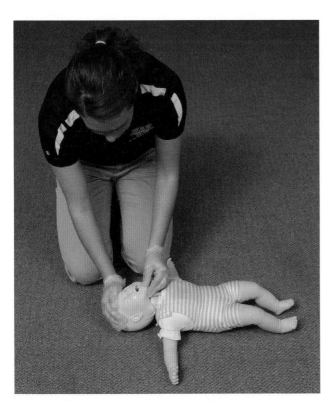

FIGURE 10.4 Opening the airway using a head-tilt/chin-lift maneuver by tilting the head to a neutral position.

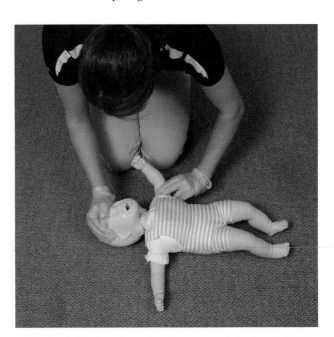

FIGURE 10.5 Identifying the brachial artery while maintaining the airway in a neutral position.

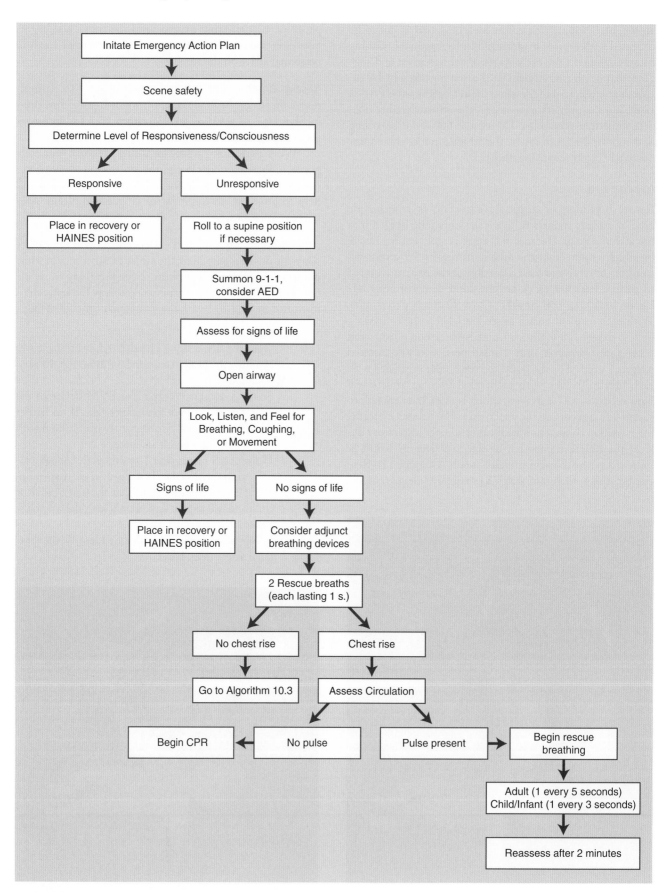

ALGORITHM 10.1 Rescue breathing for an adult, child, or infant.

SKILL 10.1

Steps for Rescue Breathing in an Adult or Child

1. Initiate the EAP.
2. Check the safety of the scene.
3. Determine the athlete's level of responsiveness by tapping his or her shoulder and shouting, "Are you all right? Are you OK?" If unresponsive, summon more advanced medical personnel and consider the need for an automated external defibrillator (AED). If the athlete is prone, immediately roll him or her to a supine position, supporting the head, neck, and back, and begin a primary assessment to determine any compromise to the ABCs (including external bleeding) by opening and adequately maintaining the airway (Fig. 10.6).
4. Airway
   - Open the airway using a head-tilt/chin-lift maneuver.
   - If a spinal injury is suspected, use a jaw-thrust maneuver.
   - Remember that opening the airway helps to move the tongue away from the back of the throat but may compromise the position of the epiglottis (Fig. 10.7).

5. Breathing
   - **LOOK, LISTEN,** and **FEEL** for signs of life for no more than 10 seconds. Signs of life or circulation include "normal breathing, coughing, or movement"[25] (Fig. 10.8).
   - Consider the use of an adjunct breathing device such as an oropharyngeal or nasopharyngeal airway to assist in maintaining the airway (Chapter 11).
   - If no breathing is detected, provide two rescue breaths. Single athletic trainers should use a resuscitation mask, whereas two athletic trainers should consider the use of a BVM (Chapter 11).[12]
6. Rescue breaths
   - Secure the resuscitation mask or BVM. If a face shield is utilized, it will be necessary to pinch the athlete's nostrils to prevent air from escaping through this opening, followed by sealing your mouth over the athlete's mouth (Fig. 10.9).

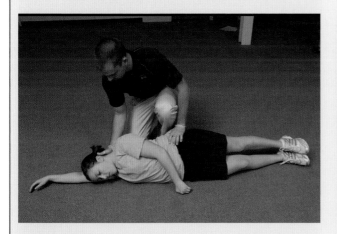

FIGURE 10.6

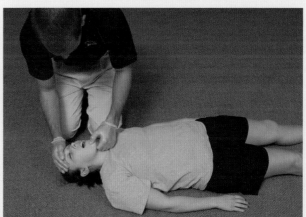

FIGURE 10.7

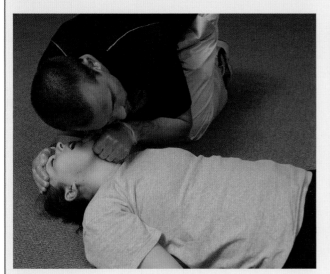

FIGURE 10.8

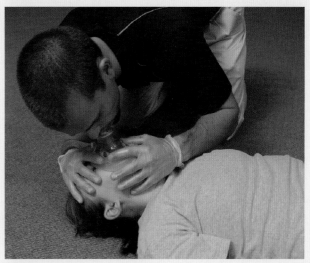

FIGURE 10.9

(Continued)

SKILL 10.1 *(Continued)*

Steps for Rescue Breathing in an Adult or Child (Continued)

- Deliver each breath over 1 second with enough volume to ensure that the chest clearly rises. If air resistance is encountered, do not force air into the athlete's lungs. Also be sure to avoid rapid or forceful breaths.
- If the chest clearly rises and falls, continue checking for signs of life.
- If, in an adult athlete, the chest does not rise and fall, retilt the head and attempt the rescue breaths again. In a pediatric athlete, reposition the head just slightly past neutral and attempt the rescue breaths again. If the chest still fails to rise, assume that the airway is obstructed. This is discussed again further on.

7. Circulation
- While maintaining the airway, find, if possible, the carotid artery in an adult or child. Remember to palpate on the side closest to you. Reaching across to palpate the opposite carotid pulse could be very disturbing to an athlete who is beginning to breathe independently.
- Palpate for a pulse for no more than 10 seconds unless you believe the athlete to be hypothermic. In that case, palpate for up to 30 to 45 seconds (Fig. 10.10)

8. Scan the athlete for any immediate threats of severe bleeding. Again, remember to maintain the airway.

9. If the athlete displays a pulse but is not breathing, begin rescue breathing by providing:
- One breath every 5 seconds ("one-one thousand, two-one thousand, three-one thousand, four-one thousand, breathe") for an adult, lasting 1 second, that makes the chest rise visibly.
- One breath every 3 seconds for child, lasting 1 second, that makes the chest rise visibly.

10. Continuing the rescue breathing while assessing for signs of adequate ventilation (i.e., chest rising and falling, normal skin color, and capillary refill) for 2 minutes or 24 breaths for an adult and 40 breaths for a child.

11. At the end of 2 minutes, remove the barrier device (if used) and reassess for signs of life.
- If a pulse is present and the athlete is still not breathing, continue rescue breathing and continue reassessing every 2 minutes.
- If there are no signs of life, including breathing and pulse, begin single- or two-person CPR (Chapter 12).
- If signs of life are present, place the athlete in the recovery or High Arm IN Endangered Spine (HAINES) position and continue to monitor the signs of life.

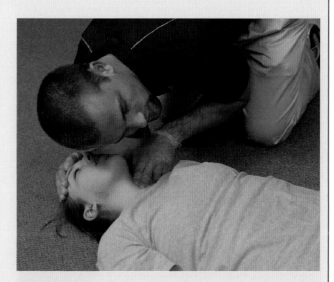

FIGURE 10.10

- Palpate for a pulse for no more than 10 seconds unless the infant is **hypothermic.** In this case, palpate for up to 30 to 45 seconds.
- If rescue breathing is indicated, administer 1 breath every 3 seconds or 40 breaths every 2 minutes.

The athletic trainer should continue with rescue breathing unless one of the following situations is encountered:

- The scene becomes unsafe for the athletic trainer.
- Another trained athletic trainer or EMS arrives to assist or take over the situation.
- The athlete begins to breathe independently.

- The athlete does not have pulse. In this case, CPR should immediately be initiated and an AED made available as soon as possible.
- The athletic trainer is too exhausted to continue providing care.
- The team physician orders the athletic trainer to stop.

Special Considerations for Rescue Breathing

There are several situations in which the athletic trainer may be required to modify the steps performed during rescue breathing. Lack of appropriate equipment, orofacial trauma, inappropriate technique, and/or other special considerations may arise during an emergency.

Lack of Appropriate Equipment   Should the athletic trainer not have a barrier device (e.g., face shield, resuscitation mask, or BVM), it may be necessary to perform mouth-to-mouth breathing. This is done by gently pinching the athlete's nose and sealing your mouth over his or her mouth. Provide one breath lasting 1 second with a visible chest rise, then remove your mouth to allow the air to escape passively. Continue until a proper barrier device or advanced medical care becomes available.

Depending on your place of employment and/or situation, as an athletic trainer you will typically have a duty to act and may be required to perform rescue breathing should someone be suffering from respiratory arrest. Failure to provide reasonable and appropriate care will most likely constitute negligence (when in question consult your legal counsel). For this reason, every attempt should be made to have the appropriate rescue equipment available on site or on your person, such as a barrier device (i.e., face shield, resuscitation mask, and a BVM) to aid in preventing the transmission of blood-borne pathogens. As Liberman and Mulder[26] point out, proper equipment is crucial in terms of managing an acute airway injury during a sporting event. Equipment should be simple, organized, and portable. A list of the recommended airway management equipment used by athletic trainers is presented in Table 10.4 and further examined in Chapter 11. Also, consider consulting your team physician in order to determine the items that should be included in the emergency airway kit (Fig. 10.11).

Orofacial Trauma   When an athlete has sustained either a direct or indirect blow to the jaw or face and the mouth cannot be opened adequately, a proper seal cannot be established during mouth-to-mouth or mouth-to-mask breathing. It may then be necessary to perform mouth-to-nose breathing.[12] To do this, begin by sealing the mouth with your lower hand and sealing your mouth over the nose. Provide one breath lasting 1 second with a visible chest rise; also allow the mouth to open so that the air can escape passively. Continue until a proper barrier device becomes available. Also, because of the orofacial trauma, blood will often be present; therefore, the use of suctioning may be required to help clear the airway.

Inappropriate Technique   Remember from the anatomy review at the beginning of this chapter that air normally enters the nose or oropharynx, then passes through the trachea and into the lungs, where it reaches the alveolar sacs. There, the oxygen–carbon dioxide exchange takes place. When rescue breaths are delivered over too long of a time period and too quickly, there is a risk that the ventilated air will pass from the trachea and enter the stomach. This can also happen when the airway is not completely open, adjunct airways are not properly inserted, and/or occasionally in the presence of a BVM.[27–29] When air enters the stomach, the stomach begins to distend, causing what is commonly known as gastric distention. Factors

TABLE 10.4	Recommended Emergency Airway Management Equipment
Personnel	**Equipment**
Athletic trainer	Manual or mechanical suction
	Yankauer tip for suction
	Oropharyngeal airways (assorted sizes)
	Nasopharyngeal airways (assorted sizes) with lubricating gel
	Appropriate size bag-valve-mask
	Oxygen source
	Oxygen tubing
	Oxygen delivery devices (nonrebreather mask, nasal cannula)
	Penlight
Physician	Properly functioning and tested laryngoscope (assorted blades)
	Topical lidocaine (Xylocaine) spray
	Endotracheal tubes (assorted sizes)
	Endotracheal tube stylet
	Adhesive tape
	Commercial percutaneous cricothyrotomy set
	Curved hemostat, Metzenbaum scissors, and Magill forceps
	Tracheal spreader
	Mounted disposable scalpel
	Shiley cuffed tracheostomy tube

Adapted from reference 24.

such as high peak pressure, short inspiratory time, large tidal volume, and incomplete airway opening (all which can occur from using a BVM improperly) can cause the pressure in the esophagus to exceed the lower esophageal

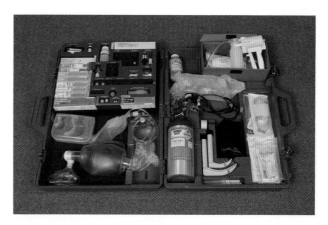

FIGURE 10.11   An emergency airway kit.

sphincter pressure, thereby allowing air into the stomach. Improperly inserted nasal and oropharyngeal adjunct airways can also impede the ability of the epiglottis to cover either the trachea or esophagus, depending on whether the athlete is breathing or swallowing. If the epiglottis cannot completely close off the esophagus, air will enter the stomach.

Gastric inflation and distention increases not only the risk of vomiting but also the **cephalad** movement of the diaphragm.[30] In fact, a vicious respiratory cycle of increasing gastric inflation and decreasing lung ventilation can develop. As already noted, as gastric distention and pressure increases, there is an associated increase in the cephalad movement of the diaphragm. This movement decreases lung movement, which increases the peak airway pressure and results in a redistribution of tidal volume from the lungs to the stomach. This leads to a further increase in gastric inflation and decreased lung ventilation.[30]

Vomiting in an unresponsive athlete increases the likelihood that the he or she will **aspirate** the vomitus. Aspiration is a serious complication and increases the risk of death. The best care to minimize the risk of gastric distention and vomiting is the placement of an advanced airway by advanced medical personnel. In all other situations, consider delivering each rescue breath over 1 second at a tidal volume sufficient to produce a visible chest rise,[12,31,32] thus ensuring proper placement of an adjunct airway device and proper positioning of the airway. Gastric distention caused by the use of a BVM is discussed in Chapter 11.

Another option for an athletic trainer is the use of cricoid pressure. Cricoid pressure, known as the Sellick maneuver, is a technique performed during resuscitation and emergency endotracheal intubation. During resuscitation it prevents air from passing through the esophagus to the stomach while being ventilated by exerting enough force on to the cricoid cartilage to occlude the esophagus. During an endotracheal intubation it allows a better view of the vocal cords, allowing for easier insertion of the tube. Cricoid pressure can also prevent solids and fluids from leaving the stomach, thereby preventing aspiration of these substances into the trachea and eventually the lungs.

This technique should be utilized by at least two *trained* individuals, one to hold pressure and one to ventilate the athlete with an adjunctive breathing device. If three athletic trainers are present, the third can assist in ventilating the athlete using a BVM. When applying pressure the use of the nondominant hand (left hand when the right hand is dominant) may be less likely to lead to error than when the dominant hand is used.[33,34] Current recommendations

---

Breakout

Contraindications to the Sellick Maneuver
The Sellick maneuver should not be used if the athlete is

1. Responsive
2. Vomiting or starts to vomit
3. A breathing tube will be placed by advanced medical personnel
4. There is trauma to the anterior neck or cervical spine

Current Research

Learning How to Perform the Sellick Maneuver

In a review of literature examining the application of cricoid pressure, Parry[35] found evidence that training and education for improving skills and preventing their decay is essential for a safe and high-quality patient care. He notes there is not enough practice in applying cricoid pressure; nevertheless, through structured education programs and training aids, practice can clearly be improved. He further states that these programs do not always have to be expensive or remove practitioners from the clinical area.[35] For example, Flucker et al.[36] found that training using a 50-mL syringe depressed to 38-mL and 30-mL, which demonstrates the correct application forces of 20 and 40 N, leads to a significant improvement in performance for 20 and 40 N, which was maintained for 1 week for both but not for 1 month. They recommend weekly training in order to maintain a level of competence to effectively provide cricoid pressure.[36]

In another study examining the theoretical knowledge and practical skills of emergency department staff (doctors and nurses) regarding the technique of cricoid pressure as well as the efficacy of two methods of cricoid pressure training (group A trained with a pressure trainer while group B was given reading materials only), researchers found 53% (n = 37) of the subjects could identify the position of the cricoid cartilage and 16% (n = 11) could identify the required pressure. Of the 70 subjects, 61% had performed cricoid pressure in practice 1 to 10 times. Immediately after training and after 4 to 6 weeks, 97% (after 4 weeks) and 70% (after 6 weeks) of group A could identify the position of the cricoid cartilage correctly, compared with 86% (after 4 weeks) and 74% (after 6 weeks) in group B, a nonsignificant difference between groups. The percentage achieving correct pressure immediately after training and 4 to 6 weeks later, 88% and 67% in group A compared with 33% and 51% in group B. The use of training devices that provided biofeedback helped the subjects to provide the correct pressure immediately after training[37]; however, as with all practical skills, continued practice is necessary to maintain competence.

suggest that 20 to 30 newtons (N) of pressure should be safe and adequate when applying cricoid pressure.

To properly apply cricoid pressure, follow the directions in Skill 10.2. Remember to check individual state laws and practice acts to determine whether the use of the Sellick maneuver is acceptable.

If the athlete does vomit, regardless of the cause, immediately roll the him or her onto the side (maintaining spinal stabilization in the presence of a head, neck, or back injury) and remove any large amount of vomitus with your gloved finger. If necessary, suction and carefully reposition the athlete onto his or her back and immediately begin providing care.

SKILL 10.2

Steps for Sellick Maneuver

1. Make sure that cricoid pressure is indicated. Consult your local and/or state protocols, facility policies and procedures, and/or medical standing orders.
   - Athlete is unresponsive
   - No suspected anterior neck or cervical spine injury
   - Athletic trainer has been properly trained

2. Application
   - Place the neck in slight extension and, using your index finger, locate the thyroid cartilage inferior to the hyoid, at approximately the level of the C4-C5 vertebral bodies (Fig. 10.12).
   - Slide your finger inferiorly until you feel the indentation below the thyroid cartilage. Be sure you are now on the cricoid cartilage and not the thyroid cartilage (Fig. 10.13).
   - Once in the proper position, apply a moderate amount of pressure (20–30 N) in an inferior and posterior (backwards) direction on the cricoid cartilage with the index and thumb, thus compressing and shutting the esophagus against the cervical vertebrae (Fig. 10.14).
   - Maintain pressure while the second athletic trainer ventilates the athlete (Fig. 10.14) but avoid excessive pressure so as not to obstruct the trachea or damage the larynx.

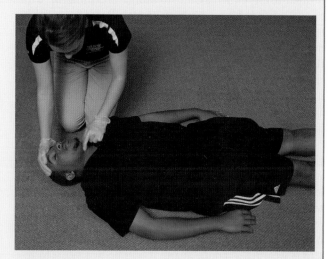

FIGURE 10.12

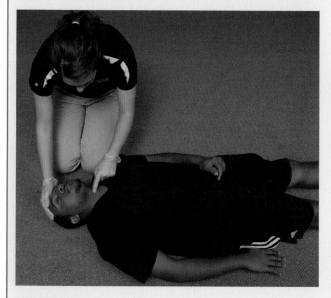

FIGURE 10.13

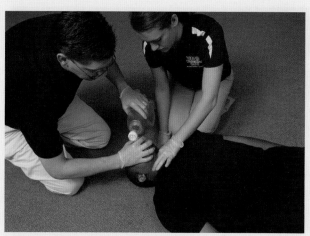

FIGURE 10.14

Special Populations   In some situations the athletic trainer may be required to provide care to an individual with a stoma or one who is wearing a mouth guard or dentures.

Mouth-to-Stoma Resuscitation   A **stoma** is an artificial opening between two cavities. A tracheal stoma, for example, is an opening at the front of the neck allowing air to pass directly into the trachea; it is often placed after an injury or illness such as the removal of the larynx. A stoma may not be readily identifiable; however, most individuals with a stoma wear a medical alert bracelet or necklace. When caring for an individual with a stoma, assess breathing over the opening of the hole rather than the mouth and nose. Rescue breathing can be accomplished using either mouth-to-stoma breathing or with the use of an infant resuscitation mask. Breaths are delivered at the same rate and depth for a mouth-to-mouth/nose or mouth-to-barrier device, but instead of breathing through the mouth or nose, the stoma will be used. It should be noted that there is no published data examining the efficacy of mouth-to-stoma breathing.[12] However, an infant resuscitation mask has been shown to create a better seal than a standard ventilation bag.[38]

When performing rescue breathing, be sure to remove your mouth from the stoma or barrier device to allow the ventilated air to escape passively. In situations where air is leaking through the mouth and/or nose, it may be necessary to seal one or both of these orifices.

Mouth Guards and Dentures   If you know that the athlete is wearing a mouth guard, it will be necessary to remove it prior to initiating care, using a gloved hand (Fig. 10.15). In sports like ice hockey, rugby, and others, you may encounter an athlete wearing dentures. Regardless of the age of the individual, if someone is wearing dentures, make every effort to leave them in place while ventilating. Leaving the dentures in place helps to maintain an adequate seal and ensure proper delivery of rescue breaths. Performing a head-tilt/chin-lift maneuver will also assist in keeping the dentures in place. If the dentures are loose and it is becoming difficult to maintain an adequate seal or provide breaths, remove the dentures using a gloved hand.

Head, Neck, or Back Injuries   If an athlete is suspected of having a head, neck, or back injury, it will be necessary to limit excessive movement of the head and neck while managing the airway. For this reason, rather than using the head-tilt/chin-lift maneuver to open the airway, it will be necessary to use a jaw thrust (with or without extension). Remember from Chapter 8 that a jaw-thrust maneuver limits the amount of movement in the cervical spine while still allowing for elevation of the hyoid bone, thus maintaining a **patent** airway by pulling the muscles away from the airway.[26] This maneuver is performed by kneeling behind the individual's head, placing your first two or three fingers behind the angle of the mandible on both sides of the jaw, and lifting the mandible upward toward the sky. This maneuver can also be performed from the side of the athlete if needed (Fig. 10.16). If the mouth remains closed during the maneuver, apply a downward pressure to the resuscitation mask on the lower jaw, using the index fingers of both your hands (Fig. 10.17). When it is performed properly, the jaw-thrust maneuver (without extension) can be used safely while maintaining cervical spine precautions in an injured individual with a possible cervical spine injury.

If a patent airway cannot be maintained, the airway injury should take precedence over any head, neck, or back injury. Therefore, it may be necessary to perform what is sometimes called a modified jaw thrust or jaw thrust with extension. In this maneuver, maintain the finger position behind the angle of the mandible on both sides of the jaw

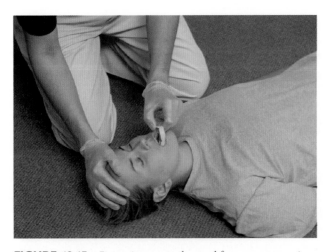

FIGURE 10.15   Removing a mouth guard from an unconscious athlete.

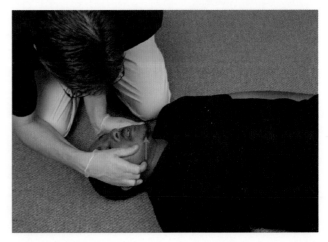

FIGURE 10.16   Jaw-thrust maneuver without extension from the side on an unconscious athlete. The arrow indicates the direction of the jaw moving upward.

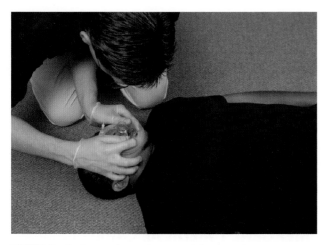

FIGURE 10.17 Applying downward force to the resuscitation mask using a jaw-thrust maneuver.

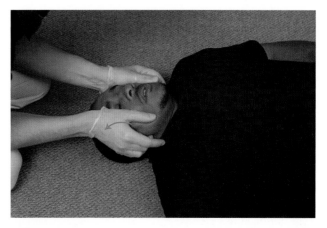

FIGURE 10.18 Jaw-thrust maneuver with extension from the top of the head in an unconscious athlete. Extend the cervical spine only far enough to allow breathes to enter the lungs. The index finger was removed to demonstrate the position on the angle of the jaw.

(Fig. 10.18) and slightly tilt the head back (extending the cervical spine) in order to help open the airway; however, tilt the head back only far enough to allow breathing.

Athletic Equipment   If an athlete is suspected of having a cervical spine injury as result of head-down contact, as in football,[39,40] or from being hit from behind or falling and hitting the crown of the head (e.g., into the ice hockey boards),[40,41] immobilization of the cervical spine is mandated. However, managing the airway properly in sports such as football, ice hockey, and lacrosse is complicated by the presence of protective headgear, mouth guards, and shoulder pads.[40–42] To gain access to the airway, the face mask of any protective helmet should be removed as soon as possible.[40,42,43] A football helmet should not be removed unless the athletic trainer is unable to gain access to the airway or if the helmet does not adequately secure the head.

Several studies cited by Waninger[40] also suggest delaying removal of the protective equipment in ice hockey until both the helmet and shoulder pads can be removed in a controlled setting or in the event that access to the airway is impossible. In one study, when the ice hockey helmet was removed, individual segmental measurements revealed a significant increase in cervical lordosis at the C6-C7 level; this was not seen when the helmet and shoulder pads

were left in place.[44] However, the presence of an ice hockey helmet, whether or not it fits properly, does result in increased movement in the sagittal and transverse planes when a prone log roll is performed.[45] Mihalik[45] points out that when an ice hockey helmet is stabilized, the head within it is not; therefore, he recommends that the helmet and face shield be removed before an emergency prone log roll is performed.

AIRWAY OBSTRUCTION

The airway can be obstructed by a mechanical obstruction (**foreign-body airway obstruction [FBAO]**) or anatomical obstruction (e.g., the tongue). In adults, airway obstructions most often occur from impacted food while eating. Airway obstructions in children occur while eating or playing.[12] Items such as chewing gum or sunflower seeds may cause airway obstruction,[46] particularly in an athletic environment. Although death from an obstructed airway is uncommon,[47] it is essential to recognize the situation and intervene immediately, while the person is still responsive.

An FBAO, sometimes referred to as a mechanical obstruction, occurs when items such as large, partially chewed food particles, marbles, toys, jewelry, mouth guards, dentures, or fluids (i.e., blood, vomit, mucus, and saliva) obstruct

Highlight

Chewing Gum Choked Teen

In 2007, a 15-year-old British teenager collapsed in his bedroom after choking on a piece of chewing gum, which lodged in his trachea. He was found by his parents, who heard him gasping for breath in his room. The youth went into cardiac arrest, requiring four paramedics to provide CPR for approximately an hour before they were able to identify a faint pulse. The teenager was taken to the hospital, where he was put on a life-support machine. However, doctors feared he would have permanent brain damage due to the lack of oxygen.[48]

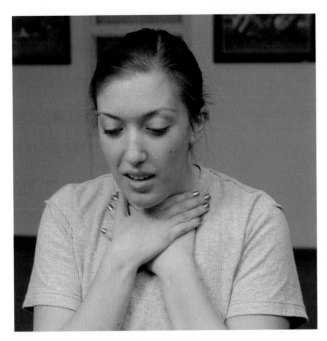

FIGURE 10.19   Universal sign of choking.

the airway. Anatomical airway obstructions occur when the tongue and/or swollen tissue blocks the upper or lower airway. Trauma to the upper and lower airway, such as a direct blow, and medical conditions, such as anaphylaxis, are the most common causes of an anatomical obstruction. In situations where an athletic trainer encounters an unconscious athlete with an airway obstruction, it has often been caused by the tongue dropping back into the athlete's throat, thus closing off the airway. This occurs as a result of muscle relaxation caused by lack of oxygen.

TABLE 10.5	Signs of an Airway Obstruction
Type	**Signs**
Partial	Clutching the neck, demonstrating the universal sign of choking
	Wheezing or high pitched sounds
	Coughing
	Ability to partially speak as air passes by the vocal cords
Complete	Clutching the neck, demonstrating the universal sign of choking
	Appears panicked due to no air exchange
	Inability to speak, silence
	Pale or cyanotic skin appearance around the mouth and nail beds

Signs of Airway Obstruction

Both foreign-object and anatomical obstructions can result in either a partially (mild) or completely (severe) obstructed airway. A partially obstructed airway results in poor air exchange and difficulty breathing, and leads to a complete airway obstruction if left untreated. A completely obstructed airway results in no exchange of air. The universal sign of choking is when an individual clutches his or her throat with the hands (Fig. 10.19). The remaining signs of a partial or complete airway obstruction are listed in Table 10.5.

EMERGENCY MEDICAL CARE FOR AIRWAY OBSTRUCTIONS

Depending on the athletic trainer's place of employment, he or she may be required to provide care to individuals of all ages. They may present with a partial or complete airway obstruction and may be conscious or unconscious, depending on the time interval between the causative event and the athletic trainer's ability to recognize that an emergency exists. This section examines how to manage an individual of any age suffering from any type of airway obstruction.

Conscious Adult and Child

Partial Airway Obstruction in an Adult and Child

A conscious adult or child suffering a partial airway obstruction will typically attempt to expel the obstruction by coughing or increasing the strength of breathing. If the athlete is coughing forcefully or attempting to breathe, do not interfere with these spontaneous efforts.[12] If the cause of the obstruction is a mouth guard, help the individual to remove it, using a gloved hand. Encourage him or her to cough in order to clear the obstruction. If the coughing continues and it appears that the individual will not be able to expel the object, consider sending a bystander to summon advanced medical personnel and be prepared to manage the obstruction.

Complete Airway Obstruction in an Adult or Child

An individual with a complete airway obstruction will be unable to breathe or speak. Approach the athlete and ask, "Are you choking?" If the person nods yes, this will verify that he or she has a complete airway obstruction is providing consent. Be sure to obtain consent from the athlete (parental consent is required for a child and infant) and begin providing care by delivering a combination of back blows and abdominal thrusts. Research has demonstrated an increase in the success rate when a combination of back blows, abdominal thrusts, and chest thrusts (when indicated) are utilized.[12] Begin care by following the directions in

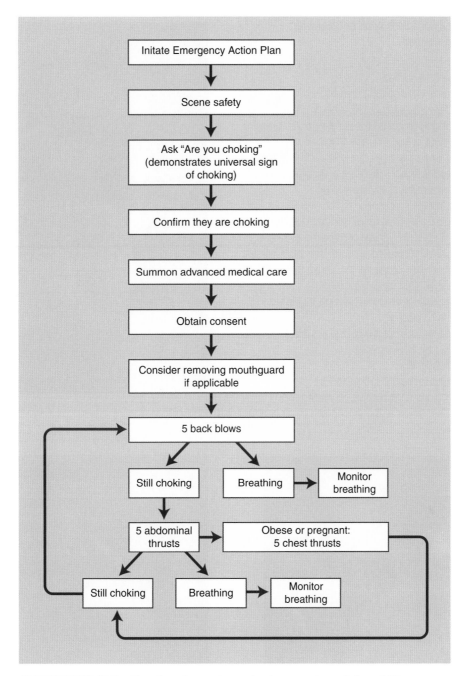

ALGORITHM 10.2   Complete airway obstruction in a conscious adult or child.

Skill 10.3 or referring to Algorithm 10.2 for an emergency action decisional algorithm.

The only difference between an adult and child (1 to 12 years of age) is that, when confronted with a child, the athletic trainer must obtain parental consent to intervene. Then the athletic trainer must stand or kneel behind the child (Fig. 10.23), depending on his or her size, and deliver the five back blows and five abdominal thrusts with less force than typically required for an adult. If the

individual is obese or in the later stages of pregnancy and the athletic trainer is unable to encircle the abdomen to perform the abdominal thrusts, it may be necessary to perform chest thrusts.[12] This is done by reaching around the individual, making a fist, and placing it in the center of the chest. Be sure the fist is not located on the xiphoid process (compressing the xiphoid process increases the risk of possible lung or abdominal trauma). Cover the fist with the other hand and provide five inward thrusts on

Steps for Managing a Conscious Adult or Child with Complete Airway Obstruction

1. Initiate the EAP.
2. Check the safety of the scene.
3. Take body substance isolation (BSI) precautions.
4. Approach the athlete, placing yourself at his or her side.
5. Place your arm diagonally across the athlete's chest, grasping the opposite shoulder to lean the individual forward.
6. Using the heel of your other hand, firmly strike the athlete five times with distinctive blows between the shoulder blades in order to dislodge the obstruction (Fig. 10.20).
7. Stand behind the athlete, placing one leg between his or hers. This will allow you to safely bring the athlete from a standing to a supine position in the event he or she becomes unresponsive.
8. Find the umbilicus with one hand and, with the other, make a fist. Place the thumb side of the fist just above the umbilicus and cover it with your other hand (Fig. 10.21).
9. Provide five quick, distinctive upward and inward thrusts in order to dislodge the obstruction.
10. Continue with a combination of five back blows and abdominal thrusts until
    - the object is dislodged.
    - the athlete begins to breathe independently.
    - the athlete becomes unresponsive, in which case you will have to lower him or her to the ground and begin care for an unresponsive obstructed airway (Fig. 10.22). Be sure to support the head and neck.

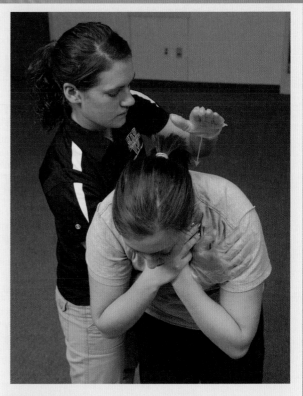

FIGURE 10.20

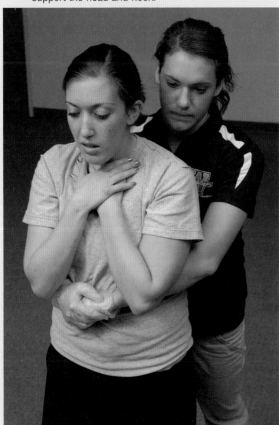

FIGURE 10.21

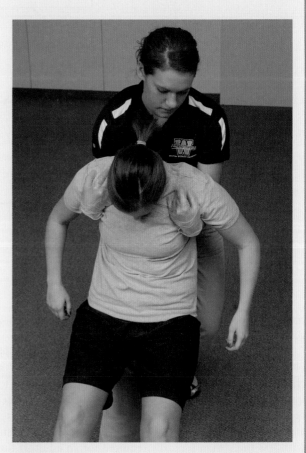

FIGURE 10.22

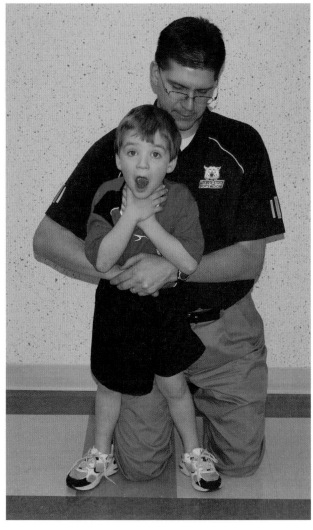

FIGURE 10.23 Treating a conscious choking child. Be sure to get down to the child's level when you are providing care.

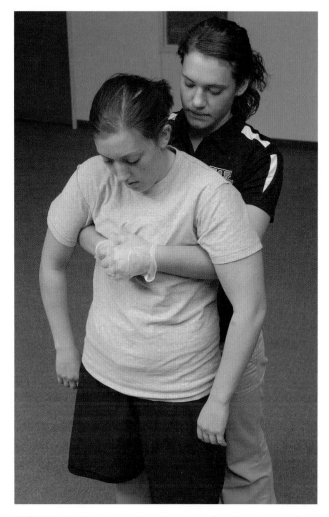

FIGURE 10.24 Proper hand position for chest thrusts for a conscious choking adult or child. The fist should be placed on the center of the sternum in a similar fashion to the abdominal thrusts.

the sternum (Fig. 10.24). Again repeat five back blows and five chest thrusts until the

1. object is dislodged.
2. athlete begins to breathe independently.
3. athlete becomes unresponsive.

Unconscious Adult or Child Athlete

An athlete who is unable to dislodge the foreign-body airway obstruction will eventually lose consciousness. Depending upon when the emergency occurred and whether there was a witness, the athletic trainer may not know the exact mechanism of the injury. Because there are many causes of loss of consciousness (e.g., airway obstruction, cardiac arrest, medical illness), the athletic trainer will have to complete a primary assessment, remembering that the airway must be cleared first before any other problems are treated.

Begin care by following the directions in Skill 10.4 or referring to Algorithm 10.3 for an emergency action decisional algorithm.

Obstructed Airway in a Conscious to Unconscious Athlete

If, during the management of an airway obstruction, the athlete becomes unconscious, immediately lower him or her to the floor, supporting the head and neck (Fig. 10.22). Open the airway by grasping the athlete's tongue and lower jaw to look for a foreign body. If a foreign body is observed, perform a finger sweep to remove the object using your index finger in an adult and your fifth (pinky) finger in a child. Perform two rescue breaths and continue with step 7 in Skill 10.4.

Obstructed Airway in an Infant

Airway obstructions in infants are a common problem, often the result of liquids,[49] foreign bodies (e.g., food, balloons,

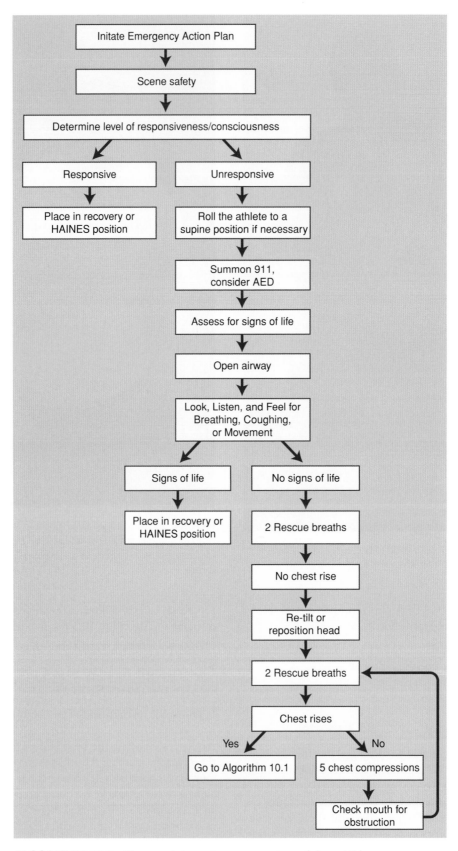

ALGORITHM 10.3   Obstructed airway in an unconscious adult or child.

SKILL 10.4

Steps for Managing an Obstructed Airway in an Unconscious Adult or Child

1. Initiate the EAP.
2. Check the safety of the scene.
3. Take BSI precautions.
4. Determine the athlete's level of responsiveness by tapping his or her shoulder and shouting, "Are you all right? Are you OK?" If he or she is unresponsive, summon advanced medical personnel and consider the use of an AED.
5. Airway
   - Open the airway using a head-tilt/chin-lift (Fig. 10.8) or jaw-thrust maneuver (Fig. 10.16).
6. Breathing (refer back to Skill 10.1)
   - Look, listen, and feel for signs of life for no more than 10 seconds.
   - Secure a breathing barrier device over the athlete's face.
   - If no adequate breathing is detected, provide two rescue breaths over 1 second with enough volume to ensure that the chest clearly rises.
7. If the two rescue breaths fail to go in or the chest does not clearly rise and fall (Fig. 10.10),
   - In an adult, tilt the head back further.
   - Reposition a child's head by retilting.
8. Reattempt two rescue breaths.
9. If the two rescue breaths fail to go in or the chest does not clearly rise and fall, prepare for chest compressions.
10. Chest compressions
    - Place the heel of one hand on the center of the athlete's chest.
    - Place the opposite hand on the top of the first hand and deliver five chest compressions at a rate of 100 compressions per minute, ensuring that each compression is a distinctive attempt to dislodge the object (Fig. 10.25).
    - Compress an adult's chest 1½ to 2 in.
    - Compress a child's chest 1 to 1½ in.
11. Open the airway by grasping the athlete's tongue and lower jaw and looking for a foreign body. If a foreign body is observed, perform a finger sweep to remove the object (Fig. 10.26).
    - For an adult, place your index finger on the inside of the cheek on the side furthest from you. Using a hooking motion, slide your finger down the cheek and sweep the object out.
    - For a child, place your fifth finger on the inside of the cheek on the side furthest from you. Using a hooking motion, slide your finger down the cheek and sweep the object out.
12. Reattempt two rescue breaths (Fig. 10.10)
    - If the two rescue breaths fail to go in or the chest does not clearly rise and fall repeat steps 10 to 11.
    - If the two rescue breath go in and the chest clearly rises and falls, continue with the primary assessment.
13. Circulation
    - While maintaining the airway if possible, identify the carotid artery.
14. Scan the athlete for any immediate threats of severe bleeding. Again, remember to maintain the airway.
15. Provide necessary care
    - If the athlete displays a pulse and is breathing, place him or her in the recovery position or the HAINES position if a spinal injury is suspected.
    - If the athlete displays a pulse but is not breathing, begin rescue breathing.
    - If the athlete displays no pulse and is not breathing, begin CPR.

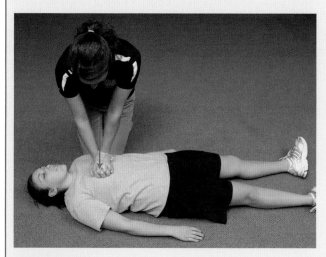

FIGURE 10.25

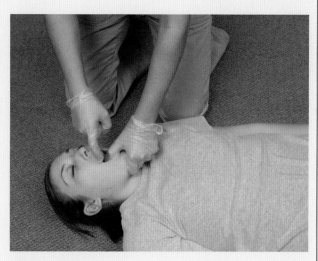

FIGURE 10.26

coins, small balls),[50] and/or other medical conditions such as croup or epiglottitis. Firm foods—such as hot dogs, nuts, and grapes to name only a few—pose the most danger because infants and young children do not grind or chew their food well. In fact, these foods are not recommended for children under the age of 4.[51] And although it is unlikely that an athletic trainer will ever have to manage an infant's obstructed airway, one never knows when this skill might be needed.

Conscious Infant with an Airway Obstruction

Unlike adults and children, infants in distress due to an airway obstruction lack the ability to communicate, making this situation potentially more dangerous. For this reason the athletic trainer should be prepared to properly manage an infant suffering from a partial or complete airway obstruction. Suspect an FBAO with a sudden onset of respiratory distress including coughing, gagging, stridor, or wheezing.[52] An infant with a complete airway obstruction cannot cry or cough and will require a combination of chest thrusts and back blows because abdominal thrusts increase the risk damage to the of liver, which is relatively large and unprotected.

Begin care by following the directions in Skill 10.5 or referring to Algorithm 10.4 for an emergency action decisional algorithm.

Unconscious Infant with an Airway Obstruction

When managing an unconscious infant with suspected airway obstruction, begin by following the directions in Skill 10.6 or referring to Algorithm 10.5 for an emergency action decisional algorithm.

Obstructed Airway in Conscious to Unconscious Infant

If, during the management of an airway obstruction in a conscious infant, the infant becomes unconscious, you should place the infant on a firm surface and immediately open the airway by grasping the infant's tongue and lower

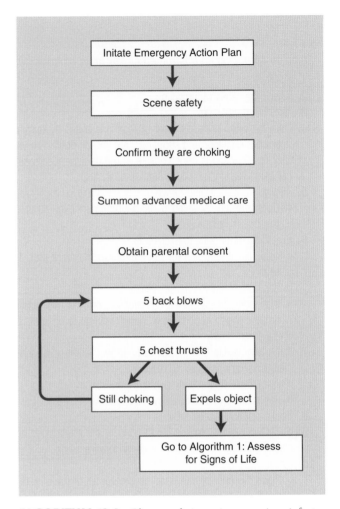

ALGORITHM 10.4   Obstructed airway in a conscious infant.

jaw and observing for a foreign body. If a foreign body is observed, perform a fifth-finger sweep (pinky sweep) beginning on the inside of the check on the side furthest from you, using a hooking motion to sweep the object of the mouth. Perform two rescue breaths and continue with step 8 in Skill 10.6.

SKILL 10.5

Steps for Managing a Conscious Infant with an Obstructed Airway

1. Initiate the EAP.
2. Obtain parental consent.
3. Take BSI precautions.
4. Place the infant in a prone position, resting on your forearm and supporting the head and neck. Rest your forearm on your thigh, keeping the infant's head lower than the body.
5. Apply five back blows between the shoulder blades (Fig. 10.27).
6. Support the infant between your forearms and roll the infant face up, again supporting the head and neck and resting your forearm on your thigh.

7. Place three fingers on the center of chest (sternum) at the nipple line, lifting your ring finger (Fig. 10.28).
8. Provide five chest thrusts, compressing approximately ½ to 1 in., keeping your fingers perpendicular to the sternum.
9. Continue repeating steps 4 to 8 until:
   - The obstruction is dislodged.
   - The infant begins to cry, cough, or breathe on his or her own.
   - The infant becomes unresponsive.

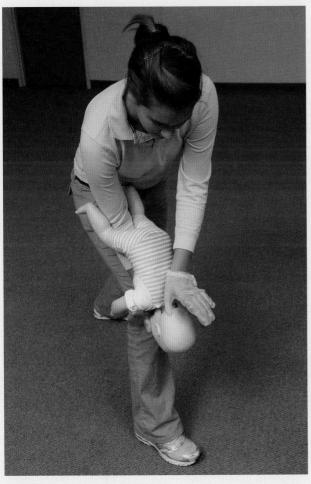

FIGURE 10.27

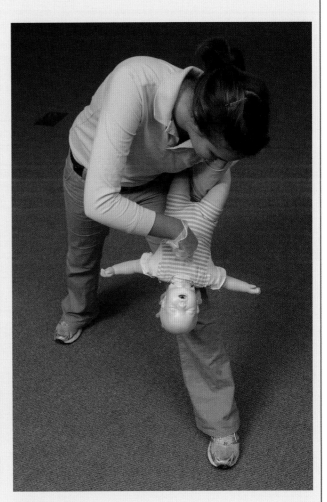

FIGURE 10.28

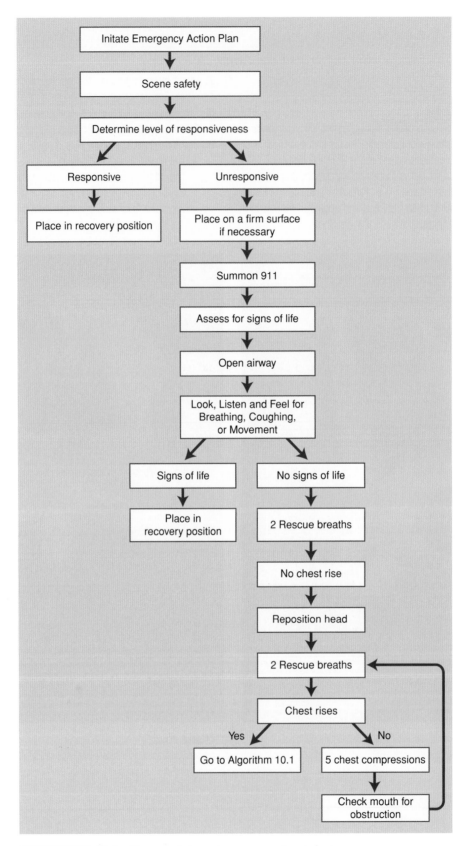

ALGORITHM 10.5   Obstructed airway in an unconscious infant.

SKILL 10.6

Steps for Managing an Unconscious Infant with an Obstructed Airway

1. Initiate the EAP.
2. Check for safety of the scene.
3. Take BSI precautions.
4. Determine the infant's level of responsiveness by tapping or flicking the feet (Fig. 10.29). If the infant is unresponsive, summon advanced medical personnel.
5. If the infant is prone, immediately place him or her in a supine position, supporting the head, neck and back, and begin a primary assessment to determine any compromise to the infant's ABCs (airway, breathing, and circulation, including external bleeding) by opening and adequately maintaining the airway.
6. Airway (Fig. 10.4)
   - Open the airway using a head-tilt/chin-lift (place in a neutral position) or jaw-thrust maneuver.
7. Breathing (Fig. 10.30)
   - Look, listen, and feel for signs of life for no more than 10 seconds.
   - Secure a breathing barrier device over the infant's face.
   - If no adequate breathing is detected, provide two rescue breaths over 1 second with enough volume to ensure that the chest clearly rises (Fig. 10.31).
8. If the two rescue breaths fail to go in or the chest does not clearly rise and fall, reposition the head by retilting.
9. Reattempt two rescue breaths.
10. If the two rescue breaths fail to go in or the chest does not clearly rise and fall, prepare for chest compressions.

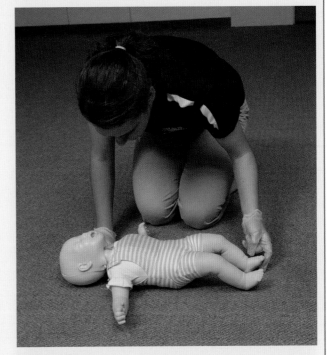

FIGURE 10.29

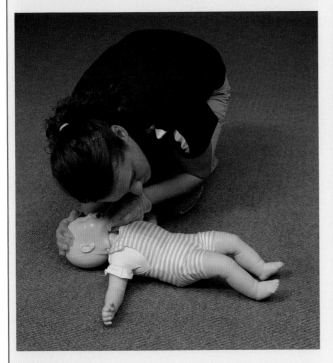

FIGURE 10.30

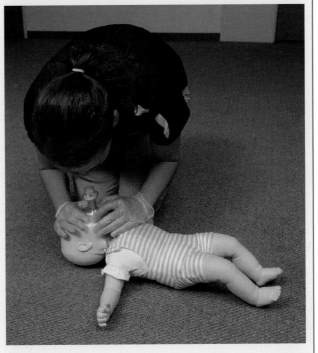

FIGURE 10.31

(Continued)

SKILL 10.6 *(Continued)*

Steps for Managing an Unconscious Infant with an Obstructed Airway (Continued)

11. Initiate chest compressions.
  ○ Place three fingers on the center of chest (sternum) at the nipple line and lift your index finger.

12. Provide five chest thrusts, compressing at a rate of 100 compressions per minute approximately ½ to 1 in. deep, keeping your fingers perpendicular to the sternum. Make sure that each compression is a distinctive attempt to dislodge the object (Fig. 10.32).

13. Open the airway by grasping the tongue and lower jaw and observing for a foreign body. If a foreign body is observed, perform a fifth-finger sweep on the inside of the cheek and sweep the object out (Fig. 10.33).

14. Reattempt two rescue breaths.
  ○ If the two rescue breaths fail to go in or the chest does not clearly rise and fall, repeat steps 11 to 13.
  ○ If the two rescue breaths go in and the chest clearly rises and falls, continue with the primary assessment.

15. Circulation
  ○ While maintaining the airway, identify the brachial artery.

16. Scan for any immediate threats of severe bleeding. Again, remembering to maintain the airway.

17. Provide necessary care.
  ○ If the infant displays a pulse and is breathing, place him or her in the recovery position.
  ○ If the infant displays a pulse but is not breathing, begin rescue breathing.
  ○ If the infant displays no pulse and is not breathing, begin CPR.

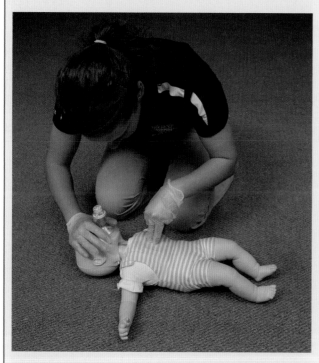

FIGURE 10.32

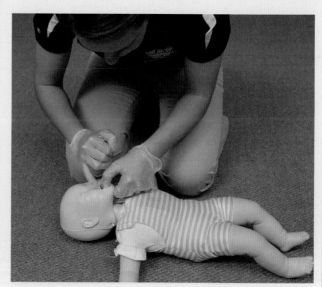

FIGURE 10.33

WRAP-UP

An athlete suffering from acute trauma or illness that impairs the function of the lungs or airways constitutes a breathing emergency. Although the athletes under your care will rarely suffer from respiratory arrest or foreign-body airway obstructions, you, as an athletic trainer, should know how to deal with such extreme emergencies. More likely, you may, on occasion, have to manage situations of less serious respiratory distress and/or inadequate breathing. This chapter focused on the role of the athletic trainer in respiratory emergencies, including the indications, contraindications, and management of athletes suffering from respiratory distress. Practicing the techniques described in this chapter periodically, most likely at the start of an athletic season or during the annual review of the EAP, will help you to remain competent in the skills required to properly manage an athlete suffering from respiratory distress or arrest. The initial care you administer may make the difference between life and death.

Scenarios

1. A female athlete competing at the regional cross-country meet finishes the race and falls to her knees. When the athletic trainer arrives on site, the athlete is responsive but complains of shortness of breath as well as numbness and tingling in her extremities, wheezing, and difficulty breathing. She has a history of exercise-induced asthma. Oxygen by partial nonrebreather mask at 15 L/min is administered.

   What is the athlete's problem?
   Describe the appropriate steps in managing this case. If the athlete became restless, combative, and/or began to present with an altered mental status, would your treatment steps change? Why or why not?

2. You are covering a collegiate ice hockey game when your star player is suddenly struck in the head with a puck. The player collapses to the ice and you and your athletic training student slide out to inspect him. The general impression indicates that a young man is lying motionless, apparently unresponsive. You immediately send your athletic training student to call 911.

   What would you do next?
   If the athlete has a pulse but is not breathing, what type of care should be administered?
   What would you do if he began breathing?

3. You are sitting at lunch with a coworker, having an enjoyable afternoon. After taking a bite of his burger, your coworker suddenly begins to cough violently.

   What should you do?
   If your coworker stopped coughing and motioned toward his throat, what would be your next step?
   If, after 30 seconds of treatment and no improvement, he lost consciousness, what would be your next step?

4. While you are covering a high school baseball game, you hear one of the parents in the crowd begin to scream. You arrive at the mother's side and realize that her 8-month-old is in distress, noting that the infant is blue but still conscious. The mother says, "I think she is choking."

   Your immediate reaction should be to provide what type of care?
   If the infant eventually lost consciousness, what steps would you take to properly manage this situation?
   At what point would you summon advanced medical care?

REFERENCES

1. Board of Certification. FAQ. http://www.bocatc.org/index.php?option=com_content&task=view&id=111&Itemid=119. Accessed June 20, 2009.
2. Pop Warner Little Scholars. About Pop Warner. http://www.popwarner.com/aboutus/history.asp. Accessed June 20, 2009.
3. American Youth Football & Cheer. About AYF. http://www.americanyouthfootball.com/about.asp. Accessed June 20, 2009.
4. American Youth Soccer Organization. A history of AYSO. http://soccer.org/Resources/RulesRegulations/. Accessed June 23, 2009.
5. United States Youth Soccer Association. Largest youth sports organization celebrates 35th anniversary. http://www.usyouthsoccer.org/aboutus/History.asp. Accessed June 20, 2009.
6. Dompier T, Powell JW, Barron M, et al. Time-loss and non–time-loss injuries in youth football players. *J Athl Train.* 2007;42(3):395–402.
7. National Safe Kids Campaign (NSKC). Injury fact: Sports injury. http://www.usa.safekids.org/tier3_cd.cfm?folder_id=540&content_item_id=1211. Accessed June 20, 2009.
8. Paluska SA, Lansford CD. Laryngeal trauma in sport. *Curr Sports Med Rep.* 2008;7(1):16–21.
9. Jewett B, Shockley W, Rutledge R. External laryngeal trauma analysis of 392 patients. *Arch Otolaryngol Head Neck Surg.* 1999;125(8):877–880.
10. Thevasagayam MS, Pracy P. Laryngeal trauma: A systematic approach to management. *Trauma.* 2005;7(2):87–94.
11. Gussack G, Jurkovich G, Luterman A. Laryngotracheal trauma: A protocol approach to a rare injury. *Laryngocope.* 1986; 96:660–665.
12. American Heart Association. Part 4: Adult basic life support. *Circulation.* 2005;112(24 Suppl):IV-19–IV-34.
13. Limmer D, Mistovich JJ, Krost W. Beyond the basics: Putting the VITAL back in vital signs. http://www.emsresponder.com/print/Emergency—Medical-Services/Beyond-the-Basics—Putting-the-VITAL-Back-in-Vital-Signs/1$8237. Accessed June 20, 2009.
14. American Heart Association. Part 10.3: Drowning. *Circulation.* 2005;112(24 Suppl):IV-133–IV-135.
15. American Heart Association. Part 10.5: Near-Fatal Asthma. *Circulation.* 2005;112(24 Suppl):IV-139–IV-142.
16. American Heart Association. Part 10.6: Anaphylaxis. *Circulation.* 2005;112(24 Suppl):IV-143–IV-145.
17. Markou NK, Myrianthefs PM, Baltopoulos GJ. Respiratory failure. *Crit Care Nurs Q.* 2004;27(4):353–379.
18. Tomlinson L, Bellingan GJ. Trauma and acute lung injury. *Trauma.* 2002;4(3):147.
19. National Highway Traffic Safety Administration, Emergency Medical Services. *National Emergency Medical Services Education Standards, Emergency Medical Responder Instructional Guidelines.* Washington, DC: U.S. Department of Transportation; 2009.
20. American Red Cross. *CPR/AED for the Professional Rescuer Participant's Manual.* Yardley, PA: Staywell; 2006.
21. Beevers G, Lip G, O'Brien E. ABC of hypertension: Blood pressure measurement. *Br Med J.* 2005;322:981–985.

22. Kraman S. Transmission of lung sounds through light clothing. *Respiration*. 2008;75(1):85–88.

23. Offner PJ, Heit J, Roberts R. Implementation of a rapid response team decreases cardiac arrest outside of the intensive care unit. *J Trauma*. 2007;62(5):1223–1227; discussion 1227–1228.

24. Perkins G, Stephenson B, Hulme J, et al. Birmingham assessment of breathing study (BABS). *Resuscitation*. 2005;64(1): 109–113.

25. Perkins G, Walker G, Christensen K, et al. Teaching recognition of agonal breathing improves accuracy of diagnosing cardiac arrest. *Resuscitation*. 2006;70(3):423–437.

26. Liberman MM, Mudler DS. Airway injuries in the professional ice hockey player. *Clin J Sport Med*. 2007;17:61–67.

27. Doerges V, Sauer C, Ocker H, et al. Smaller tidal volumes during cardiopulmonary resuscitation: Comparison of adult and paediatric self-inflatable bags with three different ventilatory devices. *Resuscitation*. 1999;43(1):31–37.

28. Doerges V, Sauer C, Ocker H, et al. Airway management during cardiopulmonary resuscitation: A comparative study of bag-valve-mask, laryngeal mask airway and Combitube in a bench model. *Resuscitation*. 1999;41(1):63–69.

29. Dorges V, Ocker H, Wenzel V, et al. Emergency airway management by non-anaesthesia house officers: A comparison of three strategies. *Emerg Med J*. 2001;18(2):90–94.

30. Wenzel V, Idris AH, Montogomery WH, et al. Rescue breathing and bag-mask ventilation. *Ann Emerg Med*. 2001; 37(4 Suppl):S36–S40.

31. American Heart Association. Part 2: Adult basic life support. *Circulation*. 2005;112(22 Suppl):III-5–III-16.

32. Dorges V, Ocker H, Hagelberg S, et al. Smaller tidal volumes with room air are not sufficient to ensure adequate oxygenation during bag-valve-mask ventilation. *Resuscitation*. 2000;44(1):37–41.

33. Cook T, Godfrey I, Rockett M, et al. Cricoid pressure: Which hand? *Anaesthesia*. 2000;55(7):648–653.

34. Andrew P. Teaching anaesthetic nurses optimal force for effective cricoid pressure: A literature review. *Nurs Crit Care*. 2009;14(3):139–144.

35. Parry A. Teaching anaesthetic nurses optimal force for effective cricoid pressure: A literature review. *Nurs Crit Care*. 2009;14(3):139–144.

36. Flucker C, Hart E, Weisz M, et al. The 50-millilitre syringe as an inexpensive training aid in the application of cricoid pressure. *Eur J Anaesthesiol*. 2000;17(7):443–447.

37. Quigley P, Jeffrey P. Cricoid pressure: assessment of performance and effect of training in emergency department staff. *Emerg Med Australas*. 2007;19(3):218–222.

38. Bhalla RK, Corrigan A, Roland NJ. Comparison of two face masks used to deliver early ventilation to laryngectomized patients. *Ears Nose Throat J*. 2004;83:414–416.

39. Heck JF, Clarke KS, Peterson TR, et al. National Athletic Trainers' Association position statement: Head-down contact and spearing in tackle football. *J Athl Train*. 2004;39(1):101–111.

40. Waninger K. Management of the helmeted athlete with suspected cervical spine injury. *Am J Sports Med*. 2004;32:1331–1350.

41. Blue J, Pecci M. The collapsed athlete. *Ortho Clin North Am*. 2002;33:471–478.

42. Swartz EE, Boden BP, Courson RW, et al. National Athletic Trainers' Association Position Statement: Acute management of the cervical spine–injured athlete. *J Athl Train*. 2009;44(3):306–311.

43. Kleiner DM, Almquist J, Bailes J, et al. *Prehospital care of the spine-injured athlete: A document from the Inter-Association Task Force for Appropriate Care of the Spine-Injured Athlete*. Dallas: National Athletic Trainers' Association; 2001.

44. Laprade R, Schnetzler K, Broxterman R, et al. Cervical spine alignment in the immobilized ice hockey player. A computed tomographic analysis of the effects of helmet removal. *Am J Sports Med*. 2000;28(6):800–803.

45. Mihalik J, Beard J, Petschauer M, et al. Effect of ice hockey helmet fit on cervical spine motion during an emergency log roll procedure. *Clin J Sport Med*. 2008;18(5):394–399.

46. Oğuz F, Citak A, Unüvar E, et al. Airway foreign bodies in childhood. *Int J Pediatr Otorhinolaryngol*. 2000;52(1):11–16.

47. Fingerhut LA, Cox CS, Warner M. International comparative analysis of injury mortality. Findings from the ICE on injury statistics. International Collaborative Effort on Injury Statistics. *Adv Data* 1998;7(303):1–20.

48. Chewing gum choked teen. *Advertiser*. 2007;40.

49. Vilke GM, Smith AM, Ray LU, et al. Airway obstruction in children aged less than 5 years: The prehospital experience. *Prehosp Emerg Care*. 2004;8:196–199.

50. Morley RE, Ludemann JP, Moxham JP, et al. Foreign body aspiration in infants and toddlers: recent trends in British Columbia. *J Otolaryngol*. 2004;33:37–41.

51. American Academy of Pediatrics. Choking prevention and first aid for infants and children. http://www.aap.org/publiced/BR_Choking.htm. Accessed November 8, 2007.

52. American Heart Association. 2005 American Heart Association (AHA) guidelines for cardiopulmonary resuscitation (CPR) and emergency cardiovascular care (ECC) of pediatric and neonatal patients: pediatric basic life support. *Pediatrics*. 2006;117:e989–e1004.

53. Assessing breath sounds. *Nursing*. 1983;13(8):68.

54. Visich MA. Knowing what you hear: A guide to assessing breath and heart sounds. *Nursing*. 1981;11(11):64–79.

55. Steadman's Concise Medical Dictionary. *Steadman's Medical Dictionary*. Philadelphia: Lippincott Williams & Wilkins; 2001.

56. Anderson M, Hall S, Martin M. Throat, thorax, and visceral conditions. *Foundation of Athletic Training: Prevention, Assessment, and Management*. Baltimore: Lippincott Williams & Wilkins; 2005:336–337.

57. Owen A. Respiratory assessment revisited. *Nursing*. 1998: 48–49.

58. Starkey C, Ryan J. *Evaluation of Orthopedic and Athletic Injuries*, 2nd ed. Philadelphia: FA Davis; 2002.

59. Frisbie JH, Sharma GVRK. Cheyne-Stokes respiration, periodic circulation, and pulsus alternans in spinal cord injury patients. *Spinal Cord*. 2005;43(6):385–388.

CHAPTER 11

Adjunct Breathing Devices and Supplemental Oxygen Therapy

CHAPTER OUTCOMES

1. Discuss the different types of breathing devices (suctioning, adjunct airways, and barrier devices) used to establish and maintain an airway and adequately ventilate an adult, child, and infant.

2. Identify the role, characteristics, and indications for the use of suction in an emergency situation.

3. Demonstrate how to prepare and administer a suction unit in an emergency situation.

4. Identify the role, characteristics, indications, and contraindications for the use of oropharyngeal (oral) and/or nasopharyngeal (nasal) airways in an emergency situation.

5. Demonstrate how to prepare, measure, and insert an oropharyngeal (oral) and/or nasopharyngeal (nasal) airway in an emergency situation.

6. Identify the role, characteristics, and indications for the use of barrier devices in an emergency.

7. Demonstrate how to prepare and administer barrier devices in an emergency situation.

8. Identify the role, characteristics, and indications for the use of a bag-valve-mask device (BVM) in an emergency situation.

9. Demonstrate how to prepare and administer a BVM for a single- or two-person rescue team.

10. Demonstrate how to establish and manage an airway using a breathing device with an athlete who has a suspected spinal injury and is wearing protective equipment.

11. Describe the role and function of supplemental oxygen therapy as an adjunct to respiratory and cardiopulmonary resuscitation.

12. Identify the indications, contraindications, and precautions for the use of supplemental oxygen in an emergency situation.

13. Demonstrate how to prepare and administer supplemental oxygen to breathing and nonbreathing athletes, using a variety of delivery devices in an emergency situation.

NOMENCLATURE

Adjunct breathing devices: devices used to assist in the resuscitation of an individual, thereby optimizing that individual's chances of survival

Artificial ventilation: when normal breathing is inefficient or has stopped, the process of supporting breathing by the application of mechanical or manual means

NOMENCLATURE *(Continued)*

Aspiration: inhalation into the airways of fluid or a foreign body (e.g., vomit)

Gag reflex: retching or gagging due to contact of a foreign body with the mucous membrane of the space between the cavity of the mouth and the pharynx

Gastric distention: expansion or bloating of the stomach, as may occur when air is forced into it

Hypoventilation: reduced alveolar ventilation relative to metabolic carbon dioxide production, so that alveolar carbon dioxide pressure increases to above normal

Hypoxemia or hypoxaemia: subnormal oxygenation of arterial blood

Hypoxia: low or below normal levels of oxygen in inspired gases, arterial blood, or tissue

Laryngospasm: spasmodic closure of the larynx in response to the introduction to water, allergens, or noxious stimuli that block the passage of air to the lungs

$PaCO_2$: arterial carbon dioxide pressure

Regurgitation: the vomiting or ejection of matter from the stomach through the mouth

Tachypnea or tachypnoea: rapid breathing

Tidal volume: volume of air taken in our out in a single breath during regular breathing

BEFORE YOU BEGIN

1. What are adjunct airway devices and why is it important to understand how to use them?

2. What are the basic steps in using a suction device? Is there a difference in suction time between an adult, child, and infant?

3. What, if any, devices can the athletic trainer utilize to help maintain an airway during an emergency?

4. What are the appropriate steps when inserting an oropharyngeal airway?

5. What is a BVM? Why are these devices more useful in providing positive-pressure ventilation than other breathing devices?

6. If an athlete with protective equipment suddenly collapsed, what strategies could be used to provide positive-pressure ventilation while attempting to remove the athlete's face mask?

7. What is supplemental oxygen? Identify the procedures for setting up and breaking down an oxygen tank.

8. What are some safety precautions one would use when working with supplemental oxygen?

Voices from the Field

Twenty years of athletic training experience has exposed me to many different types of athletic injuries. These injuries have ranged from sprains, strains, and contusions to the extremities to more serious injuries such as head injuries, neck injuries, heart conditions, and airway problems. Fortunately, these more serious injuries do not occur on a daily basis; in some sports occurrences might even be years apart. Even though they might rarely occur, it is critical for us to be well prepared when they do.

My experience with life-threatening injuries and conditions has impressed upon me the absolute necessity to be as well trained as our profession will allow in airway management and oxygen administration. This training begins as simply as with a head tilt–chin lift, as a part of the primary survey, and continues to oxygen administration, oral and nasal pharyngeal airways, and even a simple assessment of lung sounds using a stethoscope.

I can remember running out on a football field to evaluate a player who had just received a devastating blow to the chest area from another player. The player was semiconscious and was having difficulty breathing. Thankfully we had oxygen on the sidelines, which I had been trained to use in an emergency situation. The administration of oxygen relieved his labored breathing. I also had been trained to insert an oropharyngeal airway in case he became unconscious and was unable to maintain an airway on his own. Without the airway, it could have become very difficult to administer oxygen. Once on the sidelines, I was able to carefully listen to each lung to make sure both were at least receiving some air. The athlete was eventually diagnosed as having a contused lung. He was hospitalized and released the next day. We can never be too prepared!

Joel Bass, MS, LAT, ATC
Head Athletic Trainer
Weber State University
Ogden, Utah

In Chapter 10, we examined how to effectively manage an athlete with a breathing emergency using no specialized equipment beyond gloves and a simple breathing device. In most cases these basic devices will be all that is required and perhaps all that is readily available in an emergency situation. However, there may be circumstances in which access to certain **adjunct breathing devices** will improve the effectiveness of resuscitation, thereby optimizing the athlete's chances of survival. This chapter describes in detail a variety of adjunct breathing devices commonly used when treating an athlete with a breathing emergency. The techniques described in this chapter do require practice to maintain clinical competence and should be reviewed annually by an athletic trainer with the emergency action plan (EAP) and other emergency procedures.

It should also be noted that the skills addressed in this chapter are derived from the *National EMS Education Standards, Instructional Guidelines for Emergency Medical Responders*[1] and are normally taught as part of an emergency medical responder course. Athletic trainers should check with individual state laws and practice acts to determine whether use of the adjunct breathing devices presented here is acceptable in their state. If necessary, organizations such as the American Red Cross, American Heart Association, and National Safety Council offer certification courses related to these skills.

FUNCTIONS OF BREATHING DEVICES

Athletic trainers may have a variety of different breathing devices available to them when assisting an athlete with a breathing emergency. Which device is selected depends upon the emergency situation, the athletic trainer's level of training and comfort with the devices, and the availability of equipment. Adjunct breathing devices can be used for all age groups using age-appropriate techniques and equipment. They have three main functions: (a) clearing and maintaining an athlete's airway, (b) providing adequate ventilation, (c) and supplying supplemental oxygen to a breathing or nonbreathing athlete. Clearing an airway is accomplished using either a mechanical or manual suction unit. Oropharyngeal (oral) and/or nasopharyngeal (nasal) airways are used to help the athletic trainer maintain an athlete's airway. Maintaining adequate ventilation in an athlete with a breathing emergency can be accomplished by one or two athletic trainers using positive-pressure ventilation (e.g., BVM). Supplemental high-flow concentrated oxygen is used for breathing and/or nonbreathing athletes in conjunction with other breathing devices (e.g., supplemental oxygen attached to a BVM).

SUCTIONING

Suctioning is the process of removing blood, fluid, pulmonary secretions, and small food particles that have collected in an airway from either a trauma or illness. Several different types of suction units are available, all of which use a negative-pressure vacuum system to remove the foreign material and body fluids from the athlete's mouth. If fluid and/or debris are allowed to collect in the mouth, they can end up in the trachea and eventually in the lungs, thus increasing the risk of **aspiration.** However, suction units, regardless of the type of device utilized, are inadequate for removing solid objects like teeth, foreign bodies, and/or large food particles. Attempting to remove large particles or debris may actually cause the suction unit to lose its suctioning ability, making it useless. This section examines the role, characteristics, and indications for the use of suction; it also demonstrates how to prepare and administer a suction unit in an emergency.

Suction Units

All suctioning units consist of three or four main components, including (a) a mounted or portable unit, (b) suction tubing, (c) suction tips/catheters, and (d) a collection container (Table 11.1). Mounted suction units are fixed wall units generating a vacuum suction from an electrical source (e.g., hospital units) or a car manifold when installed in an ambulance. These, however, are not practical for an athletic trainer on the playing field. Portable suction units, on the other hand, can be carried on-field and create a vacuum suction similar to that of wall-mounted units. They can be used either mechanically or manually (Fig. 11.1).

Portable mechanical suction units generate vacuum suction pressure via an electrical source, battery, or oxygen-powered device. Some portable suction units can run off of all three, making them reliable tools anywhere. All suction units regardless of type (mounted or portable) must generate a negative vacuum suction pressure greater than 300 mm Hg when the suction tube is clamped and be powerful enough to provide an airflow greater than 40 L/min at the end of the suction tubing.[2] Mechanical suction units can generate a negative pressure much larger than the minimum 300 mm Hg required of all units (some manufacturers report a suction pressure as high as 700 mm Hg). They have higher-capacity collection containers (300+ mL) than portable handheld units but are also bulkier, require an energy source, and normally cost significantly more than a portable handheld unit. Mechanical suction units also do not store as well in an athletic training kit because of their size; such a unit often requires its own storage bag.

Manual portable suction units include commercial devices, bulb syringes, and even the good ol' turkey baster. Commercial devices such as the V-VAC Manual Suction Unit (Laerdal Medical, Wappingers Falls, NY) and Ambu Res-Cue Pump (Ambu Inc., Glen Burnie, MD) are compact, lightweight devices that take up little space in an athletic training kit. They generate more than 380 mm Hg of negative pressure when a handle/trigger is compressed manually; this, in turn, moves a plunger within the barrel.[3] Most units can be adjusted for adult and child suctioning by changing the stroke volume, thus decreasing the vacuum suction. For example, the Ambu Res-Cue Pump generates

TABLE 11.1	Components, Purpose, and Characteristics of a Suction Unit	
Component	**Purpose**	**Characteristics**
Suction tubing	Attaches to the suction unit; allows for the passage of body fluids and small foreign materials to the collection container.	Clear, plastic, nonkinking tube with a wide-diameter opening.
Rigid suction tip (also known as a Yankauer tip or tonsil sucker)	Attaches to the suction tubing; aids in removing the foreign material and body fluids, such as vomit and thick secretions in an unconscious athlete.	Larger opening than in a flexible catheter; may stimulate a gag reflex when inserted into the back of the mouth.
Flexible catheter	Attaches to suction tubing; aids in removing the foreign material and body fluids; used when a rigid tip cannot be used, as when suctioning through a nasopharyngeal airway or in an intubated athlete.	Clear, flexible plastic ranging in size from an 8 F to 16 F. (F or fr. stands for "French" and is a measurement of size. The larger the number, the larger the catheter.)
Collection container	Container used to collect the foreign material and body fluids.	Clear, nonbreakable plastic container that can be disposed of and/or easily removed from the suction unit and decontaminated or replaced.
Water	Used to clear the suction tubing when kinked; water is drawn into the tubing, forcing the clogged material to be drawn into the collection chamber. Used more frequently with a mechanical suction unit.	Sterile water is preferred; however, any water will work.

450 mm Hg of negative pressure at 100% stroke volume and 225 mm Hg at 50% stroke volume and is a versatile hand-powered emergency pump. The disposable collection canister also allows for easy disposal of the foreign materials and body fluids in an appropriate biohazard receptacle. The devices can then be disinfected according to the manufacturer's directions.

Using a Suction Unit

Suctioning is indicated when a gurgling sound is heard during breathing or positive pressure ventilations; when ventilations are impeded by vomitus, blood, body fluids, respiratory secretions, and/or small particles; and/or when the recovery or HAINES position and finger sweep are ineffective at clearing the airway. If fluid or vomit accumulates during ventilations, immediately stop ventilating and quickly suction the airway. Remember to observe body substance isolation (BSI) precautions, particularly when performing a finger sweep. When attempting to suction fluid, a soft suction tip/catheter is recommended. When the athlete is unresponsive or requires the removal of vomitus or thick secretions, a hard or rigid suction tip is most effective.

To use a suction device, follow the general directions in Skill 11.1 and always refer to the manufacturer's directions for specific usage information.

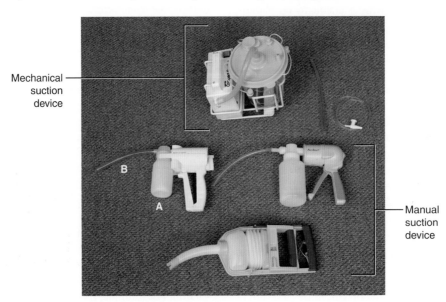

Mechanical suction device

Manual suction device

FIGURE 11.1 Portable manual and mechanical suction units. **A.** Collection canister. **B.** Suction tip/catheter.

Highlight

The Ambu Res-Cue Pump is one of the most versatile hand-powered suction pumps. It is a cost-effective alternative, offering convenience and performance and a wide range of features and benefits:

- Compact and lightweight—small and handy unit—takes up very little space
- Easy to squeeze—requires extremely little force
- Adjustable vacuum (100%, adult or 50%, children)—a wide range of application
- Fast and powerful—offering superior performance
- No regular maintenance—low-cost operation
- No special storage conditions—stores easily in most emergency kits
- Overfill protection—prevents contamination inside the pump/handle and eliminates need for flush-through procedures; prevents inconvenient exhaust splashing of liquids
- Disposable collection container—no cleaning/sterilization required
- Vacuum max: 450 mm Hg
- Disposable collection container volume: 300 mL
- Stroke adjustment: 100% or 50% vacuum
- Dimensions: 185 by 64 by 168 mm
- Weight: 230 g

SKILL 11.1

Using Suction

1. Take BSI precautions.
2. Attach the suction tubing to the suction device (if applicable) (Fig. 11.2).
3. Attach the suction tip/catheter to the suction tubing.

4. Turn the head to the side if no head, neck, or back injury is suspected (Fig. 11.3). If a head, neck, or back injury is suspected, suctioning may be accomplished with the athlete on his or her back. If a spine board is being used, tilt the board to the side. If a spine board is not being used and suctioning on the back is not working, provide manual stabilization and logroll the athlete to his or her side with assistance from other athletic trainers or rescuers. Remember never to delay suctioning over immobilization of the spine.

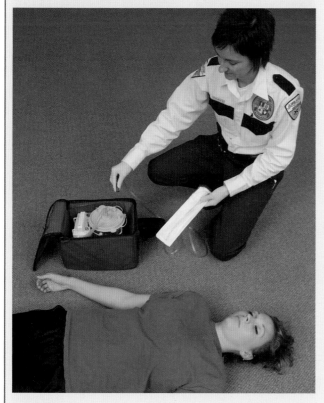

FIGURE 11.2

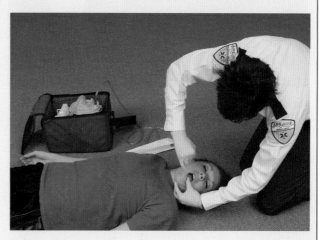

FIGURE 11.3

(Continued)

SKILL 11.1 *(Continued)*

Using Suction (Continued)

5. Open the athlete's mouth with a gloved hand.
6. Grasp the tongue and jaw and remove any solid material and/or large volumes of body fluid using a finger sweep (Fig. 11.3).
7. Measure the distance of insertion of the suction tip/catheter from the athlete's earlobe to the corner of the mouth (Fig. 11.4)
8. Insert the suction tip/catheter into the back of the mouth, using your measurement as a guide (Fig. 11.5). Do not insert the tip of the suction catheter deeper than the base of the tongue or further than what can be seen. Remember that insertion of a rigid tip/catheter may stimulate the gag reflex or may cause a decrease in the athlete's heart rate if the vagus nerve is stimulated.
9. Suction from the back of the throat outward, using a circular motion, never losing sight of the suction tip/catheter.

For an adult athlete, suction no longer than 15 seconds (10 seconds for a child and 5 seconds for an infant). Remember that suctioning limits the amount time the athletic trainer is ventilating the athlete and the longer an athletic trainer suctions, the more oxygen-deprived the athlete becomes.

10. Monitor the athlete's response to suctioning and provide necessary interventions such as positive-pressure ventilation using a BVM. If the athlete begins to gag, withdraw the suction tip/catheter until he or she stops gagging and then restart suctioning.
11. Once suctioning is complete, carefully detach the suction tubing and remove the collection container. Place the contaminated container and tubing in an appropriate receptacle.
12. Document items such total suctioning time, consistency, color, quantity, and any noticeable odors of body fluids.

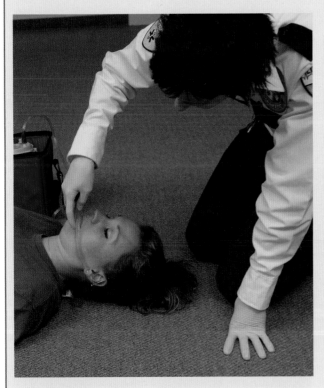

FIGURE 11.4

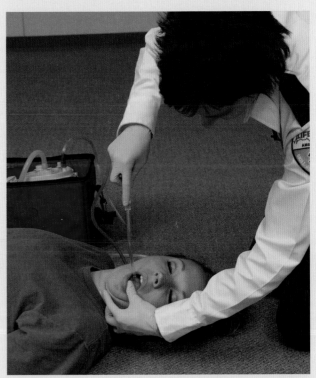

FIGURE 11.5

Special Considerations for Suctioning

There are several things to consider when suctioning an athlete. First is the need to deliver supplemental oxygen. Because the individual requiring suctioning may be in respiratory or cardiac arrest, it will be necessary to limit the amount of suctioning in order to adequately ventilate the athlete. Second, suctioning not only limits positive-pressure ventilation but also removes oxygen from the airway,[4] requiring the athletic trainer to consider hyperventilating (artificially ventilating at a faster rate than normal) the individual prior to suctioning to compensate for the loss of oxygen during suctioning. Day et al.[5] conducted a review of the literature examining the current research recommendations for suctioning and found that hyperoxygenation and hyperinflation prior to suctioning helps to prevent **hypoxemia**. Third, avoid jabbing the suction tip/catheter into the mouth and also avoid continuous contact with any tissues, so as to minimize soft tissue damage. Finally, if brain tissue is visible in the pharynx because of a skull fracture or other head trauma, avoid suctioning in that area.[6]

ADJUNCT AIRWAYS

Once an airway has been established during the primary assessment, it is imperative to maintain it. Adjunct airway devices such as an oropharyngeal airway (OPA) or nasopharyngeal airway (NPA) can assist in this process (Fig. 11.6). The tongue is often responsible for obstructing the airway when an athlete is unconscious. In such a case, the muscles relax and the tongue may fall backward into the throat, covering the trachea. Anchored as it is to the floor of the mouth, the tongue is pulled away from the trachea when the head-tilt/chin-lift and/or jaw-thrust maneuver is employed during the primary assessment.

However, when the airway cannot be maintained, as when performing cardiopulmonary resuscitation (CPR), it is possible for the tongue to slip back and obstruct the airway. Adjunct airway devices, while not the perfect solution, do help to maintain the airway by preventing the tongue from sliding over the trachea.

Two types of adjunct airway devices are commonly used by athletic trainers, depending on the situation. OPAs, as the name implies, are inserted into the mouth. The NPA is placed in the athlete's nostril. Each device has specific indications and contraindications and directions regarding its use. The following sections examine the role, characteristics, indications, and contraindications for the use of adjunct airways as well how to insert such an airway in an emergency.

OPAs

An OPA is made of a plastic material forming the letter "J." It typically has a flange at its end, which rests on the athlete's lips when properly sized and inserted (Fig. 11.7). OPAs range in size from infant to adult large (40 to 110 mm) and are normally stored in a kit. All devices contain either a hole in the center or grooves along the sides and allow air to pass into the trachea and lungs and are used on athletes with a breathing emergency.

Because an OPA is inserted into the back of the throat, it is possible for the athletic trainer to stimulate the **gag reflex** or **laryngospasm** in a conscious athlete.[7] This may induce vomiting, thus further obstructing the airway and causing the athlete to aspirate. Therefore, an OPA cannot be used on a conscious athlete.[2] It must be used only in an unconscious athlete. If the athlete begins to gag during insertion, the OPA must immediately be removed and possibly reinserted at a later time, usually once the athlete's level of consciousness has deepened. An OPA is also contraindicated in the presence of orofacial trauma, since this

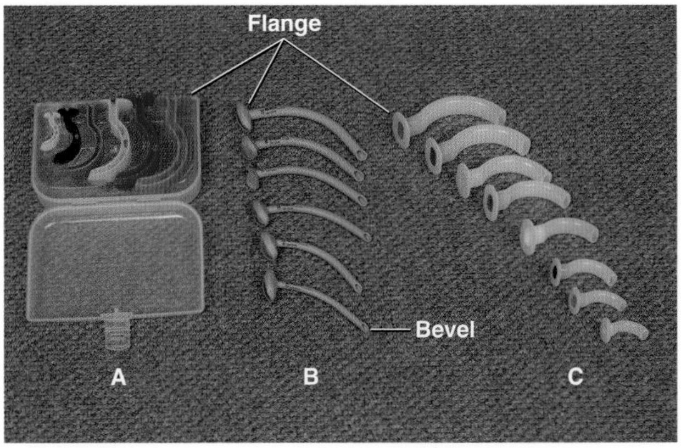

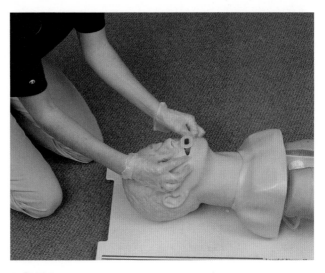

FIGURE 11.6 Oropharyngeal airway (OPA) and nasopharyngeal airway (NPA). **A.** Berman airway kit includes 6 sizes (43 mm, 60 mm, 80 mm, 90 mm, 100 mm, 110 mm) in compact carry case. **B.** Robertazzi nasopharyngeal airways from 20–36 fr. **C.** Guedel airways kits include 8 sizes (40 mm, 50 mm, 60 mm, 70 mm, 80 mm, 90 mm, 100 mm, 110 mm).

FIGURE 11.7 Proper resting position of an OPA. A properly sized and inserted OPA will sit with the flange on the lips.

would make the device more difficult to insert. When using an OPA, be prepared to suction the athlete as necessary and be sure that, once the airway has been inserted, it does not push the tongue backward into the throat.[2]

Using an OPA

To insert an OPA, follow the directions in Skill 11.2 and always refer to the manufacturer's directions for specific usage information.

SKILL 11.2

Inserting an OPA

1. Take BSI precautions.
2. Establish the athlete's level of consciousness. If he or she is conscious, consider an alternative method of maintaining the airway.
3. Establish an initial airway using a head-tilt/chin-lift or jaw-thrust maneuver (with or without extension) if a cervical spine injury is suspected. Remember that managing the airway must take precedence over managing other injuries.

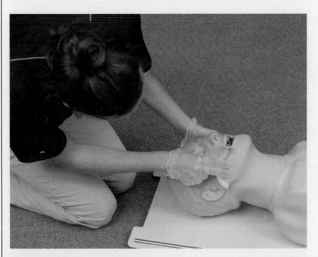

FIGURE 11.8

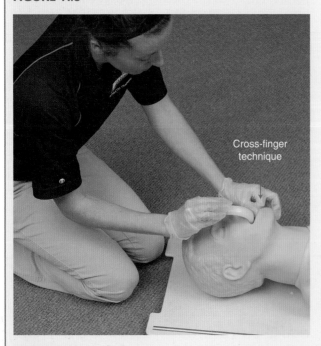

Cross-finger technique

FIGURE 11.9

4. Once the airway is established, insert the correctly sized OPA (Fig. 11.8).
   - To size the OPA, measure from the corner of the athlete's mouth to the tip of the earlobe. An alternative approach is to measure from the center of the mouth to the angle of the jaw.
5. Open the mouth, using the cross-finger technique (Fig. 11.9). Cross the index finger and thumb and place them on the upper and lower teeth, then spread them to open the mouth.
6. Place the tip of the OPA so that it rests on the roof of the mouth (Fig. 11.9).
7. Gently slide the OPA down until resistance of the soft palate is noted. Rotate the airway 180 degrees so that its tip is now pointing down into the throat (Fig. 11.10). In an adult, rotating the tip helps to prevent the tongue from being pushed further into the throat.
8. Continue inserting the OPA until the flange rests on the athlete's lips (Fig. 11.7). If the OPA falls past the lips or does not rest on the lips, it is sized incorrectly and must be removed and resized. An OPA that is too large will increase the risk of blocking the airway and prevent proper placement of ventilation device, whereas an OPA that is too small may cause the tongue to block the airway.
9. Prepare the athlete for positive-pressure ventilation.
10. Monitor the athlete and be prepared to suction. Remove the OPA if the athlete begins to gag.
11. To remove the OPA, simply withdraw the OPA following the contour of the throat.

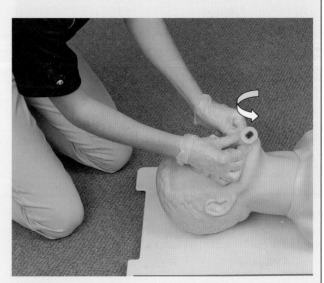

FIGURE 11.10

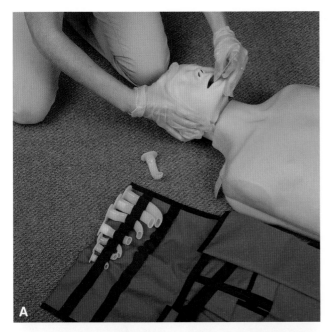

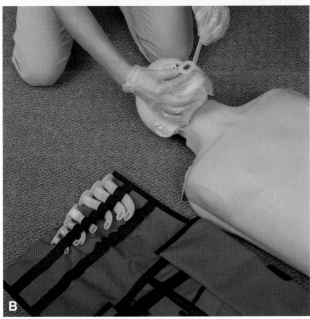

FIGURE 11.11

If the OPA must be inserted in an individual younger than 12 years of age, follow the same guidelines as in an adult except for the following:

1. Insert a tongue blade (tongue depressor) into the mouth and hold the tongue in place (Fig. 11.11A).
2. Insert the OPA with the tip point in the final resting position and follow the contours of the throat (Fig. 11.11B).

NPAs

NPAs also help to maintain the airway. These devices are made of a soft, flexible latex material and are inserted into the athlete's nostril. Like an OPA, an NPA also has a flange at its end that rests on the athlete's nostril. NPAs differ from OPAs in that NPAs are indicated in situations where the athlete is conscious with an intact gag reflex, has sustained orofacial trauma,[8] or has a clenched jaw.[2] NPAs, however, are used less frequently than OPA in the prehospital setting. One reason for this limited use is that NPAs are contraindicated in the presence of a basal skull fracture.[8]

Using an NPA

To insert an NPA, follow the directions in Skill 11.3 and always refer to the manufacturer's directions for specific usage information.

POSITIVE-PRESSURE VENTILATION DEVICES

As discussed in Chapter 10, athletes presenting with breathing or cardiac emergencies may require the use of different breathing devices to ensure adequate ventilation. Remember, ambient air contains approximately 21% oxygen and is a vital component needed to ensure adequate perfusion of the vital organs. **Artificial ventilation** or positive-pressure ventilation, therefore, is the process of manually or mechanically delivering air to an individual

---

Current Research

Contraindications to the Use of an NPA

Establishing a clinical diagnosis of a basal skull fracture in the prehospital setting is difficult because many of the signs of such a condition do not readily present themselves during an on-field assessment (e.g., bruising behind the ear, or Battle's sign) or such a diagnosis requires special equipment (e.g., testing for the presence of cerebrospinal fluid). In fact, the evidence for avoiding the use of NPAs in the prehospital setting appears solely based upon two case reports.[9,10] Securing the airway, therefore, should take precedence over the possible presence of a basal skull fracture.[8] In any case, caution should be exercised in the treatment of athletes with severe craniofacial or head injuries. With proper training and practice, however, NPAs can be safely inserted, with minimal risk of causing further trauma.

SKILL 11.3

Inserting an NPA

1. Take BSI precautions.
2. Establish the athlete's level of consciousness.
3. Establish an initial airway using a head-tilt–chin-lift or jaw-thrust maneuver (with or without extension) if a cervical spine injury is suspected. Remember that managing the airway must take precedence over managing other injuries.
4. Once the airway is established, correctly size the NPA (Fig. 11.12). The correct length of an NPA is based on the length of the device. Evidence demonstrates a relationship between the length of the NPA and the athlete's height.[8]
   - To size the NPA, measure from the tip of the nostril to the tip of the earlobe. An alternative method is to measure from the nostril to the angle of the jaw. The diameter of the NPA should be no larger than that of the nostril.
5. Coat the NPA with a water-soluble lubricant (e.g., K-Y jelly) (Fig. 11.13). Lubricating the latex makes it easier to insert the device and decreases the risk of damage to the nasal mucosa.
6. Lift the nares to reveal the airway and place the beveled edge of the NPA against the inner wall of the right nostril (Fig. 11.14).
7. Gently insert the NPA parallel to the nasal floor, following the contour of the nasal passage. Avoid lifting the NPA upward.

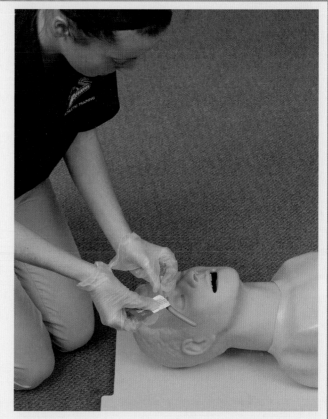

FIGURE 11.13

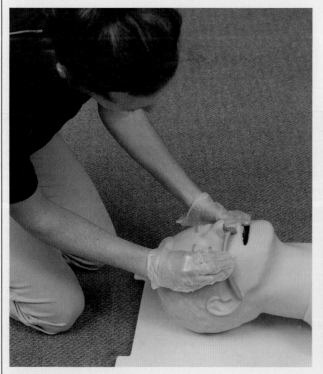

FIGURE 11.12

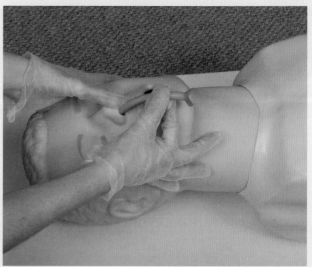

FIGURE 11.14

SKILL 11.3 *(Continued)*

Inserting an NPA *(Continued)*

8. Continue inserting the NPA until the flange rests on the nostril (Fig. 11.15). If correctly placed, the NPA will lie approximately 10 mm above the epiglottis, separating the soft palate from the posterior wall of the oropharynx.[11] An airway that is too long increases coughing and the gag reflex, which increases the risk of regurgitation and aspiration. If it is too short, the device will not separate the soft palate and pharynx.

9. If resistance is felt during insertion, avoid damage to the soft tissues by not forcing the NPA. Remove the NPA and reattempt insertion in the opposite nostril. If resistance is still felt, discontinue and continue providing care.

10. Prepare the athlete for positive-pressure ventilation.

11. Monitor and prepare to suction the athlete if he or she vomits.

12. To remove the NPA, simply withdraw the device following the contour of the nostril.

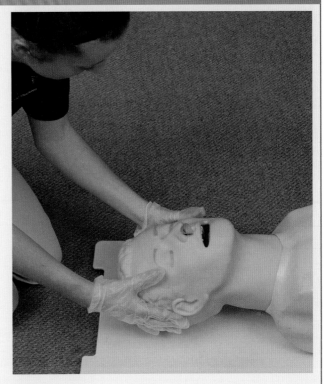

FIGURE 11.15

who is not breathing or is breathing inadequately. The positive pressure forces air into the athlete's trachea and down into the lungs. Several different positive-pressure ventilation devices, including (a) face shields, (b) resuscitation masks, and (c) BVMs are readily available to athletic trainers.

Positive-pressure ventilation devices not only assist an athlete who is not breathing or breathing inadequately but are also designed to minimize contact between the athletic trainer and athlete, thereby reducing the risk of exposure to respiratory secretions, blood, and other potentially infection materials. When used in conjunction with supplemental oxygen, positive-pressure ventilation devices can also improve oxygenation levels, delivering up to 100% oxygen in some cases. Positive-pressure ventilation devices should be standard components of all athletic training kits and should be readily available to all athletic trainers during an emergency. The following sections examine the role, characteristics, and indications for the use of barrier devices commonly used by athletic trainers in an emergency.

Face Shield

A face shield is a type of portable breathing device often carried on an athletic trainer's person (Fig. 11.16) because their cost, size, ease of use, and portability make these devices ideal to carry on a key chain, in a pocket, or in an athletic training kit. Normally composed of clear plastic (to facilitate the observation of **regurgitation,** fluid, and lip color), a face shield is placed over an athlete's face, thus limiting contact between the athletic trainer and the athlete.

Although face shields do reduce the risk of infection, contamination is still possible from the side of the shield.[12] Some face shields include a hard plastic tube or "bite block" with an airway tunnel. This tunnel is inserted into the mouth between the teeth, helping to maintain an open airway when the head-tilt–chin-lift maneuver is being performed. When placing the tube or tunnel into the mouth, be sure not to push or jam the device so far that it causes the tongue to obstruct the airway. Other face shields are secured to the athlete with an elastic band over the athlete's ears. Regardless of the face shield selected, the athletic trainer will be required to place his or her mouth over the athlete's mouth and perform mouth-to-barrier breathing while sealing the nose.

A face shield does help to prevent athletic trainer–athlete contact and is a better choice than performing mouth-to-mouth resuscitation alone; however, when possible, the athletic

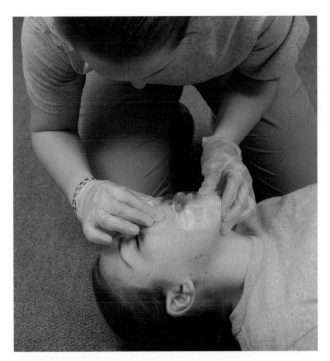

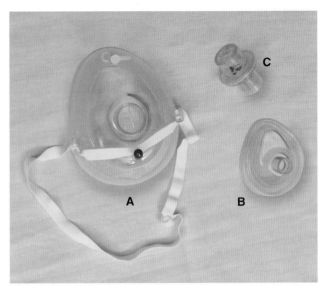

FIGURE 11.17   Resuscitation masks. **A.** Adult mask with oxygen inlet valve, **B.** Infant mask, **C.** Universal one-way value for adult or infant mask.

FIGURE 11.16   Using a face shield. When using a face shield be sure to pinch the nostrils to prevent air from escaping with each breath.

trainer should consider using another type of breathing device, such as a resuscitation mask or BVM, as soon as one becomes available.[13]

Resuscitation Mask

A resuscitation mask or pocket mask should be the first line of defense when managing a breathing emergency as a single athletic trainer (Fig. 11.17). These can be carried on an athletic trainer's person or in an athletic training kit. Resuscitation masks are made of a clear, soft, pliable plastic that contours to an athlete's face, providing a physical barrier between the athletic trainer and the athlete. The clear mask allows the athletic trainer to identify any possible regurgitation and fluid accumulation. A disposable one-way

valve allows for adequate positive-pressure ventilation but prevents the passively exhaled air from passing through the valve; instead, it escapes from a small slit on the underside of the valve. The valve can also be replaced with a BVM, as both devices typically have a standard 15/22-mm respiratory fitting.

Many resuscitation masks also are equipped with an oxygen inlet valve. When this is connected to supplemental oxygen, the athletic trainer can increase the delivered oxygen concentration from 16% to 17% (exhaled air) to approximately 30% to 45% in a nonbreathing athlete and 50% to 60% in a breathing athlete at a flow rate between 10 and 15 L/min. The oxygen concentration is lower in the nonbreathing athlete due to the mixing of supplemental oxygen and exhaled air from the athletic trainer during mouth-

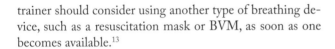

Current Research
Efficacy of Face Shields

An examination of the effectiveness of three commonly used face shields found that all three tested demonstrated adequate delivery of the recommended **tidal volume** (0.5 to 0.6 L) according to the current American Heart Association standards,[13] American Society for Testing and Materials,[12] and the European Resuscitation Council.[14] Another study examining three methods of ventilation by lay responders found that mouth-to-face shield ventilations generated a mean tidal volume of 694 mL, which is higher[15] than current recommendations. Airflow resistance has also been reported with face shields, increasing the difficulty of ensuring adequate ventilations.[13]

to-mask resuscitation. In a breathing athlete, the mask can be secured to cover the mouth and nose, using the attached elastic strap. If no strap is available, ask the athlete to hold the mask in place.

Using a Resuscitation Mask

To use a resuscitation mask, follow the directions in Skill 11.4 and always refer to the manufacturer's directions for specific usage information.

SKILL 11.4

Using a Resuscitation Mask

1. Take BSI precautions.
2. Establish the athlete's level of consciousness.
3. Establish an initial airway using a head-tilt–chin-lift or jaw-thrust maneuver if a cervical spine injury is suspected. Remember that managing the airway must take precedence over managing other injuries.
4. Properly insert an OPA or NPA depending on the athlete's level of consciousness and trauma. If an OPA or NPA is not readily available, do not delay care while waiting for one.
5. Assemble the resuscitation mask following the manufacturer's directions (Fig. 11.18).
6. Attach the supplemental oxygen tubing to the oxygen inlet valve and set the flowmeter to a minimum flow rate 10 to 12 L/min, up to a maximum of 15 L/min (Fig. 11.19).[13]
7. Position yourself at the top of or side of the athlete's head.
   a. If at the top of the head (suspected cervical spine injury or two athletic trainers):
      i. Place the base or the flat end of the resuscitation mask between the athlete's chin and lower lip, retracting the lower lip so that the mouth remains open. Place the apex or pointed end over the bridge of the nose. Place your thumbs over the mask to hold it in place on the athlete's cheeks and place your fingers on the angle of the jaw. Lift the angle of the jaw upward to open the airway and seal the mask. If necessary, slightly tilt the head back to until the airway has opened (Fig. 11.20).

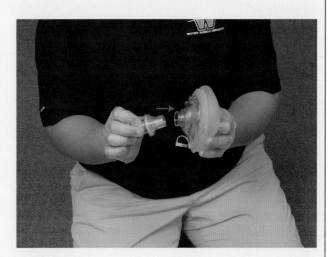

FIGURE 11.18

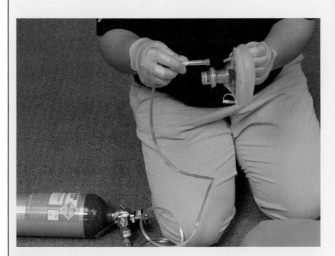

FIGURE 11.19

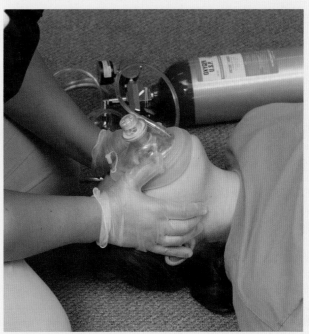

FIGURE 11.20

(Continued)

SKILL 11.4 *(Continued)*

Using a Resuscitation Mask (Continued)

b. If you are at the side of the head (no evidence of cervical spine injury) (Fig. 11.21).

   i. Kneel next to the athlete and place the base or flat end of the resuscitation mask between the athlete's chin and lower lip, retracting the lower lip so that the mouth remains open. Place the apex or pointed end over the bridge of the nose. Secure your top hand with your thumb and index finger around the top of the resuscitation mask and the palm of your hand on the athlete's forehead. With the other hand, slide your first two fingers into position under the bony part of the athlete's chin. Apply a downward pressure on the lower edge of the mask with your thumb to seal the mask. Lift the chin and tilt the head back.

   ii. An alternative method from the side of the head is to form a diamond with your fingers. Place the center of the diamond over the resuscitation mask and place the base or the flat end of the resuscitation mask between the athlete's chin and lower lip, retracting the lower lip so the athlete's mouth remains open. Place the apex over the bridge of the nose. Apply a downward pressure on the lower edge of the mask while tilting the head back.

8. Place your mouth over the one-way valve and exhale into the valve for approximately 1 second to achieve rise of the chest.

9. Remove your lips from the valve to allow for passive exhalation. Remain close to the valve.

10. If the athlete regurgitates, remove the mask and clear the airway and mask with a gloved finger. Monitor and suction as necessary.

11. Remember always to change masks when you come into contact with another athlete.

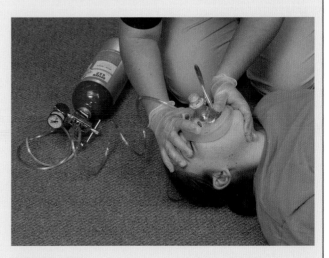

FIGURE 11.21

If the chest fails to rise while using the resuscitation mask, consider the following:

1. Repositioning the head.
2. Ensuring an adequate seal between the mask and athlete's face.
3. Repositioning the mask and your hands.

BVM

A BVM, like a resuscitation mask, is used to ventilate an athlete in case of a breathing emergency; however, a BVM is more effective, particularly when used by two trained athletic trainers.[13] They can work together to ventilate a nonbreathing athlete or an athlete who is breathing inadequately. BVMs are available in various sizes that fit neonates to adults. A variety of systems are available; however, all devices consist of three main components: (a) a self-inflating ventilation bag, (b) a one-way valve system, and (c) a mask similar to a resuscitation mask[16] (Fig. 11.22 and Table 11.2). These should work satisfactorily under a variety of environmental conditions and extreme temperatures.[13] The American Heart Association also recommends that all BVMs should have either no pressure relief valve or a pressure valve system that can be bypassed.[13] A pressure relief valve is normally found on older devices and is designed to open or "pop" off when a certain ventilation pressure is obtained; however, pop-off valves may prevent adequate ventilation.[6]

A BVM supports oxygenation and ventilation when the self-inflating bag is squeezed, forcing air through the one-way valve into the athlete's trachea and lungs, causing a visible rise of the chest. When used alone, a BVM can deliver an oxygen concentration of 21% as the device draws in room air. Connecting supplemental oxygen to the oxygen inlet valve with no oxygen reservoir bag and setting the flowmeter to a minimum flow rate of 10 to 12 L/min

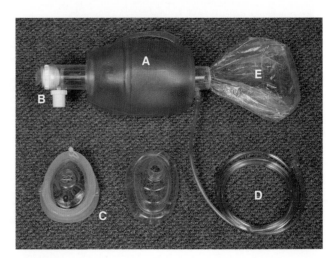

FIGURE 11.22 Bag-valve-mask device. **A.** Self-inflating ventilation bag, **B.** One-way valve system, **C.** Delivery devices, **D.** Oxygen tubing, **E.** Oxygen reservoir.

TABLE 11.2	Components, Purpose, and Characteristics of a Bag-Valve-Mask	
Component	**Purpose**	**Characteristics**
Self-inflating ventilation bag*	Holds air, which is delivered to the athlete when squeezed.	Easily disinfected or disposable; refills spontaneously within 1 second; holds 1,000 to 1,600 mL of air for an adult, 1,200 mL for a large child or adolescent, and 750 mL for an infant or small child
One-way valve*	When squeezed, allows air to flow from the bag to the athlete and diverts his or her exhaled air away from the athletic trainer during exhalation.	Similar to a resuscitation mask; 15-mm respiratory fitting; disposable; has a port allowing exhaled air to escape
Mask*	Acts as a connection between the bag and athlete; prevents contact between the athletic trainer and the athlete; allows for quick identification of regurgitation.	Clear, plastic, pliable dome that seals well to the face and covers the nose and mouth; 22-mm respiratory fitting; easily disinfected or disposable
Oxygen inlet valve	Attachment for supplemental oxygen.	Nonjam valve; delivers supplemental oxygen up to 15 L/min
Oxygen reservoir bag	Storage bag for supplemental oxygen; when the bag is squeezed, the inlet valve closes to deliver oxygen; when open during spontaneous refill, draws in oxygen, allowing for the delivery of higher oxygen concentrations.	Clear plastic bag attached to the supplemental oxygen inlet tube

*Considered necessary components of a BVM.

(up to 15 L/min) increases the oxygen concentration to approximately 40% to 60%. Adding an oxygen reservoir bag increases the oxygen concentration delivered to the athlete to greater than 90%, nearing 100%,[13] and decreases the required tidal volume necessary to maintain adequate oxygenation and ventilation.[17] The increase in oxygen concentration occurs because once the self-inflating bag is released to allow for passive exhalation, supplemental oxygen is drawn through the oxygen tubing to the oxygen reservoir bag. The next time the self-inflating bag is squeezed, the stored oxygen is delivered to the athlete.

To deliver oxygen therapy to a breathing athlete, place the mask over the athlete's nose and mouth and ask him or her to breathe normally. If the athlete is breathing at a rate less than 8 to 10 or greater than 24 to 30 breaths per minute, the athletic trainer may have to assist in the delivery of supplemental oxygen by squeezing the bag.

Using a BVM

To use a BVM, follow the directions in Skill 11.5 and always refer to the manufacturer's directions for specific usage information.

If the chest fails to rise while using the BVM as a single athletic trainer, consider the following:

1. Repositioning the head.
2. Ensuring an adequate seal between the mask and athlete's face.
3. Repositioning the mask and hands.

If the chest still fails to rise, seek an alternative method such as a resuscitation mask to ventilate the athlete.

Special Considerations for Using a BVM

BVMs are not without their disadvantages. Problems such as air leakage from around the mask, **gastric distention**,[17,19,20] regurgitation,[2] inadequate tidal volume delivery,[17,21] and inadequate fraction of delivered oxygen[22] have been reported. A poor seal between the mask and the face also causes a decrease in the total tidal volume delivered to the lungs, causing insufficient oxygenation and/or inadequate ventilation.[21] Gastric distention (which can lead to regurgitation and aspiration) occurs when air is forced down the esophagus rather than the trachea. Factors such as high peak pressure, short inspiratory time, large tidal volume, and incomplete airway opening (all of which occur when a BVM is used improperly) causes the pressure in the esophagus to exceed the lower esophageal sphincter pressure, thereby allowing air into the stomach. To decrease the risk of gastric distention, the athletic trainer should deliver each breath over 1 second to achieve a visible chest rise,[23] producing tidal volume of approximately 500 to 600 mL[2] at a rate of 10 to 12 breaths per minute with a expiratory time greater than 1:2 (inspiration:expiration). Mazzolini and Marshall's[22] examination of 16 BVMs found that all the devices examined generated the required tidal volume (with single-hand technique) necessary to decrease gastric distention and generate adequate ventilations. One device did generate a slightly larger tidal volume with a two-handed squeeze, thereby increasing the risk of gastric distention.

SKILL 11.5

Using a BVM

1. Take BSI precautions.
2. Establish the athlete's level of consciousness.
3. Establish an initial airway using a head-tilt–chin-lift or jaw-thrust maneuver (with or without extension) if a cervical spine injury is suspected. Remember that managing the airway must take precedence over managing other injuries.
4. Properly insert an OPA or NPA depending on the athlete's level of consciousness and trauma. If an OPA or NPA is not readily available, do not delay care while waiting for one.
5. Assemble the BVM following the manufacturer's directions.
6. Attach the supplemental oxygen tubing to the oxygen inlet valve on the flowmeter and set the flowmeter to a minimum flow rate of 10 to 12 L/min, up to 15 L/min. When possible, use an oxygen reservoir bag to achieve delivery of 100% oxygen. Higher oxygenation levels improve arterial oxygen saturation, thereby improving oxygen delivery when cardiac output is limited during cardiac arrest.[2]
7. Ensure proper positioning of the athletic trainers.
   a. Single athletic trainer (Fig. 11.23)
      i. Place the base or flat end of the mask between the athlete's chin and lower lip, retracting the lower lip so that the mouth remains open. Place the apex over the bridge of the nose. Place your thumb over the nose and one or two fingers across the lower half of the mask, forming a "C." Place the remaining two to three fingers under the jaw forming an "E". Grip the mask and chin tightly, applying pressure to the upper mask with the thumb and to the lower mask with the index finger. Tilt the head and lift the chin with two or three fingers. Ventilate by squeezing the BVM with one hand while maintaining the airway and mask seal or by placing the bag against your thigh.
   b. Two athletic trainers (Fig. 11.24)
      i. One athletic trainer is positioned at the top of the head and the other at the side of the head.
      ii. **Athletic trainer 1,** at the side of the head, assembles the BVM and places the mask over the athlete's face.
      iii. **Athletic trainer 2,** at the top of the head, places the base or the flat end of the resuscitation mask between the athlete's chin and lower lip, retracting the lower lip so that the mouth remains open. The apex of the mask is placed over the bridge of the nose. Place your thumbs over the mask to hold it in place on the athlete's cheeks and place your fingers on the

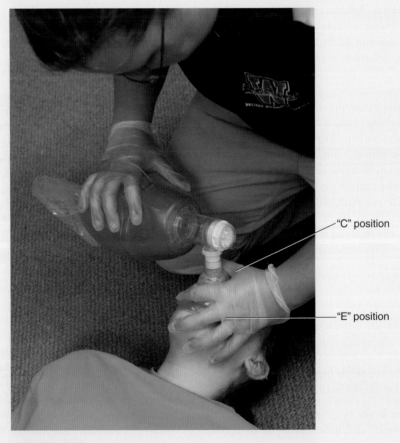

"C" position

"E" position

FIGURE 11.23

SKILL 11.5

Using a BVM (Continued)

angle of the jaw. Lift the angle of the jaw upward to open the airway and seal the mask. If necessary, tilt the athlete's head back to assist in opening the airway.

   iv. **Athletic trainer 1** then ventilates the athlete by squeezing the BVM with one or both hands.

8. Provide positive-pressure ventilation by squeezing the BVM while maintaining the airway and mask seal or by placing the bag against your thigh.

   a. Rate
      i. Adult: every 5 seconds (12 breaths per minute)
      ii. Child or infant: every 3 seconds (20 breaths per minute)

   b. Tidal volume
      i. Adult
         (1) If a good seal has been achieved, adequate tidal volume can be delivered by squeezing a 1-L adult bag about one-half to two-thirds its volume, watching for a visible rise of the chest.
         (2) If an adult 2-L bag is used, squeeze the bag about one-third of the volume.[13]
      ii. Pediatric
         (1) If a good seal has been achieved, adequate tidal volume can be delivered by squeezing a 750-mL bag about two-thirds its volume, watching for a visible rise of the chest.[18]

9. Allow the bag to self-inflate.

10. If the athlete regurgitates, remove the mask and clear the airway and mask with a gloved finger. Monitor and suction as necessary.

11. Always change masks when coming into contact with another athlete.

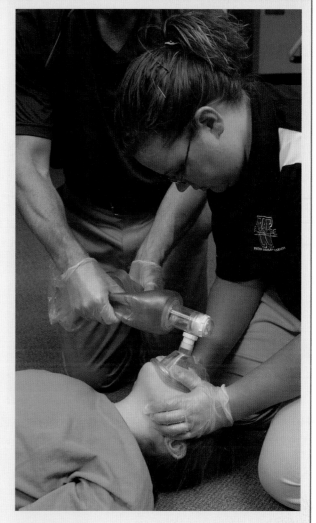

FIGURE 11.24

ESTABLISHING AN AIRWAY USING A BREATHING DEVICE IN AN ATHLETE WEARING PROTECTIVE EQUIPMENT

Athletic trainers working with athletes who may have sustained trauma to the cervical spine while wearing protective equipment (e.g., helmet and shoulder pads) must be ready to expose, prepare, and manage an airway in a short period of time with very little movement of the cervical spine. The Inter-Association Task Force for Appropriate Care of the Spine Injured Athlete and National Athletic Trainers' Association Position Statement on acute management of cervical spine injuries clearly recommends the immediate removal of a football face mask because the point at which an athlete stops breathing becomes critical[24,25] and any further delay in care could have significant consequences. However, if after a reasonable period of time the face mask cannot be

removed on-field, it will be necessary to remove the whole helmet in order to gain access to the athlete's airway, taking care to remove the shoulder pads at the same time.[24] It will also be necessary to remove an athletic helmet if the helmet interferes with establishing an airway or ventilating an athlete.[24,25]

Previous research has demonstrated that inserting a resuscitation mask under a football face mask is possible and allows for a quick initiation of positive-pressure ventilation in an athlete with a breathing emergency.[26,27] By placing the resuscitation mask between the chin and lowest portion of face mask or through the face mask's eye holes, the athletic trainer can place a resuscitation mask over the athlete's mouth and nose (Fig. 11.25). The one-way valve is then inserted between the face mask bars in order to begin ventilating the athlete using a jaw-thrust maneuver (with or without extension),[26,27] assuming that the one-way valve is long enough. Although inserting a resuscitation mask through the face mask's eye

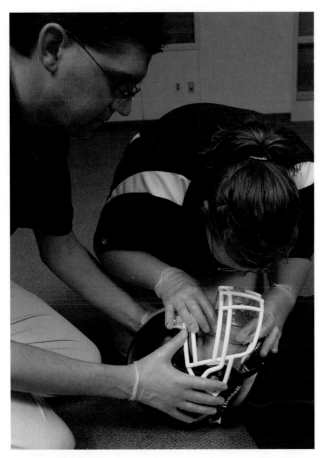

FIGURE 11.25   Inserting a resuscitation mask under a football face mask.

SUPPLEMENTAL OXYGEN THERAPY

Remember from previous discussions that adequate ventilation and oxygenation is necessary to sustain perfusion of the body's vital organs. In healthy athletes, the normal concentration of oxygen in the air (21%) is more than adequate to sustain life. During a traumatic injury or illness though, the body does not function properly and often requires additional oxygen to provide adequate perfusion to the injured body cells to prevent **hypoxia**.

Hypoxia is a decrease or insufficient supply of oxygen in inspired gases, arterial blood, or tissues and can lead to conditions such as cardiac arrhythmias, tissue and cell damage, renal damage, and eventually cerebral damage.[32] Significant hypoxia for more than 4 to 6 minutes can cause sudden cardiorespiratory arrest and leads to irreversible damage to the brain and vital organs.[33]

By administering supplemental oxygen therapy to an athlete demonstrating signs of hypoxia, the amount of oxygen delivered to the cells is increased, thereby optimizing the individual's chances of survival during an emergency. For example, an athlete in cardiac arrest will require some form of supplemental breathing. Mouth-to-face shield or mouth-

holes is slightly quicker than inserting it under the face mask, neither method completely eliminates extraneous movement of the cervical spine.[26,27] In fact, neither method should be considered a stand-alone technique.

Replacing the one-way valve with a BVM may also be possible, as these breathing devices are interchangeable. The use of a BVM may also assist in hyperventilating an athlete to compensate for loss of oxygen while removing either the face mask or the helmet, according to the accepted practice standards.[24]

Current Research

Using a Resuscitation Mask under the Face Mask in an Emergency

Ray et al.[27] suggest that both resuscitation mask insertion techniques offer a speed advantage over the complete removal of the face mask with traditional loop straps. In their study, insertion of the resuscitation mask through the eye hole averaged 13 seconds, compared with the 31.9 seconds it took to remove the two side-loop straps and retract the face mask upward with a manual screw.[27] Studies examining the use of cutting tools to remove football helmet loop straps have demonstrated it may take between 90 and 250 seconds to retract the face mask,[28–30] depending on the cutting tool used. This is in comparison with studies examining retraction of the face mask with a cordless screwdriver, which have demonstrated the ability to retract the face mask quickly (27 to 36 seconds) and with less head movement[31] and torque.[32] Therefore, although inserting a resuscitation mask under the face mask is not considered the gold standard when managing a cervical spine injury, if an athlete is not breathing and an electric screwdriver is not readily available, the ability to quickly initiate positive-pressure ventilation is critical until the face mask can be safely removed.[25]

Breakout

Indications for the use of supplemental oxygen therapy include:

- Altered mental status
- Cardiac distress (chest pain) or arrest
- Drug overdose
- Fractures
- Head, chest, or abdominal trauma
- Respiratory arrest
- Respiratory distress (e.g., asthma, chronic obstructive pulmonary disease, pneumonia, pneumothorax, pleural effusion)
- Shock (e.g., cardiogenic, hypovolemic, hemorrhagic, neurogenic)
- Stroke
- This list is not all-inclusive; any athlete presenting with signs of hypoxia can be treated with supplemental oxygen therapy.

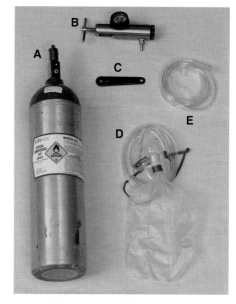

FIGURE 11.26 Components of supplemental oxygen therapy delivery system. **A.** Medical grade oxygen, **B.** Pressure regulator and flowmeter assembly, **C.** Oxygen tank wrench, **D.** Nonrebreather mask, **E.** Nasal cannula.

to-mask only provides 16% to 17% oxygen. For a healthy adult, this may be fine, but because CPR delivers only 25% to 33% of the normal cardiac output, the cells of the body are receiving the bare minimum of oxygen necessary to sustain life.[2] Therefore, the athletic trainer should provide 100% inspired oxygen during basic life support as soon as it becomes available to improve arterial oxygen saturation and arterial content when cardiac output is limited during cardiac arrest. Remember, though, *do not delay* providing care while waiting for supplemental oxygen.

Indications for the use of supplemental oxygen therapy can be found in the Breakout box above. There are no absolute contraindications to the use of supplemental oxygen therapy in an athlete presenting with signs of hypoxia. In fact, if an athlete presents with a chief complaint of shortness of breath or difficulty breathing, do not wait for specific signs of hypoxia to occur. Immediately treat the individual with supplemental oxygen therapy to prevent the condition from worsening. There are some situations in which high-flow oxygen should be used with caution.

Supplemental Oxygen Therapy Delivery System

To deliver supplemental oxygen therapy during an emergency, the athletic trainer will need to have the following (Fig. 11.26):

- Oxygen cylinder
- Pressure regulator with flowmeter
- Delivery device

Oxygen Cylinders

An oxygen cylinder or tank holds medical-grade oxygen under pressure. When full, an oxygen cylinder, which is made of steel or an alloy, is under approximately 2,000 pounds of pressure per square inch (psi). Such a cylinder is easy to recognize by its green tank or green tank top and yellow diamond placard indicating oxygen, and the United States Pharmacopoeia (USP) label (Fig. 11.27). They come in various sizes, identified by a letter (Table 11.3).

Current Research

High-Flow Oxygen: To Use or Not

Athletes exposed to high-flow oxygen for too long a time may develop oxygen toxicity or collapse of the air sacs. An athlete suffering a severe asthma attack may benefit more from short-term supplemental oxygen therapy at 28% versus 100%. An examination of short-term 28% and 100% oxygen therapy on **PaCO₂** and peak expiratory flow rates in the acute asthma patient found an increase in $PaCO_2$ with 100% oxygen after 20 minutes.[34] Therefore, severe acute asthmatics may benefit from short-term supplemental oxygen at 28% or at a level that maintains a pulse oximeter target value greater than 92% in adults and 95% in children.[34] Athletic trainers may also come into contact with athletes suffering from chronic obstructive pulmonary disease (COPD). It was previously believed that high-flow oxygen would affect the hypoxic drive, increasing blood oxygen levels and shutting off the drive to breathe.[6] To prevent worsening of the condition, the current recommendation for treating COPD patients is not to restrict access to high-flow oxygen therapy.[32,33]

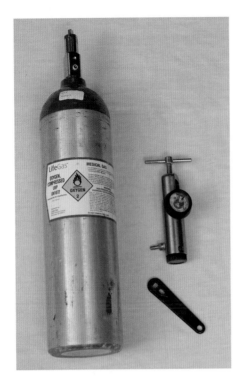

FIGURE 11.27   Oxygen tank and USP label.

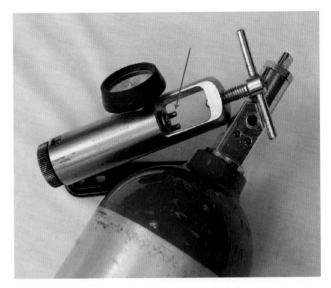

FIGURE 11.28   Oxygen tank valve stem assembly. The metal prongs (arrow) must be inserted into the corresponding holes on the cylinder's valve stem.

All cylinders should be hydrostatically tested every 5 years to avoid leaking or rupturing of the cylinder. Athletic trainers should also be sure never to allow the tank to fall below the safe residual level (less than 200 psi). Allowing this to occur may prematurely damage the cylinder and affect the ability to properly and adequately deliver supplemental oxygen therapy to an athlete in need.

Pressure Regulator with Flowmeter

Remember that oxygen in a full cylinder is under a pressure of 2,000 psi; this can be observed by reading the pressure regulator. Delivering oxygen under 2,000 psi of pressure would certainly injure an athlete, which is why a pressure regulator

is attached to the oxygen cylinder's valve stem. The pressure regulator functions to reduce the pressure of the cylinder to a manageable and safe level (less than 70 psi) in order to deliver oxygen at a rate of 1 to 15 L/min.

Portable D and E tanks have been designed with a safeguard to prevent anyone from accidentally placing a pressure regulator on a cylinder with unknown gases. A yoke assembly with three metal prongs must be inserted into the corresponding holes on the cylinder's valve stem (Fig. 11.28). The center prong on the pressure regulator should also have a donut-shaped gasket, known as an O-ring. If no O-ring is present, check the valve stem for an O-ring. The O-ring functions to provide a tight seal between the pressure regulator and cylinder. If there is no O-ring, the cylinder will leak and not function properly.

The flowmeter is connected to the pressure regulator and controls the flow of oxygen to the athlete. The Bourdon

TABLE 11.3	Cylinder Sizing for Supplemental Oxygen Therapy			
		Duration of Flow*		
Cylinder Type	**Capacity (L)**	**4 L/min**	**10 L/min**	**15 L/min**
D†	350	72	28	19
E†	625	126	50	33
M	3,000	702	280	187
G	~5,300	1,084	433	289
H	~6,900	1,413	565	376

*Based on a 2,000-psi pressure regulator reading and a 200-psi safe residual level. Determined by the following formula:

Cylinder Pressure − 200 (safe residual) × Cylinder Constant Factor / Flow Rate (L/min) = Minutes of Oxygen

Cylinder Constant Factors; D tank = 0.16, E tank = 0.28, M tank = 1.56, G tank = 2.41, H tank = 3.14.
†Portable tanks; the remaining tanks are fixed units.

TABLE 11.4	Delivery Devices for Supplemental Oxygen Therapy*		
Device	**Flow Rate (L/min)**	**Oxygen Concentration (%)**	**Type of Athlete**
Nasal cannula	1	24	Breathing
	2	28	Breathing
	3	32	Breathing
	4	36	Breathing
Resuscitation mask	10 to 15	30 to 45 and 50 to 60[†]	Nonbreathing and breathing
Nonrebreather mask	10 to 15	80 to 95	Breathing
BVM	10 to 15	40 to 60 and 90 to 100[‡]	Nonbreathing and breathing

*Delivery system should be adjusted to maintain an oxygen saturation level greater than 90% based on a pulse oximeter reading.[33]
[†]30% to 45% in a nonbreathing athlete because of the mixing of supplemental oxygen and exhaled air from the athletic trainer during mouth-to-mask resuscitation; 50% and 60% in a breathing athlete.
[‡]Without a reservoir bag, oxygen concentration will be between 40% and 60%; with a reservoir bag, it will be greater than 90%, nearing 100%.

Gauge Flowmeter is the most commonly used device because it works well at all angles. Flowmeters normally deliver a flow rate of 1 to 15 L/min, with newer units providing as much as 25 L/min. Other flowmeters, such the pressure-compensated flowmeter, must remain upright to work correctly; this is a disadvantage in the prehospital setting. Oxygen tubing is then connected to the oxygen inlet on the flowmeter and to the delivery device.

Delivery Devices

Several types of delivery devices are used when administering supplemental oxygen therapy (Table 11.4), depending on the situation. Some devices can deliver oxygen to a breathing athlete, nonbreathing athlete, or both. Supplemental oxygen therapy delivered by a nasal cannula and/or nonrebreather (NRB) mask is used with breathing athletes. Resuscitation masks and BVMs are used on both breathing and nonbreathing athletes. All devices must be attached to the flowmeter oxygen inlet.

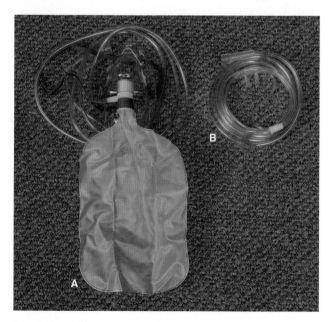

FIGURE 11.29 Nonrebreather mask (**A**) and nasal cannula mask (**B**).

Nonrebreather Mask   The NRB mask (Fig. 11.29) is the most widely used delivery device in the prehospital setting to deliver high-concentration oxygen to conscious athletes. The NRB is a clear plastic mask that fits snugly over the athlete's nose and mouth. Attached to the mask is a reservoir bag designed to hold oxygen. When the athlete inhales, oxygen from the reservoir bag passes through a one-way valve to the trachea and lungs. When the athlete exhales, the one-way valve closes, preventing the exhaled air from mixing with the oxygen in the reservoir. Flutter valves on either side of the mask allow the exhaled air to escape but close during inhalation to ensure delivery of the highest oxygen concentration possible. An NRB mask is used with the flowmeter set at no lower than 10 L/min, up to 15 L/min, delivering an oxygen concentration of up to 90% to 100%.

To ensure the highest level of oxygen concentration, the NRB mask must be secured snugly to the athlete's face. The metal nosepiece and strap should be snug enough to prevent air from escaping through the sides. The reservoir bag should always contain oxygen so that it does not deflate and limit the delivery of oxygen. Remember that the NRB mask works only if the athlete is breathing efficiently. Continually monitor the athlete's breathing and vital signs to ensure adequate ventilation and prevent the development of hypoxia.

Nasal Cannula   A nasal cannula is also used to administer supplemental oxygen to a breathing athlete. It is a flexible plastic delivery device with two prongs, which are inserted in the athlete's nostrils. Unlike an NRB mask, a nasal cannula delivers low-concentration oxygen between 24% and 36%, depending on the flow rate. Rates higher than 4 L/min may increase the risk of headaches and nosebleeds because the airflow causes the mucous membranes in the nostrils dry out.

Because most of the athletes you are called upon to treat will likely be suffering from conditions such as respiratory distress, fractures, shock, and the like, they may require high-concentration oxygen therapy; therefore, nasal cannulas will be used very little during an on-field emergency. The only time an athletic trainer may use a nasal cannula during an emergency situation is when the NRB mask causes the athlete to feel claustrophobic and there is a need for oxygen therapy. Athletic trainers may, however, come across individuals using a nasal cannula, particularly those suffering from conditions such as emphysema, congestive heart failure, or chronic bronchitis. Therefore, being familiar with these devices and their associated conditions is worthwhile.

Administering Supplemental Oxygen Therapy

To administer supplemental oxygen therapy, follow the directions in Skill 11.6 and always refer to the manufacturer's directions for specific usage information.

SKILL 11.6

Administering Supplemental Oxygen Therapy

1. Establish the athlete's level of consciousness and the need for supplemental oxygen therapy.
2. Select the desired oxygen cylinder and check to be sure that it is labeled "oxygen" (green top, yellow diamond with USP markings).
3. Place the cylinder upright in a portable stand or in the cylinder case on its side.
4. If a new cylinder is being used, remove the wrapping or cap protecting the valve stem outlet (Fig. 11.30).
5. Using an oxygen wrench, slightly open the cylinder (sometimes called "cracking the tank") for approximately 1 second to remove dirt or debris in the outlet. If an O-ring is present on the valve stem outlet, remove it, set it aside, purge the cylinder, and then reinsert it (Fig. 11.31).
6. Select the desired pressure regulator; be sure it is labeled "oxygen."
7. Inspect the pressure regulator. If the cylinder does not have an O-ring, check to be sure that the pressure regulator is equipped with one.
8. Attach the pressure regulator by matching up the male prongs on the regulator with the female outlets on the valve stem. Hand-tighten the regulator until it is snug (Fig. 11.32).

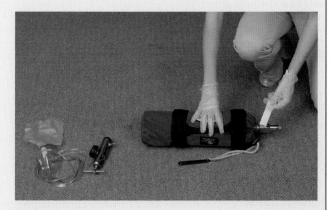

FIGURE 11.30

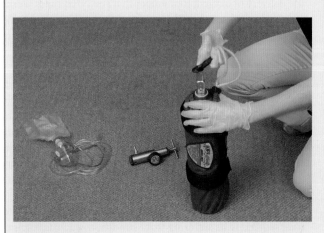

FIGURE 11.31

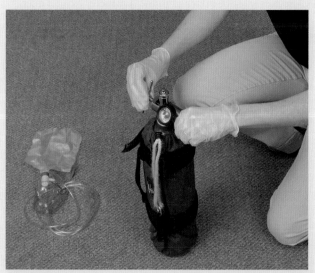

FIGURE 11.32

SKILL 11.6 *(Continued)*

Administering Supplemental Oxygen Therapy *(Continued)*

9. Using the oxygen wrench, open the cylinder one full turn (Fig. 11.33).
10. Inspect the regulator to determine how much pressure is in the cylinder.
11. Attach the oxygen tubing and delivery device.
12. Explain to the athlete the need for oxygen therapy.
13. Turn the flowmeter to the desired setting.
14. Verify that oxygen is flowing.
15. Apply the delivery device.
    a. NRB mask (Fig. 11.34)
        i. Select a mask of the appropriate size (adult, child or infant).
        ii. Place your thumb over the valve between the reservoir bag and mask to allow the bag to fill with oxygen.
        iii. Grasp the mask in one hand and the elastic band in the other. Place the mask over the athlete's mouth and nose, securing with the metal nose clamp.
        iv. Place the elastic band over the athlete's head.
    b. Nasal cannula (Fig. 11.35)
        i. Gently insert the two nasal prongs into the nostrils so they rest on the floor of the nostrils.
        ii. Drape the tubing over and behind the ears and secure under the chin.
    c. Resuscitation mask
        i. See resuscitation mask instructions (Skill 11.4).
    d. BVM
        i. See BVM instructions (Skill 11.5).
16. Adjust flow rate as necessary.
17. Monitor flow of oxygen and pressure regulator; document the athlete's condition.

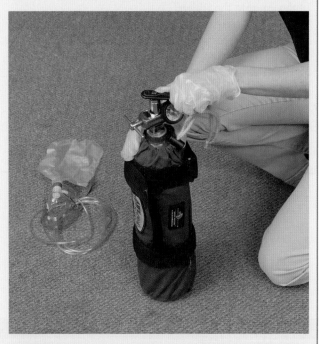

FIGURE 11.33

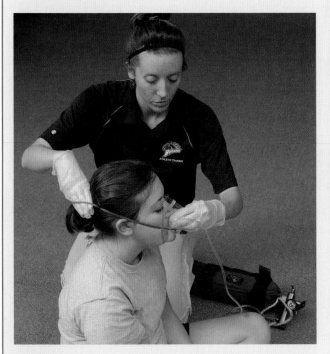

FIGURE 11.34

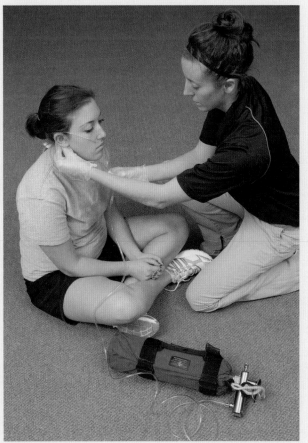

FIGURE 11.35

To disassemble supplemental oxygen equipment, follow these directions:

1. Turn of the flow meter and remove the oxygen delivery device from the athlete.
2. Close the pressure regulator using the oxygen wrench.
3. Remove the delivery tubing from the flowmeter.
4. Bleed the flowmeter of the residual oxygen.
5. Remove the pressure regulator.

Special Considerations for Using Supplemental Oxygen Therapy

The athletic trainer administering supplemental oxygen therapy should keep the following safety precautions in mind:

1. Do not use an oxygen cylinder near open flames or smoke. Although oxygen does not ignite fires, it will cause a fire to burn more rapidly.
2. Never use petroleum products (e.g., oil, grease) on the oxygen cylinder valve stem, pressure regulator, or delivery device under pressure. Oxygen does not mix well with petroleum products and may cause the cylinder to explode.
3. Never leave an oxygen cylinder upright unless it is secured in a portable stand; consider placing the tank on its side. If the cylinder falls over and the valve stem assembly is damaged, the cylinder may become a projectile because of the compressed oxygen.
4. Never expose an oxygen cylinder to temperatures of more than 120°F (49°C).
5. Never use a pressure regulator not specifically designed for the supplemental oxygen cylinder being used.
6. Periodically inspect your supplemental oxygen delivery system to make sure that all of the necessary components are functioning appropriately. If the O-ring is worn, change it immediately to avoid leakage of oxygen from the pressure regulator.
7. Be sure that the delivery devices are latex-free to avoid causing an allergic reaction in a latex-sensitive athlete.

Scenarios

1. An athlete is struck in the neck with a hockey puck. When the athletic trainer arrives on site, the athlete is unresponsive but is breathing and shows signs of life. As the athletic trainer begins his assessment, he notices a gurgling sound in the athlete's throat. When he looks into the mouth, a large pool of blood is noted.

   What adjunct breathing device could he use to remove the blood?
   Which piece of equipment would be best to remove the blood?
   Describe the steps in managing this case based on the breathing device you selected.

2. You are covering a collegiate volleyball tournament when all of a sudden there is lot of commotion coming from the stands. It is apparent that a fan has collapsed and you and your athletic training student begin to attend to the woman. The general impression reveals a middle-aged woman lying motionless and apparently unresponsive. You immediately send your athletic training student to call 911 and to get your emergency breathing kit.

   As you begin your primary assessment, what piece of emergency equipment could be used prior to the arrival of the emergency breathing kit?
   Why did you select this piece of equipment?
   Once the athletic training student arrives with the breathing kit, what could you use to help maintain the airway you have established?
   Describe how you would measure and insert this device.
   What would happen if the woman began to regain consciousness?

3. While you are covering a high school baseball game, you notice that the pitcher has a ball hit back at him. The ball strikes the pitcher in the chest and he collapses to the ground. You arrive at his side and determine that he has no signs of life. You activate your EAP by having the coach call 911 and retrieve the AED from the school's administrative office. The visiting team's athletic trainer realizes the seriousness of the injury and comes out to assist. Your emergency trauma kit contains the following: a face shield, a resuscitation mask, a BVM, OPAs, and a blood pressure cuff.

   Given the supplies in your kit, design an EAP to care for this athlete.

4. Tim, a 160-lb collegiate wrestler, is at wrestling practice when his opponent performs a single-leg tackle. Tim, who is not prepared for this attack, falls to the mat, trying to brace himself. He immediately begins screaming, the referee calls injury time, and you, as the athletic trainer, run out onto the mat. Tim has clearly dislocated his elbow and you and Sue, the athletic training student, begin to manage the situation. While you are immobilizing the elbow, you notice that Tim is becoming a little restless and is breathing rapidly. You ask Tim how he is feeling. Tim says that he is feeling a bit nauseous and as though he is going to vomit. You instruct Sue to finish immobilizing the elbow.

   What type of adjunct therapy is warranted here? Why?
   Discuss how you would manage this situation.
   If Tim stopped breathing, how would you and Sue manage the situation?

WRAP-UP

Breathing devices and supplemental oxygen therapy are necessary adjuncts to managing an athlete in respiratory or cardiac distress or arrest. Athletic trainers, though, are fortunate in that most of the athletes in their care rarely suffer from respiratory or cardiac conditions requiring the use of breathing devices or oxygen therapy. Being able to understand the role, indications, contraindications, and proper use of the devices discussed in this chapter can serve to maximize athlete outcomes if a breathing or cardiac emergency should arise, especially if asked to assist emergency medical services. Athletic trainers should also be reminded that manufacturers of breathing devices have their own recommended methods of using their equipment, which may supersede what has been discussed in this chapter.

Therefore, take the necessary time to read through the device's instruction manual to ensure its proper use in an emergency. Also, athletic equipment varies between manufacturers, and what works well with one piece of equipment may not work with another.

By practicing the techniques described in this chapter periodically and with all of your available athletic equipment, most likely at the start of an athletic season or during the annual review of the EAP, you will remain competent to intervene should you be presented with a trauma or illness requiring the use of adjunct breathing devices and/or supplemental oxygen therapy.

Also remember to check individual state laws and practice acts to determine whether the use of the adjunct breathing devices presented in this chapter are acceptable. If necessary, you can also contact organizations such as the American Red Cross, American Heart Association, and National Safety Council, which offer certification courses related to these skills.

REFERENCES

1. National Highway Traffic Safety Administration, Emergency Medical Services. *National Emergency Medical Services Education Standards, Emergency Medical Responder Instructional Guidelines*. Washington, DC: U.S. Department of Transportation; 2009.
2. American Heart Association. Part 7.1: Adjuncts for airway control and ventilation. *Circulation*. 2005;112(24 Suppl):IV-51–IV-57.
3. Simon EJ, Davidson JAH, Boom SJ. Evaluation of three portable suction devices. *Anaesthesia*. 1996;48:807–809.
4. Hatlestad D. Clearing the airway. *EMS Responder.com*. http://publicsafety.com/article/article.jsp?id=2371&siteSection=16. Accessed June 18, 2007.
5. Day T, Farnell S, Wilson-Barnett J. Suctioning: A review of current research recommendations. *Intensive Crit Care Nurs*. 2002;18:79–89.
6. Limmer D, O'Keefe MF, Grant HD, et al. *Emergency Care*, 9th ed. Upper Saddle River, NJ: Prentice Hall; 2001.
7. Sumner SM, Lewandowski V. Guidelines for using artificial breathing devices. *Nursing*. 1983;13(10):54–57.
8. Roberts K, Whalley H, Bleetman A. The nasopharyngeal airway: Dispelling myths and establishing the facts. *Emerg Med J*. 2005;22(6):394–396.
9. Schade K, Borzotta A, Michaels A. Intracranial malposition of nasopharyngeal airway. *J Trauma*. 2000;49:967–968.
10. Muzzi DA, Losasso TJ, Cucchiara RF. Complication from a nasopharyngeal airway in a patient with a basilar skull fracture. *Anesthesiology*. 1991;74:366–368.
11. Stoneham M. The nasopharyngeal airway. Assessment of position by fibreoptic laryngoscopy. *Anaesthesia*. 1993;48(7):575–580.
12. Simmons M, Deao D, Moon L, et al. Bench evaluation: Three face-shield CPR barrier devices. *Respir Care*. 1995;40(6):618–623.
13. American Heart Association. Part 4: Adult basic life support. *Circulation*. 2005;112(24 Suppl):IV-19–IV-34.
14. Wenzel V, Idris AH, Montogomery WH, et al. Rescue breathing and bag-mask ventilation. *Ann Emerg Med*. 2001;37(4 Suppl):S36–S40.
15. Paal P, Falk M, Sumann G, et al. Comparison of mouth-to-mouth, mouth-to-mask and mouth-to-face-shield ventilation by lay persons. *Resuscitation*. 2006;70(1):117–123.
16. Pruitt WC. Manual ventilation by one or two rescuers. *Nursing*. 2004;34(11):43–45.
17. Dorges V, Ocker H, Wenzel V, et al. Emergency airway management by non-anaesthesia house officers: A comparison of three strategies. *Emerg Med J*. 2001;18(2):90–94.
18. American Heart Association. Part 11: Pediatric basic life support. *Circulation*. 2005;112(24 Suppl):IV-156–IV-166.
19. Doerges V, Sauer C, Ocker H, et al. Smaller tidal volumes during cardiopulmonary resuscitation: Comparison of adult and paediatric self-inflatable bags with three different ventilatory devices. *Resuscitation*. 1999;43(1):31–37.
20. Doerges V, Sauer C, Ocker H, et al. Airway management during cardiopulmonary resuscitation: A comparative study of bag-valve-mask, laryngeal mask airway and Combitube in a bench model. *Resuscitation*. 1999;41(1):63–69.
21. Dorges V, Ocker H, Hagelberg S, et al. Smaller tidal volumes with room-air are not sufficient to ensure adequate oxygenation during bag-valve-mask ventilation. *Resuscitation*. 2000;44(1):37–41.
22. Mazzolini DG, Marshall NA. Evaluation of 16 adult disposable manual resuscitators. *Respir Care*. 2004;49(12):1509–1514.
23. American Heart Association. Part 6: CPR techniques and devices. *Circulation*. 2005;112(24_suppl):IV-47–IV-50.
24. Kleiner DM, Almquist J, Bailes J, et al. *Prehospital care of the spine-injured athlete: A document from the Inter-Association Task Force for Appropriate Care of the Spine-Injured Athlete*. Dallas: National Athletic Trainers' Association; 2001.
25. Swartz EE, Boden BP, Courson RW, et al. National Athletic Trainers' Association Position Statement: Acute management of the cervical spine–injured athlete. *J Athl Train*. 2009;44(3):306–311.
26. Ray R, Luchies C, Bazuin D, et al. Airway preparation techniques for the cervical spine-injured football player. *J Athl Train*. 1995;30(3):217–221.

27. Ray R, Luchies C, Frens MA, et al. Cervical spine motion in football players during 3 airway-exposure techniques. *J Athl Train.* 2002;37(2):172–177.

28. Swartz EE, Armstrong CW, Rankin J, et al. A 3-dimensional analysis of face-mask removal tools in inducing helmet movement. *J Athl Train* 2002;37(2):178–184.

29. Swartz EE, Norkus SA, Armstrong CW, et al. Face-mask removal: Movement and time associated with cutting of the loop straps. *J Athl Train.* 2003;38(2):120–125.

30. Jenkins HL, Valovich TC, Arnold BL, et al. Removal tools are faster and produce less force and torque on the helmet than cutting tools during face-mask retraction. *J Athl Train.* 2002;37(3):246–251.

31. Decoster LC, Shirley CP, Swartz EE. Football face-mask removal with a cordless screwdriver on helmets used for at least one season of play. *J Athl Train.* 2005;40(3):169–173.

32. Murphy R, Driscoll P, O'Driscoll R. Emergency oxygen therapy for the COPD patient. *Emerg Med J.* 2001;18: 333–339.

33. Murphy R, Mackway-Jones K, Sammy I, et al. Emergency oxygen therapy for the breathless patient. Guidelines prepared by North West Oxygen Group. *Emerg Med J.* 2001;18: 421–423.

34. Rodrigo GJ, Verde MR, Peregalli V, et al. Effects of short-term 28% and 100% oxygen on $PaCO_2$ and peak expiratory flow rate in acute asthma. *Chest.* 2003;124(4):1312–1317.

Recognition and Management of Cardiac Emergencies

CHAPTER OUTCOMES

1. Identify and describe the major structures of the cardiovascular system.

2. Describe each link in the cardiac chain of survival and how each relates to the emergency medical service system.

3. Define cardiac distress.

4. Describe how cardiac distress develops.

5. Identify and describe the signs and symptoms of cardiac distress.

6. Demonstrate how to care for an athlete suffering from cardiac distress.

7. Define sudden cardiac death and indentify its causes in athletes.

8. Define sudden cardiac arrest and identify how sudden cardiac arrest develops.

9. Identify and describe the signs and symptoms of sudden cardiac arrest.

10. Identify and describe the required components and skill necessary to adequately perform cardiopulmonary resuscitation (CPR).

11. Demonstrate how to care for an individual suffering from cardiac arrest, including the performance of single- and two-person CPR for an adult, child, and infant.

12. Identify possible complications of CPR.

13. Demonstrate how to care for an athlete with a special consideration, including protective equipment, delayed access, airway, playing surface, lack of equipment, and inappropriate skills.

14. Describe the indications for the use of an automated external defibrillator (AED).

15. Identify and describe the characteristics of an AED.

16. Identify and describe the precautions to be taken when using an AED.

17. Demonstrate how to properly use an AED on an adult and pediatric athlete.

NOMENCLATURE

Angina pectoris: paroxysmal, severe constricting pain in the chest due to myocardial ischemia; typically radiates from the precordium to one or both shoulders as well as the neck or jaw; often precipitated by exertion, exposure to cold or emotional excitement

Arrhythmia: a loss of rhythm or irregularity in the heartbeat, which can affect blood flow to the brain

Aspiration: inhalation of any foreign matter, such as food, saliva, or stomach contents into the airway

Asystole: absence of contractions of the heart's atrioventricular node as the trunk of the atrioventricular bundle and passes through the right atrioventricular fibrous ring to the membranous part of the interventricular septum, where the trunk divides into two branches, the right and left crura of the atrioventricular bundle; the two crura ramify in the subendocardium of their respective ventricles

Arteriosclerosis: stiffening/hardening of the arterial wall resulting from increased calcium deposits that causes the blood vessel to lose it elasticity, thus changing blood flow and increasing blood pressure

Atherosclerosis: buildup of fatty deposits on the inner walls of the arteries

Atrioventricular (AV) bundle: bundle of fibers that are located within the septum of the heart that transmits cardiac impulse from the AV node to the ventricles causing them to contract

Atrioventricular (AV) node: small node of modified cardiac muscle fibers located near the coronary sinus; it gives rise to the atrioventricular bundle of the heart's conduction system

Bradycardia: slowness of the heartbeat, at less than 60 beats per minute

Cardiac distress: first sign of a possible life-threatening cardiac condition, demonstrating pain, pressure, or discomfort in the chest or upper abdomen, difficulty breathing (respiratory distress), and a sudden onset of sweating and nausea and/or vomiting

Cardiac arrest: complete cessation of cardiac activity; either electrical, mechanical, or both

Coronary artery disease (CAD): medical condition where there is build up over time of excessive plaque on the inner walls of the coronary arteries of the heart

Diaphoretic: relating to, or causing, perspiration; sweating

Embolism: obstruction or occlusion of a vessel by an embolus

Emesis: vomiting

Hemoglobin (Hb): red respiratory protein of erythrocytes, consisting of approximately 3.8% heme and 96.2% globin, which, as oxyhemoglobin (HbO_2), transports oxygen from the lungs to the body tissues

Lingual: relating to the tongue or any tongue-like part

Myocardial infarction (heart attack): changes occurring in the heart muscle due to interruption of its blood supply. Results in deprivation of oxygen to a portion of the heart muscle (ischemia) and, if the oxygen supply is not restored within a few minutes, ultimately the death (necrosis) of a portion of the heart muscle

Myocardial necrosis: localized death of heart muscle

Nitroglycerin: prescription medication indicated for the acute relief of a heart attack or acute prophylaxis of angina pectoris due to coronary artery disease through the dilation of the coronary arteries

Occlusion: act of closing or the state of being closed

Palpitations: forcible or irregular pulsations of the heart, perceptible to the athlete, usually with an increase in frequency or force, with or without irregularity in rhythm

Plasma: liquid portion of the blood containing water, proteins, electrolytes, lipids, nutrients and vitamins, hormones, and metabolic waste prodcuts

Purkinje fibers: interlacing fibers formed of modified cardiac muscle cells with central granulated protoplasm containing one or two nuclei and a transversely striated peripheral portion; they are the terminal ramifications of the conducting system of the heart and are found beneath the endocardium of the ventricles

Septum: thin wall dividing two cavities or masses of softer tissue

Sinoatrial (SA) node: the mass of specialized cardiac muscle fibers that normally acts as the "pacemaker" of the cardiac conduction system; it lies under the epicardium at the upper end of the sulcus terminalis

Tachycardia: rapid beating of the heart, conventionally applied to rates of more than 100 per minute

Thrombus: a clot in the cardiovascular system formed from constituents of blood; it may be occlusive or attached to the vessel or heart wall without obstructing the lumen

Thrombolytic medications: medications used to break up or dissolve a thrombus (clot)

Transdermal: through the skin

Sudden cardiac death (SCD): abrupt, unexpected death of cardiovascular cause, in which the loss of consciousness occurs within 1 to 12 hours of onset of symptoms of an otherwise normal, clinically healthy status

Sudden cardiac arrest (SCA): unexpected loss of heart function, breathing, and consciousness, usually resulting from an electrical disturbance in the heart

BEFORE YOU BEGIN

1. Describe the anatomy of the heart. Why is adequate blood flow a vital process?

2. Describe the different stages in the adult cardiac chain of survival. Why is the cardiac chain of survival important? What are some things an athletic trainer can do to strengthen the chain?

3. What is the difference between cardiac distress and cardiac arrest? What are some of the likely causes of these conditions?

4. Identify the signs and symptoms of an athlete suffering from cardiac distress. What are the signs and symptoms an athlete may display?

5. Describe the appropriate steps to care for an adult suffering from cardiac distress.

6. Define sudden cardiac death (SCD) and identify its causes in athletes.

7. Describe the appropriate steps to care for an adult suffering from sudden cardiac arrest.

8. What, if any, complications may arise when caring for an adult suffering from sudden cardiac arrest?

9. What type of emergency equipment should an athletic trainer carry to properly manage an athlete suffering a cardiac emergency?

10. What is an automatic external defibrillator (AED)? Describe how these devices work.

11. Describe the appropriate steps for using an AED when caring for an adult and pediatric patient.

12. Identify the precautions required when using an AED.

Voices from the Field

The athletic trainer has many responsibilities when providing care. One of the most important responsibilities is responding to emergencies, particularly life-threatening conditions such as sudden cardiac arrest (SCA). The SCA emergency response is outlined in this chapter. It is important that the athletic trainer be aware of SCA care. As an athletic trainer with more than 30 years of experience, I have seen SCA twice and am still preparing to respond to future episodes. As an invited speaker who helped develop the National Athletic Trainer Association's Consensus Statement, Inter-Association Task Force Recommendations on Emergency Preparedness, and Management of Sudden Cardiac Arrest in High School and College Athletic Programs, I was asked to share my story of handling an SCA episode of an official at a college football game. I will share an abbreviated version of this story for this chapter, which emphasizes the preparedness and training that give the athlete the best chance at surviving SCA.

On September 29, 2001, Syracuse University was playing East Carolina in a football game at the Carrier Dome in Syracuse, New York. With nearly 40,000 in attendance, Conference USA Official Gerry Bram collapsed at midfield during a play. Seeing Mr. Bram collapse, I immediately instructed my graduate assistant athletic trainer to get the AED from our bench and sprint to Mr. Bram as I and our team physician ran onto the field to make an assessment. As Mr. Bram was being rolled over from a prone position, he was not breathing; I was attempting to detect a pulse. Immediately our team physician, Dr. Irving Raphael, inserted an airway as I informed him that Mr. Bram had no pulse. While all of this was occurring, the AED was being opened, saving valuable time. My associate, Brad Pike, ATC, was given the pads to place on Mr. Bram's chest, which was exposed by cutting his shirt. The AED was turned on. It analyzed Mr. Bram's cardiac rhythm and detected ventricular fibrillation. A "shock advised" order then came from the AED. Upon the command "shock now," I delivered a charge to Mr. Bram's heart, which restarted.

From the time Mr. Bram fell unconscious with SCA to the moment of his AED shock, less than a minute elapsed. With a hushed crowd watching, reportedly with many fans in their seats joining the two teams huddled on their sidelines in prayer, Mr. Bram survived his SCA. After spending several days in a local Syracuse hospital, Mr. Bram returned to his family in Philadelphia. Syracuse University Sports Medicine had just received the AED 6 weeks prior to its use on Mr. Bram, and annually we rehearse many emergency scenarios, including SCA. The staff preparation in emergency planning and training were instrumental in Mr. Bram's survival.

Actually, the event that day felt like a training session except that it was for real. Ironically, that September 29, 2001, game was a makeup of the games canceled from the weekend of September 15, 2001. Had that East Carolina game been played after the attacks of September 11, 2001, Mr. Bram would not have been in the Carrier Dome that day and would have been working a high school game in Philadelphia where an AED was not available. As fate would have it, Mr. Bram was able to work the rescheduled game on September 29. According to Mr. Bram, his SCA could not have happened at a better place and time than on that September day.

Each year on September 29, Mr. Bram calls to pass along his thanks to me, Dr. Raphael, and the fine staff of athletic trainers who responded to his SCA that day.

I think of September 29 each day as I prepare to care for athletes, because it reminds me and others that emergencies can and do occur when one least expects them.

Timothy Neal, MS, ATC
Assistant Director of Athletics for Sports Medicine
Syracuse University, Syracuse, NY

Although cardiac emergencies in the athletic environment are rare, athletic trainers working in other settings (i.e., outpatient rehabilitation, industrial, and corporate) may be interacting with patients at risk for cardiac emergencies. The two types of cardiac emergencies athletic trainers need to be able to recognize and properly manage are **cardiac distress** and **cardiac arrest.** Caused by a variety of traumas (e.g., blunt force chest trauma, penetrating chest injury, loss of blood) and/or illnesses (e.g., cardiovascular disease, drowning, suffocation, drugs, electrocution, congenital heart defect, Marfan's syndrome, etc.), cardiac emergencies lead to the inadequate delivery of oxygen-rich blood to the heart muscle and/or cause an interruption of the heart's electrical system. When the heart is deprived of oxygen or suffers from an interruption of the electrical signal, the result is the body's inability to deliver adequate oxygen to the body cells and vital organs. Without oxygen, vital organs, including the heart and brain, begin to suffer damage within minutes and eventually death if left untreated.

This chapter identifies and describes how to properly manage an athlete suffering from cardiac distress and arrest; it also demonstrates the importance of the cardiac chain of survival. The techniques described in this chapter, like all clinical skills, require periodic review, practice, and formal testing to maintain clinical competence. The skills presented in this chapter should be reviewed annually or semiannually by athletic trainers along with their emergency action plan (EAP) policies and other emergency procedures. Finally, because the science behind emergency cardiac care (ECC) is re-evaluated every 5 years, athletic trainers need to remain diligent to make sure that they are receiving the most accurate information. Remember too that, according to the Board of Certification, all certified athletic trainers must maintain and demonstrate proof of a valid ECC or cardiopulmonary resuscitation (CPR) certification every year or two, depending upon the certification body.[1] Though all attempts have been made to make sure that the information presented in this chapter is accurate and based on current science (2005 ECC Guidelines), agencies granting certification may have slightly different interpretations of the International Consensus on Cardiopulmonary Resuscitation and Emergency Cardiovascular Care with Treatment Recommendations as the science does change.[2-5]

THE CARDIOVASCULAR SYSTEM

The cardiovascular system is comprised of the heart, blood vessels, and blood, all of which work together to supply the body with oxygen-rich blood and to remove carbon dioxide by pumping deoxygenated blood to the lungs. Remember, any trauma or illness affecting the heart or blood vessels threatens the delivery of oxygen-rich blood and predisposes an athlete to a cardiac emergency. Therefore, the athletic trainer must have a thorough understanding of the anatomy and function of the circulatory system. The following section provides a brief review of the anatomy and physiology of the cardiovascular system.

Anatomy

A discussion of the cardiovascular system must begin with the heart, a four-chamber organ approximately the size of a fist. It is located under the sternum and slightly to the left, between the lungs. The upper two chambers are the atria and the lower two are the ventricles. The ventricular walls contain more muscle and are, therefore, thicker than the atria and can withstand higher blood pressures; they also generate more force than the atria when they contract. The walls of the left ventricle are also thicker than those of the right ventricle because it is responsible for pumping blood to the whole body; the right ventricle, on the other hand, is responsible for pumping blood only as far as the lungs. The right and left sides of the heart are divided by a supporting structure know as the **septum.** Located on the outside of the heart are the two coronary arteries (right and left), which supply the heart muscle with blood and oxygen. As the heart pumps, the backflow of blood into the chambers and vessels is prevented by the heart's valves. These are the aortic, tricuspid, pulmonary, and mitral valves (Fig. 12.1).

Connected to the heart's two atria and ventricles are two arteries and three veins. Connected to the right atrium are the inferior and superior vena cava. The inferior vena cava receives deoxygenated blood from the lower body, while the superior vena cava receives blood from the upper body. Connected to the right atrium is the pulmonary artery. Remember, arteries typically carry oxygenated blood; however, the pulmonary artery is the only artery in the body that carries deoxygenated blood, in this case to the lungs. Oxygenated blood from the lungs is transported back through the pulmonary vein into the left atrium. Finally, oxygenated blood from the left ventricle is transported to the body via the aortic artery. The right and left coronary arteries supply the heart muscle from a branch off of the aorta.

The final component of the cardiovascular system is blood. Blood is a mixture of two components, 45% solids, or cells (i.e., red blood cells [RBCs], white blood cells, and platelets) and 55% **plasma** (i.e., the liquid portion of the blood). Plasma is mostly water and contains proteins, nutrients, hormones, antibodies, and dissolved waste products. The average 150-pound adult has approximately 5 to 6 quarts of blood, which account for 7% to 8% of his or her body weight. Blood is a very important component of the human body and has several functions. However, the main function of concern in this chapter is the ability of the RBCs to transport oxygen from the lungs throughout the rest of the body to maintain adequate tissue perfusion. This

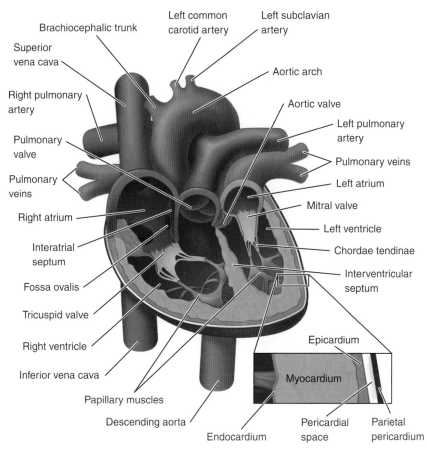

FIGURE 12.1   Anatomy of the heart. (From Anderson MK, et al. *Foundations of Athletic Training: Prevention, Assessment, and Management*, 4th ed. Baltimore: Lippincott Williams & Williams; 2009.)

is accomplished by a protein called **hemoglobin,** which is carried by the RBCs. RBCs also assist in the removal of carbon dioxide (CO_2) from the body.

Physiology

The main physiological function of the complex relationship between the heart, blood vessels, and blood is

Breakout

Functions of Blood

- Buffering to help maintain appropriate pH balance of body fluids
- Regulation of body temperature
- Prevention of blood loss through blood clotting
- Protection against toxins and microorganisms
- Transportation of oxygen, nutrients, and hormones and removal of metabolic wastes (CO_2, nitrogenous wastes, and heat)

to ensure adequate delivery of oxygenated blood to all the body's tissues. Remember, however, that the success of this system also depends on respiratory system's ability to supply the body with an adequate amount of oxygen and remove CO_2 through the process of ventilation.

Heartbeat

A normal healthy adult's heart beats anywhere between 60 and 100 times per minute. This translates into 3,600 to 6,000 beats per hour, 86,400 to 144,000 beats per day, or 31,536,000 to 52,560,000 beats per year. This ability to contract billions of times in a lifetime depends on a specialized electrical conduction system within the heart, which sends electrical impulses down the center of the heart to the left and right ventricles.

The electrical impulse begins in the upper wall of the right atrium, where specialized cells (called pacemaker cells) are gathered in a small area called the sinus node. When the **sinoatrial (SA) node** (Fig. 12.2) fires, it generates a nerve impulse chain reaction that travels

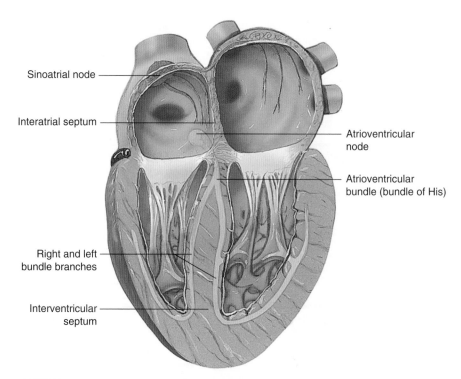

Sinoatrial node

Interatrial septum

Atrioventricular node

Atrioventricular bundle (bundle of His)

Right and left bundle branches

Interventricular septum

FIGURE 12.2 Electrical circuits of the heart. When the sinoatrial node fires, it generates a chain reaction of nerve impulses that travel throughout the heart wall, stimulating the atria to contract. This reaction travels from the atria to the ventricles as the electrical impulses pass through a junction called the atrioventricular node. (Courtesy of Anatomical Chart Co.)

throughout the heart wall, stimulating the atria to contract. This chain reaction continues from the atria to the ventricles as the electrical impulse passes through a junction called the **atrioventricular (AV) node.** The AV node lies on the right side of the septum, near the bottom of the right atrium. The main function of this junction is to slow down the electrical impulse for about a tenth of a second, so that the mechanical contraction of the atria will give the ventricles the time required to fill with blood. The right atrium, which has received deoxygenated blood from the superior and inferior vena cava, pumps blood to the right ventricle. The left atrium, which has received oxygenated blood from the pulmonary vein, pumps blood to the left ventricle.

The impulses continue traveling down the **atrioventricular bundle,** located between center of the septum, which branches into the right and left bundle branch to supply impulses to the right and left ventricles. Once these impulses have reached the base of the atrioventricular bundle they further subdivide into the **Purkinje fibers.** These are the terminal part of the heart's electrical conduction system; when they are triggered, the ventricles contract. The right ventricle, which has received deoxygenated blood from the right atrium, pumps blood through the pulmonary artery to the lungs, so that the alveoli can ex-

change carbon dioxide for newly inhaled oxygen. The left ventricle, which has received oxygenated blood from the left atrium, pumps blood up the ascending aorta to transport the oxygen throughout the body. Some of this blood, however, is diverted from the aorta to the coronary arteries, which carry oxygenated and nutrient-filled blood to the heart muscle. Inadequate perfusion of the heart muscle due to blockage of the coronary arteries leads to death of the muscle and increases an individual's risk of having a heart attack.

When the ventricles have completed a contraction and are relaxed, the atrium contracts again, having received a new impulse from the SA node. This cycle is repeated throughout life unless it is interrupted by trauma or illness.

ADULT CARDIAC CHAIN OF SURVIVAL

In Chapter 1, we discussed the "chain of survival" as a series of events that, when implemented, increases the likelihood that an ill or injured individual will survive with minimal adverse consequences. These events are an essential component of

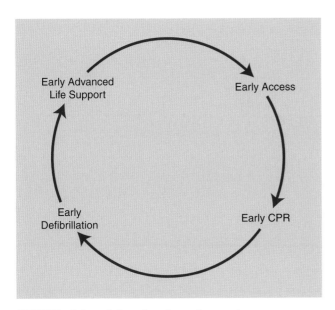

FIGURE 12.3   Adult cardiac chain of survival.

prehospital care and, when put into motion, reduce the mortality associated with injury or illness. The **cardiac chain of survival** is another series of events that, when implemented, increases the likelihood of survival from **sudden cardiac arrest** (SCA)[6–8] (Fig. 12.3). These events are critical to the survivability of an individual, because the time between the identification of an athlete in SCA, initiation of the EAP, and arrival of emergency medical services (EMS) is normally longer than 5 minutes.[9,10] Therefore, the ability of the athletic trainer to properly perform cardiopulmonary resuscitation (CPR) and apply an automated external defibrillator (AED) is critical.

The adult cardiac chain of survival consists of four parts:

1. Early access
2. Early CPR
3. Early defibrillation
4. Early advanced life support

Early Access

As in the case of any other serious trauma or illness, the ability of bystanders and/or others to access trained personnel is the first step in ensuring survivability. As athletic trainers and health care providers, we have a unique advantage because we often have the opportunity to witness the collapse of an athlete and are able to activate the EAP and initiate CPR within 30 to 60 seconds after SCA.[11] In other settings where athletic trainers work, the ability of coworkers and bystanders to recognize the signs of SCA will also be critical to an individual's survival. This is why the development of a well-organized CPR and AED program in high schools and colleges (as well as all work settings with at-risk athletes) is essential and should be reviewed on an annual basis. For further information on establishing an AED program in the high school and college setting, we recommend reviewing the article by Drezner et al.,[9] listed in the references.

Early CPR

SCA is the unexpected loss of heart function, breathing, and consciousness, usually resulting from an electrical disturbance in the heart and disrupting the heart's ability to circulate blood throughout the body and perfuse body tissues. The ability to initiate early CPR and continue the delivery of care before the arrival of an AED serves as a holding action to provide blood and oxygen to the vital organs for a short time. Early CPR has been shown to double or triple the individual's chances of survival.[12–14] Interestingly enough, an individual in SCA is more likely to receive CPR when the event is witnessed by bystanders unknown to the individual than if the arrest is witnessed by friends or family.[15,16]

Early Defibrillation

The third link in the cardiac chain of survival is considered one of the most important interventions affecting survival from SCA.[17,18] In most cases of adult SCA, the heart is in an abnormal rhythm called ventricular fibrillation (V-fib or VF). This can be reversed only by delivering an electrical shock with an AED. CPR should be provided until an AED or manual defibrillator (used by advanced EMS personnel) is available. However, as the length of time between the onset of SCA and defibrillation increases, the chances of restoring a normal heartbeat and full recovery decrease. In fact, for every minute that passes between the onset of an SCA event and the delivery of an electrical shock, the probability of survival decreases somewhere between 7% and 10% percent; after 10 minutes, the probability of survival is extremely low.[19]

Today, public access defibrillation (PAD) laws have increased the accessibility of AEDs in places where large groups or high-risk populations congregate, giving both minimally trained and trained responders access to immediate defibrillation rather than waiting for an EMS unit to arrive. Studies have shown that PAD programs improve cardiac arrest survival rates through rapid defibrillation by nonmedical personnel (bystanders) using an AED.[17,20,21] In one study, intervals of no more than 3 minutes from collapse to defibrillation were necessary to achieve the highest survival rates.[21]

SCA is one of the leading causes of death among young athletes. Because of this, increasing the presence of AEDs and timely access to them at sporting events has been recommend by the Inter-Association Task Force.[18] The development of an action plan to provide a means for early defibrillation and the potential for effective prevention of sudden cardiac death (SCD; death resulting from cardiac arrest) in high school and college athletes should be a responsibility of all athletic trainers. However, regardless of the amount of planning and preparation that takes place and the availability of an AED, not all athletes who experience an SCA will survive.[11]

Early Advanced Life Support

The final part of the cardiac chain of survival is early advanced life support. This includes the first three links mentioned above plus the care provided by an advanced emergency medical technician (AEMT). The AEMT responding to the athlete has the ability to administer drugs, implement advanced airway procedures, and take other necessary steps prior to the athlete's arrival at an advanced care facility.

PEDIATRIC CARDIAC CHAIN OF SURVIVAL

The pediatric cardiac chain of survival varies slightly from the adult chain in part because the major causes of death in infants and children (under the age of 8) are unintentional injuries, respiratory failure, sudden infant death syndrome, and sepsis.[22] As a result of these differences, the pediatric cardiac chain of survival emphasizes prevention, basic CPR, prompt access to the EMS system, and prompt pediatric advanced life support[23] (Fig. 12.4).

CARDIAC EMERGENCIES

Cardiac Distress

An athlete suffering pain, pressure, or discomfort in the chest or upper abdomen, difficulty breathing (respiratory distress), and a sudden onset of sweating (**diaphoresis**) and nausea and/or vomiting may be experiencing cardiac distress—sometimes referred to as cardiac compromise (a blanket term describing any problem with the heart) or, in most cases, **myocardial infarction** (MI). Laypeople commonly refer to this condition as a heart attack. Cardiac com-

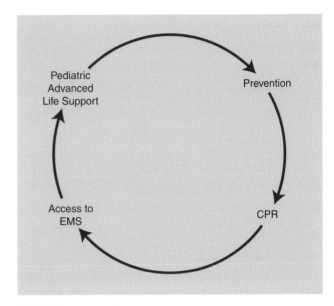

FIGURE 12.4   Pediatric cardiac chain of survival.

promise in the general population occurs more frequently and for many more reasons than what is often experienced in the athletic population.

Causes of cardiac distress in the general population are many and include narrowing or blockage of the coronary artery, often due to **coronary artery disease** (CAD). CAD is due to a buildup of fatty deposits of plaque on the inner walls of the coronary arteries, the blood vessels responsible for providing blood and oxygen to the heart itself. This buildup of plaque leads to the development of **atherosclerosis** (Fig. 12.5) and causes narrowing of the coronary arteries and, as a result, reduced blood flow. Over time, this reduction in blood flow means that the heart muscle is increasingly deprived of oxygen, resulting in the death of irreplaceable heart muscle cells. Also, as time passes, calcium deposits begin to accumulate at the plaque site, causing the arteries to harden and resulting in **arthrosclerosis.** The stiffening or hardening of the arterial wall also causes the blood vessels to lose their elasticity, leading to a further decrease in blood flow and increased cell death in the heart muscle while also increasing the athlete's blood pressure.

Eventually, the plaque thickens, increasing the risk that a **thrombus** (blood clot) will form as blood cells adhere to the roughened surface of the plaque. As the

Current Research

Heart Disease as the Leading Cause of Death

The National Center for Injury Prevention and Control suggests that, from 1996 to 2006, heart disease was the leading cause of death for all races, both sexes, and for those above age 65; it accounted for 31.4% of all deaths. Heart disease was also the leading cause of death for all races, both sexes, and all ages, accounting for 28.2% of all deaths. In comparison, heart disease accounted for 3.2% of all deaths in the 15- to 24-year-old age range.[24]

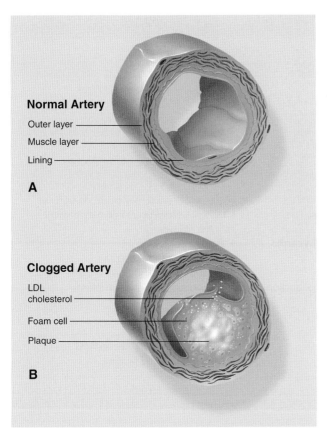

Normal Artery

Outer layer

Muscle layer

Lining

A

Clogged Artery

LDL
cholesterol

Foam cell

Plaque

B

FIGURE 12.5 Atherosclerosis: normal and clogged artery. **A.** When the level of cholesterol in the bloodstream is normal, arterial walls remain smooth and slippery. **B.** When cholesterol levels are high, excess cholesterol accumulates in the arterial walls, reducing blood flow. LDL, low-density lipoprotein.

clot grows, there is a further reduction of blood flow, or **occlusion** of the vessel, and the heart muscle's supply of oxygen is further reduced. In some cases, a section of the clot breaks off, resulting in an **embolism.** This free-floating clot travels in the bloodstream until it reaches a smaller vessel, where it becomes lodged and partially or completely blocks blood flow to the structures distal to the clot. If the clot becomes large enough to cut off most or all of the blood flow through the coronary arteries, a heart attack or stroke (if the blockage occurs in the brain) occurs. As the heart muscle dies, the tissue is replaced with scar tissue and further increases the stress on the heart. The heart chamber most often affected by the reduction in blood flow is the thickened wall of the left ventricle. The left ventricle, remember, is responsible for delivering blood throughout the body, and any decrease in its ability to contract will affect all body tissues. And although CAD is just one cause of cardiac emergencies (specifically a heart attack), as an athletic trainer, you must be familiar with other cardiovascular disorders that may lead to compromise of the heart (Table 12.1).

Signs and Symptoms of a Heart Attack

Have you ever observed an individual who was showing signs and symptoms of a heart attack? Would such a person know what the signs and symptoms were so that they could be report their emergency to EMS or an athletic trainer? Hopefully, the answer to the first question is no—you have never observed an individual demonstrating signs and symptoms of a heart attack. The answer to the second question is actually a little more concerning. Although a large majority of the U.S. population is well aware of some of the signs and symptoms of a heart attack,[26] such as chest pain,[27] only about a third of individuals are aware of the five major warning signs. This is concerning, considering that 17% of heart attacks reported in 2004 were fatal,[26] with the Centers for Disease Control and Prevention reporting that almost half of those experiencing a heart attack die from it.[28]

The five main signs and symptoms of a heart attack are shown in the Signs & Symptoms box, below. However, not all heart attacks present as they do in the movies, with obvious crushing chest pain. In fact, many individuals experiencing a heart attack encounter only mild discomfort in the center of the chest[29]; in some cases they may not experience any chest pain.[30] When chest pain or discomfort is present, most individuals describe the pain/discomfort as being felt in the center of the chest and as lasting for more than a few minutes, or that it goes away and comes back.[29] They say that the pain does not change with each breath. Some individuals may deny having pain but may admit to the presence of chest pressure.

Individuals may also report discomfort that feels like an uncomfortable pressure, squeezing, or fullness. Left neck and arm pain has also been widely reported by individuals as a symptom of a heart attack. The truth is that this pain/discomfort can in fact be found in one or both arms or in the back, neck, jaw, or even the stomach. Other signs and symptoms often experienced may include (a) a sudden onset of nausea, (b) **emesis,** (c) diaphoresis, and (d) changes in vital signs: pulse rate (rapid and weak) and blood pressure, as well as pale, bluish (cyanotic), or moist skin. Some individuals will report

Signs & Symptoms

Heart Attack[25,28,31]

- Chest pain, pressure, or discomfort that is often crushing or squeezing and that does not change with each breath
- Pain or discomfort in one arm (normally the left) or both arms or shoulders
- Pain or discomfort in the lower jaw, neck, abdomen, and/or back
- Weakness, light-headedness, or feeling faint
- Dyspnea

TABLE 12.1	Common Cardiovascular Disorders	
Disorder	**Description**	**Signs and Symptoms**

Aneurysm	• Circumscribed dilation of an artery (anywhere in the body) or a cardiac chamber due to an acquired or congenital weakness of the wall of the artery or chamber, causing a dilation or ballooning of the vessel. Over time, this weakening can rupture, causing rapid, life-threatening internal bleeding.	• Aortic aneurysm may cause no symptoms until the aneurysm begins to leak or grow.
		• Signs or symptoms may include:
		  • Pain in the jaw, neck, upper back (or other part of the back), or chest
		  • Coughing, hoarseness, or trouble breathing

Arrhythmia*	• A loss of rhythm or irregularity in the speed of the heartbeat that can affect blood flow to the brain, heart, and other vital organs.
	• A heartbeat that is too fast is referred to as **tachycardia,** whereas a heartbeat that is too slow is called **bradycardia.**
	• These conditions are normally the result of a malfunction in the heart's electrical system.
		• Many arrhythmias may cause no signs or symptoms. However, some may present with the following:
		  • **Palpitations**
		  • Bradycardia (<60 bpm)
		  • Tachycardia (>100 bpm)
		• More serious signs and symptoms include:
		  • Anxiety
		  • Weakness
		  • Dizziness and light-headedness
		  • Fainting or nearly fainting
		  • Sweating
		  • Shortness of breath
		  • Chest pain

Angina pectoris	• Paroxysmal severe constricting pain in the chest due to myocardial ischemia, often as a result of CAD or arterial spasms.	• Typically radiates from the precordium to one or both shoulders, the neck, or the jaw. • Often precipitated by exertion, exposure to cold, or emotional excitement. • Usually lasting 3 to 8 minutes, rarely longer than 15 minutes • Considered a *warning sign* of a possible heart attack. • Individuals with a history of this condition will be prescribed nitroglycerin.

Congestive heart failure	• Condition of excessive fluid buildup in the lungs and/or other organs because of inadequate pumping of the heart.
	• Develops over time as the pumping of the heart grows weaker; can affect the right side of the heart only or both the left and right sides.
		• Most common signs and symptoms of heart failure include:
		  • Shortness of breath or difficulty breathing
		  • Fatigue (tiredness)
		  • Swelling in the ankles, feet, legs, abdomen due to the buildup of fluid in the body
		  • Weight gain
		  • Frequent urination
		  • Cough that's worse at night and when lying supine

*Arrhythmias are addressed further in the cardiac arrest and AED portions of this chapter.[25]

high levels of anxiety and possibly a sense of impending doom, as if they knew something was wrong. It should be noted that although men and women have similar signs and symptoms, women are less likely than men to believe that they are having a heart attack and more likely to delay seeking emergency treatment.[32] However, there is no need here to differentiate heart attack symptoms between women and men.[33]

A cardiac emergency may be exacerbated by an individual's age and his or her medical history, increasing mortality and morbidity rates.[34] For example, an older athlete with a history of **angina pectoris** (chest pain due to myocardial ischemia precipitated by exertion, exposure to cold, or emotional excitement), CAD, diabetes mellitus, high blood cholesterol, and smoking may present with signs and symptoms more quickly and with little ability to compensate as compared with a healthy high school or college athlete. Therefore, in an athletic trainer's work setting, it may be necessary to consider potential risk factors in order to identify those at greatest risk. If an individual is considered to be "at risk," appropriate referral to a health care provider for further medical intervention is warranted, possibly, before beginning any type of strenuous activity or rehabilitation program.

Remember that the symptoms experienced by an athlete in cardiac distress are subjective and may not accurately reflect the extent of his or her condition. Fear, anxiety, and uncertainty may all cause the athlete to overreact to the situation, particularly if it is exacerbated or influenced by the overreaction of a coach, teammates, and/or parents. In fact, an individual experiencing breathing difficulty may display either adequate or inadequate breathing, depending on his or her reaction. For this reason, the athletic trainer must complete a thorough assessment to determine the severity of the emergency. The findings of the primary assessment will then determine the required interventions.

Breakout

Risk Factors for Heart Attack[35]

- Male gender, older than 45 years of age
- Female gender, older than 50 years of age (after menopause)
- Family history of heart disease
- Diabetes mellitus
- High blood cholesterol
- High blood pressure (often associated with CAD)
- Cigarette smoking
- Overweight
- Physical inactivity

Sudden Cardiac Death

An individual suffering from some form of heart disease (either diagnosed or undiagnosed) or cardiac distress where he or she did not receive an appropriate level of intervention may fall victim to SCD. As the name implies, the time and mode of death are unexpected.[36] When cardiac arrest occurs, there is a complete cessation of cardiac activity—electrical, mechanical, or both. As a result, blood stops flowing to the brain and other vital organs, eventually resulting in death if not treated within minutes. The athlete in cardiac arrest is unconscious, demonstrates no signs of life (no breathing or pulse) during the primary assessment, and will remain in that condition until the heart begins beating again.

Most causes of SCA are related to an **arrhythmia,** which is a loss of the normal heart rhythm or an irregularity in the speed of each heartbeat. Arrhythmias affect blood flow to the brain, heart, and other vital organs, with V-fib being noted in about 40% of out-of-hospital cardiac arrests,[37] followed by ventricular tachycardia (V-tach).[36] In V-fib, the heart experiences chaotic, rapid depolarization and repolarization. This causes the heart muscle to quiver and lose its ability to pump blood effectively.[9] In V-tach, the heart does beat, but too quickly, which does not allow the left ventricle enough time to fill; thereby reducing the amount of blood delivered to the organs. In the general population, factors such as CAD, severe physical stress, inherited genetic disorders, and structural changes to the heart are just some of the factors causing the development of an arrhythmia. Other causes of cardiac arrest include drowning, suffocation, electrocution, cardiac trauma, untreated respiratory arrest, poisoning, allergic reactions, and stroke. In some cases, cardiac arrest can be due to an extreme slowing of the heart, known as bradycardia.[36]

Sudden Cardiac Death in the General and Athletic Population

Although 400,000 to 460,000 individuals in the United States experience SCA yearly,[3] it accounts for approximately 325,000 deaths per year (incidence of 0.1% to 0.2% per year in the adult population) and is responsible for approximately 50% of deaths from CAD.[38] In the athletic population, SCA is considered the leading cause of death among young athletes[9,39–41] despite preparticipation physical examinations and emergency planning, including the availability of AEDs on site at athletic events.[9]

SCD in the athletic population has been defined as "an abrupt unexpected death of cardiovascular cause, in which the loss of consciousness occurs within 1 to 12 hours of onset of symptoms."[42] SCD is the result of a nontraumatic, nonviolent, unexpected event. Most cases of SCD (56%) in young athletes (younger than 35 years old) are directly related to some type of cardiovascular disease, particularly hypertrophic cardiomyopathy.[39,40,42-44] SCD appears to occur more frequently during physical exertion in competition/training[43]; however, physical exertion is not a prerequisite. Of the cardiovascular diseases, hypertrophic cardiomyopathy and congenital coronary artery anomalies account for approximately 36% and 17% of deaths, respectively, among athletes who died suddenly (or survived cardiac arrest).[43]

The following table[25,31,43-50] provides a general description of some of the cardiac causes of sudden death in athletes.

Pathology	Etiology	Clinical Features
Hypertrophic cardiomyopathy (HCM)	HCM is congenital disorder characterized by abnormal thickening of the left ventricular wall, which develops prior to the age of 20.	The thickened ventricular wall leads to electrical problems and arrhythmia, including V-fib.
Congenital coronary artery anomalies	Congenial variations in right or left coronary anatomy often recognized in association with structural forms of congenital heart disease. The most common abnormality consists of a wrong origin of the left main coronary artery.	These are considered the second most common cause of sudden death from cardiovascular disease. These anomalies are usually diagnosed by echocardiography, magnetic resonance imaging, and/or coronary angiography.
Myocarditis	Inflammation of the muscular walls of the heart resulting from a bacterial or viral infection, normally viral in athletics.	Sudden death in this case is attributed to changes in the heart muscle that lead to degeneration or death of the muscle and result in electrical instability and arrhythmias.
Arrhythmogenic right ventricular cardiomyopathy (ARVC)	ARVC is an inherited heart muscle disorder where damaged heart muscle is gradually replaced by scar tissue and fat.	ARVC may cause abnormal electrical heart rhythms and weakening of the pumping action of the heart. Symptoms include palpitations and fainting after physical activity. ARVC normally affects teens or young adults.
Mitral valve prolapse (MVP)	In MVP, the heart's mitral valve does not work properly. When the left ventricle contracts, one or both flaps of the mitral valve flop or bulge back (prolapse) into the left atrium, thereby preventing the valve from forming a tight seal. Blood is allowed to flow backward from the ventricle into the atrium.	Mitral valve backflow can cause arrhythmias. An athlete with MVP may present with chest pain, dyspnea, palpitations, and fatigue with exertion.
Commotio cordis (CC)	Derived from Latin and meaning "disturbance of the heart," CC events are a result of low-impact, nonpenetrating blows to the chest wall, which are generally not of sufficient force to cause any significant structural damage to the ribs, sternum, or heart.	The likely cause of death in CC is V-fib, which is initiated by a low-impact chest wall blow occurring within a narrow window of the cardiac cycle, just before the peak of the T wave. It had been thought that CC could be prevented by the use of a protective chest barrier. However, a recent study found that despite the use of such a barrier, a blow to chest was fatal in 32 of 85 competitive athletes.[49]
Marfan's syndrome (MS)	MS is an autosomal dominant hereditary disorder affecting many of the body's organ systems by reducing the tensile strength of the supportive connective tissue. Typically, the disorder is characterized by structural abnormalities of the cardiovascular, musculoskeletal, and ocular systems with variable clinical expressions in about 85% of patients.	Cardiac abnormalities are the leading cause of premature death in individuals with MS and include four main cardiac manifestations: aortic aneurysm, aortic insufficiency, mitral valve prolapse, and dysrhythmias. For further information see the National Marfan Foundation (http://www.marfan.org/marfan)

Current Research

Cardiac Causes of Sudden Death

The most recent study examining SCD in athletes identified 1,866 cardiovascular, trauma-related, and other sudden death events in young competitive athletes younger than 39 years of age through the U.S. National Registry of Sudden Death in Athletes. This registry "is a largely autopsy-based data set that encompasses events over a 27-year period in 38 organized sports performed at several competitive levels and provides insight into the number of such events that occur in trained athletes."[43]

Of the 1,866 sudden deaths reported in the registry, 1,049 (56%) were judged to be probably or definitely due to cardiovascular causes. Of these, 690 cases could be reliably attributed to 44 different documented primary cardiovascular diseases with hypertrophic cardiomyopathy being the most common cause. Of the remaining 817 cases, 44% of sudden deaths were attributed to trauma or some other cause, including blunt trauma (n = 416, or 22%), miscellaneous (n = 182, or 10%), unresolved cases (n = 54, or 8%), and commotio cordis (n = 65, or 3%). Of the miscellaneous cases, 2% (n = 46) were attributed to heat stroke.

EMERGENCY MEDICAL CARE FOR CARDIAC EMERGENCIES

Cardiac Distress

The signs and symptoms of many cardiac emergencies, including heart attack or angina pectoris, may or may not always be obvious and will require an athletic trainer to complete a thorough primary assessment and determine the status of the airway, breathing, and circulation (ABCs). This will be followed by a secondary assessment (physical examination and SAMPLE history) as well as the appropriate intervention (e.g., CPR, AED, assisting with medication). Delaying recognition of the problem and appropriate interventions, including advanced out-of-hospital medical care, decreases the individual's chances of receiving **thrombolytic medications** (i.e., clot-busting drugs), surgery, or other life-saving medical procedures. Regardless of the events leading to the cardiac distress, the athletic trainer should begin care by following the directions in Skill 12.1 or referring to

SKILL 12.1

Cardiac Distress

1. Initiate the EAP.
2. Check the safety of the scene.
3. Take body substance isolation (BSI) precautions.
4. Complete a primary assessment to determine any compromise in the athlete's ABCs (including external bleeding) by opening and adequately maintaining the airway if necessary. An individual responding to your questions has an airway and demonstrates signs of life (breathing and circulation) (Fig. 12.6).
5. Complete a SAMPLE history, focusing on questions based on the mnemonic OPQRST (see the Breakout box later in this chapter). Determine if the individual has a history of cardiac emergencies, risk factors, and whether or not he or she has been prescribed nitroglycerin or chewable aspirin; if so, ask whether he or she has taken the medication prior to your arrival.

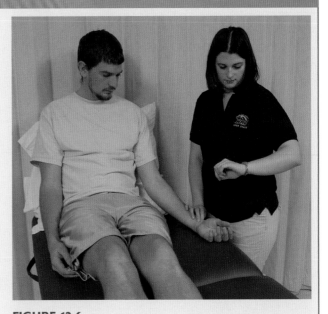

FIGURE 12.6

(Continued)

Cardiac Distress (Continued)

6. Summon advanced medical personnel for all athletes suffering chest pain. Distinguishing between cardiac conditions such as a heart attack and angina pectoris is not part of the athletic trainer's scope of practice. Therefore, any individual suffering chest pain should be treated as though he or she were having a heart attack and require initiation of EMS.

7. Place the individual in a position of comfort in order to assist breathing and relieve discomfort. Many athletes of cardiac distress find lying in a semirecumbent position more comfortable than being supine (Fig. 12.7). Loosen athletic equipment or clothing such as belts, shirt collars, to assist breathing. Consider limiting the number of bystanders (i.e., coaches, teammates) involved in order to reduce the athlete's anxiety and fear.

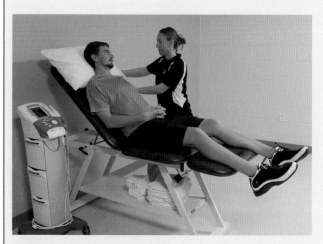

FIGURE 12.7

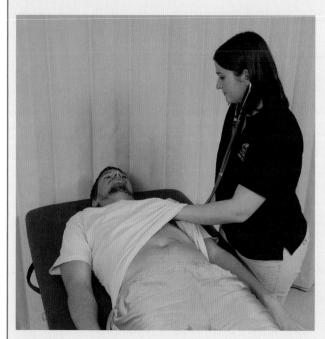

FIGURE 12.8

8. Complete a focused physical examination.
   a. Assess for dismissed or absent breaths and/or fluid in the lungs by auscultation (Fig. 12.8). Assess for unequal and/or inadequate chest expansion, inadequate or shallow tidal volume, and breathing effort (i.e., use of accessory muscles, nasal flaring, etc.).

9. Complete your assessment of baseline vital signs (Fig. 12.9).
   a. Respirations
      i. Normal or possibly rapid, shallow or labored if presenting with dyspnea and/or if congestive heart failure is present.
   b. Pulse
      i. Rapid, irregular pulse due to arrhythmias.
   c. Blood pressure
      i. Most athletes present with normal or increased blood pressure. In cases where the left ventricle is affected, a decreased blood pressure may be noted due to failure of the left ventricle to pump effectively.
   d. Skin color, temperature, and condition
      i. The skin will normally be ashen gray or bluish due to poor tissue perfusion; it will also be cool, and moist.

10. Assist the individual with medications such as a nitroglycerin and/or chewable aspirin (acetylsalicylic acid, 325 mg) if there are no known allergies and the medication has been prescribed (e.g., nitroglycerin) and recommended by the team physician or medical director.

11. Assist the athlete with the use of supplemental oxygen if allowed and you are trained to do so. Apply 15 L/min by nonrebreather mask. Supplemental oxygen should be applied immediately after the primary assessment.

12. Perform an ongoing assessment. Observe changes in level of consciousness, airway, breathing, and circulation. Repeat assessment of all vital signs, particularly in situations where medication has been administered. Reassess interventions and consider performing another focused physical examination.

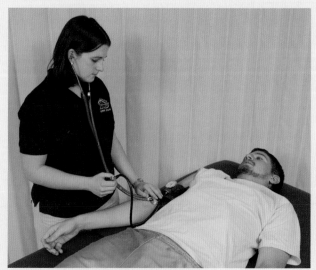

FIGURE 12.9

Algorithm 12.1 below for an emergency action decisional algorithm.

If at any time the athlete's respiration rate is less than 8 or more than 24 breaths per minute (adult), he or she will need positive-pressure ventilation using a bag-valve-mask (Chapter 11) with supplemental oxygen (if available). If the athlete loses consciousness, reassess his or her condition and provide appropriate care based on the current signs and symptoms.

Cardiac Arrest

An athlete in cardiac arrest during the primary assessment or who goes into cardiac arrest because of improper management

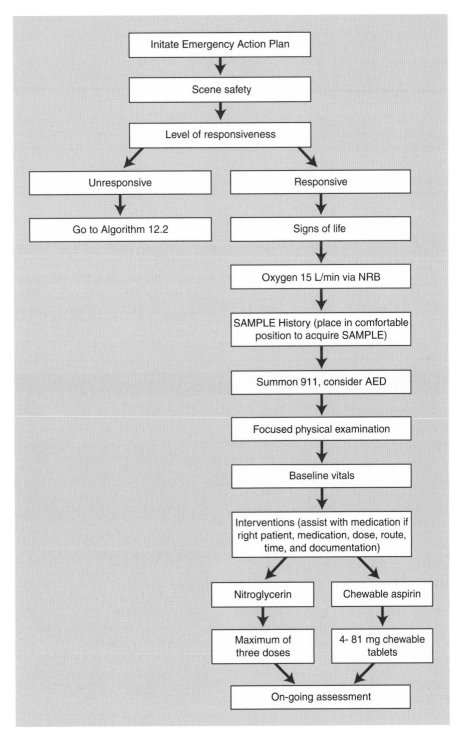

ALGORITHM 12.1 Cardiac distress.

Highlight

Administering Nitroglycerin and Aspirin during a Cardiac Emergency

Evidence suggests that the administration of chewable aspirin (acetylsalicylic acid, 325 mg) in the pre-hospital setting is safe and that the earlier aspirin is given, the greater the reduction in risk of mortality.[51] Individuals with a history of aspirin allergy or signs of active or recent gastrointestinal bleeding should not be given aspirin.[52] However, **do not delay** providing care while waiting to administer aspirin.

Individuals with a known cardiac condition may have a prescription for nitroglycerin. It is most commonly used in the treatment of angina[25] and is administered either orally (**lingually**), by placing a pill under the tongue, or by using a liquid spray. Nitroglycerin acts by dilating the blood vessels (i.e., the coronary arteries), allowing more blood to flow to the heart, while reducing its workload. Occasionally, an individual may have a nitroglycerin patch to prevent attacks of angina.[25] An individual who is conscious, has a prescription, and is exhibiting signs and symptoms of a cardiac emergency should be encourage to administer his or her medication as long as he or she is hemodynamically stable (systolic blood pressure more than 90 mm Hg), pulse rate between 50 and 100 beats per minute,[52] with no signs of increased cranial pressure, and no history of the use of Viagra or similar medications. The nitroglycerin should take effect within a couple of minutes; however, if there is no relief of chest pain after 5 minutes, the individual may use another dose, up to three total doses. Be sure to document the individual's response to the medication and the number of doses, as EMS will need this information when they arrive on scene.

Remember, *always consult* your individual state laws and practice acts, facility policy and procedure manuals, and/or standing medical orders to determine how and when these medications can and should be administrated during a cardiac emergency situation.

of another condition will (a) be unconscious/unresponsive, (b) demonstrate no signs of breathing, and (c) show no signs of life (pulseless). In this case the athletic trainer will initiate the cardiac chain of survival, beginning with early activation of EMS.[9] Except in the presence of a do not resuscitate order, CPR should be begun immediately while awaiting the arrival of an AED. However, CPR alone will not help an individual suffering from sudden cardiac arrest due to V-fib or V-tach. CPR as a technique functions to provide a small but critical amount of blood flow

Breakout

Assessing Cardiac Distress Using OPQRST

OPQRST is a mnemonic often used in emergency medicine to help guide the S (signs and symptoms) of the SAMPLE history by allowing the athletic trainer to ask certain pertinent questions about the individual's condition. OPQRST stands for:

- Onset—When did the problem start?
  - Angina pectoris usually occurs at times when the heart requires large amounts of oxygen, as during physical or emotional stress, after a large meal, or with sudden fear. As the demands for oxygen diminish, so does the pain.
  - Heart attacks can occur during periods of increased oxygen demand as well when no increased demands are placed on the heart.
- Provocation—What makes the symptoms better or worse?
  - If an individual took his or her prescribed medication, such as nitroglycerin, has it helped to alleviate some of the discomfort?
  - Positioning may increase or decrease symptoms.
- Quality—What does it feel like? Can you describe the pain and/or symptoms?
  - Angina pectoris presents with a crushing or squeezing pain that normally subsides within 3 to 8 minutes.
  - Heart attacks present also present with a crushing or squeezing sensation that does not changes with each breath. Remember that about one third of individuals experiencing a heart attack may not report any chest pain at all.
- Radiation—Where do you feel your pain? Does it travel to another location of your body?
  - Heart attacks often present with referred pain or discomfort in lower jaw, neck, and arm (normally the left side), abdomen, and/or back.
- Severity—How bad is it on a scale from 0 to 10? Zero being no pain and 10 being the worst pain ever experienced.
- Time—Has there been a change in the pain or symptoms over time?
  - Heart attacks do not resolve quickly; in fact, they may last from 30 minutes to several hours.

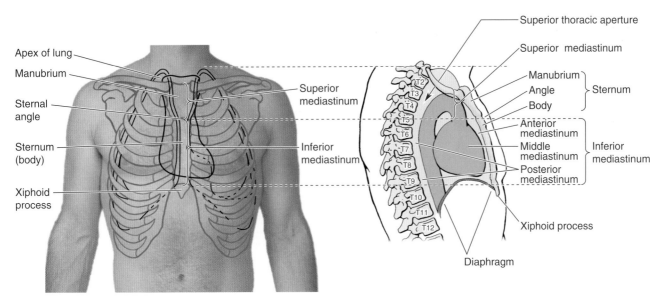

FIGURE 12.10   Position of the heart between the spine and the sternum. (From Moore KL, Dalley AF II. *Clinically Oriented Anatomy*, 4th ed. Baltimore: Lippincott Williams & Wilkins; 1999.)

(approximately one third of normal) to the heart and brain; during SCA, it can increase the likelihood of a successful defibrillation with an AED in time to prevent neurological damage.[9] Remember that the heart is located between the sternum and the spine (Fig. 12.10). Thus, chest compressions increase intrathoracic pressure and compress the heart each time the chest is compressed, producing a moderate blood flow.

In cases where SCA is witnessed and early CPR is initiated by a bystander; rather than experiencing a 7% to 10% per minute decline in survivability for every minute defibrillation is delayed, the decline survivability is now 3% to 4% per minute for every minute defibrillation is delayed.[19,53] Unfortunately, bystander CPR is initiated in less than one third of cases of witnessed SCA[54,55] and is often preformed incorrectly, normally as a result of improper chest compressions.[56] Even in situations where SCA is witnessed by an athletic trainer and immediately addressed, there is no guarantee of survival.[11]

The athletic trainer may also encounter an individual who demonstrates agonal breathing—an irregular gasping or shallow type of breathing that should not be confused with normal breathing. In fact, agonal breathing is a common sign of the early stages of cardiac arrest and suggests that death is imminent. It is often mistaken by lay responders as a sign of life and can lead to the withholding CPR.[57]

Cardiopulmonary Resuscitation Techniques

CPR used by a professional rescuer (i.e., athletic trainer) involves three basic skills; these involve management of the ABCs, or signs of life. In earlier chapters, the basic skills of airway management and breathing were addressed. As a reminder, depending on the mechanism of injury, either a head tilt–chin lift or jaw thrust (with or without extension) will be utilized to open and maintain an adequate airway. If solid materials are visible (e.g., food or a mouthguard) in the oropharynx upon opening the airway, a finger sweep may be performed to remove the object (see Fig. 10.26). To manage breathing, look, listen, and feel for the chest to rise and fall for no longer than 10 seconds (30 to 45 seconds in the presence of hypothermia). If the individual is not breathing, deliver two rescue breaths, each lasting for about 1 second, with a visible rise and fall of the chest. If the two rescue breaths go in, the athletic trainer should check for signs of life (pulse) for no more than 10 seconds while quickly scanning for severe bleeding. If no breathing or signs of life (pulse) are present, the athletic trainer will immediately begin CPR chest compressions.

Performing Appropriate Chest Compression

For CPR to be effective and to improve the athlete's chance of survival by delivering critical blood and oxygen to the heart and brain, chest compressions must be performed correctly. They can also increase the likelihood that a successful shock can be delivered when the AED arrives. The components of chest compressions that can alter effectiveness include the following[3]:

- Hand position
- Position of the athletic trainer
- Position of the athlete
- Depth, rate, and duty cycle of compressions
- Decompression

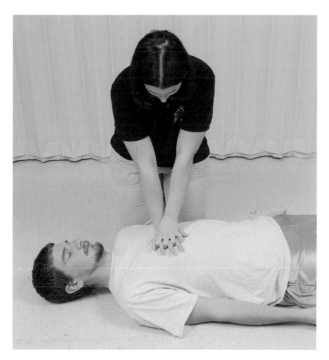

FIGURE 12.11 Correct hand placement for adult CPR. Hands should be positioned in the center of the chest, with the heel of the dominant hand on the bottom.

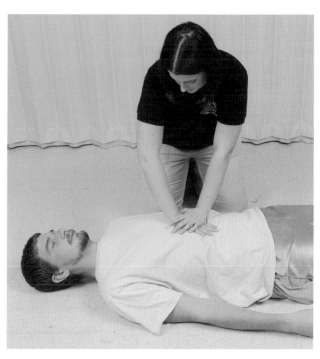

FIGURE 12.12 Incorrect hand placement for adult CPR. Incorrect hand positions increase the risk of injury and ineffective compressions.

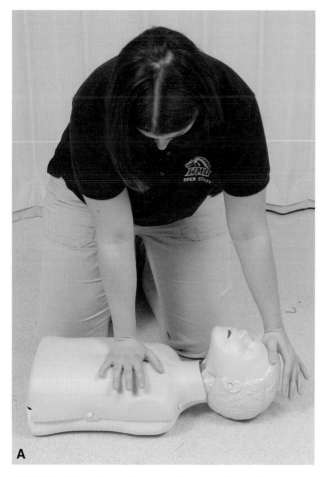

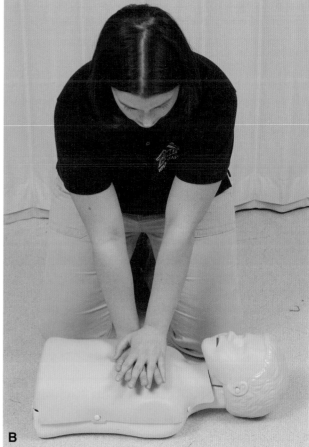

FIGURE 12.13 Hand placement for child CPR. **A.** Single-hand technique. **B.** Two-hand technique.

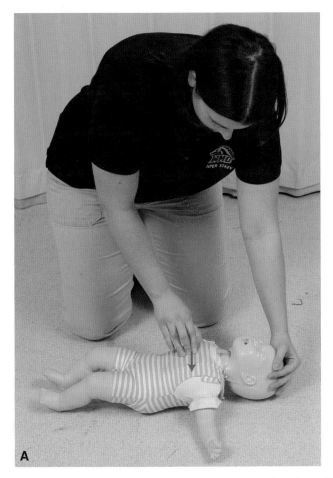
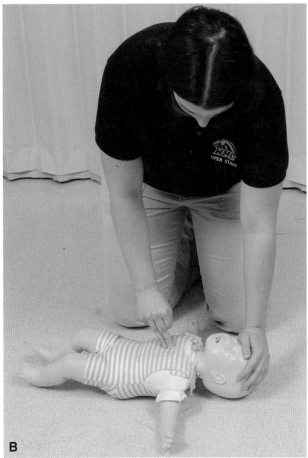

FIGURE 12.14   Hand placement for infant CPR. **A.** Place the middle and ring fingers next to the index finger and lift the index finger at the nipple line. **B.** Lift the index finger and compress the sternum straight downward using the middle and ring fingers while maintaining the infant's airway with the other hand.

Hand Placement   When treating an adult, the athletic trainer's hands should be positioned in the center of the athlete's chest, with the heel of the dominant hand on the bottom. Studies have shown that use of the dominant hand increases the quality of the chest compressions.[58] The nondominant hand is then placed on top of the dominant hand, interlocking the fingers (Fig. 12.11). Attempts should be made to prevent the interlocked fingers from resting on the chest. When the hands are allowed to rest on the chest (Fig. 12.12), there is an increased chance of incomplete or inadequate chest compression and decompression as well as trauma to the ribs and sternum.

Treating a child (from 1 to 12 years of age) is similar to treating an adult. Locate the center of the chest, placing heel of the dominant hand on the sternum (two-hand technique). The nondominant hand can be placed on top of the dominant hand. In some situations, the dominant hand alone (one-hand technique) can deliver sufficient force to perform chest compressions. Either technique is acceptable.[5,59] While performing CPR, attempts should also be made to maintain the airway (Fig. 12.13).

Treating an infant (younger than 1 year of age) is slightly different. Begin by drawing an imaginary line between the infant's nipples. Place your index finger on this imaginary line. Then place your middle and ring fingers next to your index finger and lift your index finger. Using the tips of the middle and ring fingers, compress the sternum straight downward while maintaining the infant's airway with the other hand (Fig. 12.14). It is also acceptable to use the index and middle fingers as long as they are placed below the nipple line as well.

Position of the Athletic Trainer   The athletic trainer should be positioned so that he or she is perpendicular to the athlete. All too often rescuers of all levels try to perform the combined skill of chest compression and providing breaths in a static position. The result is an increase in energy expenditure as the athletic trainer must constantly perform the skills at an angle. Fatigue can set in early, increasing the athletic trainer's risk of tiring and performing the skill ineffectively. The athletic trainer's elbows should also remain extended (Fig. 12.15), with much of the compression force coming from the hips as the athletic trainer rocks forward and backward.

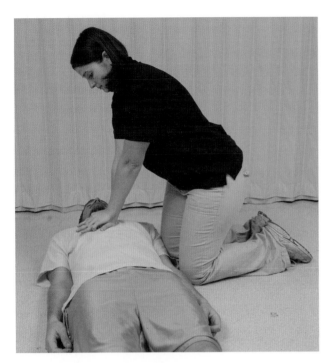

FIGURE 12.15 Correct body position in performing CPR. Elbows should remain straight while pressing straight downward on the sternum.

Position of the Athlete   To perform CPR correctly, the athletic trainer should place the athlete on a flat, hard surface with adequate space. In athletics, some of the playing surfaces or apparatus an athlete may collapse on will not allow for adequate performance of chest compressions. Therefore, it may be necessary to log roll an athlete onto a spineboard, which can increase the depth of chest compressions during CPR.[60] In an outpatient rehabilitation setting, a patient may experience SCA while lying on a treatment table. In this case it may be necessary to perform CPR standing rather than kneeling. Although the kinematics of CPR then differ, the differences do not seem to affect compression force, depth, or frequency when performed by an experienced provider[61] (Fig. 12.16). When treating an infant, the athletic trainer may place the infant on a solid surface such as the floor or a table.

Depending upon the location of the cardiac emergency, it may be necessary to create space to perform CPR effectively. A space of roughly 3 to 4 ft in all directions will allow two athletic trainers to change position and give advanced medical personnel enough space in which to work. Coaches, teammates, and other bystanders should quickly be removed from the area. If the individual collapses in and around rehabilitation equipment and playing apparatuses, quickly but safely drag him or her into an area that provides more room. If a bystander collapses in the stands, more effort may be needed to drag him or her to a space that is large enough to perform CPR. Remember, if the collapse

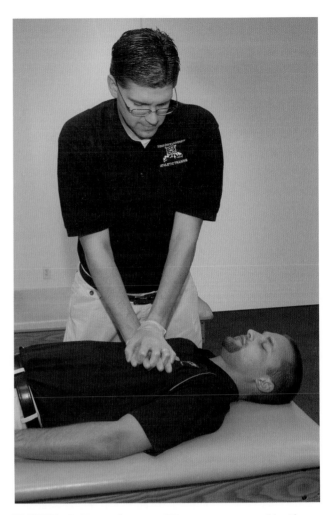

FIGURE 12.16 Performing CPR on a treatment table. If necessary, the athletic trainer can kneel on the table next to the athlete.

was unwitnessed, be sure to protect the spine while dragging the individual.

Chest Compression Depth, Rate, Decompression, and Compression–Ventilation Ratio

Depth   The depth of the chest compressions varies by age. The following are the recommended compression depths according to the 2005 ECC guidelines.

- Adults—Compress the center or the sternum 1½ to 2 inches straight down.[2,3,59]
- Children—Compress the center of the sternum approximately one third to one half the depth of the chest[5] or on the center of the sternum about 1 to 1½ inches straight down.[59]
- Infants—Compress the sternum 1 fingerbreadth below the nipple line approximately one third to one half the depth of the chest[5] or about ½ to 1 inch.[59]

Current Research

Keeping the Beat with "Stayin' Alive"

To keep pace and ensure the proper rate of chest compression, consider counting out loud, "One and two and three" or singing the song "Stayin' Alive" while doing chest compressions. Research suggests that the song contains 103 beats per minute, similar to the 100 chest compressions per minute recommend by current guidelines.[62]

Always allow the chest to return completely to its normal position (i.e., decompress, or fully recoil) following each compression. Also, pay particular attention to the depth of your chest compressions during CPR. Studies of pre-hospital and in-hospital providers find that insufficient depth of compression was observed during CPR when compared with currently recommended depths.[3]

Rate   Rate is defined as the "number of compressions delivered per minute."[3] Regardless of the age of the athlete, chest compressions should be delivered at a rate of at least 100 compressions per minute.

Decompression   Decompression is the ability of the chest to recoil fully after compression. To ensure proper tissue perfusion, the athletic trainer compresses the chest to the appropriate depth and allows the chest to return to the original starting position. Lifting the hand slightly but not completely off the chest during decompression has been shown in manikin studies to allow for full chest recoil.[63]

Compression–Ventilation Ratio   For a single athletic trainer, the current ECC guidelines recommend the use of a 30:2 compression–ventilation ratio when treating an infant, child, or adult. There is insufficient evidence that any specific compression–ventilation ratio is associated with improved outcome in individuals suffering cardiac arrest.[3]

When two athletic trainers are available, the current ECC guidelines recommend the use of a 30:2 compression–ventilation ratio only when treating an adult. When caring for a child or infant, a 15:2 compression–ventilation ratio should be utilized.[5,59]

Single-Person CPR

Depending on his or her work setting, the athletic trainer may be required to provide CPR care by themselves. Although this skill can be tiring, remember to maintain your composure, act as a professional, use your bystanders when appropriate, and provide the best care possible under the circumstances. This section outlines the steps in care that are to be taken by a single athletic trainer.

Single-Person Adult CPR   To perform adult CPR, begin care by following the directions in Skill 12.2 or referring to Algorithm 12.2 for an emergency action decisional algorithm.

Single-Person Child CPR   To perform single-person CPR on a child, follow the same steps as when providing care to an adult (Algorithm 12.2) except for the following differences:

1. Locate the center of sternum and place one hand on the sternum for a small child and two hands for a larger child (see Fig. 12.13).
2. Compress the center of the sternum approximately one third to one half the depth of the chest[5] or on the center of the sternum about 1 to 1½ in. straight down[59] at rate at least 100 compressions per minute followed by two effective breaths.
3. When an AED arrives on scene and if the child meets the criteria for its use, immediately stop and connect the AED, following the AED unit's instructions.

Single-Person Infant CPR   Depending upon the facility, work setting, or situation, it may be necessary for the athletic trainer to perform CPR on an infant. Remember that an infant is defined as anyone younger than 1 year of age. The steps required to effectively perform CPR on an infant are again similar to those in treating an adult or a child. The differences are as follows:

1. The airway in an infant is more fragile and easily obstructed and needs to be opened only to a neutral position.
2. In an infant, locate a pulse at the brachial artery (see Fig. 10.5), on the inside of the arm closest to the athletic trainer, rather than the carotid artery.
3. To perform chest compressions, imagine a horizontal line drawn between the infant's nipples. Place your index finger in the center of this line. Then place your middle and ring fingers next to the index finger. Lift the index finger and, using a straight downward

SKILL 12.2

Single-Person Adult CPR

1. Initiate EAP.
2. Check the safety of the scene.
3. Take BSI precautions.
4. Determine the individual's level of responsiveness by tapping the shoulder and shouting "Are you all right? Are you OK?" If the athlete is unresponsive, summon more advanced medical personnel and request an AED.
5. If the athlete is prone, immediately roll him or her to a supine position, supporting the head, neck, and back, and begin a primary assessment to determine any compromise to the ABCs (including external bleeding) by opening and adequately maintaining the airway (Fig. 10.6 and 10.7).
6. Airway
   - Open the airway using a head-tilt–chin-lift maneuver.
   - If a spinal injury is suspected, use a jaw-thrust maneuver (with or without extension) (Fig. 10.16 or 10.18)
7. Breathing (Fig. 10.8)
   a. Look, listen, and feel for signs of life for no more than 10 seconds. Signs of life or circulation include "normal breathing, coughing, or movement."[57]
   b. Consider the use of an adjunct breathing device, such as an oropharyngeal or nasopharyngeal airway, to assist in maintaining the airway (Chapter 11).
   c. If no adequate breathing is detected, provide two rescue breaths. Single athletic trainers should use a resuscitation mask.
   d. If the chest clearly rises and falls, continue checking for signs of life.
   e. If the chest does not rise and fall, retilt the head and attempt the rescue breaths again.
8. Circulation (Fig. 10.10)
   - While maintaining the airway, if possible, identify the carotid artery.
   - Palpate for a pulse for no more than 10 seconds unless the athlete is believed to be hypothermic. In this case, palpate for up to 30 to 45 seconds.
9. Scan the athlete for any immediate threats of severe bleeding. Again, remember to maintain the airway.
10. If the individual displays no signs of life (breathing or pulse), begin CPR (Fig. 12.11).
   - Place your dominant hand on the center of the chest and place the other hand on top of it. Perform a series of 30 chest compressions, 1 ½ to 2 in. deep at a rate at least 100 compressions per minute followed by two effective breaths.
   - To increase the effectiveness of the compressions, count out loud, "One and two and three."
11. Continue CPR without interruption as long as possible and attempt to limit any interruptions except in the case of the following:
   - The scene becomes too unsafe to continue providing care.
   - You are too exhausted to continue providing care.
   - The athlete demonstrates spontaneous signs of life.
   - Another athletic trainer or trained person (with equal or greater qualifications) arrives and care is transferred to that person or he or she begins to assist you.
   - EMS arrives and care is transferred to them so that advanced medical care can be provided.
   - An AED arrives.

motion (Fig. 12.14B), compress the center of the sternum with your middle and ring fingers. Keep your fingers as vertical as possible to help provide effective chest compressions.

4. Compress the sternum one fingerbreadth below the nipple line approximately one third to one half the depth of the chest[5] or about ½ to 1 inch[59] at a rate of at least 100 compressions per minute followed by two effective breaths.

Two-Person CPR

In some cases, depending upon the sporting event, size of the medical staff, and the availability of other trained responders, a second athletic trainer may be available to assist in performing CPR. During two-person CPR, one athletic trainer is responsible for chest compressions while the other is responsible for ventilations. Together, they can perform more fluently and with fewer interruptions, and the skill now becomes less tiring. One way of preventing exhaustion is for the athletic trainers to switch roles about every five cycles or every 2 minutes. This switch should take less than 5 to 10 seconds to make, thus minimizing the interruption of chest compressions and ventilations from changing places.

Two-Person Adult CPR

To perform two-person adult CPR, begin by following Skill 12.3 or referring to Algorithm 12.3 for an emergency action decisional algorithm.

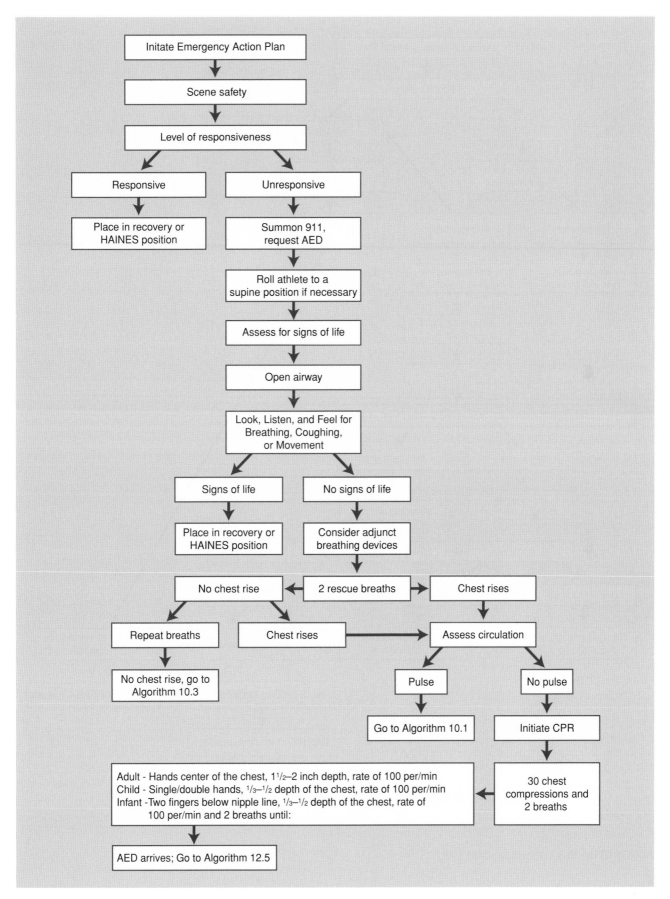

ALGORITHM 12.2   Single-person adult, child, and infant CPR.

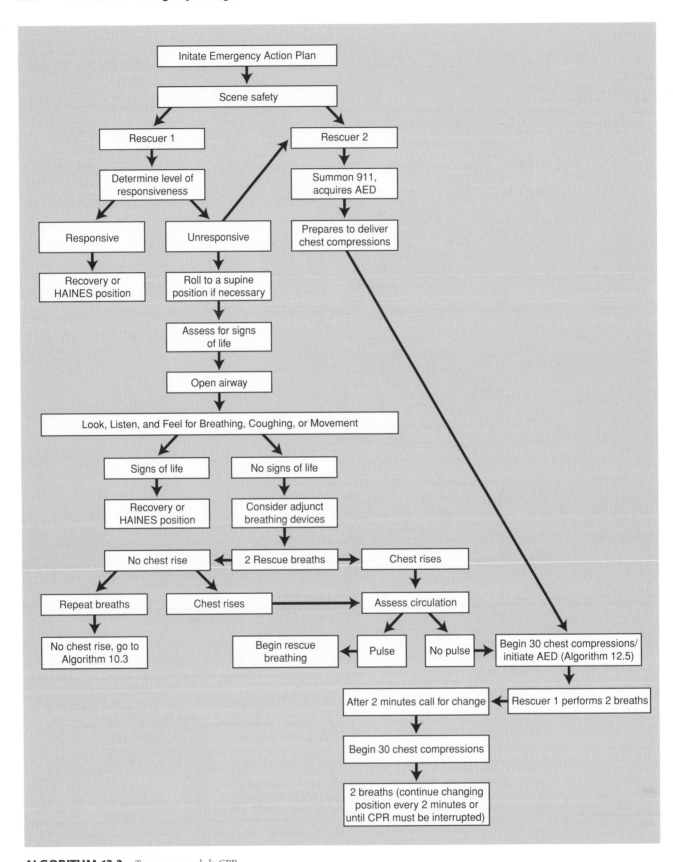

ALGORITHM 12.3 Two-person adult CPR.

SKILL 12.3

Two-Person Adult CPR

1. Initiate the EAP.
2. Check the safety of the scene.
3. Take BSI precautions.
4. **Athletic trainer 1** will determine the individual's level of responsiveness by tapping the shoulder and shouting "Are you all right? Are you OK?" If the athlete is unresponsive, **athletic trainer 2** will summon more advanced medical personnel and retrieve an AED if no bystanders are around to do so.
5. If the athlete is in the prone position, **athletic trainer 1** will immediately roll him or her to a supine position, supporting the head, neck and back, and begin a primary assessment to determine the ABCs (including external bleeding) (see Fig. 10.6).
6. Airway (see Fig. 10.7).
   ○ Open the airway using a head-tilt–chin-lift maneuver.
   ○ If a spinal injury is suspected, use a jaw-thrust maneuver (with or without extension).
7. Breathing (see Fig. 10.8)
   ○ Look, listen, and feel for signs of life for no more than 10 seconds. Signs of life or circulation include "normal breathing, coughing, or movement."[57]
   ○ Consider the use of an adjunct breathing device, such as an oropharyngeal or nasopharyngeal airway, to assist in maintaining the airway (Chapter 11).

8. *Rescue breaths* (see Fig. 10.9).
   ○ If no adequate breathing is detected provide two rescue breaths.
   ○ Two athletic trainers should consider the use of a bag-valve-mask device[3] (Fig. 12.17).
9. Circulation
   ○ While maintaining the airway, identify the carotid artery if possible.
   ○ Palpate for a pulse for no more than 10 seconds unless the athlete is believed to be hypothermic. In this case palpate for up to 30 to 45 seconds.
   ○ **Athletic trainer 2** will position himself or herself at the chest to prepare for chest compressions or will begin preparing the AED if it has arrived.
10. Scan the athlete for any immediate threats or signs of severe bleeding. Again, remember to maintain the airway (Fig. 12.18).
11. If the athlete displays no breathing or pulse, **athletic trainer 1**, in a loud voice, will say to **athletic trainer 2**, "Begin CPR."
    ○ Care will consist of 30 chest compressions and two effective breaths. During the breaths, **athletic trainer 2** may leave his or her hands on the chest; however, remember not to restrict upward movement of the chest during the breaths.

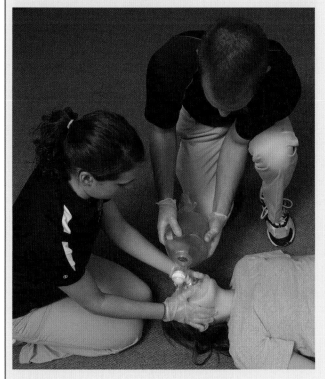

FIGURE 12.17

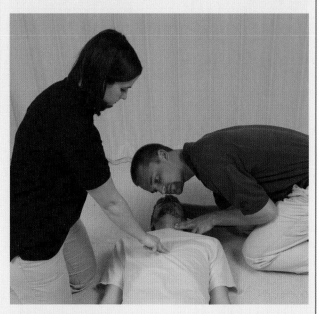

FIGURE 12.18

(Continued)

SKILL 12.3 *(Continued)*

Two-Person Adult CPR *(Continued)*

12. After five cycles or 2 minutes of care, **athletic trainers 1 and 2** will change position. **Athletic trainer 2** will indicate the change to athletic trainer 1 by saying, "Change and 2 and 3 and 4," or "28 and change and 30."
13. **Athletic trainer 1** will slide down to the athlete's chest after providing 2 breaths and begins chest compressions while **athletic trainer 2** moves up to the head and prepares to ventilate the athlete (Fig. 12.19) and (Fig. 12.20).
14. The athletic trainers will continue CPR without interruption as long as possible and try to limit any interruptions except if the following should occur:

- The scene becomes too unsafe to continue providing care.
- You are too exhausted to continue providing care.
- The athlete demonstrates spontaneous signs of life.
- Another athletic trainer or trained person (with equal or greater qualifications) arrives and care is transferred to him or her.
- EMS arrives and care is transferred to them so that advanced medical care can be provided.
- An AED arrives.

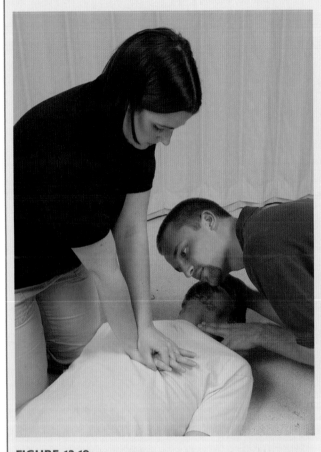

FIGURE 12.19

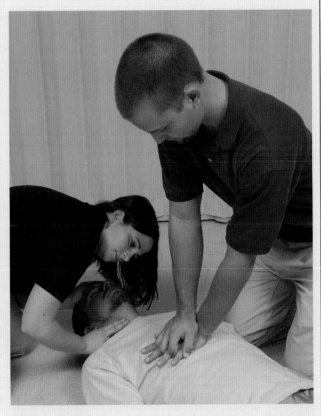

FIGURE 12.20

Check the Effectiveness of CPR During two-person CPR, athletic trainers can check the effectiveness of CPR by observing or assessing for the following:

1. During chest compressions, does athletic trainer 1 detect an artificial carotid pulse as the heart is being compressed?
2. During ventilations, does athletic trainer 2 detect upward and downward movement of the chest during ventilations?
3. Does the athlete's color improve from blue to pink?

Spontaneous Signs of Life If the athlete begins to demonstrate spontaneous signs of life, both athletic trainers should cease CPR and the athletic trainer at the head should begin to reassess the ABCs, providing appropriate care based on the presence or absence of breathing or circulation (pulse). If the athlete is unconscious but breathing and a pulse are present, place the athlete into the recovery or "High Arm IN Endangered Spine" (HAINES) position if a cervical spine injury is suspected to prevent aspiration.

Second Athletic Trainer Arrives on Scene while CPR Is in Progress   In situations where a second athletic trainer arrives on scene after CPR has been initiated, follow these steps:

1. Athletic trainer 2 in a loud voice states, "My name is [name]. I am trained in CPR. Has 911 been called?" This will be followed by, "Is someone getting an AED?" Any answer other than YES means that athletic trainer 2 is responsible for performing those steps first.
2. If 911 has been called and an AED is on the way, athletic trainer 2 should position himself or herself at the chest and begin chest compressions after athletic trainer 1 completes two breaths.

Two-Person Child CPR   Remember that a child is defined as anyone between the ages of 1 and 12. The basic principles of two-person child CPR are very similar to those of two-person adult CPR with one major difference. The compression–ventilation ratio is now 15 compressions to two breaths (15:2) rather than the 30:2 performed during one-person child CPR. The question most often asked then is: Why not keep a 30:2 ratio or the old 5:1 ratio? The answer comes from scientific data collected during a review of the 2005 ECC Guidelines, which found insufficient data to

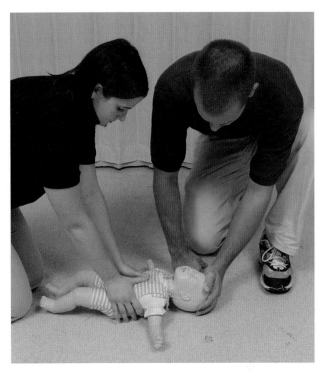

FIGURE 12.22   Thumb position of two-person infant CPR. Thumb should rest on the sternum while the hands encompass the body. Note that the athletic trainer delivering the breaths would normally be at the top of the head while doing so.

identify an optimal compression–ventilation ratio for child CPR. A mathematical model, on the other hand, supported compression–ventilation ratios higher than 5:1 for infants and children.[5] Also, similar to two-person child CPR, either the one- or two-hand technique is acceptable for chest compressions in children. To perform two-person child CPR, refer to Figure 12.21 or Algorithm 12.4 for an emergency action decisional algorithm.

Two-Person Infant CPR   Remember that an infant is anyone under 1 year of age. As in two-person child CPR, the compression–ventilation ratio is also 15 compressions to two breaths (15:2), rather than the 30:2 performed during one-person infant CPR. The other major difference lies in the hand placement for compressions. Rather than placing two fingers below the infant's nipple line, the athletic trainer will perform the two-thumb chest-encircling compression technique with a circumferential thoracic squeeze (Fig. 12.22). This technique has been shown to produce higher coronary perfusion pressures and to correct the depth and force of compression more consistently.[5] Furthermore, infants receiving treatment with this technique demonstrated higher systolic and diastolic arterial pressures compared with the two-finger technique.[64,65] However, it should be noted that the two-finger technique remains an acceptable alternative method of chest compression for two athletic trainers.[5] When performing this technique, it will be necessary to place a folded towel under the infant's shoulders (Fig. 12.23).

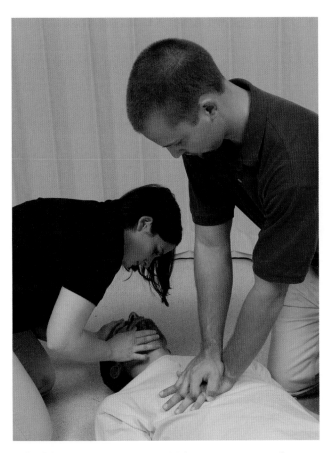

FIGURE 12.21   Two-person child CPR. Positioning for two-person child CPR is consistent with adult CPR except for the depth of compression and the compression:ventilation ratio.

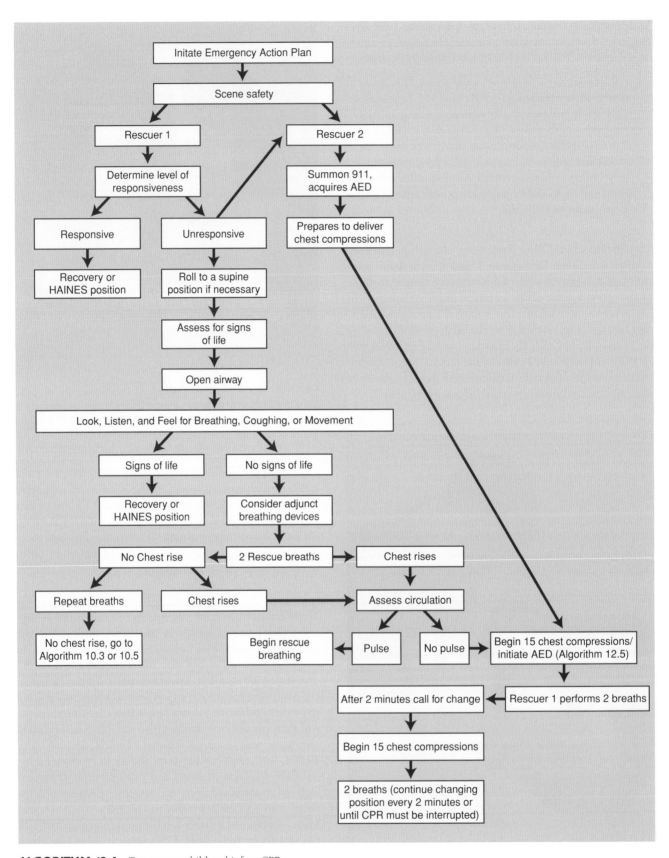

ALGORITHM 12.4   Two-person child and infant CPR.

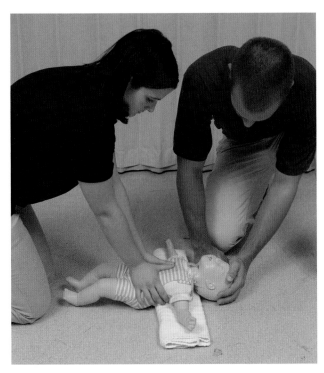

FIGURE 12.23 Towel placement under the shoulder for two-person infant CPR. Note that the athletic trainer delivering the breaths would normally be at the top of the head while doing so.

To perform two-person infant CPR, refer to Figure 12.22 or Algorithm 12.4 for an emergency action decisional algorithm.

COMPLICATIONS OF CPR

Although CPR has the potential to save lives, it also has the potential for further injury to an athlete. Several complications may arise while performing CPR, including (a) bruising and abrasions to the face and neck, (b) fractures of the hyoid bone and thyroid cartilage, (c) airway injuries, (d) vomiting, (e) aspiration, (f) retinal and subarachnoid hemorrhage, (g) fractures of ribs and the sternum, and (h) injuries to the gastrointestinal tract (lacerations, ruptures, hemorrhage) and cardiopulmonary system. However, with proper training and following proper procedures, the athletic trainer will be able to limit secondary injury. This section outlines some of the common complications encountered by an athletic trainer while performing CPR.

Trauma to the Lungs, Thorax, and Internal Organs

Proper hand placement is critical when performing chest compressions during CPR. Proper hand placement not only ensures adequate depth and decompression of the chest but also reduces the risk of trauma to structures such as the ribs, sternum, and lungs. In adults, rib and sternal fractures are a recognized complication of CPR,[66,67] whereas rib fractures in children are much rarer.[68] Rib fractures do not normally cause significant complications unless the ribs are fractured in several places, which cause a flail chest and/or dislocation.[67] Potential soft tissue trauma associated with projecting rib and/or sternal fragments includes (a) hemo- and pneumothorax, (b) lung herniation, (c) aortic injury, and (d) intra-abdominal injuries.[67,69–72]

While performing CPR, if you should hear a crack and begin to feel crepitus while compressing the chest, stop and reassess your hand position. Be sure your hands are positioned in the center of the chest, with the heel of the dominant hand on the bottom. Your hand placement will often determine the location of secondary trauma. For example, a high hand placement may cause a fracture of the first or second rib or fracture of the sternum at the third and fourth intercostal spaces. This is in comparison to a low hand placement, which may result in a fracture of ribs 6 through 11 or a sternal fracture between the fourth and sixth intercostal spaces.[70] Do not discontinue CPR; continue until advanced medical care arrives. Some fractured ribs are better than death.

Gastric Distention

Remember from Chapter 11 that there is a risk that positive-pressure ventilated air will pass from the trachea and enter the stomach.[73] When air enters the stomach, it begins to distend it, resulting in what is commonly referred to as gastric distention. This causes the abdomen to increase in size, thereby elevating the diaphragm, restricting proper lung movement (i.e., full inflation), and decreasing respiratory

Highlight

Causes of Gastric Distention[71,74–76]
- Rescue breaths are delivered over too long a time period.
- Rescue breaths are delivered too quickly.
- Airway is not completely open.
- Adjunct airways are not properly inserted.
- Inappropriate use a bag-valve-mask device.
- Incorrect intubation—tube placement into the esophagus rather than the trachea.

system compliance. Improper use of the bag-valve-mask device or poor intubation not only results in gastric distention but also increases the risk of gastric mucosal lacerations or ruptures, with bleeding into the stomach and abdominal cavity.[71]

If gastric distention is suspected, place the individual in the recovery position and gently compress the stomach to push the air of out the stomach. Though this maneuver may relieve the distention, it is likely that the athlete may vomit. Be prepared to remove any vomitus from the mouth manually or with the use of suction if available. This should be performed only if ventilation is becoming difficult. *Do not delay care* to rid an individual of gastric distention.

Vomiting

Regurgitation or vomiting is also a possible complication of CPR,[73,77,78] often as a consequence of gastric distention. During cardiac arrest, there is a decrease in the tone of the athlete's lower esophageal sphincter. This is significant because the decreased muscle tone can no longer contain the food in the stomach. In the presence of gastric distention, the relaxed lower esophageal sphincter cannot prevent regurgitation of the backed-up food in the stomach. In some instances, even if there is no food in the stomach, the athlete may still vomit blood and dark brown stomach and intestinal fluids due to severe trauma.

If vomiting occurs while you are providing CPR, immediately roll the individual to his or her side (remember to protect the neck when cervical spine trauma is suspected) to allow the vomitus to drain out of the mouth. Using your gloved hand, remove the larger vomitus particles. If a suction device is available, consider its use. However, ***do not delay care*** waiting to rid the airway of vomitus with suction. Once the large vomitus particles have been removed, continue providing appropriate care.

When the airway is not cared for immediately, there is a risk that the athlete may aspirate vomitus.[77] **Aspiration** is defined as the inhalation of any foreign matter—including food, saliva, or stomach contents—into the airway. Individuals surviving cardiac arrest who have aspirated during CPR have an increased chance of developing pneumonia and, in the worst case, developing lethal adult respiratory distress syndrome.[79] There is little an athletic trainer can do once an individual has aspirated, which is why clearing the airway immediately after vomiting is essential.

SPECIAL SITUATIONS WHEN PERFORMING CPR

There are several situations in which an athletic trainer may be required to modify or at least add additional steps to the procedure in order to perform CPR adequately. Most of these cases will occur in the athletic environment and are the result of the athlete's protective equipment, playing surfaces, inappropriate skill technique, and/or other special

considerations that may arise during an emergency situation that are not predictable. This section outlines some of situations that may be encountered by an athletic trainer.

Protective Equipment

When covering sports such as football, men's lacrosse, men's and women's ice hockey, as well as others, the athlete's protective equipment will make performing CPR more challenging. This is because when an athletic trainer arrives at the scene of injury or illness, he or she cannot, as a rule, conclusively determine whether there may be a spinal injury, making the situation more complicated. Current guidelines[80] suggest that any athlete suspected of having a spinal injury should not be moved and should be managed as though a spinal injury exists, even in the presence of SCA.

The athletic trainer will need to decide whether to remove both the helmet and shoulder pads or leave them in place once no signs of life have been found. If the decision to remove the helmet and shoulder pads is made, remember that both must be removed following established protocols. If they are to be left in place, the face mask should be removed as quickly but also as safely as possible. Refer to Chapter 17 for helmet and shoulder pad removal.

Delayed Access to the Airway

In situations where access to the airway is delayed owing to lack of appropriate equipment (loop-strap removal equipment, resuscitation mask, bag-valve-mask) or medical assistance, the athlete suffering cardiac arrest should receive compression CPR only once the chest has been exposed. The current science advisory from the American Heart Association suggests that "When an adult suddenly collapses, trained or untrained bystanders should—at a minimum—activate their community emergency medical response system (e.g., call 911) and provide high-quality chest compressions by pushing hard and fast in the center of the chest, minimizing interruptions."[81] Compression-only CPR, though intended for laypersons who are unable or unwilling to provide rescue breaths, is indicated in this situation because of the inability to access the airway. Continue with compression or hands-only CPR until an access to the airway is established, the AED arrives and is ready for use, or EMS arrives and can assist in removing the helmet and shoulder pads.

Playing Surfaces

Though most playing surfaces are rigid enough to perform chest compression in the event of SCA, some sports such as gymnastics, field events (pole vault and high jump), wrestling, swimming, and crew may offer challenges because of a lack of a rigid surface. In sports where mats (Fig. 12.24) are used to absorb impact forces consideration needs to be made whether or not to move the athlete to a rigid surface such as the floor or ground or whether or not to immediately

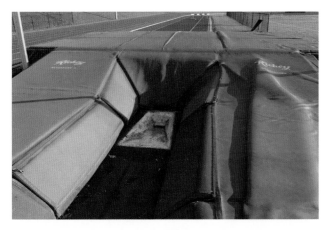

FIGURE 12.24 Pole vault landing mat. A soft surface such as a pole vaulting mat will not allow for adequate delivery of chest compressions.

Breakout

Common Errors during CPR[82,83]

Common errors encountered during CPR include:

- Slow chest compression rates (a rate of 100 compressions per minute is required)
- Inadequate chest compression depth
- Hyperventilation during breaths
- Long pauses in CPR before shock delivery
- Delivery of electrical defibrillation for nonshockable rhythms

logroll the athlete onto a spine board. In sports like crew, an emergency plan to quickly transfer an athlete to a rescue boat capable of managing SCA is critical. The aquatic environment also poses a challenge, particularly if cardiac arrest is suffered while the athlete is practicing or competing in the water. Again, an EAP must be established to determine how to quickly remove the athlete from the water in order to ensure immediate care.

Lack of Appropriate Equipment

As previously discussed in other parts of this text, an athletic trainer who is not prepared to treat an athlete suffering SCA may be at risk for negligence. For this reason, every attempt should be made to have the appropriate rescue equipment available on site or on one's person during an athletic contest or, more importantly, during practice. Recommended SCA management equipment for use by athletic trainers is

presented in the Signs & Symptoms box, below. Consider consulting your team physician in order to determine his or her needs when compiling the emergency SCA kit.

Inappropriate Technique

For CPR to be effective and to improve the athlete's chance of survival by delivering critical blood and oxygen to the heart and brain, the chest compressions must be performed correctly. The concept of high-quality chest compressions by pushing "hard and fast" in the middle of the athlete's chest, with minimal interruption, is ideal, assuming that this is done competently. Over time, CPR psychomotor skills may deteriorate if not used regularly, which is why retraining should be offered periodically. Also, during emergency situations and when working as a team, if the team has not rehearsed and/or an individual is unfamiliar with his or her role, a delay in care and/or poor technique may occur.

Highlight

Recommended Emergency SCA Management Equipment for Key Personnel

Athletic Trainer

- Adult/Pediatric AED*
  - Towel to clean chest, electrodes, razor
- Manual or mechanical suction with catheters
- Oropharyngeal airways (assorted sizes)
- Nasopharyngeal airways (assorted sizes) with lubricating gel
- Appropriate size bag-valve-mask device with oxygen reservoir
- Oxygen
  - Tubing
  - Pressure regulator with flowmeter
  - Delivery device
- Blood pressure cuff

Physician

- Properly functioning and tested laryngoscope (assorted blades)
- Topical lidocaine spray
- Endotracheal tubes (assorted sizes)
- Endotracheal tube stylet
- Adhesive tape
- Commercial percutaneous cricothyrotomy set
- Curved hemostat, Metzenbaum scissors, and Magill forceps
- Tracheal spreader
- Mounted disposable scalpel
- Shiley cuffed tracheostomy tube

*Early access to defibrillation is a necessary component of the cardiac chain of survival.

Breakout

Reasons Why Early Defibrillation Improves Survival from SCA[19]

1. The most frequent initial rhythm in witnessed SCA is V-fib.
2. V-fib can be reversed only by delivering an electrical shock provided by an AED.
3. The likelihood of a successful defibrillation diminishes rapidly over time.
4. If left untreated while waiting for EMS, ventricular fibrillation tends to deteriorate to **asystole** within a few minutes.

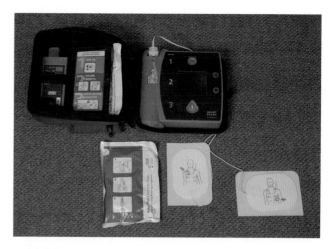

FIGURE 12.25   AED units and self-adhesive electrodes.

AUTOMATED EXTERNAL DEFIBRILLATOR

Remember the third link in the cardiac chain of survival—early defibrillation. This is considered a vital link in determining an athlete's chances of surviving SCA. Early defibrillation is essential to surviving SCA, which explains why PAD laws have increased the accessibility of AEDs in communities where large groups of individuals congregate or high-risk populations are commonly found. Access to the AEDs gives both minimally trained and trained responders access to immediate defibrillation rather than having to wait for an EMS unit to arrive. In athletics, although the prevalence of SCA is lower than in the general population, immediate access to and proper use of an AED is still essential because the athletic trainer is often the first responder to reach the athlete who has collapsed.[9] This section reviews the guidelines for proper defibrillation with an AED in adult and pediatric athletes.

AED Purpose

AEDs are sophisticated, computerized devices that use voice and visual prompts to guide the athletic trainer to safely set up and defibrillate an arrhythmia (normally V-fib) experienced during SCA.[4] Remember from earlier discussions that V-fib is a condition where the heart's electrical signal, which normally induces a coordinated heartbeat, suddenly becomes chaotic (disorganized). This disorganization results in quivering of the heart's ventricles, limiting or disrupting blood flow. V-tach, the other shockable arrhythmia, occurs when the heart beats too quickly and does not allow the chambers to fill with enough blood between beats to produce blood flow sufficient to meet the body's needs, especially the needs of the brain.

AED Characteristics

AEDs are often made of a lightweight, rigid, padded casing with a computer microprocessor designed to analyze the

heart's sinus rhythm and determine the type of electric shock necessary to depolarize the heart's muscle cells and thus eliminate V-fib and V-tach (Fig. 12.25). Units commonly used by athletic trainers are classified as automatic or automated units. All the athletic trainer needs to do is depress a button once a shockable rhythm has been established. In some cases, the athletic trainer may encounter a semiautomatic unit. These units have the automated capabilities of the AED but also feature an electrocardiogram display and a manual override, where the user (e.g., paramedics) can make his or her own decisions, either before or instead of the unit.

Depending on the unit, the athletic trainer may be required to depress a button to begin interpreting the heart's electrical rhythm; in other cases, the unit will automatically begin analyzing the heart once the electrodes have been attached.

AED Design

AED Waveforms

Today, AEDs are classified according to two types of waveforms: monophasic and biphasic. In a monophasic waveform, the electrical current flows in only one direction and varies in the speed with which the waveform returns to the zero voltage point—either gradually (damped sinusoidal) or instantaneously (truncated exponential).[84] In comparison, a biphasic waveform delivers a current that first flows in a positive direction for a specified duration and then reverses the current flow in negative direction (Fig. 12.26). Although monophasic waveform defibrillators were the first to be introduced, many have been replaced by biphasic waveform defibrillators.

AED Energy

Commercially available biphasic AEDs are manufactured to deliver either fixed or escalating energy (measured in Joules [J]) levels using one of two different biphasic waveforms (truncated exponential or rectilinear). A biphasic AED using a fixed energy level maintains a constant energy level after the initial and subsequent shocks. Units using an escalating energy level allow for an increase in the energy delivered after the initial shock until the unit reaches its maximal energy delivery. The optimal biphasic waveform energy level needed for the first or subsequent shocks is not precisely known.[4] The ideal shock dosage is one that falls within the range that has been documented to be effective for that manufacturer's unit. The current recommendation suggests the use of energies between 150 J to 200 J with a biphasic truncated exponential waveform or 120 J when using a rectilinear biphasic waveform for the initial shock in treating an adult and 2 J/kg for a child.[4,85] Subsequent shock energy levels will be determined based on the parameter established by the manufacturer.

As an athletic trainer, you will have little or no ability to modify or select the initial or subsequent energy level delivered to an athlete in SCA. However, you do need to be aware of the range of energy levels and features offered by your unit, as not all units operate alike or offer the same features. Shop around, learn what features are offered by each of the AEDs, and determine what meets the needs of your facility and population prior to any purchase.

AED Electrode Pads

Without electrodes (pads), an AED unit is useless. Though AED pad–cable systems will vary between manufacturers, all systems are designed to be one-time disposable medical devices. Adult AED electrodes are constructed with a self-adhesive backing and a recommended minimal electrode size of 50 cm² for each individual electrode. Defibrillation success is thought to be higher when using 12-cm self-adhesive electrodes compared with 8-cm electrodes.[4] Smaller self-adhesive electrodes (4.3 cm) are thought to be potentially harmful, resulting in possible **myocardial necrosis.**[86]

For best results, adult electrodes should be placed on the athlete's exposed, dry, bare chest in a sternal–apical (anterolateral) position. The right (sternal) electrode pad is placed on the right superior–anterior (infraclavicular) chest wall and the apical (left) electrode is placed on along inferior–lateral left chest, lateral to the left breast (see Fig. 12.30). In large-breasted athletes, it is acceptable to place the left electrode lateral to or underneath the left breast once any underwire bra has been removed. An accepted alternative pad placement includes placing the electrodes on the lateral chest wall on the right and left sides (biaxillary) of the chest wall (Fig. 12.27) or the left pad in the standard apical position and the right pad on the right or left upper back.[4]

Pediatric electrodes are smaller than adult electrodes and are designed to reduce the amount of energy from the AED unit to a smaller "dose" of energy that is more appropriate for a child. Recommended pediatric electrode pad placement is the same as an adult. When the pads do not fit well on the chest the recommended electrode placement is on the center of the anterior (front) chest wall and center of the back, using cervical spine precautions if a spinal injury is suspected. Depending on the manufacturer, pediatric electrodes are reversible, meaning either pad can be placed on the child's chest or back.

Maintenance

Most AEDs are easy to maintain and come with warning indicators when a problem with the unit or battery occurs.

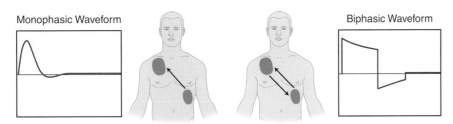

FIGURE 12.26 Defibrillation waveform. A biphasic waveforms delivers a current that first flows in a positive direction for a specified duration and reverses the current flow in negative direction while a monophasic waveform delivers a current that flows only in one direction.

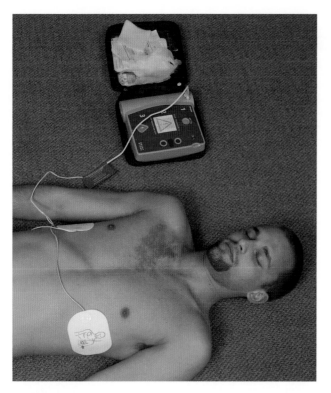

FIGURE 12.27 Alternative AED biaxillary electrode position.

Depending upon the athletic trainer's work setting, it may be necessary to check the status and battery indicator on a daily basis, as well as checking for cracks and loose components (i.e., cables, battery). If the AED does display a systems error, you will need to notify the manufacture to determine where the unit can be serviced by an authorized provider. Consult your AED user's manual to determine your unit's specific maintenance requirements.

Prior to any athletic event, remember always to check the battery and make sure that the unit is equipped with the necessary supplies, including AED electrodes, gloves, and a resuscitation mask.

Using an AED—Adult

In the event of recognized SCA in an adult, immediately activate the cardiac chain of survival, including activation of EMS, early CPR, early defibrillation, and early advanced care by EMS professionals. If cardiac arrest was witnessed and the athlete is unresponsive, breathless, and pulseless (no signs of life for more than 10 seconds), begin the AED procedures. If cardiac arrest was *not* witnessed, perform five cycles of CPR (about 2 minutes) before initiating the AED procedures.

To perform early defibrillation, begin care by following the directions in Skill 12.4 or referring to Algorithm 12.5 for an emergency action decisional algorithm.

SKILL 12.4

Using an Adult AED

1. Initiate the EAP.
2. Check the safety of the scene.
3. Take BSI precautions.
4. Determine the individual's level of responsiveness by tapping the shoulder and shouting "Are you all right? Are you OK?" If the athlete is unresponsive, summon more advanced medical personnel and request an AED.
5. If the athlete is prone, immediately roll him or her to a supine position, supporting the head, neck, and back, and begin a primary assessment to determine any compromise to the ABCs (including external bleeding) by opening and adequately maintaining the airway (see Figs. 10.6 and 10.7).
6. Determine whether the individual is unresponsive, breathless, and pulseless (no signs of life for more than 10 seconds) (see Fig. 10.10).
7. AED on scene.
   - Expose the individual's chest.
   - Turn on the AED and follow the unit's directions by:
     i. Removing the electrodes from the packaging.
     ii. Ensuring that the athlete's chest is dry.
     iii. Peeling away protective plastic backing from the electrodes (Fig. 12.28).

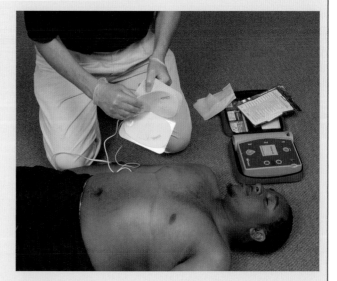

FIGURE 12.28

SKILL 12.4 *(Continued)*

Using an Adult AED (Continued)

iv. Placing one pad (WHITE) on the upper right side of the athlete's chest, above the nipple and below the collarbone (Fig. 12.29)

v. Placing other pad (RED) around the lower left side of the athlete's chest, below the nipple (Fig. 12.29).

vi. Connecting the electrodes to the AED unit (Fig. 12.30).

vii. Pressing the ANALYZE button (note that some units will automatically begin to analyze the heart rhythm once the electrodes have been attached to the AED).

viii. Advising other to STAND CLEAR by waving your hand over the body and say I'M CLEAR, YOU'RE CLEAR, WE'RE ALL CLEAR in a loud, clear, confident voice (Fig. 12.31).

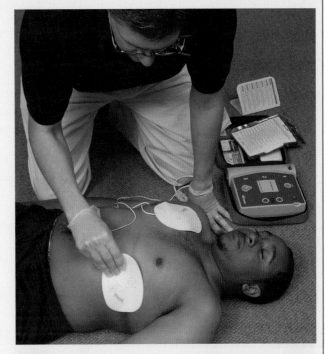

FIGURE 12.29

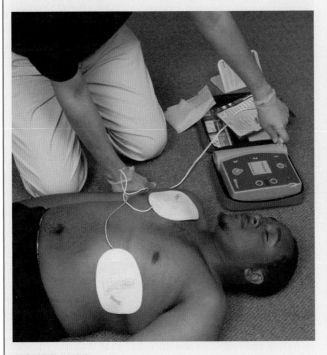

FIGURE 12.30

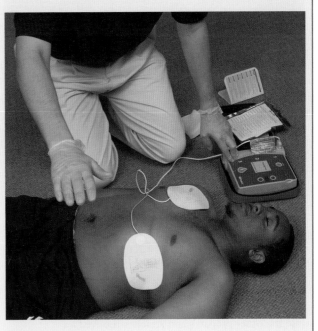

FIGURE 12.31

(Continued)

SKILL 12.4 *(Continued)*

Using an Adult AED (Continued)

(1) If a shockable rhythm (V-fib and V-tach) is advised, depress the SHOCK button (Fig. 12.32). Be sure that no one is touching the athlete by waving your hand over the body and saying SHOCKING in a loud, clear, confident voice. After one shock is delivered, immediately begin CPR (Fig. 12.33).

    a. Perform 2 minutes of CPR (about 5 cycles), starting with chest compressions (Fig. 12.33).

(2) If the AED indicates NO SHOCK ADVISED, immediately begin CPR.

    a. Perform 2 minutes of CPR for five cycles (about 5 cycles), starting with chest compressions.

    b. At the end of 2 minutes or once commanded by the AED (some units will automatically count down 2 minutes), stop CPR, stand clear of the unit, and press ANALYZE again if indicated.

- Continue following the unit's voice prompts until EMS arrives. Note the number of shocks and CPR time so this information can be passed on to EMS.
- If signs of life are noted at this point, stop and check the individual's pulse for at least 10 seconds. If a pulse and breathing are present, support the athlete as necessary. Consider placing him or her in the recovery position.

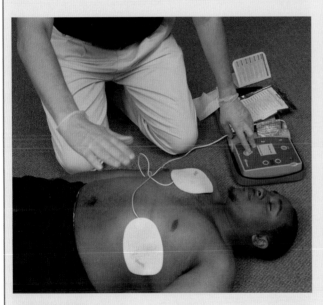

FIGURE 12.32

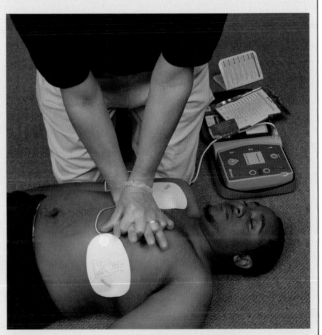

FIGURE 12.33

If an AED is not immediately available on scene, begin CPR. Once the AED arrives and is ready to use, stop CPR, confirm that the individual has no signs of life, and follow the procedures identified in step 7.

If two athletic trainers or emergency responders are present, one individual should continue performing CPR while the other prepares and attaches the AED.

Using an AED—Pediatric

Current ECC guidelines now allow for the use of an AED in the event of cardiac arrests in a child. AED use on pediatric athletes is based on Food and Drug Administration approval of these devices. A pediatric athlete is considered to be between the ages of 1 and 8 or weighing less than 55 pounds. If you are unable to determine a precise age or weight, do not delay care and use your best judgment in determining age. Currently there is insufficient information to recommend for or against the use of an AED in infants younger than 1 year of age.[5]

It is preferable to use an AED that includes the electrode-cable system specially designed for pediatric athletes.[4] Some AED models are equipped with a pediatric adapter, which allows a user to treat either an adult or a pediatric athlete with the turn of a key or flip of a switch. A pediatric pad–cable system or AED with a key or switch allows a smaller dose of energy to be delivered to the athlete. If a pediatric AED or adapter is not available, you may use an

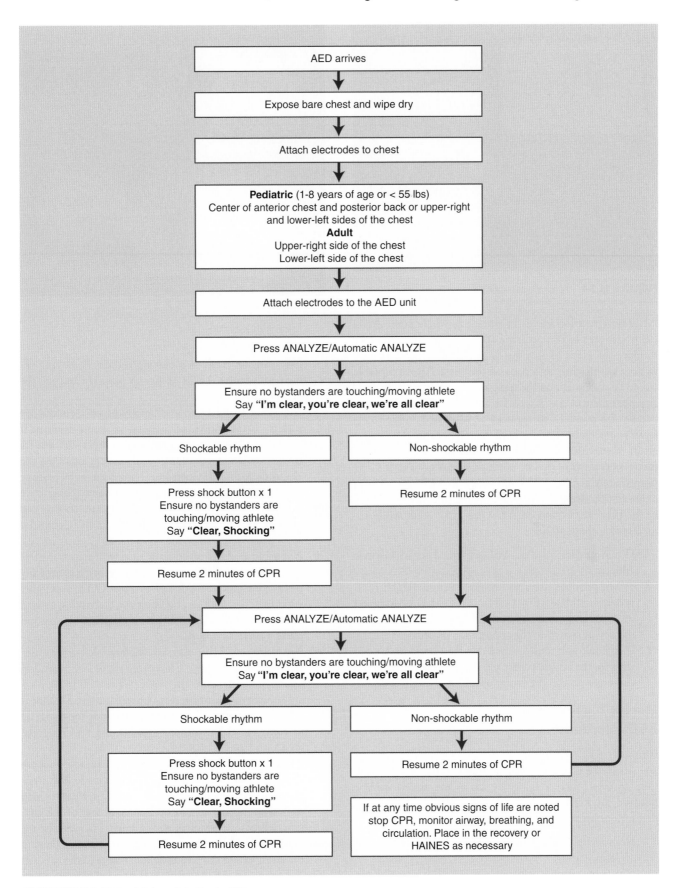

ALGORITHM 12.5   Adult and Pediatric AED.

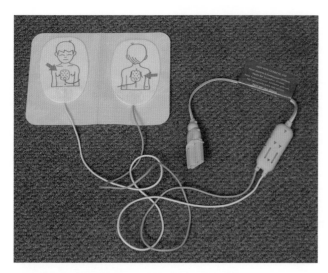

FIGURE 12.34 Pediatric pad-cable system.

AED designed for adults. In situations where adult AED electrodes are used on pediatric athletes, it may be necessary to place the electrodes in the center of the chest and back rather than placing both pads on the chest. Also acceptable would be placement on the right and left chest walls (biaxillary placement).[4]

In the event of recognized or witnessed sudden collapse of a pediatric athlete, immediately activate the cardiac chain of survival and secure an AED. In situations where there is an unwitnessed or nonsudden collapse, start CPR immediately, activate EMS, and secure an AED. To perform defibrillation using an AED, follow the directions outlined in the previous section on AED use in an adult while remembering these points:

1. When possible, use an AED designed for a pediatric athlete.
2. When possible, use a pad cable system designed for a pediatric athlete. (Fig. 12.34). If the AED is designed for both adult and pediatric athletes, be sure to move the key or switch to the appropriate position.
3. If an adult unit must be used and the electrodes are too large for the athlete's chest, place one on the center of the chest and one on the center of the back (Fig. 12.35).

AED Precautions

Although AEDs are relatively simple to use, there are several situations where the athletic trainer must take precautions to avoid further injury to self or the athlete and/or to avoid interfering with the function of the AED. These precautions are as follows:

1. Not touching an individual while the AED is analyzing or defibrillating.
2. Not using alcohol wipes to dry or clean the athlete's chest.
3. Not using an AED around flammable materials.

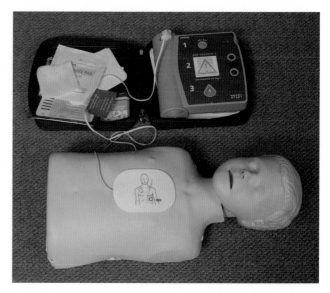

FIGURE 12.35 Appropriate pad placement for a pediatric athletes using adult electrodes.

4. Not using an AED in a moving vehicle. A moving vehicle affects the AEDs ability to properly analyze the heart's rhythm.
5. Not using an AED on a athlete lying on a conductive surface. If the individual is lying in or on water or if the athlete is covered with water, remove the athlete from water and wipe the chest dry before attaching the electrode pads. If the person is lying on a metal plate or metal bleachers, remove him or her to a nonconductive surface before defibrillating. If the athlete has exposed metal as part of his or her athletic equipment, consider appropriate removal of the equipment.
6. Not using an AED on an individual wearing a transdermal medication patch (e.g., nitroglycerin). Remove any medication patches with a gloved hand and thoroughly wipe the chest before attaching the electrodes, since a patch could block the delivery of electrical energy and cause a small skin burn.
7. Not using an AED over an implantable medical device (e.g., pacemaker). Electrodes should be placed at least 1 in. away from the device. If the individual has an implantable cardioverter defibrillator (ICD) that is delivering shocks, allow 30 to 60 seconds for the ICD to complete the treatment cycle before attaching the AED.
8. Removing excessive chest hair. An excessively hairy chest results in poor contact of the electrode pad, trapping air between the electrode and skin, thus causing electrical impedance and occasional arcing of the current, which can result in a skin burn. Hair can be removed by briskly removing an electrode pad or shaving the chest where the electrode must be placed.
9. Not using an AED within 6 ft of a cellular phone or portable radio transmitter. It is believed that the electromagnetic fields created by cell phones and portable

radios interfere with the AED's ability to analyze the heart rhythm. Although it has been difficult to confirm this, studies have shown that digital cell phones may cause distortion of the voice prompts.[87,88]

ESTABLISHING AN AED PROGRAM

Although cardiac emergencies in the athletic environment are rare, athletic trainers in other work settings may be dealing with athletes at risk for cardiac emergencies. For this reason, immediate access to an AED is essential. All athletic trainers regardless of work setting should have developed a clearly defined AED protocol as part of the facility's EAP. Because the U.S. Food and Drug Administration require a prescription to purchase an AED, medical oversight from a team or designated physician will be necessary.

When determining the need for implementation of an AED program, Drezer et al.[9] identified several time-sensitive intervals and criteria that must be addressed in order to increase the likelihood of SCA survival based on recommendations from the American Heart Association. When the "EMS call-to-shock interval of less than 5 minutes cannot be reliably achieved with a conventional EMS system and a collapse-to-shock interval of less than 5 minutes can be reliably achieved

(in more than 90% of cases)"[9] with an AED program—not only by the athletic trainer but also others such as coaches, administrators, and lay responders—then implementing such a program should be highly considered. Regular training and/or a mock SCA collapse/event with local EMS personnel will also allow the athletic trainer to establish whether or not these time-sensitive intervals can be met.

AED programs should also be considered when working with children or adults who are known to be at risk for SCA or in situations where the frequency of cardiac arrest is such

Breakout

Time-Sensitive Intervals during SCA

1. The time from collapse to activation of EMS. The target goal should be less than 1 minute.
2. The time from collapse to initiation of CPR. The target goal should be less than 1 minute.
3. The time from collapse to delivery of the first AED shock. A target goal of time from collapse to first shock should be 3 to 5 minutes.
4. The time from collapse to arrival of EMS personnel at the athlete's side.

Scenarios

1. While covering a high school football game, you note that one of the sideline referees is struggling to maintain his position on the field to make the right call. During a time out, you approach the referee and note that he is having difficulty breathing and appears diaphoretic. When you question him, he reports feeling that he is about to be sick. You quickly approach the head referee and inform him of the situation.

   What is the sideline referee suffering from? Identify the potential signs and symptoms associated with the referee's condition.
   Describe the appropriate steps to manage this case.
   If the referee were an athlete, how would care be different?

2. Mary, an athletic trainer at an outpatient rehabilitation center, was exercising during lunch with a coworker. Tim, a 55-year-old man, was on a Stairmaster when he began clutching his chest. He suddenly lost consciousness and fell off the unit. Mary quickly assessed the situation and determined that Tim was suffering from cardiac arrest. Reacting immediately, she initiated the facility's EAP by calling 911 and began performing CPR.

   In performing CPR, what are the essential components of chest compressions?
   Because Tim collapsed by the Stairmaster, what may Mary need to do before beginning CPR?
   A second athletic trainer arrives; what instructions should Mary provide to him?

3. You are covering a middle school basketball game when you suddenly hear a scream coming from the opponents' bench. An 11-year-old child has collapsed and appears to be unconscious.

   What should your immediate action be?
   The 11-year-old demonstrates no signs of life. What would you next step be?
   One minute later, another athletic trainer arrives with an AED. What would your next step be, now that the AED has arrived and there are two athletic trainers?
   At what point do you stop providing care?

4. Sam, a recent college graduate and newly certified athletic trainer, has taken his first job at a local high school. During his first 2 weeks on the job, he assesses the overall athletic training program, which was handed over to him by the previous athletic trainer. One area of concern is the lack of an adequate EAP for dealing with an athlete in cardiac arrest, in particular the lack of early access to an AED. The athletic director instructs Sam to design a proposal that outlines why the high school needs an AED or an EAP. Sam's immediate reaction is to outline several key areas of discussion, including defining SCA, describing the cardiac chain of survival, and identifying the purpose and necessity of having an AED on site.

   If you were Sam, how would describe/discuss the key areas outlined above?

that there is a reasonable probability of AED use within 5 years of athletic trainer training and AED placement. For further information on establishing an AED program and management of SCA in high school and college athletes, we recommend reviewing the article by Drezner et al.,[9] listed in the references.

WRAP-UP

As an athletic trainer you are fortunate that most of the athletes under your care will rarely suffer from SCA. However, at some point in your career, you may be placed in situation where you will be required to manage an individual suffering from SCA. Remaining calm, maintaining a high level of professionalism, and reacting based on your training may make the difference between saving and not saving a life. Understanding the vital role you and your actions and preparation play in the cardiac chain of survival is critical to improving athlete outcomes. Reviewing, practicing, and keeping your ECC skills up to date will allow you to remain competent and ready to manage an athlete in SCA successfully. Like many of the emergency trauma or medical skills discussed thus far, the initial and subsequent care you administer may be the difference between life and death.

REFERENCES

1. Board of Certification. FAQ. http://www.bocatc.org/index.php?option=com_content&task=view&id=111&Itemid=119. Accessed June 20, 2009.
2. American Heart Association. Part 3: Overview of CPR. *Circulation.* 2005;112(24 Suppl):IV-12–IV-18.
3. American Heart Association. Part 4: Adult basic life support. *Circulation.* 2005;112(24 Suppl):IV-19–IV-34.
4. American Heart Association. Part 5: Electrical therapies: Automated external defibrillators, defibrillation, cardioversion, and pacing. *Circulation.* 2005;112(24 Suppl):IV-35–IV-46.
5. American Heart Association. Part 11: Pediatric basic life support. *Circulation.* 2005;112(24 Suppl):IV-156–IV-166.
6. American Heart Association. Part 12: From science to survival: Strengthening the Chain of Survival in every community. *Resuscitation.* 2000;46(1–3):417–430.
7. Goldberger J, Cain M, Hohnloser S, et al. American Heart Association/American College of Cardiology Foundation/Heart Rhythm Society Scientific Statement on Noninvasive Risk Stratification Techniques for Identifying Patients at Risk for Sudden Cardiac Death: A Scientific Statement From the American Heart Association Council on Clinical Cardiology Committee on Electrocardiography and Arrhythmias and Council on Epidemiology and Prevention. *J Am Coll Cardiol.* 2008;52(14):1179–1199.
8. Olasveengen TM, Lorem T, Samdal M, et al. Strengthening weak parts of the local chain of survival after out-of-hospital cardiac arrest. *Resuscitation.* 2008;77(Suppl 1):S50–S50.
9. Drezner J, Courson R, Roberts W, et al. Inter-Association Task Force recommendations on emergency preparedness and management of sudden cardiac arrest in high school and college athletic programs: A consensus statement. *J Athl Train.* 2007;42(1):143–158.
10. Nichol G, Stiell I, Laupacis A, et al. A cumulative meta-analysis of the effectiveness of defibrillator-capable emergency medical services for victims of out-of-hospital cardiac arrest. *Ann Emerg Med.* 1999;34(1):517–525.
11. Drezner J, Rogers K. Sudden cardiac arrest in intercollegiate athletes: Detailed analysis and outcomes of resuscitation in nine cases. *Heart Rhythm.* 2006;3(7):755.
12. Holmberg M, Holmberg S, Herlitz J, et al. Survival after cardiac arrest outside hospital in Sweden. *Resuscitation.* 1998;36:29–36.
13. Cobb L, Fahrenbruch C, Walsh T, et al. Influence of cardiopulmonary resuscitation prior to defibrillation in patients with out-of-hospital ventricular fibrillation. *JAMA.* 1999;281:1182–1188.
14. Nordberg P, Hollenberg J, Herlitz J, et al. Aspects on the increase in bystander CPR in Sweden and its association with outcome. *Resuscitation.* 2009;80(3):329–333.
15. Casper K, Murphy G, Weinstein C, et al. A comparison of cardiopulmonary resuscitation rates of strangers versus known bystanders. *Prehosp Emerg Care.* 2003;7(3):299–302.
16. Hollenberg J, Herlitz J, Lindqvist J, et al. Improved survival after out-of-hospital cardiac arrest Is associated with an Increase in proportion of emergency crew-witnessed cases and bystander cardiopulmonary resuscitation. *Circulation.* 2008;118(4):389–396.
17. Capucci A, Aschieri D, Piepoli M, et al. Tripling survival from sudden cardiac arrest via early defibrillation without traditional education in cardiopulmonary resuscitation. *Circulation.* 2002;106(10):1065–1070.
18. Drezner J, Courson R, Roberts W, et al. Inter-association task force recommendations on emergency preparedness and management of sudden cardiac arrest in high school and college athletic programs: a consensus statement. *Heart Rhythm.* 2007;4(4):549–565.
19. Larsen M, Eisenberg M, Cummins R, et al. Predicting survival from out-of-hospital cardiac arrest: a graphic model. *Ann Emerg Med.* 1993;22:1652–1658.
20. Becker L, Gold L, Eisenberg M, et al. Ventricular fibrillation in King County, Washington: A 30-year perspective. *Resuscitation.* 2008;79(1):22–27.
21. Valenzuela T, Roe D, Nichol G, et al. Outcomes of rapid defibrillation by security officers after cardiac arrest in casinos. *N Engl J Med.* 2000;343(17):1206–1209.
22. Centers for Disease Control and Prevention. Web-based Injury Statistics Query and Reporting System (WISQARS) (Online): 10 leading causes of death, United States, Ages <1 to 8. *National Center for Injury Prevention and Control, Centers for Disease Control and Prevention.* www.cdc.gov/ncipc/wisqars. Accessed July 19, 2009.
23. American Heart Association. Part 6: Pediatric basic and advanced life support. *Circulation.* 2005;112(22 Suppl):III-73–III-90.
24. Centers for Disease Control and Prevention. Web-based Injury Statistics Query and Reporting System (WISQARS) (Online): 10 leading causes of death, United States, All ages. *National Center for Injury Prevention and Control, Centers for Disease Control and Prevention.* http://www.cdc.gov/injury/wisqars/index.html. Accessed July 19, 2009.

25. National Heart Blood and Lung Institute. Diseases and conditions index. *National Heart Blood and Lung Institute*. Accessed July 2009.

26. Fang J, Keenan N, Dai S, et al. Disparities in adult awareness of heart attack warning signs and symptoms – 14 States, 2005. *MMWR Morb Mortal Wkly Rep.* 2008;57(7):175–179.

27. Heart attack: Do you know the signs? *People's Medical Society Newsletter.* 1999;18(3):5.

28. Centers for Disease Control and Prevention. Know the signs and symptoms of a heart attack. http://www. cdc.gov/DH-DSP/library/fs_heartattack.htm. Accessed July 2009.

29. Ornato JP, Hand MM. Warning signs of a heart attack. *Circulation.* 2001;104(11):1212–1213.

30. Canto JG, Shlipak MG, Rogers WJ, Malmgren JA, Frederick PD, Lambrew CT, Ornato JP, Barron HV, Kiefe CI. Prevalence, clinical characteristics, and mortality among patients with myocardial infarction presenting without chest pain. *JAMA.* 2000;283(24):3223–3229.

31. Smith BW. Cardiovascular disorders. In: Cuppett M, Walsh KM, eds. *General Medical Conditions in the Athlete*. St. Louis: Elsevier; 2005:95–126.

32. National Heart Blood and Lung Institute. Women and heart attack. http://www.nhlbi.nih.gov/actintime/haws/women.htm. Accessed July 19, 2009.

33. National Heart Blood and Lung Institute. Heart attack symptoms in women: Are they different? *National Institutes of Health News.* http://www.nih.gov/news/pr/dec2007/nhlbi-10. htm. Accessed July 19, 2009.

34. Rosamond W, Flegal K, Furie K, et al. Heart disease and stroke statistics—2008 update: A report from the American Heart Association Statistics Committee and Stroke Statistics Subcommittee. *Circulation.* 2008;117(4):e25–e146.

35. National Heart Blood and Lung Institute. What are heart disease risk factors? http://www.nhlbi.nih.gov/health/dci/ Diseases/hd/hd_whatare.html. Accessed June 1, 2010.

36. American Heart Association. Sudden cardiac death. http:// www.americanheart.org/presenter.jhtml?identifier=4741. Accessed July 19, 2009.

37. Rea T, Eisenberg M, Sinibaldi G, et al. Incidence of EMS-treated out-of-hospital cardiac arrest in the United States. *Resuscitation.* 2004;63:17–24.

38. Sovari AA, Kocheril AG, McCullough PA. Sudden cardiac death. *eMedicine.* 2006. http://emedicine.medscape.com/ article/151907-overview

39. Maron BJ. Heart disease and other causes of sudden death in young athletes. *Curr Probl Cardiol.* 1998;23(9):480–529.

40. Maron BJ. Sudden death in young athletes. *N Engl J Med.* 2003;349(11):1064–1075.

41. Van Camp S, Bloor C, Mueller F, et al. Nontraumatic sports death in high school and college athletes. *Med Sci Sports Exerc.* 1995;27:641–647.

42. Maron BJ, Roberts W, McAllister H, et al. Sudden death in young athletes. *Circulation.* 1980;62(2):218–229.

43. Maron BJ, Doerer JJ, Haas TS, et al. Sudden deaths in young competitive athletes: Analysis of 1866 deaths in the United States, 1980–2006. *Circulation.* 2009;119(8):1085–1092.

44. Maron BJ, Maron MS, Lesser RL, et al. Sudden cardiac arrest in hypertrophic cardiomyopathy in the absence of conventional criteria for high risk status. *Am J Cardiol.* 2008;101:544–547.

45. Anderson M, Hall S, Martin M. Cardiovascular disorders. *Foundation of Athletic Training: Prevention, Assessment, and Management.* Baltimore: Lippincott Williams & Wilkins; 2005:621–640.

46. Bezold LI. Coronary artery anomalies. *eMedicine.* 2009. http://emedicine.medscape.com/article/895854-overview. Updated Jan. 2010.

47. Koester MC. A review of Sudden Cardiac Death in young athletes and strategies for preparticipation cardiovascular screening. *J Athl Train.* 2001;36(2):197–204.

48. Madias C, Maron BJ, Weinstock J, et al. Commotio cordis: sudden cardiac death with chest wall impact. *J Cardiovasc Electrophysiol.* 2007;18(1):115–122.

49. Doerer JJ, Haas TS, Estes NAM, et al. Evaluation of chest barriers for protection against sudden death due to commotio cordis. *Am J Cardiol.* 2007;99(6):857–859.

50. Lopez R, Berg-McGraw J. Marfan syndrome in a female collegiate basketball player: A case report. *J Athl Train.* 2000; 35(1):91–95.

51. American Heart Association. Part 5: Acute coronary syndromes. *Circulation.* 2005;112(22 Suppl):III-55–III-72.

52. American Heart Association. Part 8: Stabilization of the patient with acute coronary syndromes. *Circulation.* 2005;112 (24 Suppl):IV-89–IV-110.

53. Valenzuela T, Roe D, Cretin S, et al. Estimating effectiveness of cardiac arrest interventions: a logistic regression survival model. *Circulation.* 1997;96:3308–3313.

54. Herlitz J, Ekstrom L, Wennerblom B, et al. Effect of bystander initiated cardiopulmonary resuscitation on ventricular fibrillation and survival after witnessed cardiac arrest outside hospital. *Br Heart J.* 1994;72:408–412.

55. Stiell I, Nichol G, Wells G, et al. Health-related quality of life is better for cardiac arrest survivors who received citizen cardiopulmonary resuscitation. *Circulation.* 2003;108:1939–1944.

56. Wik L, Kramer-Johansen J, Myklebust H, et al. Quality of cardiopulmonary resuscitation during out-of-hospital cardiac arrest. *J Am Med Assoc.* 2005;293:299–304.

57. Perkins GD, Walker G, Christensen K, et al. Teaching recognition of agonal breathing improves accuracy of diagnosing cardiac arrest. *Resuscitation.* 2006;70(3):432–437.

58. Kundra P, Dey S, Ravishankar M. Role of dominant hand position during external cardiac compression. *Br J Anaesthesiol.* 2000;84:491–493.

59. American Red Cross. *CPR/AED for the Professional Rescuer Participant's Manual.* Yardley, PA: Staywell; 2006.

60. Andersen L, Isbye D, Rasmussen L. Increasing compression depth during manikin CPR using a simple backboard. *Acta Anaesthesiologica Scandinavica.* 2007;51(6):747–750.

61. Chi C, Tsou J, Su F. Effects of rescuer position on the kinematics of cardiopulmonary resuscitation (CPR) and the force of delivered compressions. *Resuscitation.* 2008;76(1):69–75.

62. 'Stayin' Alive' helps people stay alive. http://www.nme.com/ news/the-bee-gees/40517. Accessed October 17, 2009.

63. Aufderheide T, Pirrallo R, Yannopoulos D, et al. Incomplete chest wall decompression: a clinical evaluation of CPR performance by EMS personnel and assessment of alternative manual chest compression-decompression techniques *Resuscitation.* 2005;64:353–362.

64. David R. Closed chest cardiac massage in the newborn infant. *Pediatrics.* 1988:552–554.

65. Todres I, Rogers M. Methods of external cardiac massage in the newborn infant. *J Pediatr.* 1975;86:781–782.

66. Powner D, Holcombe P, Mello L. Cardiopulmonary resuscitation-related injuries. *Crit Care Med.* 1984;12(1):54–55.

67. Lederer W, Mair D, Rabl W, et al. Frequency of rib and sternum fractures associated with out-of-hospital cardiopulmonary resuscitation is underestimated by conventional chest X-ray. *Resuscitation.* 2004;60(2):157–162.

68. Maguire S, Mann M, John N, et al. Does cardiopulmonary resuscitation cause rib fractures in children? A systematic review. *Child Abuse Negl.* 2006;30(7):739–751.

69. Sprague LD, Ferrigni FJ. Lung herniation after cardiopulmonary resuscitation. *N Engl J Med.* 2004;351(7):695–695.

70. Sommers MS. The shattering consequences of CPR: How to assess and prevent complications. *Nursing.* 1992;22(7).

71. Hashimoto Y, Moriya F, Furumiya J. Forensic aspects of complications resulting from cardiopulmonary resuscitation. *Leg Med.* 2007;9(2):94–99.

72. Ali B, Zafari AM. Narrative review: Cardiopulmonary resuscitation and emergency cardiovascular care: Review of the current guidelines. *Ann Intern Med.* 2007;147(3):171–179.

73. Oschatz E, Wunderbaldinger P, Sterz F, et al. Cardiopulmonary resuscitation performed by bystanders does not increase adverse effects as assessed by chest radiography. *Anesth Analg.* 2001;93:128–133.

74. Doerges V, Sauer C, Ocker H, et al. Smaller tidal volumes during cardiopulmonary resuscitation: Comparison of adult and paediatric self-inflatable bags with three different ventilatory devices. *Resuscitation.* 1999;43(1):31–37.

75. Doerges V, Sauer C, Ocker H, et al. Airway management during cardiopulmonary resuscitation: A comparative study of bag-valve-mask, laryngeal mask airway and combitube in a bench model. *Resuscitation.* 1999;41(1):63–69.

76. Dorges V, Ocker H, Wenzel V, et al. Emergency airway management by non-anaesthesia house officers: A comparison of three strategies. *Emerg Med J.* 2001;18(2):90–94.

77. Virkkunen I, Ryynänen S, Kujala S, et al. Incidence of regurgitation and pulmonary aspiration of gastric contents in survivors from out-of-hospital cardiac arrest. *Acta Anaesthesiol Scand.* 2007;51(2):202–205.

78. Virkkunen I, Kujal S, Ryynänen S, et al. Bystander mouth-to-mouth ventilation and regurgitation during cardiopulmonary resuscitation. *J Intern Med.* 2006;260(1):39–42.

79. Rello J, Diaz E, Roque M, et al. Risk factors for developing pneumonia within 48 hours of intubation. *Am J Respir Crit Care Med.* 1999;159:1742–1746.

80. Swartz EE, Boden BP, Courson RW, et al. National Athletic Trainers' Association Position Statement: Acute management of the cervical spine–injured athlete. *J Athl Train.* 2009;44(3):306–311.

81. Sayre MR, Berg RA, Cave DM, et al. Hands-only (Compression-Only) cardiopulmonary resuscitation: A call to action for bystander response to adults who experience out-of-hospital sudden cardiac arrest: A science advisory for the public from the American Heart Association Emergency Cardiovascular Care Committee. *Circulation.* 2008;117:2162–2167.

82. Abella B, Edelson D. Resuscitation errors: A shocking problem. *Agency for Healthcare Research and Quality.* http://www.webmm.ahrq.gov/case.aspx?caseID=155. Accessed December 29, 2008.

83. Brennan R, Braslow A. Skill mastery in public CPR classes. *Am J Emer Med.* 1998;16(7):653–657.

84. Cummins RO, Hazinski MF, Kerber RE, et al. Low-energy biphasic waveform defibrillation: Evidence-based review applied to emergency cardiovascular care guidelines : A statement for healthcare professionals from the American Heart Association Committee on Emergency Cardiovascular Care and the Subcommittees on Basic Life Support, Advanced Cardiac Life Support, and Pediatric Resuscitation. *Circulation.* 1998;97(16):1654–1667.

85. Hazinski MF, Nadkarni VM, Hickey RW, et al. Major changes in the 2005 AHA guidelines for CPR and ECC: Reaching the tipping point for change. *Circulation.* 2005;112(24 Suppl):IV-206–IV-211.

86. Dahl C, Ewy G, Warner E, et al. Myocardial necrosis from direct current countershock: Effect of paddle electrode size and time interval between discharges. *Circulation.* 1974;50:956–961.

87. Trigano A, Blandeau O, Dale C, et al. Clinical testing of cellular phone ringing interference with automated external defibrillators. *Resuscitation.* 2006;71(3):391–394.

88. Kanz K, Kay M, Biberthaler P, et al. Effect of digital cellular phones on tachyarrhythmia analysis of automated external defibrillators. *Eur J Emerg Med.* 2004;11(2):75–80.

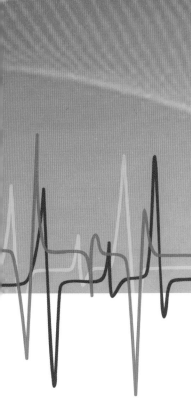

CHAPTER · 13

Recognition and Management of Hypoperfusion

CHAPTER OUTCOMES

1. Identify and explain how blood and fluids travel through the body.
2. Determine how to calculate cardiac output.
3. Identify the differences between systolic and diastolic blood pressure and the device normally used to measure blood pressure.
4. Identify the differences between perfusion and hypoperfusion.
5. Describe how the body reacts to sudden losses in blood/fluid volume and what mechanisms the body undergoes to compensate for such processes.
6. Identify postural hypotension and a method used to assess the condition.
7. Identify the major signs and symptoms of shock.
8. Identify the steps and processes in order to use an antishock garment to manage severe cases of shock.
9. Identify the differences between the major types of shock, their signs and symptoms, and overall general management.

NOMENCLATURE

Cardiac output: the volume of blood being pumped by the heart in 1 minute

Diastolic blood pressure: the lowest pressure in the arteries when the heart is not pumping or is at rest

Evisceration: removal of viscera

Hypoperfusion: inadequate delivery of oxygen and nutrients to the cells of the body as a result of decreased blood flow

Hypotension: low blood pressure

Hypovolemia: decreased blood volume or volume of blood plasma

Perfusion: the delivery of oxygen and nutrients to body cells via the blood vessels

Postural hypotension: a sudden fall in blood pressure that occurs when a person assumes a standing position, often called orthostatic hypotension

NOMENCLATURE *(Continued)*

Pulse pressure: the systolic blood pressure minus the diastolic blood pressure

Sphygmomanometer: a device with an inflatable sleeve used to cut off/restrict blood flow and measure blood pressure

Stroke volume: the volume of blood pumped by the left ventricle in one contraction

Systolic blood pressure: the maximal pressure of the arteries while the heart is beating

BEFORE YOU BEGIN

1. What happens to blood pressure as a result of shock?
2. What are the different types/classifications of shock?
3. How is shock generally managed in the athletic setting?
4. What are the major signs and symptoms of shock?
5. Are there any management steps that the athletic trainer can use to prevent shock?

Voices from the Field

Assessment of injury is successful when an efficient recognition and response to signs and symptoms occurs. When assessing any injury, regardless of cause, the certified athletic trainer must consider the possibility of shock. A failure to recognize the signs and symptoms of shock can turn a common injury such as a fracture into a life-threatening condition. An advanced understanding of the circulatory system—including blood flow, cardiac output, and blood pressure—is critical in recognizing shock. In addition to the anatomy and physiology of circulation, an athletic trainer must be familiar with the various types of shock as well as their unique signs and symptoms. A complete understanding of shock is essential for appropriate and rapid emergent care of an injured person or athlete. It is simply not enough to recognize the traditional signs and symptoms of shock: vomiting or nausea, dilated pupils, cyanosis, decreased blood pressure, increased heart and respiration rates, a weak pulse, cool clammy skin, and an alteration in mental status. While these signs and symptoms are critical, they are not always consistent with the numerous types of shock. Failure to recognize these conditions may result in mismanagement of an injured person, causing permanent disability or possibly death.

Recognition of shock, regardless of cause, must be followed by appropriate management of the airway, breathing, circulation, and severe bleeding, and then any other conditions found. If your primary survey indicates a serious threat to life, then immediate steps to alert emergency medical services (EMS), minimize blood loss, and initiate CPR must begin. If the initial assessment does not indicate an immediate life threat, then a more systematic evaluation of the vital signs is indicated and appropriate steps to manage shock and injury must be initiated. It is critical that these lifesaving skills of immediate recognition and management be practiced logically and effectively. Cardiopulmonary resuscitation (CPR) is one of the first skills many health care providers learn, and some may take these skills for granted as a result. When teaching and learning the steps to manage shock, one must practice with diligence to understand the mechanisms, types, signs and symptoms, and management of this life-threatening condition. Students should have the mindset that these recognition and management skills may be necessary to save a life. In order for students to truly develop competence and perform these skills proficiently, athletic training educators should instruct their students and test their ability to perform these skills under a variety of scenarios, with a progression of difficulty and urgency. This will allow athletic training students to gain confidence in their skills and allow them to gradually increase their involvement with emergency care under the supervision of a qualified clinician. Confidence in one's skills and abilities ensures preparedness for the life-threatening situation, no matter where or when it happens.

Mack D. Rubley, PhD, ATC, LAT, CSCS
Director, Athletic Training Education
University of Nevada, Las Vegas

Athletes will be injured multiple times throughout their careers. Many of these injuries will not be life-threatening; they will mainly be sprains or strains that heal relatively quickly. Some injuries, however, can be more serious, resulting in a condition called shock. Shunting of blood during shock can be very dangerous and may lead to death if not properly managed by trained personnel. Therefore, athletic trainers must be knowledgeable and prepared to manage situations when their athletes suffer from injuries or illnesses that may lead to shock. In this chapter, we will cover the major types of shock, their specific etiologies, and the various treatments for shock.

An overview of the circulatory system is needed to fully understand how blood is carried through the body. A brief description is included here but you may refer to Chapter 12 for a more complete review. The red blood cells, or more specifically the hemoglobin within them, carry oxygen from the lungs to all body systems. Oxygenated blood leaves the lungs via the pulmonary veins, which carry it to the left atrium of the heart and into the left ventricle, to be pumped out of the heart via the aorta. The blood then travels throughout the body and eventually returns to the right atrium of the heart, through the right ventricle, and back to the lungs to be oxygenated. On its way throughout the body, the blood moves through a series of vessels called arteries, smaller vessels called arterioles, and still smaller ones called capillaries. Deoxygenated blood is sent through the venous system back again to the heart. The smooth muscle in the walls of these vessels can change the vessels' diameter to accommodate differences in blood flow.

The heart pumps blood throughout the body; the rate and extent of this pumping varies depending upon physiological stresses imposed on the body. The amount of blood (volume) pumped per beat is called the **stroke volume.** The total amount of blood pumped per minute is called the **cardiac output.** To calculate the total cardiac output, multiply the stroke volume by the heart rate:

$$CO = SV \times HR^1$$

The amount of pressure exerted on the vessels depends upon the volume of blood pumped and the resistance to blood flow. **Systolic blood pressure** is the pressure exerted against the vessel walls when the heart pumps; **diastolic blood pressure** is the pressure against the vessel walls when the heart is not pumping. It is read with the help of a **sphygmomanometer.** The difference between these two pressures is called the **pulse pressure;** it is determined by the difference in the numeric values of the systolic and diastolic pressures (e.g., 120/80, for a pulse pressure of 40). High pulse pressure values may cause more artery damage and increase the stress on the heart.

The dilation and constriction of the blood vessels plus the cardiac output from the heart play an important part in determining an individual's blood pressure and the overall **perfusion** or delivery of blood and oxygen to the body. When an inadequate amount of blood is delivered or there is blood loss, the body is in a state of **hypoperfusion.** The exact causes of hypoperfusion are multifaceted but predominantly stem from the loss of fluid, changes in vessel size, or irregularities in the heartbeat that affect the heart's pumping function. When the heart fails to pump or does not pump properly to keep the tissues oxygenated, shock ensues.

SHOCK

To compensate for the loss of blood/fluid, or hypoperfusion, the body reacts defensively in several ways. To begin, blood flow is shunted from the extremities to the major organs to maintain blood pressure and supply the organs

Signs & Symptoms

Shock

- Vomiting or nausea
- Dilated pupils
- Listless pupils
- Bluish lips or nails (from lack of oxygen)
- Decreased blood pressure
- Increased respirations and heart rate
- Weak pulse
- Cool skin
- Altered mental status
- Thirst
- Delayed capillary refill

with the vital nutrients and oxygen they need to survive. As a result, there is less blood flow to the skin, which becomes cool and pale. As the blood flows to the internal organs, the sudden rush of blood to the digestive system can cause the individual to become nauseated or vomit. Other physiological processes, including brain function, can be affected by the lack of blood and oxygen. The brain requires a constant supply of oxygen and can survive for only a few minutes if that supply is cut off. As the heart tries to pump more blood, the pulse rate increases, with a concomitant increase in the rate of respiration. If shock worsens or lasts too long, respiration can become very labored and shallow. A late sign of shock is a drop in blood pressure due to the loss of blood volume.

The overall severity of shock depends on its mechanisms; it may be classified as compensated, decompensated, or irreversible. *Compensated* shock is due to the body's effort to "compensate" for a decrease in tissue perfusion or inadequate removal of metabolic wastes. In early shock, the heart beats faster, respirations increase, and the blood vessels of the extremities become constricted. Compensated shock results from the body's efforts to redirect or divert blood flow to the major organs and maintain blood pressure. Thus, the extremities become cool and pale, while cardiovascular responses increase. Capillary refill is used as a measure of perfusion for the diagnosis of compensated shock in infants and children. That is, after being compressed and becoming pale, the nail beds should normally return to their normal color (refill with blood) within 2 seconds; when this fails to occur, the child may be in shock. Capillary refill is not recommended as a diagnostic measure in adults, since other metabolic or physical conditions can affect perfusion in older individuals. In *decompensated* shock, the body cannot adjust for the loss of blood, fluid, or inadequate perfusion; thus, systolic blood pressure decreases, usually to less than 90 mm Hg, with the distal pulses difficult to find. Decompensated shock can lead to organ failure and must be managed immediately. Finally, *irreversible* shock results when the body can no longer attempt to correct or adjust for blood loss or cannot maintain adequate perfusion of the major organs. Hypoxia then causes tissues to die and irreversible organ damage ensues.

Individuals who are in shock can suffer from **postural hypotension.** This means that when the individual stands up suddenly, the lowered blood pressure will cause him or her to feel dizzy or faint. Postural hypotension occurs because the blood pools in the lower extremities with diminished flow to the brain. An athlete can be assessed for postural hypotension with the *tilt test*, which is performed by monitoring the athlete's vital signs (i.e., blood pressure, pulse, respirations) as the athlete is gradually moved from a supine position to a more vertical position. A positive tilt test results when the heart rate is raised by more than 20 beats, the athlete feels dizzy or light-headed, and the systolic blood pressure drops more than 20 mm Hg (Fig. 13.1).

General Management of Shock

If an athlete is experiencing shock or shock-like symptoms, several management steps must be taken to limit the severity (Algorithm 13.1 and Skill 13.1). First, an initial assessment is performed followed by a detailed physical exam (Chapter 8) to find immediate life-threatening conditions. If blood loss is the causative factor, it must be controlled immediately to limit bleeding. Appropriate splints or management techniques for fractures are then applied. The athlete's airway is maintained and if there is no suspicion of serious spinal injury his or her legs should be elevated 8 to 12 in. to help blood flow back to the major organs. Respiratory and heart rates are monitored and recorded for reexamination over time. The athlete should be covered with a blanket or towels to keep him or her warm. Vital signs are reassessed periodically and the athlete is either transported to a medical facility or arrangements for transport via EMS are made if necessary. Finally, it is important not to give anything by mouth.

If the athletic trainer is certified as an emergency medical technician (EMT) or has experience and physician approval, he or she may apply military antishock trousers (MAST) or a pneumatic antishock garment (PASG) to help increase blood pressure. These are inflatable devices similar to intermittent compression devices; either one of these garments may be placed on the lower extremities and lower abdomen, secured, and then inflated with air to increase pressure. A MAST or PASG should be used only by a person

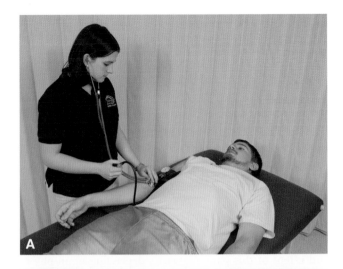

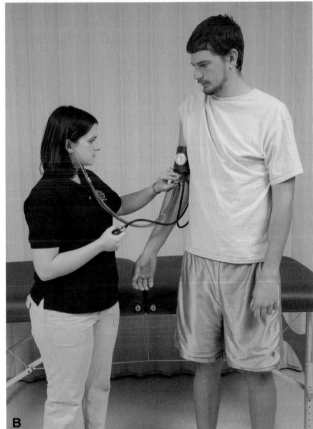

FIGURE 13.1 Tilt-test procedure. **A.** Conducting the tilt test while the athlete is lying down. **B.** Conducting the tilt test while the athlete is standing.

SKILL 13.1

Shock Management

1. Assess vital signs
2. Control any loss of fluids
3. Maintain open airway (supplemental oxygen may be necessary)
4. Place athlete in a supine position (if no suspected spinal injury)
5. Elevate the legs
6. Keep the athlete warm
7. Monitor vital signs
8. Transport the athlete to a medical facility

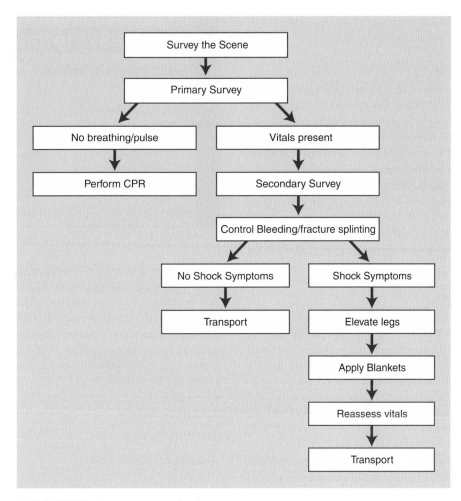

ALGORITHM 13.1   Managing shock.

who has been properly trained to do so. It is appropriately applied only when the athlete's systolic blood pressure has fallen below 50 mm Hg or when bleeding is occurring in the areas covered by the device. Do not use such a device if the individual has cardiogenic shock, abnormal lung sounds, penetrating thoracic injury, pulmonary edema, **evisceration,** or lower extremity fractures, or if the individual is pregnant.

Types of Shock

There are several types of shock, and the athletic trainer must be cognizant of these. Each type can be treated similarly, but there may be instances in which special care must be rendered. If the athletic trainer is not sure of the specific type of shock, he or she should follow the general shock management steps outlined previously and summon EMS for transport to a medical facility.

Hypovolemic Shock

Hypoperfusion occurs when there is a loss of body fluids. The total amount of fluid in the body will fall below normal values, which is referred to as **hypovolemia,** and can be caused by dehydration, vomiting, or blood loss. As a result, the body attempts to move fluids from intracellular and interstitial cells into the vasculature, resulting in a decrease in blood pressure along with other symptoms. When there is low blood volume, damage to the kidneys or brain can

Signs & Symptoms

Hypovolemia

- Low blood pressure
- Pale skin
- Diminished pulse
- Dizziness
- Fainting
- Inadequate capillary refill
- Nausea
- Thirst

follow, potentially resulting in death. When shock caused by hypovolemia occurs, it is termed *hypovolemic shock*.[2]

Hemorrhagic Shock

Shock caused by the loss of blood and the oxygen-carrying capacity of the blood is called *hemorrhagic shock*. Excessive bleeding internally (due to blunt trauma) and externally are the main causes of hemorrhagic shock. In such situations, the total amount of blood/fluid loss is extremely difficult to ascertain; therefore, the athletic trainer should examine the clothes and surrounding areas for blood/fluid loss. Categories for hemorrhagic shock based upon the volume of blood lost are listed in Table 13.1. The management of hemorrhagic shock should begin with controlling blood loss immediately and then following the general guidelines for managing shock.

Anaphylactic Shock

Anaphylactic shock results from the body's reaction to an allergen (see Chapter 20 for the specific mechanisms of allergic reactions). As the body reacts to an allergen, the local blood vessels dilate and chemical reactions occur so that plasma leaks from the vessels, resulting in edema or swelling. Although anaphylactic reactions may cause only local redness, itching, or hives, severe reactions may produce such extensive edema that the airways become constricted. This, in turn, may lead to wheezing and difficulty breathing, or respiratory emergency. Hives and localized redness may also result from the release of histamine, which causes the blood vessels to leak fluid into the surrounding tissues, lowering the total blood volume and resulting in shock. As the dilation of vessels becomes widespread, the pressure within the vessels drops suddenly, and perfusion is compromised. Symptoms can occur over an extended period of time, but they can also arise quickly, depending on the severity of the reaction.[4]

Treatment of Anaphylactic Shock If an athlete is suspected of suffering from anaphylactic shock, immediate attention is necessary to prevent a collapse of the respiratory system and to minimize the low blood pressure or

Signs & Symptoms
Anaphylactic Shock

- Hives
- Redness of the skin
- Itching
- Diarrhea
- Vomiting
- Difficulty breathing
- Low blood pressure
- Fainting
- Swelling of the lips, face, and neck

hypotension that usually accompanies an anaphylactic reaction. As mentioned in Chapter 12, the most common and best treatment is to administer epinephrine (adrenaline). Epinephrine dilates the airways and relieves the histamine-induced constriction; however, it provides only temporary relief of symptoms. Therefore, it is important to continue monitoring the airway and provide rescue breathing if necessary, and local EMS should also be contacted. In addition, if an athlete has a history of anaphylaxis, the Asthma and Allergy Foundation of America recommends that an "allergy action plan" be created and posted in athletic training settings for action steps and management, including appropriate medical referral.

Septic Shock

Septic shock arises from severe infection, which can cause the blood vessels to dilate, lowering the blood pressure and causing hypoperfusion. In severe cases, septic shock can lead to organ failure and death. Septic shock usually occurs when bacteria or fungi trigger the release of chemical mediators that increase capillary permeability, dilate vessels, and produce hypotension, resulting in tissue hypoxia. The cardiovascular system, specifically the heart, tries to make up for this loss by pumping harder and faster, which can eventually lead to myocardial dysfunction. Septic shock must be diagnosed by medical personnel, with evidence of blood cultures for signs

TABLE 13.1	Classification of Hemorrhagic Shock[3]
Classification	**Description**
Compensated	Less than 1,000 mL blood loss, minimal to no changes in heart and respiratory rate and blood pressure
Mild	Approximately 1,000 to 1,500 mL blood loss with tachycardia, anxiety, increased respiration
Moderate	Approximately 1,500 to 2,000 mL blood loss with alterations of mental status, significant decrease in blood pressure, tachypnea
Severe	Greater than 2,000 mL blood loss with altered mental status, significant decrease in blood pressure, heart rate over 140 bpm, tachypnea, or respiratory collapse. Considered as a life-threatening situation

Signs & Symptoms

Septic Shock

- Red skin
- Flushed face/neck
- Hyperventilation
- Low blood pressure
- Fever
- Confusion

Signs & Symptoms

Cardiogenic Shock

- Altered mental status
- Hypotension
- Rapid, weak pulse
- Cool, clammy skin
- Diminished urine output (oliguria)
- Hyperventilation
- Jugular vein distention

of infection, a high white blood cell count, hyperventilation, and a systolic pressure below 90 mm Hg or mean arterial pressures below 60 mm Hg.[5] Treatment should follow the general shock management guidelines as well as the inclusion of corticosteroids,[6] surgical excision of the infection site, or drainage of any pus, completed by medical personnel.

Neurogenic Shock

Neurogenic shock is a sudden loss of function in the autonomic nervous system, such as a spinal cord injury. In some cases, neurogenic shock may also be induced by fear, horror, and hypothermia, which interrupts autonomic control of the vessels. The signs and symptoms are similar to those of other of shock. Management of neurogenic shock calls for the same procedures used to treat general shock, as outlined in Skill 13.1.

Cardiogenic Shock

When the heart does not work properly, circulation of the blood is compromised. The heart's dysfunction affects its ability to pump blood, which may lead to cardiogenic shock.[7] Cardiac damage is commonly due to myocardial infarction, arrhythmia, valvular dysfunction, or other abnormalities. In most cases, cardiogenic shock occurs after a myocardial infarction, where blood output is greatly diminished. If cardiogenic shock is suspected, treatment would include an assessment of vital signs, provision of supplemental oxygen, possible CPR, and transportation to a medical facility.

Hypoglycemic (Insulin) Shock

Athletes with diabetes are susceptible to changes in blood sugar. When athletes do not consume enough food or take too much oral or injected medication, their level of blood sugar may fall below normal, causing hypoglycemia. This can lead to insulin shock, a potentially a life-threatening condition. Treatment includes ingestion of soda or fruit juice or other foodstuffs. If the individual does not respond after 15 to 20 minutes, medical referral and general treatment for shock is recommended. Chapter 19 outlines more specific steps for the treatment and control of hypoglycemia.

Psychogenic Shock

Psychogenic shock can occur when an athlete is suddenly exposed to fear, joy, anger, or grief. The emotional state quickly dilates the vessels, leading to a decline in the blood pressure. As a result, there is a temporary lack of blood flow and oxygen to the brain and other body tissues. Fainting may then occur. When an athlete suffers from psychogenic shock, the general management steps outlined previously should be followed.

WRAP-UP

In this chapter, the basic physiological processes, types, and management associated with shock have been outlined. The role of the athletic trainer is to be able to recognize the major signs of symptoms of shock, especially in regard to athletic

Signs & Symptoms

Neurogenic Shock

- Hypotension
- Venous pooling
- Inadequate cardiac output
- Bradycardia
- Nausea
- Vomiting
- Cold/clammy skin
- Shallow, rapid breathing

Signs & Symptoms

Insulin Shock (Hypoglycemia)

- General weakness
- Confused, drowsy, or dizziness
- Hunger
- Headache
- Increase perspiration
- Tachycardia
- Irritability
- Difficulty breathing

Scenarios

1. During soccer practice, Rachel, the team's starting forward, goes to head the ball and collides with another teammate's head. She falls to the ground holding her head with her hands. As Tom runs over to the scene, he notices that her head is bleeding profusely. It appears that Rachel has a severe scalp laceration. Tom applies a bandage over the site to control bleeding. EMS is activated and arrives 10 minutes later, but the bleeding is still not controlled. Rachel's mental status appears to be changing as a result.

   What type of shock do you suspect and what are its major signs and symptoms?

2. At an outdoor cross-country practice on a beautiful spring day, one of the runners is stung by an unidentified insect. His skin at the bite site begins to swell and turn red. As you walk him to the athletic training facility, the athlete becomes worse, showing signs of labored breathing and dizziness. When you arrive to the athletic training facility, it is apparent that he is having a more severe reaction than you had anticipated.

   What type of shock is the athlete experiencing and what are the appropriate management steps?

3. One of your athletes appears to have a dizzy spell every time she stands up quickly. You suspect that she has postural hypotension.

   What test can you perform to confirm this and what are some steps she could take to help alleviate this situation?

4. During a football practice, a defensive lineman is injured when another player falls on top of him. As you evaluate the injury, you suspect that the lineman has a nondisplaced tibial fracture. As you are splinting the leg, you notice that the lineman is becoming unresponsive and sweaty. He is apparently suffering from shock due to the trauma to his leg.

   What should you do as you wait for EMS to arrive?

injuries or metabolic conditions. Quick management and activation of EMS when shock occurs can minimize complications and improve the outcomes of these potential life-threatening situations.

REFERENCES

1. Powers SK, Howley ETE. Circulatory responses to exercise. In: *Exercise Physiology: Theory and Application to Fitness and Performance*, 6th ed. New York: McGraw-Hill; 2007.
2. Kelley DM. Hypovolemic Shock: An Overview. *Crit Care Nurs Q*. 2005;28(1):2–19.
3. Martel MJ. Hemorrhagic shock. *J Obstet Gynaecol Can*. 2002; 24(6):504–511.
4. Asthma and Allergy Foundation of America. http://www.aafa.org/display.cfm?id=4. Retrieved April 29, 2008.
5. Tslotou AG, Sakorafas GH, Anagnostopoulos G, et al. Septic shock: Current pathogenetic concepts from a clinical perspective. *Med Sci Monit*. 2005;11(3):RA76–RA85.
6. Sligl WI, Milner DA Jr, Sundar S, et al. Safety and efficacy of corticosteroids for the treatment of septic shock: A systematic review and meta analysis. *Clin Infect Dis*. 2009;49(1): 93–101.
7. Gowda RM, Fox JT, Khan IA. Cardiogenic shock: Basics and clinical considerations. *Int J Cardiol*. 2008;123:221–228.

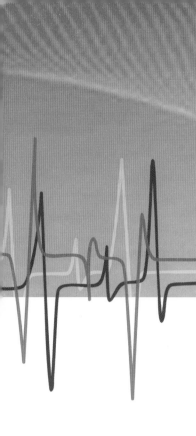

C H A P T E R • 14

Recognition and Management of Soft Tissue Injuries

CHAPTER OUTCOMES

1. Identify the types of open and closed soft tissue injuries.

2. Recognize the signs and symptoms of open and closed soft tissue trauma.

3. Identify the components and procedures of a primary and secondary survey.

4. Properly assess and manage soft tissue injuries.

5. Describe cleansing, debridement, and dressing techniques for acute open wounds.

6. Properly manage and control external hemorrhage.

7. Understand the signs and symptoms of soft tissue trauma that warrant referral and/or activation of the emergency action plan.

8. Understand the importance of universal precautions in the management of soft tissue trauma.

NOMENCLATURE

Antimicrobial: substance used to prevent or kill microorganisms

Angle recession glaucoma: type of glaucoma caused by blunt trauma

Approximate: bring together

Asphyxia: ineffective oxygen intake

Auscultation: listening to sounds

Beck's triad (acute compression triad): signs of cardiac tamponade

Blebs: blisters in the lung or elsewhere

Clean: environment absent of gross contamination (not sterile) or technique to reduce or eliminate microorganisms

Complex lacerations: trauma to the medial canthus, lacrimal apparatus, levator aponeurosis, and/or lid margin of the eye as well as to or other areas

Cytotoxic: damaging to cells

Dehiscence: opening of wound

Denuded: an area where skin or soft tissue has been removed

NOMENCLATURE *(Continued)*

Diplopia: double vision

Eschar: scabbing

Floaters: protein deposits or cells floating in the vitreous humor and seen in the field of vision

Flora: plants; but in this context internal and external microorganisms found on animals

Hematuria: blood in the urine

Hyphema: trauma-induced bleeding into the anterior chamber of the eye

Kiesselbach's plexus (Little's area): anteroinferior nasal septum, with a rich supply of capillaries

Orbital hematoma: black eye

Periwound: area of skin around a wound bed

Photophobia: sensitivity to or avoidance of light

Semiocclusive and occlusive dressings: dressings that seal a wound from the external environment

Sharp debridement: use of sterile scissors and tweezers to remove nonviable tissue

BEFORE YOU BEGIN

1. What is contained in the primary and secondary survey for an athlete who sustains a soft tissue injury?

2. Demonstrate appropriate cleansing, debridement, and dressing techniques for open soft tissue injuries.

3. What are the signs and symptoms of wound infection?

4. Describe the signs and symptoms of external arterial bleeding and the appropriate steps to control it.

5. What are some signs and symptoms of trauma to the thorax that would require you to activate the emergency action plan and immediately refer the athlete to emergency medical services?

6. What local and systemic signs and symptoms can be associated with thermal, chemical, and electrical burns?

Voices from the Field

During the first half of an away football game, an offensive lineman was struck in the left low back with a helmet while blocking for a running play. The athlete was removed from play and an evaluation was performed on the sideline by an athletic trainer. The initial evaluation revealed tenderness over the left low back region. The athlete showed no signs or symptoms of nausea, vomiting, pain with inspiration, or pain radiating into the lower extremities. The athlete was allowed to return to play. At halftime, a re-evaluation by the athletic trainer produced signs and symptoms of a contusion to the left low back. The athlete was fitted with a protective pad and allowed to finish the game without further injury or development of signs and symptoms of serious trauma.

After returning to campus, 24 hours after injury, the athlete noticed a small amount of blood in his urine. An evaluation by the athletic trainer noted that the tenderness over the left low back area had significantly increased. The athlete was immediately referred to team physicians for further evaluation. Plain radiographs were negative. Further diagnostic imaging demonstrated a left kidney contusion. Urinalysis revealed slightly elevated levels of blood in the urine. Four days after the injury, ecchymosis was present over the area, extending distally into the buttocks and proximally into the torso. The athlete was restricted from all activity.

A follow-up urinalysis 6 days after the injury was normal. Seven days after the injury, the athlete was allowed to participate in a game without injury or complications. Nine days after the injury, an evaluation by team physicians revealed a resolving hematoma and ecchymosis at the point of impact with mild induration of the surrounding tissue. Urinalysis was negative.

The absence of signs and symptoms initially highlights the importance of monitoring the condition of the athlete. Early recognition and prompt evaluation of the subsequent kidney contusion allowed the athlete to return to play the following week without associated trauma.

Doug Frye, BS, LAT, ATC
Head Athletic Trainer
Jacksonville University
Jacksonville, Florida

Trauma to soft tissue structures may involve the skin, muscles, tendons, ligaments, and organs. The majority of injuries to these structures do not result in an emergency event but require proper assessment and management to lessen further complications. Injuries that are potentially life-threatening require activation of the emergency action plan (EAP).

OPEN AND CLOSED WOUNDS

Soft tissue injuries are classified as open or closed wounds. An open wound is a break or tear in the skin involving the epidermis, dermis, and/or subcutaneous tissues. Open wounds include abrasions, avulsions, blisters, incisions, lacerations, and punctures. Abrasions are caused by a shear force against a rough surface (concrete, artificial grass, or dirt), commonly in one direction. Avulsions are due to a tearing force, with the removal of skin and/or soft tissue from its normal anatomical location. Blisters are caused by uni- or multidirectional shear forces with the presence of moisture; they lead to the collection of fluid between the epidermis and dermis. Incisions result from a sharp tensile force, producing a clean or regular break in the skin. Lacerations are caused by the application of tension and shear, resulting in an irregular tear in the skin. Punctures result from tensile loading and penetration of a sharp object into the skin.

A closed wound is described as an injury to soft tissues without the presence of a break or tear in the skin; closed wounds include contusions, lacerations, ruptures, and hematomas. Contusions are the result of a blunt force and cause hemorrhage underneath the skin. Closed lacerations and ruptures are caused by direct trauma, producing tension and shear to the soft tissues. A hematoma results from a blunt force, causing a localized collection or pooling of blood within the soft tissues.

Signs and Symptoms of Soft Tissue Injuries

The signs and symptoms of soft tissue injuries depend on the severity of trauma and the open or closed nature of the wound. Open wounds have an acute onset with pain typically concentrated around the area of damaged skin. Trauma to surrounding soft tissue may produce other areas of pain. Observation may reveal erythema; external hemorrhage; **denuded,** scraped, or torn skin or soft tissue; debris in the wound bed; and shock. The level of pain and amount of hemorrhage will depend on the depth of tissue involvement, with deeper wounds producing greater levels of pain and bleeding. The athlete's passive and active range of motion may be limited by pain when there are open wounds over joints such as the knee and elbow and when inappropriate dressing techniques have been used.

Closed wounds also have an acute onset, with localized pain over the trauma site. Referred pain may also be present. Observation may demonstrate ecchymosis and swelling over the site, unresponsiveness, shock, nausea, vomiting, abnormal vital signs, and difficulty breathing. Internal hemorrhaging may be present but requires advanced diagnostic testing for proper evaluation. Passive and active range of motion can be affected by pain, internal hemorrhage, and shock.

Assessment of Soft Tissue Injuries

Assessment of soft tissue injuries is conducted through primary and secondary surveys; most are performed on-field during practices and competitions. The primary survey serves to identify life-threatening trauma, which can be present with some open and closed wounds. Assessment of cardiovascular and respiratory systems, the head and spinal column, excessive or uncontrolled hemorrhage, fractures, dislocations, nerve injury, and other soft tissue trauma should be performed initially.[1]

If a life-threatening injury does not exist, a secondary survey should be conducted to determine the extent of soft tissue damage. The survey should include a history, inspection, and palpation as well as range-of-motion and neurological testing.[1] With the majority of soft tissue injuries, the athlete will remain conscious, and a history can be obtained without complications. Questions regarding the mechanism of injury, location of pain, presence of numbness or tingling, and sensations or sounds felt or heard upon receipt of the injury can indicate the level of tissue damage and associated trauma. A bilateral inspection should be performed to assess the integrity and color of the skin, swelling and deformity of soft tissue, hemorrhage, and presence of debris in an open wound. External hemorrhage is likely with open wounds and is categorized as capillary, venous, or arterial. Superficial abrasions demonstrate capillary bleeding with oozing and bright red blood. Venous bleeding is dark red, with a steady flow; it is seen with lacerations, incisions, and avulsions. Severe lacerations and avulsions can produce arterial bleeding with bright red blood in a squirting flow. Capillary, venous, and arterial bleeding is present with most closed wounds but cannot be assessed visually. Deformities such as flaps of skin, cavities, and complete removal of soft tissue may be present with avulsions, blisters, incisions, and lacerations. Debris and contaminants in open wounds may lead to infection and should be removed through proper management techniques.[2,3] Palpation of soft tissues for swelling and location of pain can indicate a closed wound. Direct contact with the surface or bed of an open wound should be avoided. Range-of-motion testing of the affected extremity with active, passive, and resistive methods and functional testing will indicate the readiness level of the athlete to return to play. Testing of neurological status is imperative with severe open and closed wounds to determine trauma to nerves, nerve roots, and the central nervous system.

Central Emergency Care

Care for open and closed soft tissue injuries should be performed with techniques guided by universal precautions. Many techniques are performed on-field whereas others require either a **clean** or sterile environment.

Management of open soft tissue injuries focuses on the immediate and follow-up care of the wound and surrounding tissues. Immediate care is performed on-field or in an athletic training facility and includes control of hemorrhage, cleansing, debridement, dressing of the wound, and possible treatment for shock. See Chapter 13 for information about the management and treatment of shock. When on-field treatment is performed, additional care is required after practice or competition in the athletic training facility or medical facility, with referral as needed. Follow-up care consists of daily assessments to determine dressing integrity and possible development of adverse reactions and wound infection.

General cleansing, debridement, and dressing techniques can be used with most open wounds. These techniques are performed using universal precautions.

Cleansing

Cleansing is the delivery of a solution or fluid to the wound surface by a mechanical force to remove foreign bodies/debris, excess exudate, and dressing residue as well as to reduce bacterial counts and rehydrate the wound.[5] Among the cleansing techniques of whirlpool baths, soaks, scrubbing, swabbing, and irrigation, irrigation is preferred. Irrigation

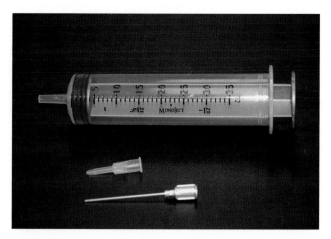

FIGURE 14.1   35-mL syringe, 19-gauge plastic cannula, and needle hub.

has been shown to achieve the general purposes of cleansing without damaging granulation and epithelial tissues.[6] Irrigation should be delivered to the wound bed between 4 and 15 pounds per square inch (psi); 8 psi is optimal.[7] A 35-mL syringe with a 19-gauge needle hub, plastic cannula, or angiocatheter delivers a solution/fluid of around 8 psi (Fig. 14.1).

Cleansing solutions should be nontoxic to tissues, reduce microorganisms, and remain active with organic material; they should also be nonallergenic, widely available, and cost-effective.[8] Sterile 0.9% saline and potable tap water have been shown to be completely safe for use on most open wounds.[9] Povidone–iodine, acetic acid, hydrogen peroxide, and sodium hypochlorite (Dakin's solution) are **cytotoxic** to human fibroblasts and macrophages and should not be used for cleansing the wound bed.[7] However, these solutions can be used to cleanse **periwound** tissues. The solution used for cleansing should be delivered to the wound bed at body temperature (98.6°F or 37°C) because cooler temperatures can slow physiological processes and delay healing.[10]

Begin cleansing the wound by placing the athlete in a seated, supine, or prone position on a table. Prepare the area with towels to catch excess body fluids and irrigation drainage. Fill the syringe with saline or tap water. Aim the syringe at the wound bed from a distance of 4 to 6 in. and depress the plunger (Fig. 14.2). Move the syringe back and forth over the wound or concentrate the irrigation over debris. Place a cupped, gloved hand above the wound bed to lessen splash-back from the irrigation stream. Continue to refill the syringe and irrigate the wound until all debris is removed. Cleanse the periwound tissues by irrigating or swabbing the area with sterile gauze. Do not touch the wound bed with the gauze. Dispose of and clean supplies and equipment following Occupational Safety and Health Administration (OSHA) standards. Wounds that are clean,

Breakout

Universal Precautions

- Wash hands with soap and water or alcohol-based gel prior to gloving.
- Use latex or nonlatex gloves at all times.
- Use of eye/face protection, mask, and gown during irrigation.
- Dispose of all contaminated supplies (disposable and sharp) in compliance with OSHA standards.[4]
- Disinfect all nonliving surfaces with appropriate cleansers following manufacturers' guidelines.
- Wash all reusable supplies with appropriate solutions and at appropriate temperatures in compliance with OSHA standards.[4]
- Wash hands following cleansing, debridement, and dressing techniques.

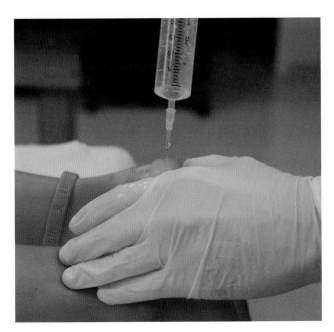

FIGURE 14.2   Irrigation of wound.

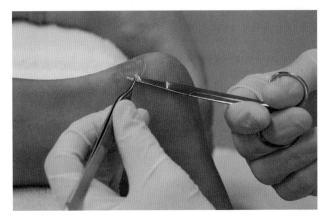

FIGURE 14.3   Sharp debridement of a blister.

granulating, and have minimal exudate can be damaged by daily, routine, or ritualistic cleansing.

Debridement

Debridement is the removal of materials from the wound bed until only normal, soft, and well-vascularized tissue is present, thus reducing bacterial growth and promoting healing.[11] Irrigation is an effective form of debridement and is sufficient for most open wounds. Autolytic debridement is the softening and digesting of necrotic/devitalized tissue and waste by the body through the action of neutrophils, lymphocytes, and macrophages in a moist environment under semiocclusive and occlusive dressings. **Sharp debridement** is necessary with other wounds, such as blisters, to remove necrotic/devitalized tissue still attached to the body.[11] With sterile instruments, sharp debridement involves the removal of nonviable tissue along the border between viable and nonviable tissues, stopping if bleeding occurs (Fig. 14.3). Nonviable, nonbleeding tissue serves as a culture medium for bacteria and requires removal as soon as possible. Prior to performing sharp debridement on athletes, athletic trainers should review applicable state practice acts to determine approval.

Dressings

Dressing is the application of materials to a wound surface to maintain an optimal (clean and moist) environment that will promote healing, reduce pain, prevent contamination and infection, contain exudate, and provide mechanical protection. The choice of a dressing is based on the type of wound and goals of the dressing. The ideal dressing should maintain high humidity at the wound–dressing interface, remove excess exudate, allow for gaseous exchange, provide thermal insulation, be impermeable to bacteria, and be free of particles, fibers, or toxic contaminants. It should allow dressing changes without additional trauma as well as being sterile, nontoxic, nonallergenic, and nonadherent; it should also remain physically strong in both dry and wet conditions.[12] Overall, three categories of dressings are available for open wounds: woven, skin tapes, and semiocclusive/occlusive.

Woven dressings, such as sterile gauze and nonadherent pads, should not be applied directly to the wound bed but can be used as secondary dressings.[13] Skin tapes are used with superficial, linear lacerations and incisions in areas of minimal static and dynamic tension, such as the face and scalp. Skill 14.1 details application guidelines for skin tape.

Semiocclusive and occlusive dressings—foams, films, hydrogels, hydrocolloids, and skin adhesives—provide a moist wound environment (Fig. 14.6). Research has demonstrated that wounds treated by occlusion heal more rapidly and are less painful, less likely to become infected, and less prone to cross-contamination.[14–16] Additional advantages of these dressings include fewer daily cleansing and dressing changes, waterproof construction, and increased compliance. Topical **antimicrobial** ointments can be used underneath semiocclusive and occlusive dressings, but they are not necessary.

Foams are used with partial- and full-thickness wounds; most require a secondary dressing such as a film to secure the foam to the wound bed. These dressings can remain on the wound bed from 3 to 7 days, requiring replacement when filled with exudate or with leakage from the secondary dressing. Films are appropriate for superficial and partial-thickness wounds and do not require a secondary dressing. Because these dressings are nonabsorbent, they should not be used with heavily draining wounds. Films can remain on the wound

SKILL 14.1

Skin Tape Application

1. Cleanse and débride the wound with irrigation, using saline or tap water, until all debris is removed (Fig. 14.2).
2. Cleanse the periwound tissues with irrigation, using saline or tap water or by scrubbing with moistened sterile gauze.
3. Dry the periwound tissues and lightly pat the wound with sterile gauze, avoiding the shedding of fibers.
4. Apply a thin coat of tape adhesive or tincture of benzoin along the outside of the wound so as to increase adherence of the strips.
5. Open the package and remove the strips.
6. Apply the strips individually or together as indicated on the package insert.
7. Anchor the strip(s) below the wound on the periwound tissues (Fig. 14.4).
8. **Approximate** the wound edges and pull the strip(s) with minimal tension across the wound.
9. Anchor the strip(s) on the periwound tissues above the wound (Fig. 14.5).
10. Continue to apply strips across the wound as described, approximately 3 mm apart, until approximation of the wound tissue is achieved.
11. Place a nonadherent sterile dressing over the strips and secure them.
12. Monitor daily for signs of infection and **dehiscence** (opening of the wound).
13. Leave the strips in place for a minimum of 5 to 7 days or until the strips have separated from the skin.

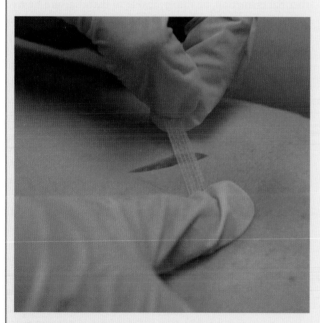

FIGURE 14.4   Initial anchor below the wound.

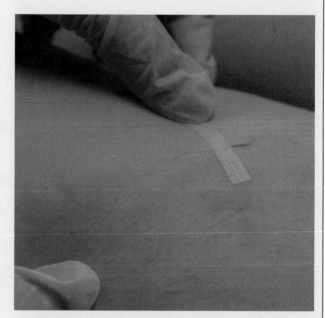

FIGURE 14.5   Anchor following tissue approximation.

bed up to 7 days if leakage does not occur, since leakage would compromise the occlusive barrier. Hydrogels are indicated for partial- and full-thickness wounds; some designs require a secondary dressing. Based on their high water content and subsequent drying, hydrogels can remain on the wound bed for only 3 days. These dressings should be changed when filled with exudate or with leakage. Hydrocolloids are used with superficial, partial-, and full-thickness wounds and can absorb moderate levels of exudate. The dressings can remain on the wound bed for up to 7 days, requiring changes only with leakage.

A secondary dressing is not required but will improve adherence to the periwound tissues. When treating open soft tissue injuries with easily approximated wound edges that occur in areas of low tension and stress, dermal adhesives may be used to replace standard wound closure devices (sutures, staples, adhesive strips, and skin tapes). Dermal adhesives can also be used in combination with subcutaneous sutures but cannot replace the latter. Sutures, staples, skin tapes, or dermal adhesives to close a wound should be used within 12 hours after injury to ensure proper healing and an acceptable cosmetic outcome.

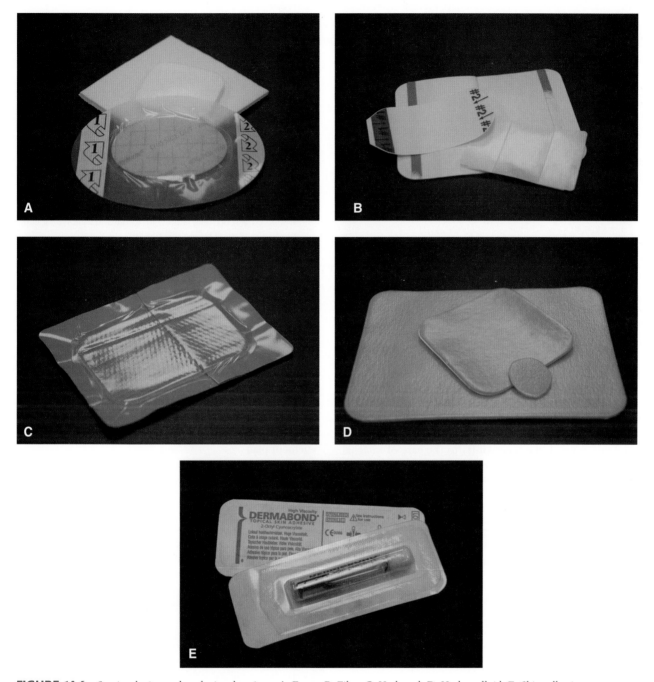

FIGURE 14.6 Semiocclusive and occlusive dressings. **A.** Foam. **B.** Film. **C.** Hydrogel. **D.** Hydrocolloid. **E.** Skin adhesive.

Skill 14.2 details the guidelines for the application of dermal adhesives.[17]

Referral and/or activation of the EAP for the treatment of open soft tissue injuries is necessary in several situations. In these cases, do not be concerned with a thorough cleansing, debridement, and dressing sequence; promptly cover the wound with sterile gauze, control bleeding, immobilize the body part, and refer. In some situations, activation of emergency medical services may be required. At a medical facility, further evaluation and treatment techniques may include cauterization or surgery to control bleeding as well as cleansing and debridement under general or local anesthesia; radiographs, magnetic resonance imaging, or computed tomography to locate embedded objects; deep and/or superficial suturing; application of staples, skin tapes, or dermal adhesives; surgical reattachment of tissue; advanced wound dressing techniques; administration of tetanus and/or antimicrobials; and admission for observation.

SKILL 14.2

Application of Dermal Adhesives

Refer to individual state practice acts for regulations regarding the use of dermal adhesives.

1. Cleanse and débride the wound with irrigation, using saline or tap water, until all debris is removed (Fig. 14.2).
2. Cleanse the periwound tissues with irrigation, using saline or tap water or by scrubbing with moistened sterile gauze.
3. Dry the periwound tissues and lightly pat the wound with sterile gauze, avoiding the shedding of fibers.
4. Remove the ampule from the package and crush it in the middle.
5. Gently squeeze the ampule to push the adhesive into the applicator tip.
6. Approximate the wound edges and apply a thin layer of adhesive with a gentle brushstroke onto the wound edges.

7. Apply a second layer after 15 to 20 seconds have elapsed.
8. Maintain tissue approximation throughout the application process and for 60 seconds following application of the final layer.
9. Maximal adhesion should be achieved at 2.5 minutes following application of the final layer.
10. A secondary dressing of sterile gauze or nonadherent pads can be applied when the adhesive is no longer tacky, normally 5 minutes after application.
11. Keep the wound dry until the adhesive has separated from the wound edges, normally after 5 to 10 days. Gentle washing of the site is allowed during this period.
12. Monitor daily for signs of infection and dehiscence.

Note: For a video demonstration of dermal adhesive application, see http://www.dermabond.com/product/how-it-works.html.

See Skills 14.3 through 14.7 for the management of abrasions, avulsions, blisters, incisions and lacerations, and punctures, respectively.

Management of closed soft tissue injuries should initially focus on the cardiovascular and respiratory systems and monitoring of vital signs. When management is established and normal, the focus shifts to the care of internal hemorrhage, inflammation, and pain in order to minimize the development of complications. Management of these injuries is conducted on-field, in the athletic training facility, and at medical facilities. The urgency of management techniques and referrals is based on the extent of trauma, the structures involved, and the overall condition of the athlete. Some closed wounds may be undetectable acutely; therefore, monitoring of the athlete is critical in the management plan.

Life-threatening closed wounds are managed with activation of the EAP, monitoring of vital signs (see Chapter 9),

Signs & Symptoms

Open Soft Tissue Injuries Requiring Referral

These include wounds involving the following:

- Uncontrolled external hemorrhage
- Moderate loss of soft tissue
- Heavy contamination
- Unsuccessful tissue approximation
- Unremovable embedded objects
- Lapse of tetanus immunization
- Deep wounds comprising subcutaneous tissue
- Presence of numbness or tingling
- Signs of infection (presence of abscess/pus, heat, edema, erythema, cellulitis, discharge [exudate with inflammation, seropurulence, hemopurulence, pus], delayed healing, discoloration, friable granulation tissue that bleeds easily, unexpected pain/tenderness, bridging of the epithelium or soft tissue, pocketing at the base of the wound, abnormal smell, and wound breakdown)[2,3] (Fig. 14.7).

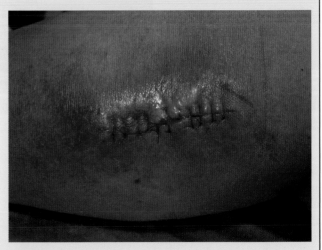

FIGURE 14.7 Infected postsurgical wound. (Courtesy of Stedman's/WoltersKluwer Health)

SKILL 14.3

Management of Abrasions

1. Cleanse and débride the wound with irrigation, using saline or tap water, until all debris is removed (Fig. 14.2).
2. Cleanse the periwound tissues with irrigation, using saline or tap water or by scrubbing with moistened sterile gauze.
3. Dry the periwound tissues with sterile gauze.
4. Dress the wound with a foam, film, hydrogel, or hydrocolloid based on wound depth and amount of exudate.

5. Center the dressing over the wound bed, leaving a minimum of 2 cm of the dressing extending from the wound margins on the periwound tissues (Fig. 14.8).
6. For athletes and active individuals, the application of Cover-Roll (BSN-Jobst, Inc., Charlotte, NC) over the dressing will further secure the dressing to the area (Fig. 14.9).
7. Monitor the wound and dressing daily for signs of infection and leakage.

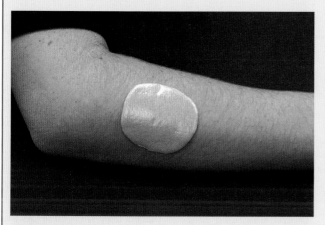

FIGURE 14.8   Abrasion dressed with hydrocolloid.

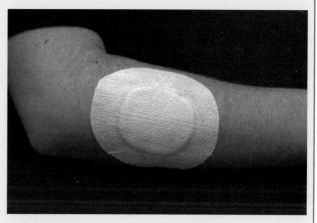

FIGURE 14.9   Application of Cover-Roll.

SKILL 14.4

Management of Avulsions

1. Cleanse and débride the wound with irrigation, using saline or tap water, until all debris is removed (Fig. 14.2).
2. Dress the wound with sterile gauze soaked in saline and wrap with additional gauze.

3. Gently irrigate completely avulsed tissue with saline. Wrap the tissue in saline-soaked gauze and place in a watertight bag. Place the bag into ice water or onto an ice bag. Do not allow direct contact of tissue with ice. Refer the athlete immediately along with the avulsed tissue.

SKILL 14.5

Management of Blisters

1. For a closed blister not affecting daily or athletic activities, place a hydrogel over the roof to reduce friction. A foam donut pad can also be used over the hydrogel for comfort. Cover with tape or Cover-Roll.
2. For a closed blister affecting daily/athletic activities, cleanse the roof and periwound tissues by scrubbing with sterile gauze soaked with povidone–iodine.
3. Make a small incision in the roof with a sharp, sterile instrument and allow the blister to drain. Refer to individual state practice acts for regulations regarding the use of this technique.
4. Remove the roof through sharp debridement (Fig. 14.3).
5. Cleanse the wound bed with saline or tap-water irrigation (Fig. 14.2).

6. Dry the periwound tissues with gauze.
7. Dress the wound with a film, hydrogel, or hydrocolloid, depending on wound depth and exudate.
8. Center the dressing on the wound bed and extend it onto the periwound tissues by 2 cm.
9. For athletes and active individuals, apply Cover-Roll to secure the dressing.
10. For an open blister, débride the roof and cleanse with irrigation.
11. Dry the periwound tissues.
12. Dress the wound with a film, hydrogel, or hydrocolloid.
13. Protect the blister and lessen friction by placing a hydrogel over the dressing. A foam donut pad can also be used.
14. Monitor daily for signs of infection and leakage.

SKILL 14.6

Management of Incisions and Lacerations

1. Cleanse and débride the wound with irrigation, using saline or tap water, until all debris is removed (Fig. 14.2).
2. Cleanse the periwound tissues with irrigation, using saline or tap water or by scrubbing with moistened sterile gauze.
3. Dry the periwound tissues and lightly pat the wound with sterile gauze, avoiding the shedding of fibers.
4. Based on wound depth and location, approximate wound edges and apply skin tape (Skill 14.1) or dermal adhesive (Skill 14.2).
5. Monitor the wound daily for infection and dehiscence.
6. Refer the athlete if venous or arterial bleeding cannot be controlled, tissue approximation cannot be achieved based on wound length or depth, or the wound is heavily contaminated.

and treatment for shock (see Chapter 13); these steps may include cardiorespiratory resuscitation (CPR), use of an automatic external defibrillator (AED), rescue breathing techniques (see Chapter 10), and control of hemorrhage. Further evaluation and treatment is conducted at the medical facility, and hospitalization is common. Management of non–life-threatening closed wounds may include the application of ice and compression, treatment for shock, and monitoring of vital signs.

External and internal hemorrhage accompanies soft tissue injuries. External hemorrhage stems from open wounds, and the amount and flow varies based on the depth of tissue trauma. External hemorrhage is controlled by direct pressure on the wound, elevation of the wound and/or body part, and pressure over points throughout the body. Internal hemorrhage stems from closed wounds and cannot be detected without diagnostic testing. Hemorrhage from some closed wounds, such as a contusion, can be controlled with compression. However, because internal hemorrhaging is not immediately recognized in most cases, other techniques are not performed.

Direct pressure entails placing sterile gauze directly over the wound with a gloved hand; then firm pressure is applied against the soft tissue and bone. Bleeding should stop within minutes with most wounds. If bleeding continues, additional gauze is placed over the gauze on the

SKILL 14.7

Management of Punctures

1. Observe the wound. If the embedded object is large and intact or broken off in the wound, apply sterile gauze around the object (Fig. 14.10). Next, immobilize the object and/or joint and refer.
2. If the embedded object is small and can be located visually, remove the object with sterile instruments. Use caution to avoid pushing the object deeper into the cavity.
3. Allow bleeding to occur, as this can serve to cleanse the wound. However, apply compression immediately to control venous or arterial bleeding.
4. Cleanse the wound and periwound tissues by irrigating it with saline or tap water (Fig. 14.2). Use caution to avoid forceful irrigation of the solution into the wound, which can push debris and contaminants into the cavity.
5. Dress the wound with sterile gauze, film, or hydrocolloid. Wounds with large cavities will require advanced dressings and follow-up care.
6. Based on the uncertainty of debris and contaminants in the cavity, closely monitor the wound daily for signs of infection.
7. Check to determine tetanus immunization. A lapse of 5 years since last tetanus booster requires referral to obtain immunization.[18]

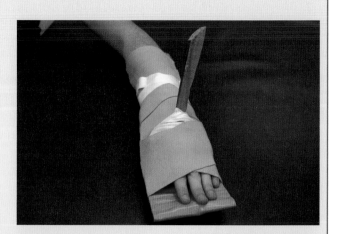

FIGURE 14.10   Dressing of a puncture wound with embedded object.

wound and continued pressure is applied. Elevation of the involved body part aids in the control of external and internal hemorrhage with the help of gravity. Elevation and direct pressure, used together, should control most cases of external hemorrhage. Pressure points, areas of the body in which a large artery is located superficially over a bone, are used for uncontrolled external hemorrhage. Apply firm pressure on the artery with the tips of the fingers or heel of the hand against the underlying bone. Pressure points can also be used with direct pressure and elevation. There are 11 such points, located over the mandible (facial artery), behind the clavicle (subclavian), at the medial upper arm (brachial), on the distal forearm at the wrist (radial and ulnar), at the midgroin (iliac), at the anterior and posterior distal lower leg (anterior and posterior tibial), on the temple (superficial temporal) and the anterior neck (common carotid), and at the cubital fossa (brachial), medial proximal thigh (femoral), and popliteal space (popliteal)[19] (Fig. 14.11).

Open and closed soft tissue injuries may lead to shock due to blood loss from external and internal hemorrhage, severe pain, excessive movement of the affected body part/area, and psychological reactions to trauma. Evaluation and monitoring for signs and symptoms of shock should be performed with all soft tissue injuries (see Chapter 13). Management techniques include maintaining the

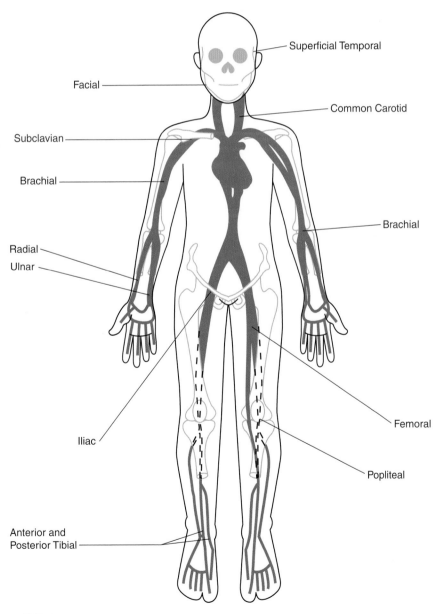

FIGURE 14.11 Pressure points.

cardiovascular and respiratory systems, controlling hemorrhage, maintaining body temperature, monitoring of vital signs, and—with wounds not involving the head and neck—elevating the lower extremities 8 to 12 in. In the case of wounds involving the head and neck, the head and neck are elevated.

ASSESSMENT AND MANAGEMENT OF SOFT TISSUE INJURIES

Open and closed soft tissue trauma can occur in any region of the body. When injuries are sustained, emergency assessment and management techniques are critical. This section details specific injuries to various body areas and discusses additional assessment and management techniques that are utilized after a history is obtained.

Face

Lacerations to the face are frequent and produce varying amounts of external hemorrhage (Fig. 14.12). After controlling the hemorrhage, assess the area for associated trauma (fracture) and the wound for severity (depth) and debris. Brain trauma can accompany facial lacerations and should be suspected and further evaluated. Cleanse and débride the wound with saline or tap water irrigation. Close the wound with skin tape (Skill 14.1) or dermal adhesive (Skill 14.2) in order to approximate the edges of the torn tissue. Although not required, the wound may be covered with nonadherent or sterile gauze pads and secured with Cover-Roll. With uncontrolled hemorrhage, unsuccessful tissue approximation, embedded objects, or other trauma, dress the wound with sterile gauze and activate the EAP or immediately

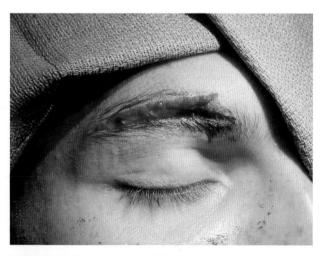

FIGURE 14.12 Laceration of the eyebrow.

refer the athlete. Cosmetic outcomes should be considered with all facial lacerations and should guide management techniques.

Human bite wounds to the facial area require a thorough assessment focusing on functional and cosmetic outcomes and the potential for infection.[20] Contamination with oral **flora** is present with these wounds and copious saline or tap water irrigation, minimal debridement, and tetanus prophylaxis are recommended.[21,22] Following cleansing and debridement, dressing techniques similar to those provided for abrasions (Skill 14.3) and lacerations (Skill 14.6) may be implemented.

In the treatment of facial bite wounds, the use of prophylactic antibiotic therapy has demonstrated no significant decrease in the incidence of infection.[23,24]

Oral Cavity and Lip

Lacerations to the oral cavity and lips will produce heavy external hemorrhage, but they heal faster than open wounds on the extremities and trunk. Excessive or uncontrolled hemorrhage from oral cavity trauma can compromise the airway, producing a life-threatening situation. Additionally, swelling of the tongue can be great in the first 48 hours after trauma and may affect the airway.[25] Control hemorrhage and carefully inspect the oral cavity and lips for pieces of teeth and other debris.[25] Cleanse and irrigate the oral cavity and lips with copious amounts of saline or tap water. Generally, small lacerations of the oral cavity do not require referral for closure or use of a dressing. Lacerations to the mucosa that interfere with the occlusal surfaces of the teeth and are deep enough to trap food particles require referral for advanced closure techniques.[25] Tongue lacerations with uncontrolled hemorrhage, flaps of tissue, or trauma to the edges or completely through the tongue should be referred for repair. Lip lacerations pose a cosmetic concern and require referral for advanced closure techniques. Following management of oral cavity and lip lacerations, including suturing, no dressing is required.

Nose

Epistaxis, or nasal hemorrhage, is a common injury normally managed with conservative techniques. However, uncontrolled hemorrhage through blood loss and pooling of blood can create a life-threatening event, potentially compromising the airway. Assessment includes visual inspection and palpation to rule out associated trauma (fracture). Saline or tap water irrigation of the nasal cavity can be used if necessary. Hemorrhage results from trauma to the anterior (referred to as **Kiesselbach's plexus** or **Little's area),** posterior, or superior nasal cavities. Most injuries occur from trauma to the anterior cavity. Skill 14.8 describes the management of epistaxis.

SKILL 14.8

Management of Epistaxis

1. Typically, the hemorrhage is self-limiting or controlled with application of direct pressure to the septal area for a minimum of 5 minutes.[26] Tilt the head forward to prevent pooling of blood within the pharynx.
2. Ice placed over the nose will assist in the control of hemorrhage.
3. Nasal packing with a commercially available nasal tampon can also be used to control hemorrhage. Lubricate the tampon as directed with sterile water, petroleum jelly, or antibiotic ointment to minimize pain during insertion.[26] Some designs allow for air inflation of a cuff to provide pressure on the damaged vessel.
4. If these techniques are unsuccessful, continue with direct pressure, ice, or nasal packing; activate the EAP; and refer the athlete immediately.

Throat and Neck

Trauma of the throat and neck can result in both open and closed soft tissue injury, frequently including contusions and lacerations. Such wounds in this area often involve damage to the trachea, jugular veins, carotid arteries, laryngeal nerves, esophagus, and cervical spine.[27] Assessment begins with inspection and observation for an open airway, breathing and speech patterns, hemorrhage, and associated trauma. Presence of an obstructed airway, respiratory distress, dyspnea, change in voice quality (hoarseness or loss of voice), inability to swallow, coughing, blood from the throat, laryngospasm, severe pain or swelling, uncontrolled hemorrhage, deformity of cricoid and thyroid cartilage, or suspicion of cervical spine trauma can be life threatening and signals activation of the EAP and immediate referral for further evaluation and treatment.[27,28] In these situations, establish an airway; initiate CPR, AED, and/or rescue breathing; control hemorrhage; monitor vital signs and watch for signs of shock; and, in the case of a possible cervical spine injury, provide in-line stabilization (see Chapter 13). In the absence of a life-threatening situation, manage a contusion or laceration of the throat and neck as described in Skill 14.9.

Eye

Although the majority of eye and orbit injuries encountered are mild, vision-threatening trauma can occur and be hidden or undetectable on the field and/or in the athletic training facility. Open and closed soft tissue trauma may include orbital hematoma, eyelid laceration, corneal abrasion and laceration, hyphema, globe rupture, and detached retina (Fig. 14.13). These injuries require careful, immediate assessment and management and, when warranted, referral to an ophthalmologist. If external hemorrhage is present, control it with direct pressure and remove glasses or contact lenses (Skill 14.10).

Inspect the periorbital area for swelling, discoloration, lacerations, and fractures and the globe and eyelid for swelling, lacerations, discoloration, and debris. Palpate the orbital area and eyelid for the presence of deformity and swelling. Assess visual acuity using a Snellen chart, newspaper, or other print media. Hold the newspaper or newspaper-size print media (10- to 11-point size) approximately 14 in. away from the athlete's face.[29] Assess each eye individually and then both together. Have the athlete wear her or his glasses or contacts, if normally worn, during the evaluation. Check pupillary size and reactivity to light bilaterally. Assess eye motility by examining the tracking of both eyes in upward, downward, left, and right directions.[1] Neurological testing should include cranial nerves II (vision), III (pupillary size and reactivity, motility, and upper eyelid elevation), IV (motility), and VI (motility). If available, compare the findings from these assessments to baseline data from the preparticipation physical examination to determine

SKILL 14.9

Management of Throat/Neck Contusions and Lacerations

Contusion

1. Apply an ice pack over the area (with no compression).
2. Monitor vital signs.
3. Carefully observe for external swelling, which may indicate internal bleeding and additional trauma.[28]

Laceration

1. Cleanse and débride with saline or tap water irrigation (Fig. 14.2).
2. With tissue approximation in areas of minimal skin tension, close the wound with skin tape (Skill 14.1) or dermal adhesive (Skill 14.2).
3. Lacerations with heavy contamination, unsuccessful tissue approximation, embedded objects, or uncontrolled hemorrhage should be dressed with sterile gauze and referred.

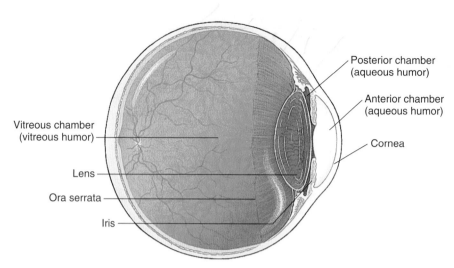

Posterior chamber
(aqueous humor)

Anterior chamber
(aqueous humor)

Cornea

Vitreous chamber
(vitreous humor)

Lens

Ora serrata

Iris

FIGURE 14.13 Sagittal section of the eye. (Courtesy of Anatomical Chart Co.)

abnormalities. The presence of several signs and symptoms indicates activation of the EAP and immediate referral. Cover the eye with sterile gauze and maintain direct pressure for external hemorrhage, avoiding application of pressure over the globe. Monitor vital signs and treat for shock.

Open soft tissue trauma may involve the eyelid and/ or cornea with abrasion and laceration injuries. Manage simple lacerations of the eyelid with control of hemorrhage, saline or tap water irrigation, wound closure with skin tape or dermal adhesive, or dress with sterile gauze and refer for possible suturing. Abrasions are managed as previously described. Tissue debridement is typically not performed, and shallow lacerations will heal properly without tissue approximation or dressing. Cosmetic outcomes should

---

SKILL 14.10

Removal of Contact Lenses

These steps can be performed by the athlete or with assistance from the athletic trainer.

1. If possible, place 1 or 2 drops of contact lens wetting solution or saline in the eyes.
2. Have the athlete look upward.
3. Pull the lower eyelid slightly down with a finger.

4. Place a fingertip on the inferior or bottom edge of the lens (Fig. 14.14A).
5. Gently move or slide the lens in a lateral/inferior direction.
6. Squeeze the lens between two fingers and remove it from the eye (Fig. 14.14B).
7. Inspect the eye for pieces of torn lens and remove them if present by irrigating with saline solution.

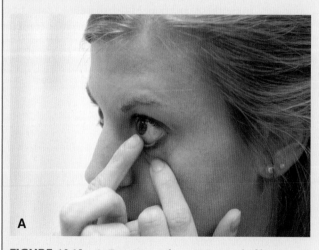

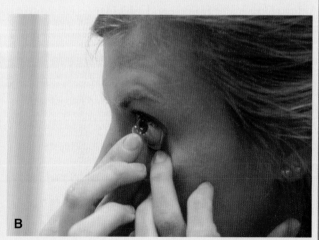

FIGURE 14.14 **A.** Fingertip on lens. **B.** Removal of lens.

Signs & Symptoms

Signs and Symptoms of Eye Trauma Requiring Referral

- Uncontrolled hemorrhage
- Severe pain
- Bony deformity
- Severe eyelid laceration
- Loss of vision
- **Diplopia**
- Blurred vision
- **Photophobia**
- **Floaters**
- Loss or restriction of eye range of motion
- Visible discoloration or defect of globe
- Unequal/irregular pupil size and/or reactivity
- Loss of active eyelid elevation
- Debris in/on the globe

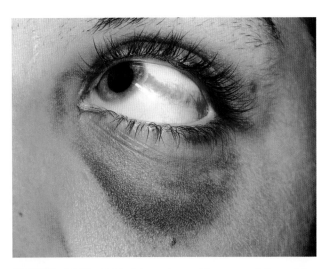

FIGURE 14.16 Orbital hematoma. (Courtesy of Dean John Bonsall, MD, FACS.)

guide management and return-to-play decisions. **Complex lacerations** require immediate referral and, in some situations, activation of the EAP (Fig. 14.15). Excessive blunt or penetrating trauma causing the laceration can mask more serious injury to the globe. Lacerations of the lid margin, lateral and medial canthal regions, and medial third of the lids can involve trauma to underlying structures.[28] Control hemorrhage, do not remove embedded objects, dress the wound with sterile gauze, and refer. Wound closure and follow-up techniques will influence the success of cosmetic and functional outcomes.

Trauma to the globe may result in closed soft tissue injuries such as orbital hematomas, hyphemas, detached retinas, and globe injuries. An **orbital hematoma** is managed with the application of ice to lessen internal hemorrhage, swelling, and pain (Fig. 14.16). Ice placed in a small plastic bag, clean latex glove, or English ice bag is applied over the area. For cold-sensitive athletes use ice water instead of ice. Lessen the recurrence of hemorrhage initially by instructing the athlete not to blow his or her nose. A **hyphema** can be initially undetectable and requires careful assessment[29] (Fig. 14.17). Over time, blood will flow into

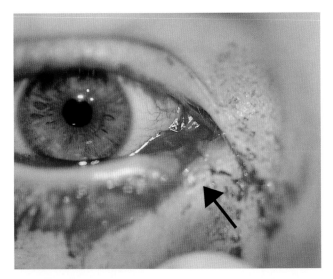

FIGURE 14.15 Laceration of the lacrimal duct. With gentle inferior traction, the full-thickness laceration and involvement of the area of the lacrimal duct become visible (*arrow*). (From Fleisher GR, Ludwig S, Baskin MN. *Atlas of Pediatric Emergency Medicine*. Philadelphia: Lippincott Williams & Wilkins; 2004.)

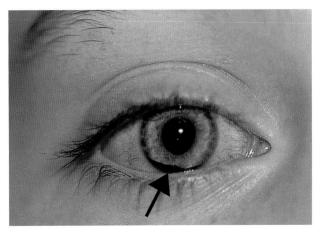

FIGURE 14.17 Hyphema. (Used with permission from Fleisher GR, Ludwig S, Baskin MN. *Atlas of Pediatric Emergency Medicine*. Philadelphia: Lippincott Williams & Wilkins; 2004:403.)

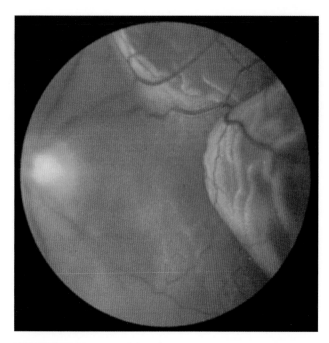

FIGURE 14.18   Retinal detachment.

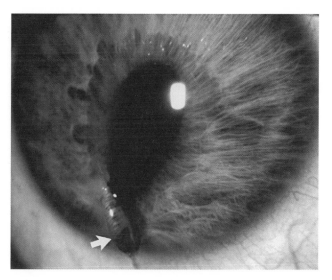

FIGURE 14.19   Elliptical/teardrop pupil. Note protrusion of iris (*arrow*). (From Fleisher GR. *Textbook of Pediatric Emergency Medicine*, 5th ed. Philadelphia: Lippincott Williams & Wilkins; 2005.)

the anterior chamber and become visible. Following assessment or with suspicion of this vision-threatening injury, manage the situation by activating the EAP and immediately referring the athlete to lessen additional trauma to the eye. Stabilize the athlete with the head elevated in a semireclining or seated position. An annual evaluation by an ophthalmologist to monitor for the development of **angle recession glaucoma** is recommended.[29]

Retinal tears and detachments resulting from trauma can be painless but are medical emergencies (Fig. 14.18). Assessment of the eye may reveal the presence of floaters, sudden loss of vision, bright flashes of light, or an expanding shadow or curtain over the field of vision.[29] Manage retinal injury with EAP activation and immediate referral. Eye patching or specific positioning of the athlete is not necessary. Excessive compression of the eye can cause a globe rupture, indicated by severe pain, by an elliptical or teardrop-shaped pupil[1] (Fig. 14.19), and possible hyphema. Manage this vision-threatening injury with activation of the EAP and immediate referral. Further evaluation by an ophthalmologist is warranted to rule out other closed trauma to the globe.

Corneal abrasions result from contact lenses, debris trapped under the eyelid, and external objects striking the cornea (Fig. 14.20). Assessment reveals a foreign-body sensation in the eye, photophobia, pain, and tearing of the eyes. Techniques to remove debris trapped under the eyelid are described in Skill 14.11. Most abrasions are not detected during initial assessment. The use of fluorescein strips and a cobalt-blue light will reveal the abrasion, changing the orange dye to a bright green color (Skill 14.12). Refer to individual state practice acts to determine use of fluorescein strips. Manage corneal abrasions by covering the eye with sterile gauze, avoiding compression on the globe, and refer-

ring the athlete to an ophthalmologist. Patching of the injured eye following diagnosis, once the standard of care, has been shown to have no effect on pain relief and healing rates and is no longer recommended for corneal abrasions.[30]

Because of rapid cell regeneration, recovery from superficial corneal abrasions is fairly brief. However, the use of contact lenses should be avoided until such an abrasion is healed.[29] Corneal lacerations are caused by direct trauma from external objects striking the cornea, producing defects of varying depth. Assess the cornea and pupil for evidence of discoloration, obvious laceration with extrusion or spilling of contents, or an elliptical or teardrop-shaped pupil. In the management of a laceration, do not attempt to cleanse or débride the wound. Dress the affected eye with sterile gauze and cover with a rigid shield

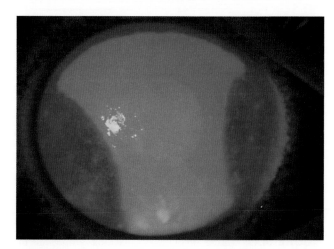

FIGURE 14.20   Large corneal abrasion indicated by cobalt-blue light following fluorescein instillation. (From Tasman W, Jaeger E. *The Wills Eye Hospital Atlas of Clinical Ophthalmology*, 2nd ed. Philadelphia: Lippincott Williams & Wilkins; 2001.)

SKILL 14.11

Removal of Debris under the Eyelid

Lower Eyelid

1. Have the athlete look upward.
2. Gently depress or pull the lower eyelid downward.
3. Remove debris with a saline-soaked sterile gauze pad or cotton tipped applicator (Fig. 14.21).
4. Release the eyelid and irrigate the eye with saline solution.

Upper Eyelid

1. Cleanse the surface of the lower eyelid with saline solution.
2. Have the athlete look downward.
3. Gently pull the upper eyelid downward onto the surface of the lower eyelid (Fig. 14.22).
4. Inspect the surface of the lower eyelid for debris and remove it.
5. If unsuccessful with removal, gently pull the upper eyelid downward.
6. Place a cotton-tipped applicator across the upper eyelid.
7. Pull the upper eyelid upward against and over the applicator (Fig. 14.23).

8. Have the athlete look downward.
9. Locate the debris and remove it with saline-soaked gauze or another applicator.
10. Release the eyelid and irrigate the eye with saline solution.

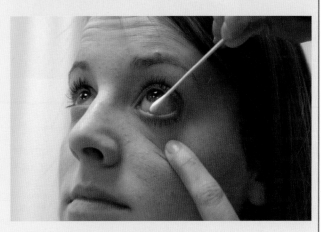

FIGURE 14.21   Removal of lower eyelid debris.

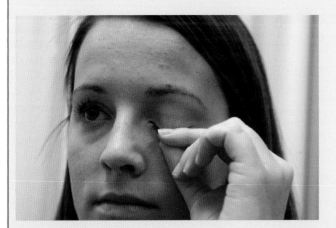

FIGURE 14.22   Upper eyelid on lower eyelid.

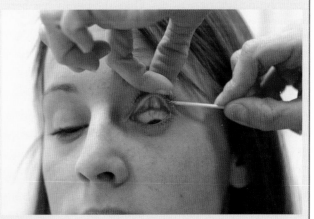

FIGURE 14.23   Upper eyelid over applicator.

SKILL 14.12

Use of Fluorescein Strips

1. Place the athlete in a seated or supine position.
2. Remove a fluorescein strip and soak it with saline solution.
3. Lightly touch the end of the strip to the conjunctiva of the lower eyelid, avoiding direct contact with the cornea.
4. Have the athlete open and close the eye several times.
5. With the lights turned off, illuminate the eye with a cobalt-blue light.
6. Abrasions will be illuminated with a bright green color (Fig. 14.24).

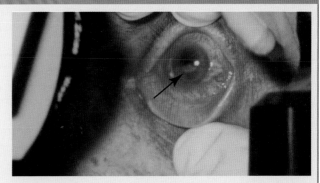

FIGURE 14.24   Green color on cornea, demonstrating abrasion. (From Berg D, Worzala K. *Atlas of Adult Physical Diagnosis.* Philadelphia: Lippincott Williams & Wilkins; 2006.)

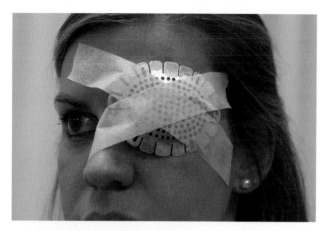

FIGURE 14.25   Shielding of the eye.

(Fig. 14.25), avoiding compression over the eye. Activate the EAP and refer immediately, keeping the athlete in a semireclining or seated position.

Ear

Open soft tissue injuries of the external and internal ear can occur during athletic activities. Once the history has been obtained, inspect the auricle for swelling, discoloration, hemorrhage, or soft tissue defects. Using an otoscope, inspect the tympanic membrane for perforations and the auditory canal for fluid (Skill 14.13). Palpate the external ear for swelling and other defects. Assess hearing and balance for deficits. Findings of uncontrolled hemorrhage, large soft tissue avulsion, excessive swelling, sudden pain or popping in the ear, perforations in the tympanic membrane, fluid in the auditory canal, loss of hearing that lasts longer than 1 hour after injury, and balance deficits require EAP activation and immediate referral. In some cases, brain trauma may be associated and further evaluation is warranted. Establish an airway, control hemorrhage, monitor vital signs, treat for

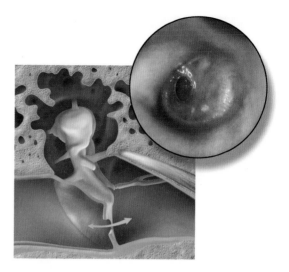

Perforation
• A hole in the tympanic membrane caused by chronic negative middle ear pressure, inflammation, or trauma

FIGURE 14.27   Tympanic membrane rupture. (Courtesy of Anatomical Chart Co.)

shock, and—with suspected brain trauma—provide in-line stabilization.

Tympanic membrane ruptures present with visible perforations of the membrane, pain following a popping in the ear, loss of hearing, and possible fluid in the auditory canal (Fig. 14.27). Manage a suspected rupture with immediate referral of the athlete to a physician. *Do not* attempt to cleanse the auditory canal or apply a dressing. Small perforations will heal without further treatment, whereas larger perforations may require surgery. Manage laceration and avulsion injuries to the ear using the same techniques as for other parts of the body. Control hemorrhage and cleanse, débride, and dress the wound as needed. Refer the athlete with uncontrolled hemorrhage, unsuccessful tissue approximation, or completely avulsed

SKILL 14.13

Use of the Otoscope

1. Place the athlete in a seated position.
2. Insert a clean speculum on the otoscope.
3. Place the end of the otoscope partially into the external auditory canal.
4. Continue to insert the otoscope into the canal with either a downward pull on the earlobe or an upward pull on the superior ear.
5. Move forward to view the auditory canal and tympanic membrane (Fig. 14.26).

Note: For an otoscopy tutorial and additional photographs of injuries to the ear, see http://www.bris.ac.uk/Depts/ENT/otoscopy_tutorial.htm.

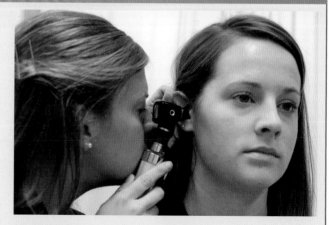

FIGURE 14.26   Otoscopic evaluation.

tissue. Closure techniques should be planned with a view to cosmetic outcome.

Thorax

Open and closed soft tissue injuries to the thorax commonly result from blunt trauma and may involve the lungs and heart. Injuries to the lungs, pneumothorax, or hemothorax; pulmonary contusion and asphyxia; and contusion of the heart, commotion cordis, and cardiac tamponade may be undetectable during initial assessment but can rapidly develop into life-threatening situations. Continual monitoring and reassessment of the athlete is recommended to identify and manage these conditions.

Inspect the thorax for structural abnormalities, external hemorrhage, and discoloration. The thorax and abdomen are divided into quadrants to guide assessment (Fig. 14.28). These quadrants represent areas of tenderness of the included structures. Assess heart and respiratory rate and blood pressure, observe breathing patterns, conduct **auscultation** of each lung, and palpate for deformity and swelling. Reevaluate vital signs and breathing patterns and sounds until emergency transportation or referral is completed. The signs and symptoms of injury that require EAP activation and immediate referral are shown in the box below. Prior to transportation, establish an airway, initiate CPR, AED,

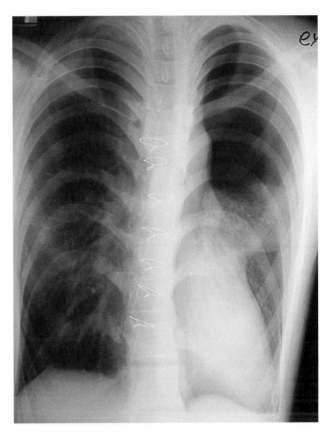

FIGURE 14.29 Radiograph of a large left pneumothorax. (From Fleisher GR, Ludwig S, Baskin MN. *Atlas of Pediatric Emergency Medicine*. Philadelphia: Lippincott Williams & Wilkins; 2004. Courtesy of Dr. Mark Waltzman.)

and/or rescue breathing, control hemorrhage, and monitor vital signs, being alert for signs of shock.

A pneumothorax is a collection of air in the pleural cavity leading to a partial or full collapse of the lung (Fig. 14.29). A spontaneous pneumothorax can occur

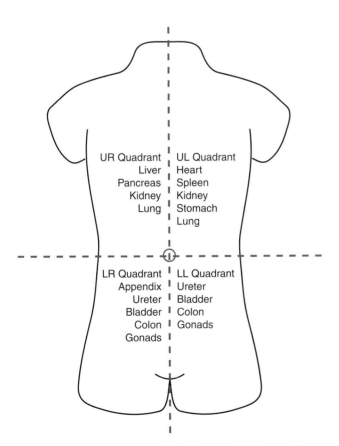

UR Quadrant	UL Quadrant
Liver	Heart
Pancreas	Spleen
Kidney	Kidney
Lung	Stomach
	Lung

LR Quadrant	LL Quadrant
Appendix	Ureter
Ureter	Bladder
Bladder	Colon
Colon	Gonads
Gonads	

FIGURE 14.28 Quadrants of the thorax and abdomen (relative to the athlete).

Signs & Symptoms

Thoracic Injuries Requiring Referral

- Gradual onset of pain
- Difficulty, pain, or absence of breathing
- Abnormal lung sounds (wheezes, stridor, crackles)

Note: For recordings of lung sounds see http://solutions.3 m.com/wps/portal/3M/en_US/Littmann/stethoscope/ education/heart-lung-sounds/

- Nausea
- Uncontrolled external hemorrhage
- Blood with coughing
- Deformity of trachea, larynx, or ribs
- Abnormalities in respiration rate, depth, or sounds, heart rate, or blood pressure
- Signs of shock

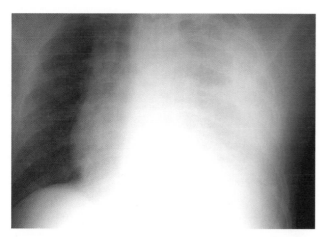

FIGURE 14.30 Radiograph of a massive left hemothorax. (From Harwood-Nuss A, Wolfson AB, et al. *The Clinical Practice of Emergency Medicine,* 3rd ed. Philadelphia: Lippincott Williams & Wilkins; 2001.)

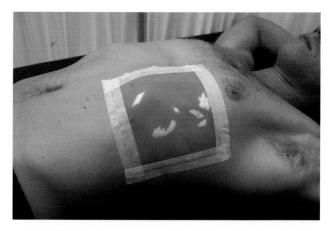

FIGURE 14.32 Initial treatment of pneumothorax.

from the rupture of **blebs,** direct trauma to the ribs, a penetrating puncture wound of the lung, abnormal breathing patterns during exercise, or disease. When air continues to enter the pleural cavity without escape, a tension pneumothorax can develop. The buildup of air and increase in pressure will collapse the involved lung and place pressure on the heart, vena cava, and uninvolved lung, compromising circulation. Direct trauma to the thorax causing a closed wound and internal hemorrhage can result in a hemothorax (Fig. 14.30), a collection of blood in the pleural cavity, pulmonary contusion (Fig. 14.31), collection of blood in the alveolar and interstitial spaces, or **asphyxia.** Assessment findings of a spontaneous or tension pneumothorax, hemothorax, pulmonary contusion, and asphyxia are summarized in the box below. Manage these conditions with EAP activation and prompt referral. Control external hemorrhage, administer rescue breathing and oxygen if needed,

monitor vital signs, and treat for shock. Manage an open pneumothorax by covering the opening with an occlusive dressing that provides a seal, thus preventing passage of air into the pleural cavity (Fig. 14.32). Secure the edges of the dressing with tape if needed. Do not attempt to remove an impaled object from an open wound.

Commotio cordis is a life-threatening heart condition resulting from a sudden, nonpenetrating blow to the anterior thorax on an otherwise healthy young athlete.[31] It is due to a blow that lands directly over the heart and that occurs just prior to the T-wave peak of the cardiac cycle, causing an arrhythmia (commonly ventricular fibrillation).[31]

At assessment, half of those who sustain this injury will immediately collapse without vital signs, whereas others

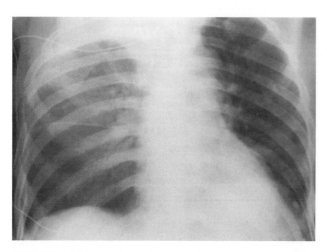

FIGURE 14.31 Radiograph of a right pulmonary contusion with edema. (From Eisenberg RL. *An Atlas of Differential Diagnosis,* 4th ed. Philadelphia: Lippincott Williams & Wilkins; 2003.)

Signs & Symptoms

Spontaneous or Tension Pneumothorax, Hemothorax, Pulmonary Contusion, and Asphyxia Requiring Referral

- Severe pain over the involved lung
- Difficulty of and/or pain with breathing
- Shortness of breath
- Rapid breathing
- Decreased or absent breath sounds
- Cyanosis
- Decrease in blood pressure
- Distention of neck veins
- Displacement of the trachea away from the side of direct trauma (tension pneumothorax)
- Frothy blood/sputum with coughing (hemothorax and pulmonary contusion)
- External hemorrhage (open pneumothorax)

may briefly perform an activity and then collapse. Manage commotio cordis with CPR/AED, monitor for shock, and activate the EAP. Successful outcomes, even with prompt CPR and AED, are rare.

Blunt or penetrating trauma to the anterior thorax can also cause cardiac tamponade, a laceration or rupture of cardiac tissue producing a flow of blood and edema in the pericardial space. With accumulation of the fluid and increased pressure, ventricular filling during diastole is reduced, which can eventually prove fatal. Assessment commonly reveals **Beck's triad,** or **acute compression,** demonstrated by distended neck veins (increased jugular venous pressure), weakness of the peripheral pulses (hypotension), and diminished heart sounds. Pulsus paradoxus, or paradoxical pulse, an abnormal (greater than 15 mm Hg) drop in systemic blood pressure during inspiration, will also be found. Management techniques should include CPR, AED, monitoring for shock, and activation of the EAP. CPR and AED techniques are often unsuccessful.

Crushing or compression trauma to the thorax may result in a myocardial or heart contusion as the heart is compressed between bony structures. The injury can cause damage or rupture of heart valves, chamber walls and tissues, internal hemorrhage, and arrhythmias. Assessment findings will include severe chest pain, shortness of breath, difficulty breathing, and an irregular cardiac rhythm. Initiate CPR, AED, and rescue breathing as needed. Activate the EAP and immediately refer the athlete.

Impalements

Impalement injuries are open soft tissue traumas caused by the penetration of an object into the body, commonly the abdomen or oral cavity. The penetrating object remains in the body and requires surgical excision. Assessment will demonstrate the obvious deformity and object penetration with accompanying external hemorrhage. Following activation of the EAP for immediate transport, maintain airway, breathing, and circulation (the ABCs), control external hemorrhage, and treat for shock. Provide in-line stabilization if needed. Do not attempt to remove, cut, or reposition the impaled object.[32] Movement or attempts at removal can result in massive hemorrhaging or breaking/splintering of the object, causing additional difficulties during surgical removal.[33] Apply sterile gauze around the impaled object and then immobilize it to lessen further trauma. Based on the high risk of contamination from oral flora and debris, tetanus prophylaxis and antibiotics are recommended.[33]

Abdomen

Abdominal trauma during athletic activities is rare but can be life-threatening when it occurs. Most injuries are the result of blunt trauma, producing open and closed soft tissue conditions such as contusions and lacerations involving the

Signs & Symptoms

Abdominal Injuries Requiring Referral

- Diffuse or localized quadrant pain
- Pain or difficulty breathing
- **Hematuria**
- Inability to urinate
- Uncontrolled external hemorrhage
- Abnormalities or absence of abdominal/bowel sounds
- Abnormal vital signs
- Rigidity of abdominal and/or back musculature
- Point or rebound tenderness in quadrants
- Abnormal percussion sounds
- Signs of shock

organs. Like trauma of the thorax, signs and symptoms of serious injury may not develop early and thus may not be detectable during the initial assessment.

Inspect the abdomen for pain, external hemorrhage, and discoloration over the upper right and left and lower right and left quadrants (Fig. 14.28). Assess vital signs and breathing patterns, auscultate the abdomen, palpate the quadrants for muscle tone and point and rebound tenderness, and perform percussions over the quadrants. Signs and symptoms that warrant EAP activation are listed in the box above. Manage these situations by maintaining the ABCs, controlling external hemorrhage with open lacerations and impalements, immobilizing impaled objects, and monitoring vital signs with the athlete in a supine position. *Do not allow the athlete to take anything by mouth, as this will reduce the chance of complications due to subsequent evaluation, treatment, and/or surgery.*

Blunt trauma to the abdomen can result in a contusion or laceration of the spleen, kidney, liver, ureter, bladder, urethra, or solar plexus. A contusion or laceration of the spleen may produce pain in the upper left quadrant and left shoulder (Kehr's sign), nausea, vomiting, signs of shock, and rebound tenderness as well as abdominal guarding from internal hemorrhage. The spleen has the ability to splint itself and control internal hemorrhage, which may hide signs and symptoms of trauma during the initial assessment. Systemic infections such as mononucleosis can enlarge the spleen and place the athlete at risk for trauma upon an aggressive return to activity. Evaluation by a physician prior to return is recommended.

Hematuria, nausea, vomiting, pain over the low back and upper right and left quadrants, contusion at the site of trauma, signs of shock, rigidity of the lower back musculature, and pain during inspiration can indicate a kidney contusion or laceration. Contusion or laceration of the liver may produce referred pain just inferior to the right scapula, pain in the upper right quadrant, signs of shock, and rebound tenderness and abdominal guarding with the presence of

SKILL 14.14

Management of Abdominal Trauma

1. Maintain the ABCs.
2. Monitor vital signs.

3. Monitor and treat for shock.
4. Activate EAP for referral.

internal hemorrhage. Some diseases, such as hepatitis, can inflame the liver and increase the risk of injury.

Trauma to the ureter, bladder, and urethra may produce general lower abdominal pain and tenderness, lower right and left quadrant pain, rigidity of the abdominal musculature, nausea, vomiting, and signs of shock. Bladder contusions and lacerations can include suprapubic and lower right and left quadrant pain, hematuria, and inability to urinate; it can be associated with pelvic fracture. Urethral trauma can present with gross hematuria, perineal pain, and leakage of blood from the urethra. Skill 14.14 describes management techniques for spleen, kidney, liver, ureter, bladder, and urethral trauma.

A contusion to the solar plexus (celiac plexus) and the resultant paralysis of the diaphragm causes an inability to inhale and visible fear and anxiety. Manage this temporary condition with airway assessment, loosening of tight clothing and equipment, and firm instructions to the athlete to "pant like a dog" and focus on long inspirations and short expirations.[1] After breathing is controlled, assess the abdomen for associated trauma and monitor vital signs.

Genitalia

Trauma to the genitalia is more common among males than females because of the external exposure of several structures. Direct trauma can cause a laceration, contusion, hematoma, or torsion injury. Assessment of these injuries should be conducted in a professional and discreet manner. Instructions and guidelines can be provided to the athlete for a self-assessment. Inspect the genitals for external hemorrhage, discoloration, and swelling (Fig. 14.33). Palpate the scrotum and testicles for tenderness, swelling, and sensation. Findings of uncontrolled external hemorrhage, inability to urinate, hematuria, swelling of the testicles and/or scrotum, persistent pain or an increase in pain, or abnormal sensation or position of the testicles requires immediate referral to a physician for further evaluation and treatment.

Open lacerations of the penis and scrotum will produce varying amounts of external hemorrhage. Control hemorrhage with direct pressure and cleanse the wound by irrigating it with saline or tap water. Dress the wound with a loosely applied nonadherent dressing or leave it uncovered. Blunt trauma to the scrotum can result in a testicular contusion, producing immediate pain and possible nausea, vomiting, and difficulty breathing. Several techniques have been illustrated in the literature to reduce pain, but there is little support for their use and effectiveness. These techniques include a sitting position with lift and drop, supine

position and knees to the chest, and kneeling position with bouncing. Manage a contusion with psychological support and reassurance to the athlete. Control swelling and pain with the application of an ice pack. Following a reduction in pain, the athlete can perform a self-assessment.

Blunt scrotal trauma may also result in the accumulation of fluid in the tunica vaginalis (hydrocele), rupture of enlarged spermatic cord veins (varicocele), or accumulation of blood in the scrotum (hematocele). These conditions produce pain and swelling of the scrotum and obvious abnormalities on palpation. Seek immediate referral to lessen the risk of permanent damage to the testicle. Torsion of the spermatic cord due to traumatic or structural abnormalities can occur and will produce intense pain and tenderness, nausea, swelling of the scrotum, and possible vomiting. Manage this situation with immediate referral to prevent potential loss of the testicle.

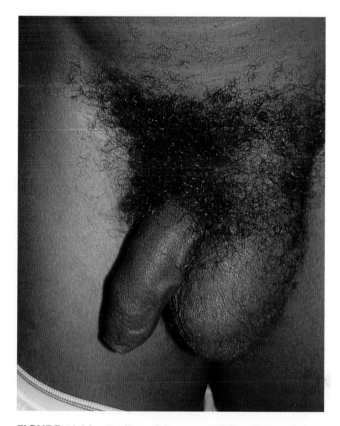

FIGURE 14.33   Swelling of the scrotum following a torsion injury. (From Fleisher GR, Ludwig S, Baskin MN. *Atlas of Pediatric Emergency Medicine*. Philadelphia: Lippincott Williams & Wilkins; 2004.)

Avulsions and Amputations

Avulsions and amputations can occur at any location on the body, but they commonly involve the upper and lower extremities, nose, and ears. Avulsion injuries, a tearing away of skin and/or soft tissue from the body, are discussed in the section on open wounds, above. These wounds typically involve small amounts of tissue removal. Amputations, a removal of tissue and/or body part, are classified as complete or incomplete and result from avulsion, crush, and guillotine (sharp cutting) mechanisms.[34] Complete amputations are total removal of the tissue/body part from the body; incomplete amputations result in some structure, skin, muscle, tendon, or ligament remaining in place, keeping the tissue/body part partially attached to the body. These injuries are frequently limb- and life-threatening and require prompt assessment, management, and transportation to a medical facility.

Begin assessment of avulsions and amputations with a determination of ABC status. Next, assess vital signs, neurological status, and degree of tissue damage. Based on the severity of these injuries, the EAP is activated in the majority of cases. The overall condition of the athlete, severity of tissue involvement and damage, and time since the injury dictate management techniques.[35] With the athlete stable or with additional personnel, conduct a search for the avulsed or amputated tissue and/or body part and attempt to determine time lapse since the injury.

Manage the overall condition of the athlete by maintaining the ABCs and monitoring for shock. Control external hemorrhage with direct pressure and elevation. In some situations, use of pressure points (Fig. 14.11) or a tourniquet may be necessary. Use of a tourniquet to control external hemorrhage is restricted to trained paraprofessionals such as emergency medical technicians. Furthermore, following application, a tourniquet should be removed only by a physician. Skill 14.15 presents management techniques for avulsions and incomplete and complete amputations.

If possible, document times of injury, tissue/body part discovery, tissue/body part dressing, and tissue/body part icing. Time is critical in the management and transportation of the athlete and avulsed/amputated tissue/body parts to a medical facility; the exact amount of time for which the tissue/body part remains viable for revascularization or reattachment is unknown.[36]

Burns

Burns are caused by thermal, chemical, and electrical sources and often result in open and closed soft tissue wounds. These injuries can occur in outdoor and indoor environments and may progress into life-threatening situations.

Thermal

Sunburn (actinic burn) is damage to the skin caused by exposure to ultraviolet (UV) light, mainly UVB (Fig. 14.34). Skin damage ranges from erythema of the outer layer of the epidermis to destruction of the epidermis, dermis, and subcutaneous tissues. Inspection of the skin may reveal erythema and edema in mild cases; erythema and blisters accompanying moderate cases; and erythema and black, brown, or gray skin color in severe cases. Erythema is visible 3 to 5 hours after overexposure; it reaches a maximum at 12 to 24 hours and fades over 72 hours.[37] Pain, fever, chills, burning and/or itching of skin, and nausea may also be present. Symptomatic treatment is recommended for the management of sunburn.[38] The use of nonsteroidal anti-inflammatory drugs, acetaminophen, hydrocortisone, aloe vera, cool compresses, and oatmeal soaks in cool water may provide relief from pain and itching/burning.[38] With the presence of blisters or discolored skin, dress the areas with saline-soaked

---

SKILL 14.15

Management of Avulsions and Amputations

Avulsions and Incomplete Amputations

1. Gently irrigate heavily contaminated tissue with saline prior to dressing.
2. Dress the wound with saline-soaked gauze and wrap with additional gauze.
3. Prevent further injury from excessive movement with immobilization of the body part.
4. If present and successfully located, gently wrap the avulsed tissue in saline-soaked gauze and place in a watertight bag.
5. Do not attempt to replace the tissue or body part.
6. Place the bag onto an ice bag or in ice water. Do not allow the tissue to come into direct contact with ice.
7. Monitor vital signs and neurological and circulation status of distal body parts until arrival at a medical facility.

Complete Amputations

1. Irrigate the stump with saline if it is heavily contaminated.
2. Dress the stump with saline-soaked gauze and cover with a gauze dressing.
3. Immobilize and elevate the stump.
4. If successfully located, gently wrap the amputated tissue and body part in saline-soaked gauze and place in a watertight bag. Do not attempt to replace the tissue or body part.
5. Place the bag onto an ice bag or in ice water. Do not allow the tissue to come into direct contact with ice.

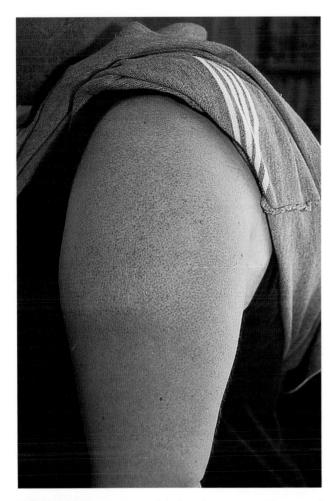

FIGURE 14.34   Sunburn of the lateral upper arm. (Courtesy of George A. Datto III, MD.)

gauze, cover, and refer to a physician. Follow the general cleansing, debridement, and dressing techniques for open wounds (abrasions [Skill 14.3] and blisters [Skill 14.5]) in the management of these injuries. Prevention of sunburn remains the most effective approach. Prevention strategies are listed in the Breakout box.

Chemical

Damage to the skin and soft tissue from chemical agents occurs through a chemical reaction rather than a thermal mechanism. The concentration of the agent and the duration of its contact with the skin determine the amount of soft tissue trauma.[39] Based on the site and mode of contact, these injuries can be life-threatening and require EAP activation and prompt referral.

Assessment of the involved skin area may reveal yellow or black/brown **eschar,** white to grayish-brown tissue, exposed dermal tissue, or edema (Fig. 14.35). Varying amounts of pain, central nervous system depression, hypotension, and respiratory difficulties during inhalation can also be present.[39] Manage most chemical burns by removing all clothing and equipment contaminated with the agent, brushing any solid or dry agent from the skin, and using copious, gentle water irrigation. Begin low-pressure irrigation (at 4 to 8 psi) immediately and continue until transportation is secured for referral. Syringe or shower irrigation is preferred to immersion.[40] With eye involvement, irrigation or immersion is used, with opening and closing of eyelids encouraged. Contain and dispose of irrigation drainage, which is likely contaminated with the chemical agent. Maintain ABCs, monitor vital signs, and treat for shock if necessary. During management, the athletic trainer

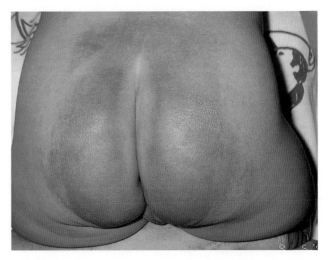

FIGURE 14.35   Chemical burn of the buttocks. (From Fleisher GR, Ludwig S, Baskin MN. *Atlas of Pediatric Emergency Medicine.* Philadelphia: Lippincott Williams & Wilkins; 2004.)

should wear two pairs of gloves and protective eyewear and clothing to prevent contact with the chemical agent.

Electrical

Electrical injuries occur from low- and high-voltage sources and cause open and closed soft tissue thermal trauma. Although open wounds such as entry and exit burns are visible during assessment, more extensive closed wounds and life-threatening injuries can initially be undetectable. Prior to beginning assessment, identify the power source and turn it off or disengage the athlete from the electrical current with a nonconducting object such as dry wood, cardboard, clothing, or rope.[41] Assessment of a low-voltage injury typically reveals a local burn to the hands of varying depth from contact with an exposed extension cord (Fig. 14.36). Additional external signs of injury may be absent. High-voltage injuries occur from an electric arc or electric current. Electric arc trauma demonstrates single or multiple circumscribed burns of varying depths at points of arc contact, commonly the hands, skull, and heels[41] (Fig. 14.37). Flashes of the arc can ignite clothing and cause additional burns. Trauma from high-voltage electric current will reveal charred, leathery, and depressed entry and explosive exit wounds with a black metallic coating on the skin. If the person is thrown away from the high-voltage current, impact injuries such as fractures, dislocations, and open and closed soft tissue trauma are likely. Evidence of closed trauma is often absent. Because electric current can affect almost every organ system in the body, unconsciousness, transient numbness and paresthesia at contact points, tachycardia, cardiac arrest, respiratory fail-

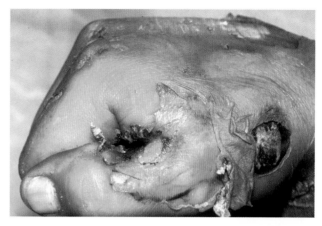

FIGURE 14.37 High-voltage electrical burn of the dorsal hand. (From Rubin E, Farber JL. *Pathology*, 3rd ed. Philadelphia: Lippincott Williams & Wilkins, 1999.)

ure, vessel rupture and thrombi, tetanic contractions, nausea and vomiting, and shock can be present during assessment.[41] Evidence of open fractures and/or dislocations; uncontrolled external hemorrhage; extreme pain; absence of ABCs; and unconsciousness warrant EAP activation. Establish an airway; initiate CPR, AED, and/or rescue breathing; control hemorrhage; and monitor vital signs.

Manage low-voltage burns without life-threatening trauma on the basis of the depth of tissue involvement: superficial, partial, or full thickness. Cleanse, débride, and dress superficial and some partial-thickness burns as described for treatment of abrasions (Skill 14.3) earlier in the chapter. Other partial- and all full-thickness burns require referral for advanced tissue care and systematic and pain treatment. Manage high-voltage trauma by maintaining ABCs; monitoring vital signs; treating for shock; dressing wounds with saline-soaked gauze; immobilizing any fractures, dislocations, and/or suspected spinal cord injury; and activating the EAP. Further evaluation to determine the presence of closed trauma and advanced soft tissue management must be done in a medical facility.

WRAP-UP

This chapter presented open and closed soft tissue trauma sustained by athletes and managed by athletic trainers. Appropriate assessment through primary and secondary surveys guides management techniques for these injuries. Care of open wounds consists mainly of cleansing, debridement, and dressing techniques; the majority of these injuries do not require immediate referral. Daily monitoring for adverse reactions and signs and symptoms of infection should be conducted. Following assessment, individuals with closed wounds require continual observation, and many conditions warrant referral and/or EAP activation. Universal precautions should be followed in the management of open and closed soft tissue trauma.

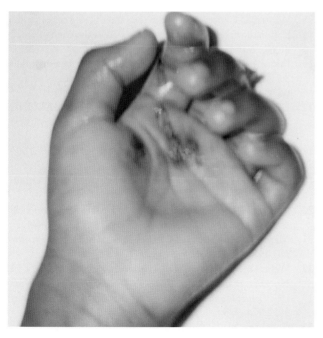

FIGURE 14.36 Low-voltage electrical burn of the palm of the hand. (From Fleisher GR, Ludwig S, Baskin MN. *Atlas of Pediatric Emergency Medicine*. Philadelphia: Lippincott Williams & Wilkins, 2004.)

Scenarios

1. In the second half, one of the soccer forwards jumps for a header against an opponent. Upon landing, the athlete begins to touch her forehead repeatedly. She continues to run down field until the referee stops the match because of the presence of blood from a small laceration on the forehead.

   What actions are required immediately on the field in the management of this case?
   What actions are necessary on the sidelines and/or in the athletic training facility?
   What actions are needed after the conclusion of the match?

2. During the fifth inning, a batter hits a pop fly that travels midway down the right-field foul line. The right fielder sprints toward the foul area near the stands and bleachers. He continues in a sprint with arms raised to catch the ball and strikes the concrete wall of the stands with his thorax, immediately falling to the ground. You proceed onto the field. When you get to the athlete, you see him coughing frothy blood and having difficulty in breathing.

   What steps should be taken to manage this situation?

3. A wide receiver catches a pass and is tackled, striking his left shoulder and helmet against the dirt infield of a converted baseball/football field. He comes to the sidelines with his right eyelid closed, complaining of pain from "something in my eye." He immediately removes his helmet and begins to rub his right eye. This athlete normally wears contact lenses for play.

   What actions are required in the management of this case?

4. Toward the conclusion of postseason strength testing, an athlete suddenly enters the athletic training facility shouting "There has been an accident!" You enter the adjacent strength and conditioning facility and observe an athlete lying prone on the ground in obvious distress, grasping his right hand. You approach the athlete and immediately notice a moderate amount of arterial blood under the right hand on the floor. Another teammate explains that the injured athlete tried to rerack two 45-lb plates and lost his grip, pinching his right third finger between the plates. The injured athlete releases his hand and reveals an incomplete amputation at the distal interphalangeal joint of the third finger.

   What actions are required in the management of this case?

REFERENCES

1. Starkey C, Ryan JL. *Evaluation of Orthopedic and Athletic Injuries*, 2nd ed. Philadelphia: FA Davis; 2002.
2. Cutting KF, Harding KG. Criteria for identifying wound infection. *J Wound Care*. 1994;3:198–201.
3. Cutting KF, White RJ. Criteria for identifying wound infection—revisited. *Ostomy Wound Manage*. 2005;51:28–34.
4. US Department of Labor Occupational Safety & Health Administration. Bloodborne Pathogens Regulation 1910.1030 (Standards—29 CFR). http://www.osha.gov/pls/oshaweb/owadisp.show_document?p_table=STANDARDS&p_id=10051. Accessed March 7, 2007.
5. Barr JE. Principles of wound cleansing. *Ostomy Wound Manage*. 1995;41:15S–21S.
6. Goldsmith SP. Wound care: Combining three classification systems to select dressings. *Home Health Care Manage Prac*. 1996;8:17–27.
7. Bergstrom N, Allamn R, Alvarez O, et al. *Treatment of Pressure Ulcers*. Clinical Practice Guidelines No. 15. AHCPR Publication No. 95-052. Rockville, MD: US Department of Health and Human Services; 1994.
8. Flanagan M. Wound cleansing. In: Morison M, Moffatt C, Bridel-Nixon J, et al., eds. *Nursing Management of Chronic Wounds*. London: Mosby; 1997.
9. Fernandez R, Griffiths R, Ussia C. Water for wound cleansing. *Cochrane Database Syst Rev*. 2002;(2):CD003861. http://www.cochrane.org/reviews/en/ab003861.html. Accessed March 22, 2007.
10. Selim P, Bashford C, Grossman C. Evidence-based practice: Tap water cleansing of leg ulcers in the community. *J Clin Nurs*. 2001;10:372–379.
11. Attinger CE, Bulan EJ. Debridement. The key initial first step in wound healing. *Foot Ankle Clin*. 2001;6:627–660.
12. Turner T. Which dressing and why? *Nurs Times*. 1982;78:1–3.
13. Casey G. Wound dressings. *Pediatr Nurs*. 2001;13:39–42.
14. Wiechula R. The use of moist wound-healing dressings in the management of split-thickness skin graft donor sites: A systematic review. *Int J Nurs Pract*. 2003;9:S9–S17.
15. Winter GD. Formation of the scab and the rate of epithelialization of superficial wounds in the skin of the young domestic pig. *Nature*. 1962;193:293–294.
16. Pirone L, Monte K, Shannon R, et al. Wound healing under occlusion and non-occlusion in partial-thickness and full-thickness wounds in swine. *Wounds*. 1990;2:74–81.
17. ETHICON product information for DERMABOND. http://www.dermabond.com/home.jhtml?_requestid=213895. Accessed March 7, 2007.
18. Goldstein EJC. Bite wounds and infection. *Clin Infect Dis*. 1992;14:633–640.
19. Pressure points. http://www.tpub.com/corpsman/144.htm. Accessed March 7, 2007.
20. Morgan JP III, Haug RH, Murphy MT. Management of facial dog bite injuries. *J Oral Maxillofac Surg*. 1995;53:435–441.
21. Marcy SM. Infections due to dog and cat bites. *Pediatr Infect Dis*. 1982;1:351–356.
22. Weber EJ, Callaham ML. Mammalian bites. In: Marx JA, Hockberger RS, Walls RM, eds. *Rosen's Emergency Medicine: Concepts and Clinical Practice*. 5th ed. St. Louis: Mosby; 2002:774–785.
23. Callaham M. Controversies in antibiotic choices for bite wounds. *Ann Emerg Med*. 1988;17:1321–1330.
24. Lindsey D, Christopher M, Hollenbach J, et al. Natural course of the human bite wound: Incidence of infection and

complications in 434 bites and 803 lacerations in the same group of patients. *J Trauma*. 1987;27:45–48.

25. Armstrong BD. Lacerations of the mouth. *Emerg Med Clin North Am*. 2000;18:471–480.

26. Viehweg TL, Roberson JB, Hudson JW. Epistaxis: Diagnosis and treatment. *J Oral Maxillofac Surg*. 2006;64:511–518.

27. Shrager JB. Tracheal trauma. *Chest Surg Clin N Am*. 2003; 13:291–304.

28. Perry M, Dancey A, Mireskandari K, et al. Emergency care in facial trauma—A maxillofacial and ophthalmic perspective. *Injury*. 2005;36:875–896.

29. Weber TS. Training room management of eye conditions. *Clin Sports Med*. 2005;24:681–693.

30. Flynn CA, D'Amico F, Smith G. Should we patch corneal abrasions? A meta-analysis. *J Fam Pract*. 1998;47:264–270.

31. Maron BJ, Gohman TE, Kyle SB, et al. Clinical profile and spectrum of commotio cordis. *J Am Med Assoc*. 2002;287: 1142–1146.

32. Ketterhagen JP, Wassermann DH. Impalement injuries: The preferred approach. *J Trauma*. 1983;23:258–259.

33. Eachempati SR, Barie PS, Reed RL II. Survival after transabdominal impalement from a construction injury: A review of the management of impalement injuries. *J Trauma*. 1999;47:864–866.

34. Blank-Reid C. Nursing. Traumatic amputations, unkind cuts. www.findarticles.com/p/articles/mi_qa3689/is_200307/ai_n9257015#continue. Accessed April 15, 2007.

35. Bledsoe B, Porter R, Shade B. *Paramedic Emergency Care*. Upper Saddle River, NJ: Brady Prentice Hall; 1997.

36. Pons P, Markovchick V. *Prehospital Emergency Care Secrets*. Philadelphia: Hanley & Belfus; 1998.

37. Hall HI, May DS, Lew RA, et al. Sun protection behaviors of the US white population. *Prev Med*. 1997;26:401–407.

38. Han A, Maibach HI. Management of acute sunburn. *Am J Clin Dermatol*. 2004;5:39–47.

39. Edlich RF, Farinholt HMA, Winters KL, et al. Modern concepts of treatment and prevention of chemical injuries. *J Long Term Eff Med Implants*. 2005;15:303–318.

40. Reilly DA, Garner WL. Management of chemical injuries to the upper extremity. *Hand Clin*. 2000;16:215–223.

41. Edlich RF, Farinholt HMA, Winters KL, et al. Modern concepts of treatment and prevention of electrical burns. *J Long Term Eff Med Implants*. 2005;15:511–532.

WEB REFERENCES

US Department of Labor Occupational Safety and Health Administration Bloodborne Pathogens. http://www.osha.gov/SLTC/bloodbornepathogens/index.html. Accessed March 7, 2007.

ITIM: NSW Institute of Trauma & Injury Management. http://www.itim.nsw.gov.au/index.cfm. Accessed March 7, 2007.

Trauma.Org. http://www.trauma.org/index.php/. Accessed April 15, 2007.

Auscultation Assistant. http://www.wilkes.med.ucla.edu/inex.htm. Accessed April 15, 2007.

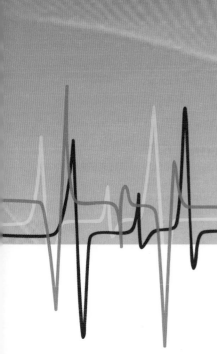
Recognition and Management of Skeletal Injuries

CHAPTER OUTCOMES

1. Define skeletal injuries.
2. Identify and describe the different types of skeletal injuries, including fractures, dislocations, and subluxations.
3. Describe the differences between open and closed skeletal injuries.
4. Identify the signs and symptoms associated with skeletal injuries.

5. Describe the indications and general guidelines for immobilizing skeletal injuries.
6. Describe the proper immobilization techniques and select appropriate splinting materials to stabilize injured joints or bones and maintain distal circulation, sensation, and movement.
7. Describe the availability, purpose, and maintenance of commonly used immobilization devices in athletic training.

NOMENCLATURE

Angulated fracture: a fracture where the two ends of the broken bone causes the extremity to deviate sharply from its normal anatomical position

Articulating surface: the ends of bones that join or connect together loosely via ligaments and a joint capsule to allow joint motion

Closed fracture: a fracture in which skin is intact at the site of fracture, also known as a simple fracture

Complete fracture: a fracture involving the entire width of the bone

Compound fracture: a fracture in which the bone ends are displaced and pierce through the dermis

Crepitus: the grating, crackling, or popping sounds and sensations experienced under the skin and joints. The sound can be created when two rough surfaces in the human body come into contact, such as two edges of a broken bone

Displaced fracture: a fracture in which the two ends of the broken bone are separated from one another and are no longer in correct anatomic alignment

Fracture: a break in the continuity of the bone and damage to surrounding tissues

Incomplete fracture: a fracture that does not extend through the full width of a bone

Immobilize: to render fixed or incapable of moving

Nondisplaced fracture: a fracture in which the two ends of the broken bone are separated from one another but continue to be in correct anatomic alignment

Open fracture: the presence of a wound on the skin surface leading down to the site of the fracture

Radiolucent: relatively penetrable by x-rays or other forms of radiation

Simple fracture: see closed fracture

Subluxation: an incomplete dislocation

BEFORE YOU BEGIN

1. Define skeletal injuries. What are some of the different types of skeletal injuries?

2. What is a joint dislocation? What are some of the causes of a joint dislocation? Why are joint dislocations dangerous?

3. Identify the signs and symptoms of skeletal fractures and joint dislocations. What are the similarities and differences between the two?

4. Identify and discuss the accepted management of a skeletal fracture.

5. What does the acronym CSM represent? When should CSM be assessed in managing a skeletal injury?

6. Identify and discuss the different types of immobilization devices available to athletic trainers.

7. Define the following: C-curve, reverse C-curve, and T-curve.

8. An athlete has suffered a right shoulder injury after falling on an outstretched hand. Describe the steps necessary to apply a sling and swathe in order to immobilize the joint.

Voices from the Field

The role of the athletic trainer is a unique one in the health care system. We are fortunate to develop relationships with our patients (student athletes) before they have a need for our services. Sometimes this can lead us to relax during the day-to-day delivery of our care. Then, within a split second, our patient is injured and our recognition and management skills come in to play. The ability to evaluate the injury and manage it appropriately is the first step in the athletic trainer's delivery of health care. Appropriate recognition and management can result in less lost time and a better outcome. These tests of the athletic trainer's skills can be as simple as a stress fracture or as complicated as an open fracture.

Sometimes the evaluation and recognition can be obvious. One morning the administrative coordinator for our sports medicine program was heading to the campus mailbox to get our mail. On her way she tripped over a dolly that had inadvertently been left in the hallway. One of my associates got to

her first and then summoned me to help. When I arrived, she was lying prone on the floor. My associate rolled her eyes as I asked her what was wrong. I looked down and realized that the lower tib-fib of the woman's right leg was rotated at 180 degrees and her foot was sticking up in the air. In this case, the recognition of a displaced tib-fib fracture was easy. The packaging and management was a little more complex. On a simpler note, understanding and recognizing stress reactions and managing them before they develop into full-blown stress fractures can take weeks off the patient's recovery time. The athletic trainer's proficiency in recognizing and managing skeletal injuries is a very important component of his or her health care delivery.

Charles Rozanski, MS, LAT, ATC
Associate Director of Athletics for Sports Medicine
North Carolina State University
Raleigh, NC

Preparing for and dealing with a traumatic emergency situation is sometimes a lengthy and arduous physical task, and when mismanaged, it can lead to negative clinical outcomes. Contact sports such as football, ice hockey, and rugby expose athletes to direct violent blows of high and low velocity, resulting in what emergency medical service (EMS) personnel refer to as painful, swollen, or deformed joint injuries. Included in this category are skeletal injuries, or what are commonly referred to as bone fractures, joint dislocations, and subluxations. Although soft tissue injuries such as external wounds can be easily managed with direct pressure and a pressure

bandage, proper emergency immobilization of skeletal injuries must be learned and practiced in order for athletic trainers to minimize the severity of the injury and ensure the safety of the injured athlete. This chapter will familiarize you with the different types and causes of skeletal injuries, various immobilization and splinting materials, and strategies to properly apply such materials. Although it does not cover every type of splint or immobilization technique, this chapter examines a variety of procedures used to immobilize painful, swollen, fractured, or deformed joints. The knowledge thus gained and specific criteria for splinting and immobilization will allow the athletic trainer to improvise or create other techniques needed to splint and immobilize specific conditions.

SKELETAL INJURIES

When the skeletal system sustains a violent blow, those forces that are not initially absorbed by the body's soft tissue are transmitted to the skeletal system, resulting in possible skeletal (bony) injuries. The mechanisms of injury for acute skeletal injuries include (a) a direct violent force/blow (e.g., being struck by an object), (b) an indirect violent force (e.g., landing on an outstretched hand), and (c) a rotational or (d) bending force (e.g., rotating around a fixed point). A direct violent force/blow, such as being struck by a blunt object or a piece of sporting equipment (e.g., baseball bat, lacrosse stick), delivers a direct external force and causes a skeletal injury at the point of contact. Areas with limited protective equipment or soft tissue may be at greatest risk for injuries (e.g., forearm, hands). An indirect violent force occurs when an external load or force is applied to the body and the energy is transmitted to a point away from the site of initial contact, causing injuries there. For example, falling on an outstretched hand may cause injuries to the bony structures of the shoulder or shoulder girdle as the external force is transmitted along the length of the ulna and humerus.[1] When a bone is twisted about itself, the excessive load causes the bone first to crack parallel to its neutral axis, followed by a second crack along the plane of maximal tensile strength, resulting in a spiral fracture.[2] Three-point

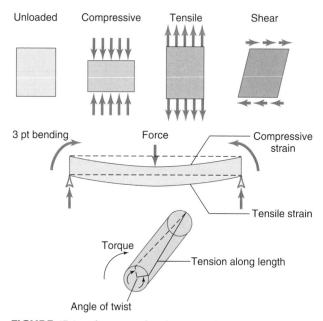

FIGURE 15.1 Three-point bending. Basic forces acting on a long bone and the deflection of the bone in response (top). Compression shortens the length, tension increases the length, shear distorts the length, bending (middle) causes it to bow, and torsion (bottom) results in twisting around the long axis. (From Bucholz RW, Heckman JD. *Rockwood & Green's Fractures in Adults,* 5th ed. Philadelphia: Lippincott, Williams & Wilkins; 2001.)

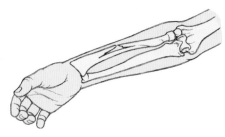

FIGURE 15.2 Incomplete closed skeletal fracture. Fracture occurs partially across the bone.

bending places a compression force at one side of the bone and a tension force at the other, resulting in injuries to the tension side (e.g., greenstick fracture) (Fig. 15.1). The purpose of this section is to identify and describe the different types of skeletal injuries, including fractures, dislocations, and subluxations, and to discuss their associated signs and symptoms.

Skeletal Fractures

A skeletal **fracture** is a break in the continuity of the bone, which occurs when a significant force has been applied to the body through a direct, indirect, or rotational mechanism of injury. Fractures are initially categorized as complete or incomplete. An **incomplete fracture** occurs when there is a partial break across the bone (Fig. 15.2), whereas a **complete fracture** occurs when the bone breaks completely, creating two distinct halves (Fig. 15.3). This may result in either a **displaced** (Fig. 15.4) or **nondisplaced fracture.** Such injuries may be further categorized as closed or open. A **closed fracture** occurs where there is no loss of the continuity between the fracture site and the dermis[1] (Fig. 15.3). These are often referred to as **simple fractures.** An **open fracture** develops when there is loss of continuity between the fracture site and dermis, resulting in an open wound and external bleeding.

It is worth mentioning that the presence of an open wound does not necessarily constitute what is often considered to be a compound fracture. A **compound fracture** occurs only when fractured[3] bone ends are displaced and pierce through the dermis (Fig. 15.5). Such an injury will normally present with a visible deformity through the skin as well as external bleeding. The open wound is now susceptible to infection (as is the bone) due to the exposure to dirt and other microorganisms, shock, and other soft tissue and

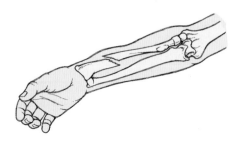

FIGURE 15.3 Complete closed skeletal fracture. Fracture occurs through the bone, creating two distinct halves.

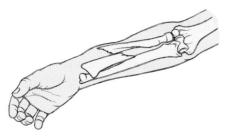

FIGURE 15.4 Displaced skeletal fracture. Fracture when two ends of the broken bone are separated from one another and no longer assume the correct anatomic alignment.

neurovascular injuries; this means that immediate medical attention is required to limit further injury.

Additionally, skeletal fractures can be described according to the shape and pattern of the fractured area, which may indicate the nature of causative force. For example, a transverse fracture (i.e., a fracture forming at a right angle with the axis of the bone) of the tibia occurs as a result of a direct force at the point of contact with the fracture site; a rotational or torsion force, on the other hand, often results in a spiral fracture away from the initial point of contact.[3] Specific examples of skeletal fractures classified by shape and pattern (e.g., linear, transverse, etc.) and by the position of the bony fragments are presented in Table 15.1.

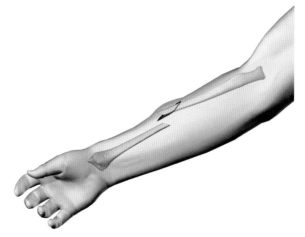

FIGURE 15.5 Open fractures. In an open, or compound, fracture, the bone ends are displaced and pierce through the dermis. (LifeART image copyright © 2010 Lippincott Williams & Wilkins.)

Joint Dislocation

A joint dislocation occurs when a sufficient force is applied to a joint to displace its articulating surface from its normal anatomical position (Fig. 15.6). This causes the joint capsule and ligaments to stretch beyond the joint's normal limits, resulting in severe stretching or rupture of the supporting

---

Current Research

To Reduce or Not? That Is the Question

The question of whether or not to reduce a joint dislocation is one that will puzzle humanity (or at least athletic trainers) for all time. You may have heard of discussions about reducing shoulder, finger, and elbow dislocations. The phrase, "It's just a finger, what harm can it do?" is one that has the potential for future repercussions, particularly if the athlete really was not a candidate for said reduction and you were functioning outside of your scope of practice. For example, reduction of a finger dislocation is contraindicated under the following circumstances:

- Digital neurovascular compromise
- Associated fracture
- Open joint dislocation
- Ligamentous or volar plate rupture
- Joint instability
- Inability to reduce the dislocation

These require a consultation with a "hand surgeon … to determine if management should be primarily surgical without a reduction attempt."[15]

At *no* time should an athletic trainer attempt to reduce a dislocated joint. Prentice[3] makes this very clear in his text when he states, in bold letters, **"DISLOCATIONS SHOULD NOT BE REDUCED IMMEDIATELY, REGARDLESS OF WHERE THEY OCCUR."**

Although joint dislocations to shoulder, elbow, hip, knee, and ankle constitute orthopedic medical emergencies and may lead to disastrous consequences if not treated immediately, improper handling of such situations can be even more disastrous. Immediate reduction or realignment should be performed only by a physician. If an athletic trainer is granted permission to perform any type of joint dislocation reduction, it must be clearly articulated and documented in the facility's standard operating procedures, identifying who is qualified and under what circumstances and normally only after receiving online medical direction.

Any situation where neurovascular compromise is suspected should be considered a "load and go" situation (Chapter 1). Perform a rapid assessment, stabilize the joint, and immediately transport the athlete to the nearest medical facility.

TABLE 15.1 Types of Skeletal Fractures

Name	Image	Description
Avulsion		Fracture causing a bone fragment to be pulled off the bone by forces from a muscle or ligament
Comminuted		Fracture causing two or more small bone fragments in addition to the upper and lower sections of a broken bone
Depressed		Fracture with displacement of the bone (normally a flat bone) inward
Displaced		Fracture in which the fragments are separated and are not in alignment
Epiphyseal		Fracture to the growth plate of a long bone in a child or adolescent
Greenstick		Incomplete fracture resulting from bending of a bone

TABLE 15.1   Types of Skeletal Fractures *(Continued)*

Name	Image	Description
Impacted		Bone fragments driven so firmly together that they become interlocked, limiting movement between the fragments
Longitudinal		Fracture running the length of the shaft
Spiral		Fracture running at oblique angles, creating a helical line in the bone
Transverse		Fracture crossing the bone at a 90-degree angle to the bone's axis
Oblique		Fracture at a 45-degree angle to the bone's axis

From Anderson MK, Parr GP, Hall SJ. *Foundations of Athletic Training: Prevention, Assessment, and Management,* 4th ed. Baltimore: Lippincott Williams & Wilkins; 2009.

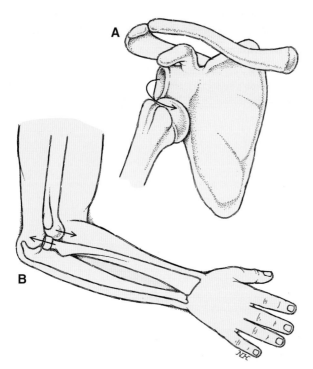

FIGURE 15.6 Joint dislocation. **A.** Subglenoid dislocation of shoulder. **B.** Dislocation of elbow. (From *Stedman's Medical Dictionary*. 27th ed. Baltimore: Lippincott Williams & Wilkins; 2001.)

soft tissue structures and increased joint instability. Joint dislocations are most commonly the result of a direct or indirect force. Among those engaged in heavy physical activity (athletes, members of the military), dislocations most often affect the shoulders,[4-6] elbows,[7-9] and fingers.[10] Injuries due to motor vehicle accidents and falls from a significant height result in dislocations to the hips, knees, and ankles; however, any joint involving two bones can become dislocated. A youth soccer player striking his opponent with a direct blow to the medial knee may dislocate the patella. A high school wrestler bracing on an outstretch hand with an elbow extended when being thrown to the mat may dislocate that elbow as the force is directed along the axis of the ulna into the elbow joint.

Dislocations not only result in a disruption of the normal articulation of the bones at the joint, but they are also associated with tendon, ligament, vascular, and neurological injuries. Arteries and nerves can be compressed between the displaced joints or when the dislocation spontaneously reduces (i.e., the joint relocates on its own), resulting in decreased or absent circulatory or neurological functions. If left untreated, this can lead to loss of limb function, permanent disability, or the loss of a limb. A dislocation of the knee is considered an orthopedic emergency and requires immediate medical attention owing to the high rate of associated injuries to the surrounding neurovascular structures.[11-14] Reduction of a joint dislocation should be attempted only by trained and qualified medical professionals under appropriate circumstances because of the risk of neurovascular compromise.

Joint Subluxations

A joint **subluxation** is an incomplete dislocation. In a subluxation, the relationship between the two joint surfaces is altered; however, the joint surfaces remain in contact with each other. Athletes sustaining dislocations may develop chronic instability of said joint, increasing the risk of further injuries in the form of joint subluxations.[16] The patella, for example, is at increased risk for subluxation after the joint has been dislocated once.[17] Subluxations present with a variety of signs and symptoms, depending on the severity of the injuries. A thorough history is often the best way of determining whether a subluxation has occurred.

RECOGNIZING SKELETAL INJURIES

Without adequate recognition and immobilization, skeletal fractures and joint dislocations can result in further injuries or may compromise vital organs, soft tissues, and neurovascular

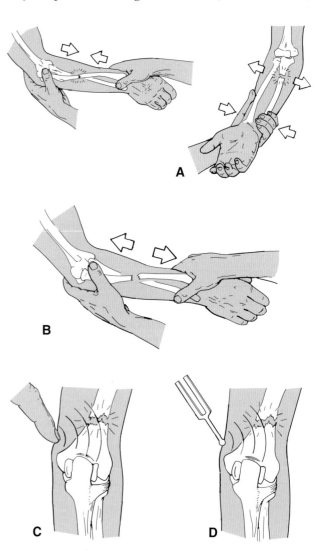

FIGURE 15.7 Determining a possible fracture. **A.** Compression (axial and circular). **B.** Distraction. **C.** Percussion. **D.** Vibration.

Signs & Symptoms

Skeletal Injuries

Signs and Symptoms	Fracture	Dislocation	Subluxations
Rapid swelling	X	X	X
Sudden pain	X	X	X
Direct tenderness	X	X	X
Loss of function	X	X	X
Possible deformity and angulation	X	X	
Crepitus	X		
False motion	X		
Delayed discoloration	X	X	X
Open wounds	X	X	
Joint locked into position	X	X	
Circulatory compromise	X	X	X
Neurological compromise	X	X	X

Note: The extent and quality of the signs and symptoms will depend upon the severity of the injury. Table 15.1 is meant to serve as a reference tool and is not an all-conclusive list of the signs and symptoms of skeletal injuries.

structures, causing a loss of function or permanent disability. The athletic trainer should begin with a thorough assessment of the scene to determine the mechanism and extent of the injury. Identification of the mechanism of injury will help to determine whether the impact forces were direct, indirect, or rotational; it may also identify the point of impact. These clues can help the athletic trainer to determine the approximate location, type, and severity of the injury. Remember from Chapter 8 that, as you arrive on scene and begin your primary assessment, you will gain a general impression of the athlete's condition. This will include observing for such things as the individual's level of consciousness (and emotional response if conscious), posture (e.g., hip dislocation presenting with a shortened, adducted, internally rotated limb), and tissue guarding (e.g., splinting the elbow by holding it close to the body). After formally establishing the individual's level of consciousness, airway, breathing, circulation (the ABCs), and bleeding, begin the secondary assessment.

During the secondary assessment, be cautious and—if you suspect a skeletal injury or joint dislocation—avoid any unnecessary movement of the joint or extremity. A conscious athlete may be anxious and concerned about his or her condition; if a deformity is present, the athlete may be panicked, aggressive, and on the verge of shock, all of which can complicate the situation. By remaining calm and reassuring the athlete, you will help to decrease his or her anxiety level while you to remain focused on managing the situation. During the physical examination, be sure to compare the extremities bilaterally (think about how the joint would

normally look and feel) using the acronym DOTS (deformity, open wounds, tenderness, and swelling). This will help you to identify the possible presence of skeletal injuries.

In an emergency situation, determining the specific type of skeletal fracture, particularly in the case of a closed fracture, is often unnecessary and in many situations not possible. Joint dislocation, on the other hand, tends to be a little easier to recognize because the disturbance and/or gross disarrangement of the joint articulations occurs on a larger scale and is normally (although not always) obvious. In the case of subluxation, it will be necessary to rely on the individual's description of the injury. The signs and symptoms of skeletal fractures, joint dislocations, and subluxations are very similar (see the Signs & Symptoms box, above) and may include minor to severe pain, swelling in or around the injury site, and/or possible deformity. Therefore, all skeletal fractures and joint dislocations—as well as severe sprains, strains, and even contusions—should be treated as painful, swollen, deformed joints until a definitive clinical diagnosis can be made. Although it is sometimes difficult to determine the type or presence of a fracture, the athletic trainer may use some common fracture assessment techniques during the secondary assessment (Fig. 15.7). Fractures can be assessed with percussion, vibration using a tuning fork, compression, and distraction. Although not an exact science for detecting breaks, these methods may alert the athletic trainer to a possible fracture and enable him or her to manage the site with appropriate splinting methods.

First-Time Dislocations

Athletic trainers should always assume the worst and treat all major musculoskeletal injuries, particularly first-time joint dislocations, as if they were skeletal fractures and—after stabilizing the athlete's ABCs—immobilize the joint or limb for further medical care. For example, a shoulder dislocation can result in a trauma to the humeral head, referred to as a Hill–Sachs or reverse Hill–Sachs lesion.[18,19] These injuries result in articular cartilage defects on the posterior (Hill–Sachs lesion) or anterior (reverse Hill–Sachs lesion) aspect of the humeral head as the humeral head dislocates in an anterior or posterior direction and the glenoid rim is impacted against the humeral head after the dislocation. These types of injuries do not typically preclude or complicate reduction in the emergency room[19]; however, unless your x-ray vision is working that day, being able to determine the type and extent of the injury will be difficult.

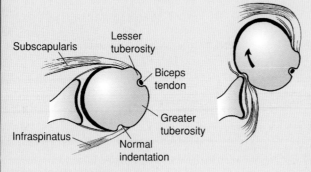

Hill–Sachs lesion associated with anterior shoulder dislocation. On dislocation, the posterior aspect of the humeral head engages the anterior glenoid rim. The glenoid rim then initiates an impression fracture, which can enlarge. (From Bucholz RW, Heckman JD, Court-Brown C, et al., eds. *Rockwood and Green's Fractures in Adults,* 6th ed. Philadelphia: Lippincott Williams & Wilkins; 2006.)

STRATEGIES FOR APPLYING IMMOBILIZATION DEVICES

Immobilizing skeletal injuries and even soft tissue injuries (i.e., sprains or strains) using improvised or commercial splinting devices requires athletic trainers to follow certain established management guidelines. When you are presented with an injury situation, begin by activating the emergency action plan and make sure that someone has notified EMS if indicated. Remember to take body substance isolation precautions and to establish and stabilize the athlete's ABCs

before beginning to immobilize a painful, swollen, and/or deformed joint (Fig. 15.8).

Prehospital Management of Skeletal Injuries

The following immobilization strategies and recommendations will enable you to manage and transport an injured athlete and to minimize further injuries:

1. First and foremost: *life before limb.* Never compromise an individual's survival to immobilize an injury. Treat

Using Tuning Forks to Detect Fractures

Compression and percussion testing is commonly utilized to elicit pain that is indicative of a possible simple fracture.[20,21] These clinical tests are particularly useful to athletic trainers when making return-to-play decisions when diagnostic tests such as radiographs are not readily available.[20] Although they are commonly described in many traditional athletic training texts[16,22,23] and are widely utilized, their reliability has not been validated. Moore[21] examined the use of a tuning fork and stethoscope versus the use of compression and percussion testing to assess possible fractures, finding that the tuning fork and stethoscope were more reliable than radiographs. Using a tuning fork at 128 Hz and auscultation, researchers attempted to detect fractures in adults (of the femoral neck) and children (of the femoral neck, shaft, and tibia), respectively.[24,25] They found that the use of a tuning fork and auscultation demonstrated a sensitivity of 91% and specificity of 81% (femoral neck) and 94% sensitivity (all areas evaluated) versus the "gold standard" of radiographs. Lesho[26] also compared the use of a tuning fork test without auscultation against a bone scan for the identification of tibial stress fractures. A 128-Hz tuning fork was applied to the anterior tibia, and the test was considered positive if the patient reported an increase in anterior shin pain. Lesho determined the sensitivity and specificity of the tuning fork test to be 75% and 67%, respectively.[26] Although the tuning fork was not sensitive enough to rule out a stress fracture, this research did suggest that in situations where the patient is at moderate to high risk of fracture, the use of a bone scan may be avoided in the presence of a positive tuning fork test. Another study comparing three tuning forks of different frequency (128, 256, and 512 Hz) to detect stress fractures found that the 256-Hz tuning fork elicited the highest pain ratings and had the greatest sensitivity (77.7% to 92.3%) in detecting stress fractures of the lower leg and foot.[27]

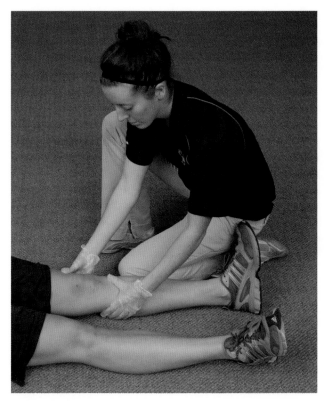

FIGURE 15.8 Immobilizing a painful, swollen, deformed joint. When stabilizing a lower extremity injury, the ground can act as a support and assist in immobilizing the injury. When stabilizing an upper extremity injury, a second athletic trainer can assist in immobilizing the joint.

all life-threatening injuries before dealing with any non–life-threatening issues.

2. Reassure the athlete and his or her family or friends that you are there to help. A demonstration of empathy will comfort the athlete.

3. Immobilize skeletal injuries before transporting the individual to minimize further injury unless there is an immediate threat to life or the scene becomes unsafe. The athletic trainer will need to use his or her best judgment as to which moving technique (Chapter 6) is appropriate. In situations where an athlete must be transported immediately (i.e., a "load and go" situation), consider stabilizing the individual on a spine board or vacuum mattress.

4. Expose the injury by removing clothing and protective equipment from the injury site. If clothing (e.g., a shoe) or protective equipment is supporting the injury, leave the clothing or equipment in place. Remember to ensure the athlete's modesty. Remove jewelry, watches, etc., to prevent constriction of the injured underlying soft tissue as the injury begins to swell.

5. Control any bleeding by applying a sterile dressing over any open wounds. In situations where there is a fracture (closed or open), you may opt to control bleeding and minimize the risk of shock by applying indirect pressure around the fracture site using a donut ring (Fig. 15.9). Covering any open wounds with a dressing (sterile if possible) will help to prevent infection.

6. Complete a thorough secondary assessment. Remember to use the acronym DOTS when completing the physical examination. Include a thorough assessment of the distal extremity's circulation, sensation, and movement (CSM). Be sure to document all pertinent findings.

7. To prevent further damage to the injury site, immobilize the extremity above and below the injured area. For example, a midshaft fracture to the radius or ulna would require you to extend the splint to the joints above and below the fractured bones. In such a case, you must stabilize the wrist and elbow to prevent any further movement of the joint. To immobilize an injury to a joint—as in a dislocation or subluxation—you

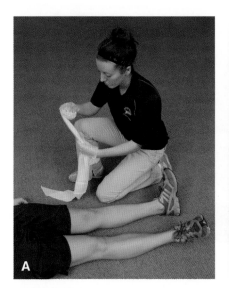
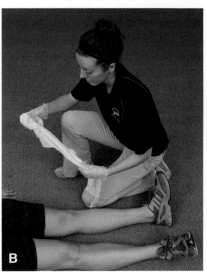
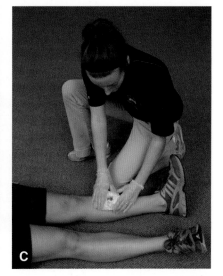

FIGURE 15.9 Donut ring. **A.** Begin by wrapping a triangular bandage around your hand. **B.** Weave the tail of the bandage in and out of the circle. **C.** Apply the donut around the open wound, being sure not to push the bone back into the body.

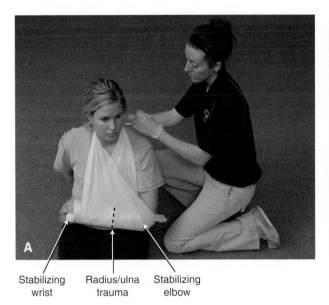
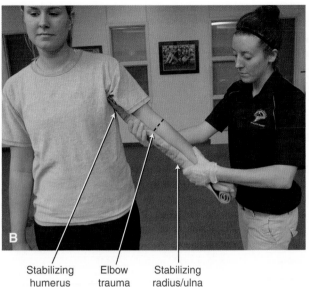

| Stabilizing wrist | Radius/ulna trauma | Stabilizing elbow | Stabilizing humerus | Elbow trauma | Stabilizing radius/ulna |

FIGURE 15.10 Appropriate splint sites for bone and joint injuries. **A.** When splinting a bone injury, as in an ulnar fracture, splint the joints above (elbow) and below (wrist) the injury site. **B.** When splinting a joint injury, as in an elbow fracture, splint the bones above (humerus) and below (radius and ulna) the injury site.

must splint the bones above and below the injured site (Fig. 15.10).

8. Prevent movement as much as possible and immobilize the injury site in a position that maintains stability and neurovascular function. Also, splint the injury only if it does not cause more pain to the athlete. If the act of splinting does increase pain, consider waiting for additional medical resources and place the individual in a position of comfort.

9. In using a rigid splint, be sure to provide adequate padding to the splint, particularly around bony prominences and to increase support to the area (Fig. 15.11). Commercial rigid splints such as the SAM Splint and some board splints come prepadded. Materials such as gauze pads, triangular bandages, or T-shirts can be used to pad improvised rigid splints. Be sure that all hollow spaces and voids are filled and prevent pressure points by padding or wrapping around all bony prominences if necessary (Fig. 15.11).

10. Avoid splinting directly over the injured area or over open wounds. Securing a bandage directly over an open wound may cause further irritation to the wound; therefore, bandages should be tied above and below wounds.

11. Recheck the distal extremity CSM once the splint has been properly secured (Fig. 15.12). This requires you to avoid covering the athlete's fingers and toes when

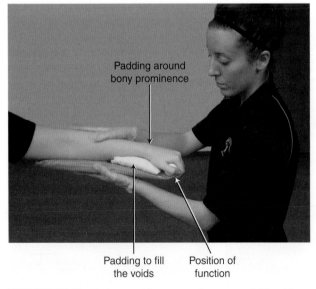

Padding around bony prominence

Padding to fill the voids   Position of function

FIGURE 15.11 Pad around bony prominences and fill voids.

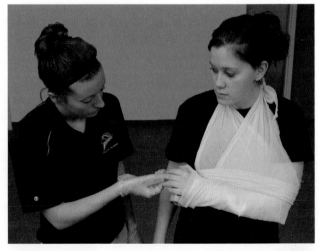

FIGURE 15.12 Assessing circulation, sensation, and movement. Capillary refill is normal when color returns within less than 2 seconds after releasing the nail bed.

PRICE Is Right

PRICE is an acronym commonly used in the treatment of skeletal and soft tissue injuries (Chapter 14) to reduce the symptoms of acute inflammation. PRICE stands for:

- *Protect (or protection)*: Protect the injury site to limit any type of unnecessary movement, using the immobilization devices and techniques described in this chapter and Chapter 16.
- *Rest or restriction from activity*: Limit activity according to the type and severity of trauma as well as according to medical advice.
- *Ice*: Apply crushed ice directly to the skin for up to 30 minutes, repeating this approximately every 1½ to 2 hours for up to 72 hours (or longer depending on the severity of the injury) to help reduce inflammation and control pain. *Do not* apply frozen gel packs to the skin without a barrier (towel) and *do not* apply ice directly to an open fracture or compound fracture. In the latter case, ice applied indirectly to the area may be beneficial.
- *Compression*: Apply an elastic wrap in a distal-to-proximal direction to limit the formation of the swelling in and around the injury site. Be sure to assess the distal neurovascular structures to ensure that the wrap is not too tight. In the case of soft tissue injuries, a horse-shoe pad can be placed around the injury site in conjunction with the elastic wrap to limit swelling.
- *Elevation*: Once the injury has been stabilized, consider elevating the extremity 6 to 10 in. above the heart to reduce swelling and limit the effects of blood pooling in the extremity. In the case of an unstable fracture, *do not* elevate the injured extremity.

possible. Any compromise to neurovascular status such as tingling, numbness, discoloration (e.g., cyanosis), or decreased skin temperature will require you to completely release the securing material and reapply the splint, this time with the bandages not quite as tight.

12. Elevate the limb and apply ice to the secured splinted area if it does not cause any discomfort and is not contraindicated (e.g., as it would be with a cervical spine injury).
13. ***Do not*** attempt to reduce dislocations of the spine, wrist, hip, knees, or open fractures.
14. ***Do not*** attempt to realign a severely deformed extremity without receiving online medical direction and only if you are trained to do so.

INJURY IMMOBILIZATION

When a skeletal injury is suspected, it must be immobilized before any additional care can be provided, such as applying ice, elevation, or even transportation to the nearest medical facility. To prevent movement and provide additional support to the injured area, immobilize the limb, using a splint or some other method of securely fixing a joint, bone, or other movable parts. Immobilizing a skeletal fracture or joint dislocation with a splint prevents the bone's sharp edges or displaced bones from damaging surrounding soft tissues and neurovascular structures and helps to reduce pain, minimize the risk of shock, and prevent further injuries (preventing closed fractures from becoming open fractures and reducing the risk of secondary tissue damage and infection).

To Realign or Not? That Is the Other Question

Making the decision to realign any skeletal injury is like making the decision to relocate a joint dislocation. It should be performed only by a physician. However, if—because of severe neurovascular compromise or the inability to properly stabilize the skeletal injuries[13,28]—and the athletic trainer has been given permission to realign a closed angulated long bone, the requirements to perform such a procedure should be well articulated and documented in facility's standard operating procedures and/or emergency action plan, identifying who is qualified and under what circumstances, and normally only after receiving online medical direction.

When dealing with an open or compound fracture, cover the wound with a sterile dressing and immobilize the limb in the position found.[13]

Before moving the affected limb, be sure to explain to the athlete what you are about to do. Longitudinal traction is applied to the affected limb; it is then moved manually to the correct anatomical position.[28] If at any time there is a significant increase in athlete's pain or tissue resistance is noted, ***immediately*** stop and immobilize the limb where it lies. Reassess the athlete's neurovascular status after the limb has been moved. If the neurovascular status has worsened, return the limb to its original position and transport immediately.[28]

Again, the decision to realign any skeletal injuries should also be identified as part of facility's standard operating procedures and/or emergency action plan. Damage caused by an athletic trainer's inappropriate action or harm suffered by the athlete may result in legal liability procedures (Chapter 3).

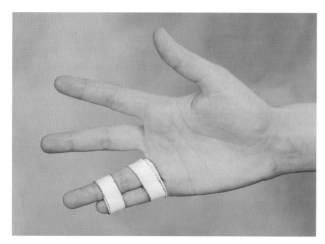

FIGURE 15.13 Anatomic "buddy" splint. (From Abell BA. *Taping and Wrapping Made Simple*. Baltimore: Lippincott Williams & Wilkins; 2010.)

A wide variety of immobilization devices are available to athletic trainers, depending upon the individual's practice setting. Based on the extent of the athlete's injury and the availability of equipment, each type of splint has its pluses and minuses, making one more or less advantageous to use over another, depending upon the situation. Although community responders often use improvised splinting devices, athletic trainers and EMS personal have access to a variety of commercial splints, such as (a) vacuum splints, (b) air splints, and (c) SAM Splints. However, regardless of the devices available, the basic strategies to ensure the proper application of the splint remain the same.

Immobilization Devices

Anatomical and Soft Splints

Immobilization devices or splints are normally categorized as either improvised or commercial. Within each category, there are numerous types of splints available to the athletic trainer. The first type, regardless of the practice setting or an athletic trainer's

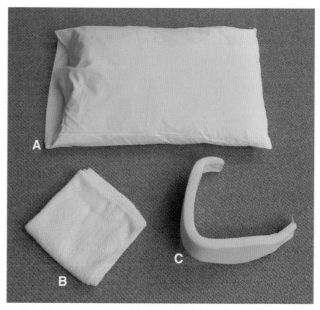

FIGURE 15.14 Soft splints. **A.** Pillow. **B.** Towel. **C.** Soft cervical collar.

experience level, is the anatomical splint. Anatomical splinting involves immobilizing one part of the body with another part of the body. Examples of anatomical splinting include splinting the arm to the chest to protect the shoulder, splinting the legs together to protect the knees, or buddy taping the fingers after a finger sprain, fracture, or spontaneous dislocation (Fig. 15.13).

Improvised soft splints are made of items such as blankets, pillows, and towels, whereas commercial soft splints include soft cervical collars. Soft splints are more adaptable than rigid splints and can conform better to some extremity injuries (e.g., ankle), but compared with rigid splints, they do not limit as much motion (Fig. 15.14).

Rigid Splints

Rigid splints are made of a variety of materials and may be improvised or commercially produced (Fig. 15.15). Items such

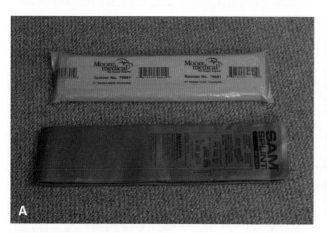

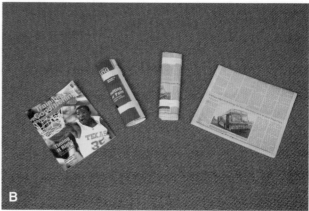

FIGURE 15.15 Commercial and improvised rigid splints. **A.** Commercial rigid splint for a wrist or hand injury. **B.** Improvised rigid splint using newspapers and magazines.

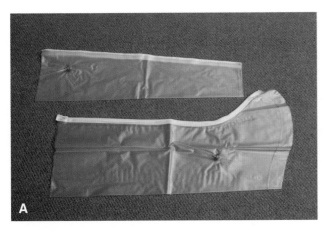
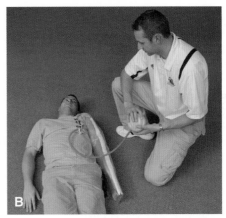

FIGURE 15.16   **A.** Air splint. **B.** To use the air splint, select the appropriate size, place the involved extremity in the splint, open the valve, blow air in the splint, and—once it is filled—close the valve.

as wooden boards, tongue depressors, cardboard, and even tree branches may be used as an improvised rigid splint. A majority of the commercially produced splints are specialty splints. Splints such as vacuum, air, ladder, and/or traction splints may require advanced training and practice beyond using basic household items. The SAM Splint, Ortho-glass splint, padded wooden boards, and aluminum finger splints are examples of commercially produced splints. The advantage of a rigid splint is that, once applied correctly, it will limit any further movement and reduce the risk of additional soft tissue or bony injuries. The disadvantage of some rigid splints is their inability to conform to injuries involving a significant deformity. Rigid splints are often used to manage nondisplaced closed fractures.

Box Splint   A box splint, for example, is a rigid splint comprised of three padded rigid boards and a U-shaped foot piece. An individual's foot is placed inside the box splint, which surrounds the entire foot, ankle, and distal tibia and fibula. Straps are then secured around the lower leg and foot. Box splints are suitable for ankle fractures, ankle dislocations, and distal fractures of the tibia and fibula. The athlete's shoe may have to be removed before applying this type of splint[28]; however, this decision will be based on the severity of the injury.

Air Splint   Air splints are easily applied, clear, inflatable plastic splints (Fig. 15.16). When inflated by mouth, they provide a uniform compressive force around the injured extremity and are **radiolucent**.[3] Air splint sets usually include a full leg, full arm, half leg, half arm, foot and ankle, and hand and wrist. Air splints do have one major disadvantage: they cannot be used on closed displaced or open fractures. The cylindrical splint requires the injury to conform to the splint rather than the splint conforming to the injury. If applied to an angulated or dislocated joint injury, such a splint may actually produce a painful manipulation of the joint or puncture due to the bone's sharp edges. Therefore, air splints should not be used on injuries where there is an increased risk of altering a deformed extremity.[3]

The newer counterpart to the traditional air splint is the PneuSplint by Laerdal Medical (Wappingers Falls, NY) (Fig. 15.17). The PneuSplint is a disposable air splint that, unlike the traditional air splint, is inflated and configured before it is applied to the injury. This splint will work for nondisplaced as well as angulated extremity injuries. It has perforations that allow the athletic trainer to conform the splint to the extremity and can be inflated using a pump. It is held in place using "quick open and close" straps. The PneuSplint is puncture-resistant and radiolucent. Skill 15.1 provides general guidelines for the preparation and application of a PneuSplint.

Vacuum Splint   Rapid-form vacuum splints are designed to aid in the stabilization of an injury while providing minimal movement to the injured area or extremity[29] (Fig. 15.18). They are composed of a strong, tough plastic containing polystyrene (Styrofoam) beads.[28] Rapid-form splints use a vacuum technology that immobilizes the injury without placing excessive pressure on it.[29] A vacuum splint, unlike a rigid splint, can be applied to angulated fractures and used on dislocations without the risk of further injuries because the splint molds itself around the injury.[29] The splint conforms to the injured

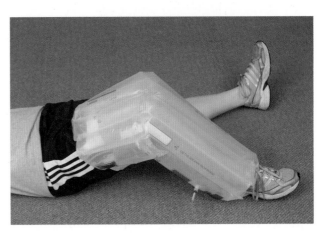

FIGURE 15.17   PneuSplint.

SKILL 15.1

Using a PneuSplint

Preparation*

1. Begin with a complete assessment of the extremity, including the distal neurovascular structures.
2. Apply appropriate dressings to all wounds in and around the injuries site.
3. Inflate the splint by pulling the inflation nozzle out.
4. Once a desired level of compression is reached, push the inflation nozzle in.

Application for Straight Immobilization

1. Continue to support and limit any excessive movement of the injured extremity as a second athletic trainer places the printed side of splint under and away from the injury.
2. Secure the splint snugly, using the hook and loop straps provided.
3. If the splint does not conform easily to the injury, adjust the amount of air in the splint until it conforms appropriately.

Application for Angled Immobilization

1. Continue to support and limit any excessive movement of the injured extremity as a second athletic trainer places the printed side of splint under and away from the injury.
2. Tear the splint along dotted lines on both sides.
3. Adjust the splint to the appropriate angle and secure it in place using the fasteners on the splint.
4. Secure snugly using the hook and loop straps provided.
5. If the splint does not conform easily to the injury, adjust the amount of air in the splint until the splint conforms appropriately.

Completion

1. Reassess the distal neurovascular structures. Any compromise to these structures requires immediate attention.

*Information based on the manufacturer's directions.

area as the athletic trainer draws the air out of the sleeve using a handheld pump.[3] The removal of the air is what gives the splint its rigidity. The polystyrene beads inside the splint also help to reduce lost body heat and are radiolucent. The vacuum splint mattress has also been used to provide total body support similar to the use of traditional backboard.[30]

Because there are a variety of vacuum splints currently on the market, Skill 15.2 provides general guidelines for the preparation, application, and evacuation of rapid-form vacuum splints.[29]

SAM Splint The SAM Splint (Sam Medical Products, Newport, OR) is a malleable commercial splint; when bent

into one of three simple curves, it becomes a rigid splint for a various extremity injuries. The strength and pliability of the splint is attributed to the thin aluminum alloy core that is sandwiched between two layers of closed-cell foam.[31] The SAM Splint is lightweight and compact; it can be rolled and/or folded for storage in an emergency trauma kit. The

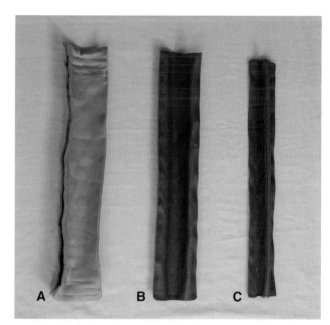

FIGURE 15.19 SAM Splint curves. **A.** C-curve is formed by creating a longitudinal bend in the center of the splint. **B.** Reverse C-curve formed using the C-curve with an additional bend of the edge of splint in the reverse direction of the C-curve. **C.** T-curve is formed by folding the outer edges of the splint together, followed by bending half of each side of the splint in the opposite direction of the original fold to create a T-shaped beam.

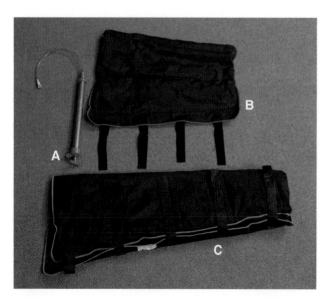

FIGURE 15.18 Vacuum splint kit. **A.** Pump. **B.** Arm splint. **C.** Leg splint.

SKILL 15.2

Using a Rapid-Form Vacuum Splint*

Preparation

1. Remove the splint from its carrying care and select the appropriate splint that will splint the joints above and below the fracture site for injuries to the bone or above and below the bone for injuries to the joint. Shoulder and hip injuries may require additional immobilization procedures and equipment.
2. Begin with a complete assessment of the extremity, including the distal neurovascular structures.
3. Apply appropriate dressings to all wounds in and around the injury site.
4. Place the splint next to the athlete with the valve side down and distribute the Styrofoam beads evenly throughout the splint.
5. Make sure that the splint has enough air within the sleeve to keep the beads from collecting at the bottom of the splint when it is lifted to the vertical position. However, too much air will make it impossible to mold the splint to the injured extremity.

Application

1. Continue to support and limit any excessive movement of the injured extremity as a second athletic trainer places the splint under the injury.
2. Position the splint so one strap is above and another below the suspected injury site.
3. Wrap the splint around the injury and, before the straps are secured, massage the beads into place to make sure that any and all voids are filled. If the splint does not conform easily to the injury, adjust the amount of air in the splint until it conforms appropriately.

4. The splint should conform easily. If not, adjust it by allowing air into the device. Splint edges should not overlap.

Evacuation

1. To evacuate the air from the splint, attach the splint's vacuum pump to the appropriate coupling device.
2. Once this is secured, begin to extract the air. As the air is removed, the splint will begin to harden. Resistance on the pump handle will indicate that enough air has been evacuated from the splint.
3. Disconnect the coupling device so the air cannot escape.
4. Place the splint straps securely around the injury site.
5. Make any necessary adjustment to ensure athlete comfort by removing or allowing air into the splint. Add additional support such as a sling or swathe.
6. Complete a thorough assessment of the distal neurovascular structures such as skin color, pulse, capillary refill, sensation, and mobility. Any compromise to these structures requires immediate attention.
7. When working with a dislocated joint, evacuate enough air to allow the splint to resemble modeling clay. Using a second athletic trainer or bystander as a model, mold the splint to his or her simulated injury and then simply transfer the splint shape to the athlete.

*Information is based on the manufactures directions for the EVAC-U-SPLINT.[29] Some units may not function exactly according to the information provided above.

Sam Splint is not affected by extremes of temperature or altitude; it is radiolucent, fastened into place using tape or wraps (elastic or cotton), and can be reused after being disinfected with standard cleaning solutions.[31]

The splints are available in several lengths: 9, 18, 36, and 3¾ in. The intended use of the splint will often determine the size selected. As previously mentioned, the strength of the splint is determined by its shape when formed to the injured body part. The SAM Splint can be made into three shapes: The first shape is the C-curve, which is created by forming a lengthwise longitudinal bend in the shape of a C (Fig. 15.19A). The reverse C-curve (Fig. 15.19B) is stronger than the C-curve and is formed using the C-curve with an additional bend of the edge of splint in the reverse direction of the C-curve. The final shape, the T-curve, is the strongest of the three splint shapes[31] (Fig. 15.19C). It is formed by folding the outer edges of the splint together followed by bending half of each side of the splint in the opposite direction of the original fold to create a T-shaped beam. Specific examples are provided in Chapter 16.

Highlight

Using the SAM Splint as a Cervical Collar

SAM Splints can serve more than just one purpose; more than 20 different immobilization techniques are outlined in the manufacturer's user's guide.[31] These do not include the many ways in which the device is used by outdoor enthusiasts—as a flame guard, flashlight holder, or canoe paddle. If such a user suffered a cervical spine injury, he or she could use the SAM Splint as a cervical collar to stabilize the spine. McGrath and Murphy[32] compared the effectiveness of the SAM Splint molded into a cervical collar with that of the Philadelphia cervical collar at limiting cervical spine movement. They found both to be equally effective in limiting five different movements.[32]

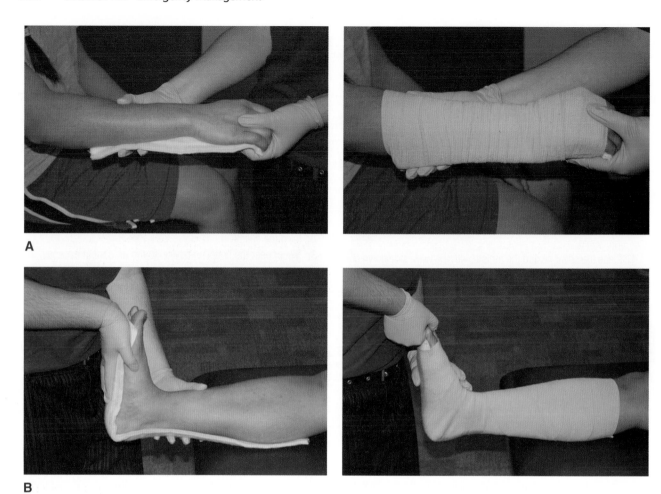

FIGURE 15.20 Ortho-Glass Splint. **A.** Volar splint for a wrist injury. **B.** Posterior splint for an ankle injury.

Orthoglass Splint Like the SAM Splint, Ortho-Glass (BSN Medical, Inc., Charlotte, NC) is a commercial splinting system. When such a splint is passed under cool water, a chemical reaction occurs that hardens the padded fiberglass insert. Though not an ideal splinting medium for an on-field injury (e.g., in football or lacrosse), Ortho-Glass works well in a controlled environment to stabilize a variety of upper-(Fig. 15.20) and lower-body injuries (Fig. 15.20B). The material comes in a variety of widths and can be cut to length and shaped around the injured extremity. Finally, because the splint can be molded to only one side of the body, it allows for an increase in joint edema and can be worn temporarily until a proper medical referral can be made.

Traction Splints

The application of a traction splint does not typically fall within the athletic trainer's scope of practice. Remember from Chapter 1 that the application of a traction splint for stabilization of a femoral fracture is an advanced skill performed by emergency medical technicians, advanced emergency medical technicians, and paramedics. Therefore, this section is intended to serve an informational purpose only. Athletic trainers should consult with their team physicians and with individual state laws and practice acts to determine

whether the use of traction splints is an acceptable form of immobilization in their area of practice.

Traction splints were designed during World War I as a method of decreasing the secondary loss of blood associated with femoral fractures. They may be used with isolated closed and open fractures of the femoral shaft[28,33] and are designed to apply a constant pull along the length of the limb to stabilize the fracture, reduce blood loss, reduce quadriceps muscle spasms, and help maintain the athlete's distal vascular supply.[34,35] Muscle spasms occur as the quadriceps and hamstrings go into protective spasms. These cause the two ends of the femur to override each other, thus increasing pain and the risk of soft tissue injuries, especially to the blood vessels (e.g., the femoral artery) and nerves (e.g., the sciatic and femoral nerves).

The placement of a traction splint requires two well-trained individuals, one to apply initial manual traction and another to set up and apply the mechanical traction. Several types of traction splints are available, including Faretec Traction Leg Splints (Faretec, Painesville, OH); Sager Traction Splints (Sager, Redding, CA); and the Kendrick Traction Device (Kendrick, Kent, OH) (Fig. 15.21). Each traction splint should be used in accordance with the manufacturer's guidelines. Remember, regardless of the type of traction

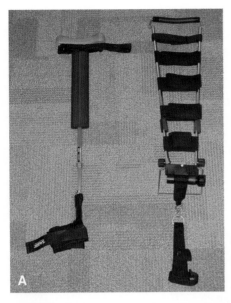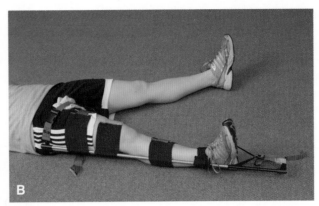

FIGURE 15.21   **A.** Traction leg splints. **B.** Application of a traction splint.

splint selected, it is necessary to assess the athlete's neurovascular status before and after applying the splint.

Support Materials for Immobilization Devices

Once the proper immobilization device is selected, the athletic trainer must then determine how to properly secure it to the body. There are several possible methods, ranging from elastic bandages to cotton roll gauze. Some devices, such as a vacuum or traction splint, come with the necessary materials for supporting the device. When preparing an emergency trauma kit, it is beneficial to have several different types of methods available. This section outlines some of the supportive devices available to athletic trainers.

Slings

A sling is a triangular bandage suspended from the neck to support an injured upper extremity (e.g., clavicular fracture, shoulder dislocation, or other injury to the upper or lower arm). It may be used alone to stabilize a skeletal injury (e.g., clavicular fracture) or in conjunction with other immobilization techniques to provide further support to the injury (e.g., humeral or forearm fracture) once it has been immobilized. A triangular bandage is ideal for fabricating a sling but strips of clothing, blankets, and even towels can also be used. When applying a sling, remember to keep the hand higher than the elbow and, whenever possible, allow the fingers to be exposed so that the athlete's neurovascular status can be monitored. In addition, the sling should support the injured area to decrease pressure on the affected limb. To tie a triangular bandage into a sling, follow the directions in Skill 15.3.

Swathes

Swathes are bands used in conjunction with a sling to supply further immobilization, particularly to an upper extremity, by binding the athlete's arm to his or her chest (e.g., anatomical splint). Cravat bandages are the most commonly used type of swathe (see Fig. 15.24). However, swathes can be improvised by using belts, sheets, shirts, and other items (Fig. 15.25).

Bandages

Bandages are used to help support limbs that have sustained a variety of injuries, including bone fractures and joint dislocations. They are also used in conjunction with sterile dressings applied directly over an open wound to control external bleeding. A triangular bandage folded into a cravat is commonly used to splint and support extremity injuries (Fig. 15.26). Triangular bandages are purchased commercially or improvised using a 40-in. square, which is folded diagonally and then cut along the fold.[36] To make a cravat, fold the triangular bandage to make a 2-in.-wide strip by folding the tip of the triangular bandage to its base. Continue this process until the desired size is achieved, usually 2 in. to 4 in. in width. Bandages may also be fabricated from many other household materials such as belts, shirts, or strips torn from clothing or blankets.

Wraps

Elastic or cotton wraps of varying sizes are commonly used to secure splints. Wraps are applied from the distal segment of the extremity to the proximal segment in a circular or spiral pattern (Fig. 15.27). When using elastic wraps, be careful to avoid applying the wrap too tightly.[37] Failure to monitor distal neurovascular status can lead to impaired distal perfusion and sensation.

SKILL 15.3

Applying a Sling and Swathe

1. Place one end of the base of the open triangle over the shoulder of the uninjured side (Fig. 15.22).
2. Allow the triangular bandage to hang in front of the chest on the opposite side with the apex behind the elbow of the injured extremity (Fig. 15.22).
3. Bend the injured arm upward 4 or 5 in. so that the hand is slightly elevated and place the injured forearm close to the chest wall over the bandage.
4. Bring up the low end of the bandage over the shoulder of the injured side and tie a knot at the uninjured side of the neck. Place a gauze pad under the knot (Fig. 15.23).
5. Twist the apex at the elbow or tuck it into the elbow.
6. Using a 2- or 3-in. cravat, secure the elbow and distal humerus to the body by tying the bandage to the noninvolved limb (swathe) (Fig. 15.24).
7. Place a gauze pad under each knot.

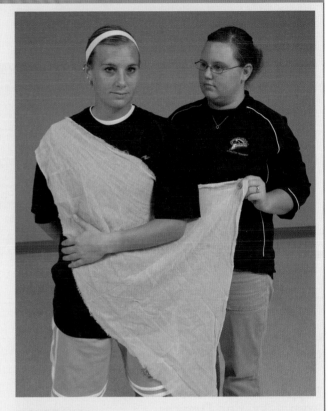

FIGURE 15.22

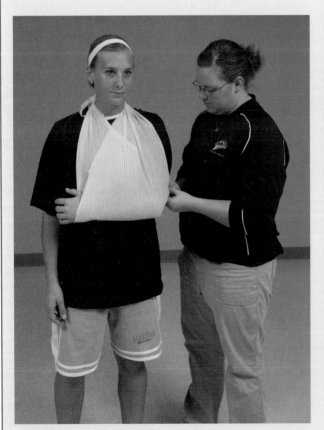

FIGURE 15.23

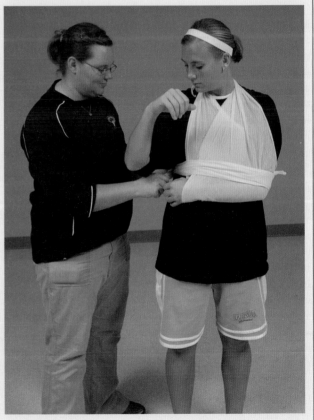

FIGURE 15.24

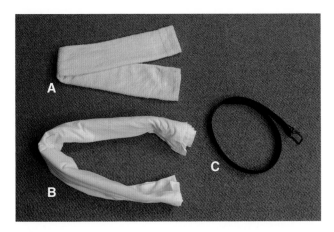

FIGURE 15.25   Improvised swathes. **A.** Towel. **B.** Sheet. **C.** Belt.

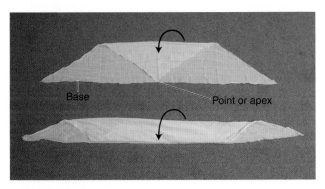

FIGURE 15.26   Folding a cravat into a triangular bandage. Fold the point (or apex) to the base and continue folding over until a 2- to 3-in. strip is formed.

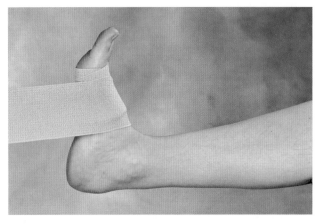

FIGURE 15.27   Applying an elastic wrap. Begin distally and wrap proximally; do not apply the wrap too tightly. (From Abell BA. *Taping and Wrapping Made Simple*. Baltimore: Lippincott Williams & Wilkins; 2010.)

Do not use a wire or cord to secure a splint in place because these materials can damage tissue by disrupting blood flow.

WRAP-UP

Skeletal injuries commonly occur in the course of physical activity, competitive sports, and life in general. Because athletic trainers are often the first individuals on site when such injuries occur, being prepared by developing a detailed emergency action plan that identifies how and when to immobilize skeletal injuries—as well as having the proper equipment readily available—will help to minimize the athlete's chances of sustaining a secondary injury. By understanding how to properly select, use, and

Scenarios

1. A high school running back is rushing down the sideline when he is hit from the side by an opposing player, forcing him into the visiting team's sideline bench. His femur strikes the bench violently. As you rush over to him, you notice that he is in severe pain and that his thigh appears to be shortened and angulated. You attempt to palpate his femur and realize that his quadriceps and hamstrings are in spasm in an effort to protect the joint.

   What type of splint should be applied and why?

2. Sally is playing basketball when a teammate passes the ball, hitting the tip of her middle finger. As Sally approaches, you notice that the middle finger of her left hand is angularly deformed.

   What type of splint may be used to immobilize the finger?
   Who should be responsible for relocating the deformed joint?
   Are there any risks if the athletic trainer tries to relocate the joint?

3. Tom, running down the court during a basketball game, collides with another player. The opposing player lands on Tom's lateral leg. Mary, the athletic trainer covering the game, runs onto the court to manage the situation. She quickly determines that Tom has a possible fracture of the fibula.

   What are some common signs and symptoms Mary may have recognized when making this clinical diagnosis?
   What type of immobilization device would you recommend and why?

4. While covering a high school softball game, Shelia is summoned onto the field to assess Samantha, an injured outfielder. Samantha reports falling on her outstretched arm while attempting to catch a pop fly. She presents with all the signs and symptoms of a clavicular fracture.

   How should Shelia attempt to stabilize this injury in order to transport Samantha to the hospital?
   How would you describe the mechanism of injury to the doctor at the emergency room?

apply the immobilization devices and techniques presented in this chapter, athletic trainers will be able to effectively stabilize and manage skeletal injuries as well as associated soft tissue injuries when they occur. Chapter 16 describes in detail the techniques for immobilizing a wide variety of skeletal injuries (and soft tissue injuries) to the extremities, thorax, and pelvis.

REFERENCES

1. Adams JC. *Outline of Fractures: Including Joint Injuries.* London: Churchill and Livingstone; 1972.
2. Nordin M, Frankel VH. *Basic Biomechanics of the Musculoskeletal System,* 3rd ed. Philadelphia: Lippincott, Williams & Wilkins; 2001.
3. Prentice WE. *Arnheim's Principles of Athletic Training,* 13th ed. New York: McGraw-Hill; 2009.
4. Baykal B, Sener S, Turkan H. Scapular manipulation technique for reduction of traumatic anterior shoulder dislocations: Experiences of an academic emergency department. *Emerg Med J.* 2005;22:336–338.
5. Owens BD, Dawson L, Burks R, et al. Incidence of shoulder dislocation in the United States Military: Demographic considerations from a high-risk population. *J Bone Joint Surg Am.* 2009;91(4):791–796.
6. Wang RY, Arciero RA, Mazzocca AD. The recognition and treatment of first-time shoulder dislocation in active individuals. *J Orthop Sports Phys Ther.* 2009;39(2):118–123.
7. Paksima N, Panchal A. Elbow fracture-dislocations: The role of hinged external fixation. *Bull Hosp Joint Dis.* 2004;62(1–2):33–39.
8. Rettig AC. Elbow, forearm and wrist injuries in the athlete. *Sports Med.* 1998;25(2):115–130.
9. Josefsson P, Nilsson B. Incidence of elbow dislocation. *Acta Orthop Scand.* 1986;57(6):537–538.
10. Rettig AC. Athletic injuries of the wrist and hand: Part II: Overuse injuries of the wrist and traumatic injuries to the hand. *Am J Sports Med.* 2004;32(1):262–273.
11. Stannard JP, Sheils TM, Lopez-Ben RR, et al. Vascular injuries in knee dislocations: The role of physical examination in determining the need for arteriography. *J Bone Joint Surg Am.* 2004;86(5):910–915.
12. Martinez D, Sweatman K, Thompson EC. Popliteal artery injury associated with knee dislocations. *Am Surg.* 2001;67(2):165–167.
13. Hubble MW, Hubble JP. *Principles of Advanced Trauma Care.* Albany, NY: Delmar Thompson Learning; 2002.
14. Henrichs A. A review of knee dislocations. *J Athl Train.* 2004;39(4):365–369.
15. Polansky RE, Kwon NS. Joint reduction, finger dislocation. *eMedicine.* 2009. Available at http://emedicine.medscape.com/article/109206-overview. Accessed May 24, 2010.
16. Schultz SJ, Houglum PA, Perrin DA. *Examination of Musculoskeletal Injuries,* 2nd ed. Champaign, IL: Human Kinetics; 2005.
17. Fithian DC, Paxton EW, Stone ML, et al. Epidemiology and natural history of acute patellar dislocation. *Am J Sports Med.* 2004;32(5):1114–1121.
18. Beeson MS. Complications of shoulder dislocation. *Am J Emerg Med.* 1999;17(3):288–295.
19. Perron AD, Ingerski MS, Brady WJ, et al. Acute complications associated with shoulder dislocation at an academic emergency department. *J Emerg Med.* 2003;24(2):141–145.
20. Kazemi M. Tuning fork test utilization in detection of fractures: A review of the literature. *J Can Chiropr Assoc.* 1999;43(2):120–124.
21. Moore MB. *The Use of a Tuning Fork and Stethoscope versus Clinical Fracture Testing in Assessing Possible Fractures.* Blacksburg, VA: Education, Virginia Polytechnic Institute and State University; 2005.
22. Konin JG, Wiksten D, Isear JA, et al. *Special Tests for Orthopedic Examination,* 3rd ed. Thorofare, NJ: Slack; 2006.
23. Starkey C, Ryan J. *Evaluation of Orthopedic and Athletic Injuries,* 2nd ed. Philadelphia: FA Davis; 2002.
24. Bache JB, Cross AB. The Barford test. A useful diagnostic sign in fracture of the femoral neck. *Practitioner.* 1984;228:305–307.
25. Misurya RK, Khare A, Mallick A, et al. Use of tuning fork in diagnostic auscultation of fractures. *Injury.* 1987;18:63–64.
26. Lesho EP. Can tuning forks replace bone scans for identification of tibial stress fractures? *Mil Med.* 1997;162(12):802–803.
27. Wilder RP, Vincent HK, Stewart J, et al. Clinical use of tuning forks to identify running related stress fractures. *Athl Train Sports Health Care.* 2009;1(1):12–18.
28. Lee C, Porter KM. Prehospital management of lower limb fractures. *Emerg Med J.* 2005;22:660–663.
29. Hartwell, Medical. EVAC-U-SPLINT Application Guidelines. http://www.hartwellmedical.com/. Accessed June 6, 2006.
30. Ahmad M, Butler J. Spinal boards or vacuum mattresses for immobilisation. *Emerg Med J.* 2001;18:379–380.
31. Scheinberg S. *SAM SPLINT User Guide.* SAM Medical Products; 2005.
32. McGrath T, Murphy C. Comparison of a SAM splint-molded cervical collar with a Philadelphia cervical collar. *Wilderness Environ Med.* 2009;20(2):166–168.
33. Bledsoe BE, Barnes D. Traction splints: An EMS relic? *JEMS.* 2004;29(8):64–69.
34. Wood SP, Vrahas M, Wedel SK. Femur fracture immobilization with traction splints in multisystem trauma patients. *Prehosp Emerg Care.* 2003;7(2):241–243.
35. Limmer D, O'Keefe MF, Grant HD, et al. *Emergency Care,* 9th ed. Upper Saddle River, NJ: Prentice Hall; 2001.
36. Karren KJ, Hafen BQ, Limmer D, et al. *First Aid for Colleges and Universities,* 8th ed. Upper Saddle River, NJ: Benjamin Cummings; 2003.
37. Meredith RM, Butcher JD. Field splinting of suspected fractures: Preparation, assessment, and application. *Phys Sportsmed.* 1997;25.

Immobilization Techniques for Extremity, Thoracic, and Pelvis Injuries

CHAPTER OUTCOMES

1. Identify the appropriate evaluation techniques to properly immobilize an extremity, thoracic, or pelvic injury during an emergency situation.

2. Describe the indications and proper techniques for removing equipment and clothing in order to evaluate and properly immobilize an extremity injury during an emergency situation.

3. Identify the mechanism of injury, signs and symptoms, and possible immobilization techniques for a variety

of extremity, thoracic, and pelvic injuries during an emergency situation.

4. Describe the proper immobilization techniques for a variety of extremity, thoracic, and pelvic injuries during an emergency situation.

5. Demonstrate the proper of immobilization techniques to stabilize a variety of extremity, thoracic, and pelvic injuries to maintain normal distal neurovascular status during an emergency situation.

NOMENCLATURE

Acromioclavicular joint: joint between the acromial end of the clavicle and the medial margin of the acromion

Anatomical snuff box: a hollow seen on the radial aspect of the wrist when the thumb is extended fully; it is bounded by the tendon of the extensor pollicis longus posteriorly and of the tendons of the extensor pollicis brevis and abductor pollicis longus anteriorly. The radial artery crosses the floor, which is formed by the scaphoid and trapezium bones

Arteriography: visualization of an artery or arteries by x-ray imaging after injection of a radiopaque contrast medium

Avascular necrosis: death or decay of tissue due to local ischemia in the absence of infection

Coaptation: joining or fitting together of two surfaces

Complex dislocation: dislocation with concomitant fractures about a joint

Concomitant: occurring simultaneously

Flail chest: condition in which two or more consecutive ribs on the same side of the chest have been fractured in at least two places, with resulting instability of the chest wall, paradoxic respiratory movements of the injured segment, and loss of respiratory efficiency

NOMENCLATURE *(Continued)*

FOOSH: falling on an outstretched hand

Glenohumeral joint: ball-and-socket synovial joint between the head of the humerus and the glenoid cavity of the scapula

Gutter splint: splint located on the radial or ulnar side of the wrist

Hemothorax: accumulation of blood in the pleural cavity (space between the lungs and the walls of the chest) caused by rupture of blood vessels due to trauma

Interosseous membrane: broad and thin plane of fibrous tissue separating many of the bones of the body

Jones fracture: transverse fracture of the proximal shaft of the fifth metatarsal

Longitudinal compression: compression of the ends of two long bones

Maceration: softening of the skin from moisture

Osteoarthritis: arthritis characterized by erosion of articular cartilage, which becomes soft, frayed, and thinned with outgrowths of marginal osteophytes; pain and loss of function result; mainly affects weight-bearing joints, is more common in women, the overweight, and in older individuals

Patella alta: patella assuming a more proximal position than anticipated when visualized on a lateral radiograph of the knee; a high-riding patella

Plafond: ceiling, especially the ceiling of the ankle joint—i.e., the articular surface of the distal end of the tibia

Pott fracture: fracture of the lower part of the fibula and of the malleolus of the tibia, with lateral displacement of the foot

Q-angle: angle formed by the line of traction of the quadriceps tendon on the patella and the line of traction of the patellar tendon on the tibial tubercle. The area is usually larger in women than in men

Maisonneuve fracture: spiral fracture of the neck of the fibula resulting from violent external rotation of the ankle

Parietal pleura: outer lining of the pleural cavity

Pneumothorax: accumulation of air/gas in the pleural cavity—may be due to trauma but can also occur spontaneously

Position of function: correct position for most upper extremity splinting. The wrist is allowed to be slightly extended and the fingers in a relaxed flexed position (sometime referred to as the "can position"), as if supporting a can

Radial nerve palsy: paralysis of the radial nerve leading to loss of function of the muscles innervated by the radial nerve

Retinaculum: retaining band or ligament that allows tendons to maintain normal anatomical position and function

Scapulothoracic joint: articulation between the scapula and the dorsal thorax; it is not a true anatomical joint because it lacks a synovial capsule and there are muscles between the anterior surface of the scapula and the thorax

Simple dislocation: dislocation without concomitant fractures about a joint

Sternoclavicular joint: synovial articulation between the medial end of the clavicle and the manubrium of the sternum and cartilage of the first rib

Translate: to change the position of figures or bodies in space without rotation

Volkmann's ischemic contracture: ischemic contracture resulting from irreversible necrosis of muscle tissue following a brachial artery injury, classically involving the forearm flexor muscles

BEFORE YOU BEGIN

1. What is the most appropriate method of immobilizing trauma to the clavicle?

2. How many different methods are there to stabilize trauma to the humeroradial, humeroulnar, or radioulnar joints?

3. Describe the appropriate steps to apply a sugar-tong splint for trauma to the forearm.

4. Why are elbow, hip, and knee dislocations so dangerous? What should be an immediate concern when attempting to stabilize these injuries?

5. What is the difference between a Cadillac splint and ankle stirrup splint? When would you apply these?

6. What is a traction splint? Are athletic trainers allowed to apply such a splint in an emergency situation? When is such a splint indicated?

7. If an athlete sustained a pelvic fracture, how would you handle it? What would be an athletic trainer's number one concern?

Voices from the Field

Proper and immediate identification of the signs and symptoms of a musculoskeletal injury is important in order to be able to competently stabilize the injury As certified athletic trainers (ATCs), we must be confident with our emergency training immobilization procedures so that we can provide swift and proper interventions in the event of an emergency.

While at an away game, our running back was hit by a defensive lineman in the hip area. The running back was tackled and landed on all fours when he was struck directly in the left hip by the lineman. When I arrived at his side, he was in severe pain, lying prone, his hip in internal rotation and knee in flexion. Our coach was adamant that the player be taken off the field, to the point of being almost violent. The player was turned supine and, after performing a primary and secondary assessment he was basket-carried off the field by athletic trainers and placed supine in a position of comfort on the sideline. The home team's physician was alerted to report to the visiting sideline, as well as emergency medical services (EMS). Interestingly enough, EMS was found by the home team's ATC in the crowd, where they were eating a snack.

Once EMS and the physician arrived on site, a paramedic began administering morphine for pain, as directed by the physician. The EMS response team questioned me as to whether a traction splint was needed. Based on the signs and symptoms presented and an understanding of how a traction splint functions, I knew that this was not the best course of action, because we had determined that the young man had sustained a hip dislocation as well as a hip fracture. He was, therefore, splinted in a position of comfort using a soft splint (pillows) to support the hip and knee. He was then spine-boarded and transported to the nearest hospital, where his hip was relocated.

The player was released after 3 days in the hospital and placed in a wheelchair, where he spent the next 6 weeks. During this period, he lost nearly 75 pounds. However, he returned to football in 10 months and, during the following season, went on to break the conference rushing single-season record.

The final diagnosis was a posterior hip dislocation with a posterior wall acetabular fracture. Surgical intervention was not needed, because the posterior wall of the acetabulum relocated on its own during the 6 weeks of the non–weight-bearing period.

This case demonstrates the necessity for proper and immediate recognition of musculoskeletal injuries. As seen in this case, if the dislocation was immediately recognized, proper treatment could have been performed on the field to eliminate excessive movement to the limb. The situation could have been further complicated had the athlete been placed in a traction splint. However, it was recognized that this was not the correct procedure. Ultimately the athlete received the necessary care and returned to competitive sports. Lesson learned: athletic trainers must be advocates for their athletes and be knowledgeable of all types of splinting devices, including the indications and contraindication to all applications of each apparatus.

Michael Hann, M.S., LAT, ATC
Head Football Athletic Trainer
Sacred Heart University
Fairfield, CT

It is critical that the airway, breathing, and circulation be monitored in every situation where a suspected fracture is present and that necessary precautions must be reviewed before a life-threatening injury occurs.

Maintaining composure during an emergency is one of the most important skills that athletic trainers possess. We must make quick and often unpopular decisions about how to manage an injury and whether or not to return an athlete to play. When a fracture or dislocation is suspected, immediate immobilization and splinting is critical. Even a simple finger fracture that would heal in 3 to 5 weeks can become displaced, requiring surgery, internal fixations, and a much longer re-covery time. Permanent deformity and/or loss of function can also result if fractures and dislocations are not recognized and managed promptly and effectively. In my 14 years as an ATC I've seen too many athletes who weren't splinted or chose not to wear their splint who ended up as surgical cases. One Division II women's basketball player I worked with jeopardized her career as a veterinary surgeon due to a displaced finger fracture.

Valerie W. Herzog, EdD, LAT, ATC
Graduate Athletic Training Program Director
Weber State University
Ogden, UT

I n Chapter 15 we examined the different types of skeletal injuries and general management procedures, including mechanisms of injury, general signs and symptoms, commonly encountered immobilization devices, and general strategies for immobilizing an injury. In this chapter we examine in greater detail a variety of skeletal trauma to the appendicular and axial skeleton, mechanisms of injury, signs and symptoms, evaluation techniques where appropriate, and, more importantly, how to apply specific types of immobilization devices to minimize further injury and disability. Immobilizing traumatic bone or joint injuries is an art form, requiring practice, so when an injury does occur, the athletic trainer is able to competently and efficiently stabilize the injury with little pain or secondary trauma to the athlete. The techniques described in this chapter are not limited to immobilizing skeletal trauma; soft tissue trauma such as ligament sprains and muscle strains can also immobilized using these techniques.

ASSESSMENT OF THE UPPER EXTREMITY AND THORAX

Prior to immobilizing the upper extremity or thorax, the athletic trainer should have already completed a scene survey, made a

SKILL 16.1

Musculoskeletal Emergency Care

1. Initiate EAP (when indicated).
2. Check the safety of the scene.
3. Take and maintain appropriate body substance isolation (BSI) precautions.
4. Begin the primary assessment. Remember "life before limb." Never compromise an individual's survival to splint what appears to be a grossly deformed, painful extremity injury unless that deformed extremity poses a risk. Femoral and pelvic fractures, for example, increase the risk of hypoperfusion secondary to the significant blood loss associated with these injuries.
5. Begin a head-to-toe assessment using the mnemonic DOTS. For an athlete wearing protective equipment, remove as necessary and with as little movement as possible in order to properly assess the extremity. If a cervical spine injury is suspected, consider applying a cervical collar.
6. Establish baseline vitals and gather a SAMPLE history.
7. Immobilize all painful, swollen, or deformed extremities. Cover all open wounds with sterile dressings and remember to check circulation, sensation, and movement (CSM) before and after immobilization of the extremity.
8. Apply ice and, once stabilized, elevate the limb if necessary to decrease edema formation.

primary assessment, and provided any necessary interventions to life-threatening conditions involving the airway, breathing, and circulation (ABCs), head, spine, and/or abdomen. The secondary assessment (Chapter 8) is the next step. Remember, during this examination the athletic trainer will inspect and palpate for signs of any potential musculoskeletal trauma that may require immobilization (i.e., deformity, open wounds, tenderness, swelling, or DOTS) (Skill 16.1). Severely deformed extremity injuries are normally obvious; however, not all extremity injuries can be easily identified because of the protective equipment and clothing worn by some athletes. A general rule of thumb when assessing any musculoskeletal injuries is to remove only necessary clothing and equipment according to the environment, severity of the injury, and the recommendations of your facility's emergency action plan (EAP).

Protective Equipment Considerations

To adequately assess the shoulder, the athletic trainer may have to perform the physical assessment under the shoulder pads. In some situations, such as a shoulder dislocation or clavicular fracture, the athletic trainer may have to remove the athlete's protective equipment.[1] Loosening the protective equipment's (e.g., football, ice hockey, lacrosse) fasteners or straps should allow for adequate room to reach under the pads to palpate and assess the joint's integrity. Football shoulder pads are designed with a hollow channel running parallel from the clavicle to the **acromioclavicular joint** (ACJ). This channel is accessible when the shoulder pad's cantilever is elevated after the shirt has been removed. Extreme caution must be used when performing any type of palpation under protective equipment because the athletic trainer is relying on feel rather than sight to assess the injury. Palpation of the shoulder joint should be discontinued if the athlete experiences any increase in pain and/or deformities are noted.

When protective equipment or clothing must be removed to access the shoulder joint, the athletic trainer must do so with as little movement as possible. This may require assistance from another individual. A loose-fitting shirt can be removed by asking the athlete to slide the uninvolved limb out first, lifting the shirt over his or her head and then sliding it down over the involved limb (Fig. 16.1). If this is unsuccessful or if the shirt is too tight or removing the shirt increases the athlete's pain, the shirt will have to be cut down one of the seams, moving from a superior to an inferior direction. Loosen the equipment's fasteners or straps and remove the protective equipment in a similar fashion to the shirt. If the protective equipment and shirt can be removed at the same time, follow the directions above.

The remaining upper extremity (i.e., elbow, forearm, wrist, and hand) is not normally covered by any protective equipment except in sports such as ice hockey and lacrosse and by goalies in team sports where a projectile is used. Ice hockey and lacrosse players are required to wear protective gloves, usually made of a stiff outer layer (leather) and contoured according to the sport. Goalies in sports such as field hockey and ice hockey wear hand-protective equipment used to deflect the projectile. Such gloves can usually be slid off with minimal difficulty but may require another athletic trainer to help support and stabilize the limb. If other types of protective equipment are being used and must be removed to access an injury, the athletic trainer should do so with as little movement as possible. Athletic trainers should practice removing any protective equipment that he or she is unfamiliar with prior to an emergency.

IMMOBILIZING THE UPPER EXTREMITY AND THORAX

Traumatic injuries to the upper extremity may result in anything from a fractured phalanx to a dislocated elbow or shoulder. The type of injury sustained is dependent upon the mechanisms of injury, location of force application, and amount of force applied. This section outlines common skeletal injuries to the upper extremity and thorax and the techniques for properly immobilizing these injuries.

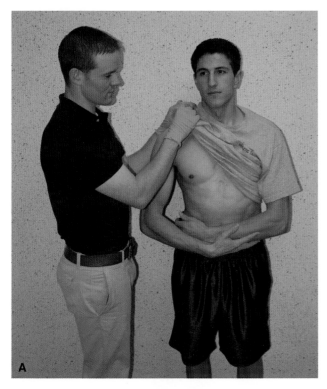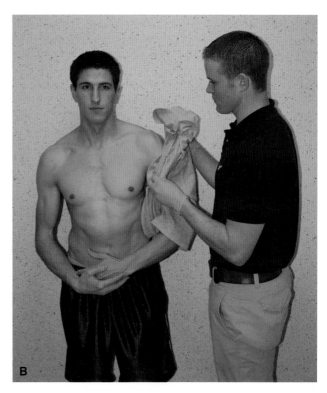

FIGURE 16.1   Shirt removal for an upper extremity injury. **A.** Slide the uninvolved limb out first. **B.** Lifting the shirt over the head, slide it down over the involved limb.

Shoulder Complex

Trauma to the shoulder joint and girdle occurs due to a direct blow to the tip or any aspect of the shoulder or shoulder girdle (e.g., being struck in the chest with a piece of playing equipment or by another opponent), falling on the tip of the shoulder, or an indirect force transmitted up the humerus from falling on an outstretched hand **(FOOSH)** or elbow. Shoulder girdle injuries such as sprains of the **sternoclavicular joint** (SCJ) are common, whereas traumatic dislocations (anterior or posterior direction) are rare occurrences because of the force required to rupture the sternoclavicular and costoclavicular ligaments[1–3] and only make up only 3% of all shoulder girdle injuries[4] and 1% of all joint dislocations.[5] Anterior SCJ dislocations are more prevalent than posterior dislocations[2,6]; however, individuals who have sustained a posterior SCJ dislocation are at greater risk for life-threatening emergencies because of the compression of the large neurovascular structures (i.e., subclavian artery and vein, and brachial plexus), trachea, and esophagus located just posterior to the joint.[2,3,7] These individuals may present with dizziness, nausea, and difficulty breathing or swallowing.

Fractures of the clavicle (collarbone) account for approximately 5% of all orthopedic fractures[8] and are most common in children.[9] The middle third of the clavicle is the most common location for these fractures.[3] If a clavicular fracture is suspected, you will have to manage the injury carefully to limit secondary damage to the neurovascular structures (i.e., the brachial plexus) posterior to the clavicle. Early immobilization and referral to appropriate medical personnel also helps to limit secondary trauma such as a **pneumothorax.**

The ACJ functions to maintain the relationship between the clavicle and scapula during the early and late stages of joint motion. The ACJ also works in conjunction with the **scapulothoracic joint** to provide the upper extremity with a connection point to the axial skeleton. Unlike injuries to the SCJ, injuries to the ACJ are very common in athletics[10]

Breakout

Acromioclavicular Joint Grades

1. Grade or type I—Minor sprain of AC ligament, intact joint capsule, intact coracoclavicular (CC) ligament, intact deltoid and trapezius
2. Grade or type II—Rupture of AC ligament and joint capsule, sprain of CC ligament but CC intact, minimal detachment of deltoid and trapezius
3. Grade or type III—Rupture of AC ligament, joint capsule, and CC ligament; clavicle elevated (up to 100% displacement); detachment of deltoid and trapezius
4. Grade or type IV—Rupture of AC ligament, joint capsule, and CC ligament; clavicle displaced posteriorly into the trapezius; detachment of deltoid and trapezius
5. Grade or type V—Rupture of AC ligament, joint capsule, and CC ligament; clavicle elevated (greater than 100% displacement); detachment of deltoid and trapezius
6. Grade or type VI (rare)—Rupture of AC ligament, joint capsule, and CC ligament; clavicle displaced behind the tendons of the biceps and coracobrachialis

because this joint is structurally weaker than the SCJ. ACJ injuries are classified into six types and are known as shoulder separations.[3,11] A sprained acromioclavicular ligament occurs with grades I and II. A grade III sprain or dislocation involves trauma to the acromioclavicular and coracoclavicular ligaments resulting in an upward displacement of the clavicle (dislocation). Grade IV to VI injuries are significant and result in greater displacement of the ACJ (i.e., clavicle); they often require surgery to repair the joint.

The mechanism of injury of a humeral fracture often determines the location of the trauma. Proximal fractures of the humerus are the second most common fracture of the upper extremity.[12] Midshaft fractures are most often caused by a direct violent force associated with falls (landing laterally) and motor vehicle accidents.[8] A direct blow to the elbow or falling on an outstretched hand results in trauma to the distal humerus. In immature patients, falling on a hyperextend wrist or repetitive overuse activities such as in throwing sports may predispose these individuals to distal humeral epiphyseal plate injuries.[13]

When a humeral fracture is suspected, the athletic trainer will have to identify any possible damage to the neurovascular structures surrounding the humerus. The peripheral nerves and vascular supply of the upper extremity arise off the brachial plexus (Fig. 16.2) and subclavian artery. These structures run parallel to the humerus. The proximity of the peripheral nerves and arteries to the bone increases the risk of secondary trauma in the presence of a traumatic injury to the humerus. Depending upon the severity and location of the trauma, damage may occur to structures such as the radial (C5-T1) and ulnar (C8-T1) nerves and the brachial artery. A displaced or open midshaft humeral fracture increases the risk of damage to the radial nerve running posteriorly to the humerus,[14,15] resulting in **radial nerve palsy.** In fact, trauma to the radial nerve is the most common nerve injury associated with midshaft humeral fractures.[14] Trauma to the distal humerus resulting in a supracondylar humeral fracture (more common in children) increases the risk of damage to the brachial artery and can result in a diminished or absent radial

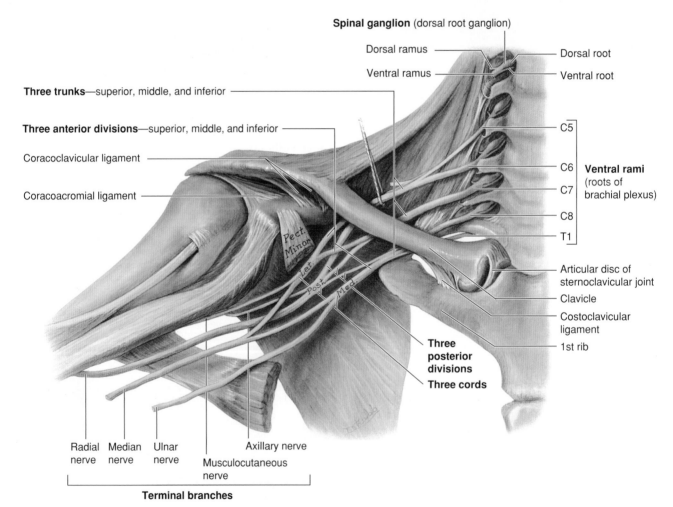

FIGURE 16.2   Formation of the brachial plexus. This large nerve network provides innervation to the upper limb and shoulder region. The brachial plexus is formed by the ventral rami of the fifth through eighth cervical nerves and the greater part of the ramus of the first thoracic nerve (the roots of the brachial plexus). Small contributions may be made by the fourth cervical and second thoracic nerves. Observe the merging and continuation of certain roots of the plexus to three trunks, the separation of each trunk into anterior and posterior divisions, the union of the divisions to form three cords, and the derivation of the main terminal branches from the cords. (From Moore KL, Dalley AF II. *Clinically Oriented Anatomy,* 4th ed. Baltimore: Lippincott Williams & Wilkins; 1999.)

pulse[16]; it also increases the risk of a **Volkmann's ischemic contracture.**

On physical examination, athletes will complain of sudden pain over and around the trauma site, swelling, crepitus, joint deformity, limited mobility and/or complete loss of joint function, false motion, and possibly altered neurovascular status distal to the injury. In the case of a dislocation (e.g., glenohumeral, ACJ, or SCJ), joint deformity should be noted. For some injuries, a further examination of the mechanism of injury and pain characteristics may help determine which portion (i.e., distal, middle, or proximal) of the involved structure has been damaged. A midshaft humeral fracture, for example, presents with a greater degree of deformity based on the location of the fracture. Fractures above the insertion of the pectoralis major cause proximal humeral shaft fractures to rotate and abduct, whereas fractures between the deltoid and pectoralis major present with the proximal humerus in an adducted position[17] (Table 16.1). However, regardless of the trauma, any painful, swollen, or deformed shoulder joint or shoulder girdle should be

TABLE 16.1	Shoulder Complex Injuries and Immobilization Techniques		
Injury	**Mechanism of Injury**	**Signs and Symptoms**	**Immobilization Techniques**
ACJ sprain/ dislocation	Direct blow to the tip of the shoulder Falling on the tip of the shoulder Indirect force transmitted along the humerus from FOOSH or posterior elbow	Pain, swelling, crepitus over ACJ Deformity (upward displacement of the acromion) Upward or horizontal movement of the distal clavicle Inability to abduct arm	Commercial or improvised sling and swathe (Fig. 16.10) Desault bandage (Skill 16.3)
Clavicular fracture	Distal fracture • Direct violent force to the shoulder joint Middle fracture • Indirect violent force such as landing on the lateral aspect of the shoulder Proximal fracture • Direct violent blow to the anterior chest	Pain, swelling, discoloration, or skin bulging over fracture site Snapping and/or popping sound Splints affected limb against the body to immobilize joint Affected shoulder presents in a downward and slightly forward position	Clavicle sling (Skill 16.2) Desault bandage (Skill 16.3)
Humeral fracture	Proximal shaft fracture • Direct violent force applied to the upper arm or indirect force traveling the length of the humerus with a FOOSH injury Midshaft shaft fracture • Direct violent force associated with falls (landing laterally) Distal shaft fracture • Direct blow to the elbow or FOOSH	Proximal shaft fracture • Present similarly to shoulder dislocations with pain along proximal humerus, up into the shoulder joint with the athlete immobilizing the upper arm close to the body Midshaft shaft fracture • Present with a greater degree of deformity based on the location of the fracture Distal shaft fracture • Present with abnormal positioning of the elbow, swelling, pain near the elbow, and a loss of motion at the elbow	Proximal and distal fractures using a posterolateral padded rigid splint (Skill 16.4) or coaptation splint (Skill 16.5) with a sling and swath. Midshaft fractures require a padded rigid splint or vacuum splint with the elbow held at a 45- or 90-degree angle.
SCJ dislocation	Anterior dislocations • Indirect force anterolateral shoulder traveling medially through the clavicle Posterior dislocations • Direct blow to the medial end of the clavicle • Indirect posterolateral force directed through the clavicle	Severe pain, crepitation, and swelling over SCJ Deformity (either anterior or posterior displacement of the medial clavicle) Loss of shoulder joint function Dizziness, nausea, difficulty breathing, or swallowing with a posterior dislocation	Commercial or improvised sling and swathe (Fig. 16.10) Desault bandage (Skill 16.3)

SKILL 16.2

Clavicle Sling

1. Assess distal neurovascular status.
2. Begin by gently placing the limb on the injured side across the athlete's chest with the fingertips almost resting on the opposite shoulder (Fig. 16.3).
3. Place a triangular bandage between the chest and the affected limb with the apex of the bandage pointing toward the elbow and one tail over the uninvolved side (Fig. 16.3).

4. Place the free tail between the axilla and the affected arm (Fig. 16.3).
5. Supporting the limb, adjust the tails of the bandage and secure (Fig. 16.4). A gauze pad is placed between the sling knot and the body for comfort (Fig. 16.4).
6. Add a swathe for additional support.
7. Reassess distal neurovascular status and document findings.

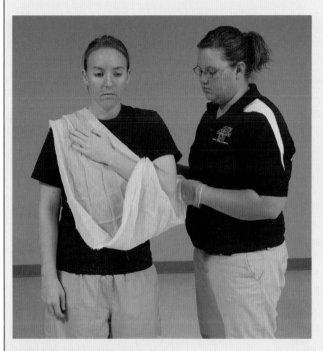

FIGURE 16.3

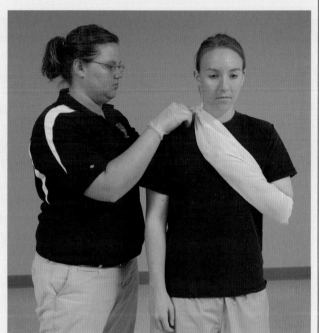

FIGURE 16.4

SKILL 16.3

Desault Bandage

A Desault bandage binds the athlete's elbow to the side of the body and is commonly used for clavicular trauma.[18]

1. Gently place the limb on the injured side across the athlete's chest with the elbow at a 90-degree angle.
2. Assess distal neurovascular status.
3. Anchor a 6-in. elastic wrap over the ACJ, moving the wrap down and around the wrist and finally back over the ACJ.
4. Moving behind the back and toward the involved shoulder, wrap the bandage around the middle of the involved humerus across the front of the body, level with the nipples, moving under and around the axilla of the uninvolved shoulder (Fig. 16.5).

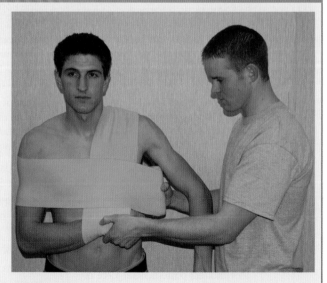

FIGURE 16.5

SKILL 16.3 *(Continued)*

Desault Bandage (Continued)

5. Continue behind the back and across the involved arm, moving the wrap downward at an angle so that it crosses below the wrist, moving under the axilla of the uninvolved shoulder (Fig. 16.6).
6. Continue behind the back, this time wrapping the bandage over the involved arm's ACJ, moving sharply down in front of the body, underneath the wrist moving around the axilla of the uninvolved shoulder (Fig. 16.7).
7. Secure with pins or tape (Fig. 16.8).
8. Reassess distal neurovascular status and document findings.

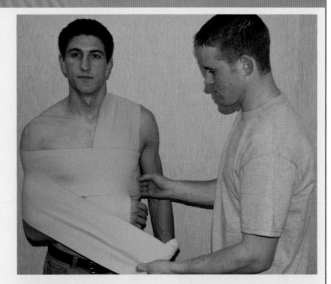

FIGURE 16.6

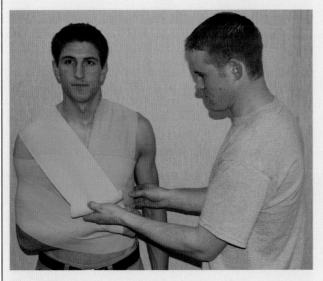

FIGURE 16.7

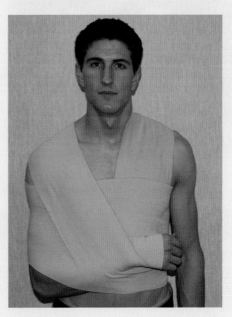

FIGURE 16.8

immobilized and referred to the appropriate medical personnel for proper care.

A bilateral comparison of neurovascular status (CSM) is warranted before and after immobilizing the trauma by assessing circulation at the radial pulse and/or assessing capillary refill. Sensation is assessed by stroking the dorsum of the hand. Motor function is tested by asking the athlete to wiggle his or her fingers or assessing grip strength. Proper immobilization using the following immobilization techniques will help to limit secondary trauma, particularly when dealing with a posterior SCJ dislocation and humeral shaft fractures.

SKILL 16.4

Posterolateral Rigid Board Splint

1. Begin by gently placing the injured limb across the chest with the fingertips almost resting on the opposite shoulder; provide additional support if needed (Fig. 16.9).
2. Assess distal neurovascular status.
3. Place a padded rigid splint on the posterolateral surface of the involved humerus (Fig. 16.9).
4. Secure the splint to the humerus using two bandages or elastic wraps (Fig. 16.9).
5. Provide additional support by using a sling and swathe (Fig. 16.10).
6. Place a gauze pad between the sling and swathes knots for comfort (Fig. 16.10).
7. Reassess distal neurovascular status and document findings.

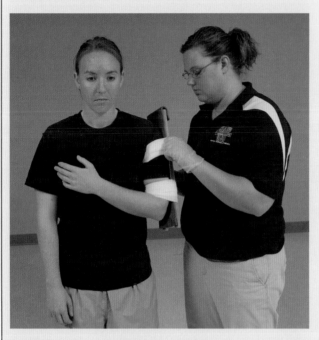

FIGURE 16.9

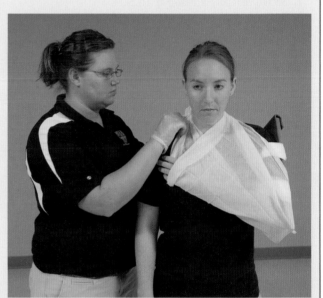

FIGURE 16.10

SKILL 16.5

Coaptation Splint using a SAM Splint

1. Stabilize and support the extremity.
2. Assess distal neurovascular status.
3. Begin by folding a 36-in. SAM Splint on itself, creating a 12-in. double-layer section.
4. Secure the double layer section using white athletic tape and then shape into a "U," forming a fishhook.
5. A C-curve is applied to the 24-in. length of the splint.
6. With the athlete in upright position, one athletic trainer stabilizes the upper extremity to prevent any excessive movement while the other places the "U" around the elbow just distal to the axilla, up along the lateral aspect of the arm and over the deltoid (Fig. 16.11).
7. Any extra material along the deltoid is folded back onto the splint (Fig. 16.11).

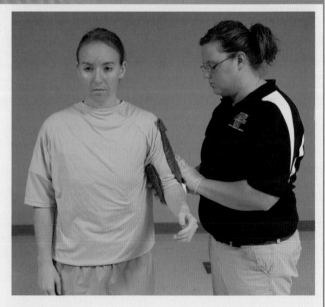

FIGURE 16.11

SKILL 16.5 *(Continued)*

Coaptation Splint using a SAM Splint (Continued)

8. Mold the splint for comfort and secure, using a wrap of choice (Fig. 16.12).

9. Fill voids and protect bony prominences (Fig. 16.12).

10. Secure the extremity to the chest by applying a sling and swathe for additional comfort and support (Fig. 16.13).

11. Reassess distal neurovascular status and document findings.

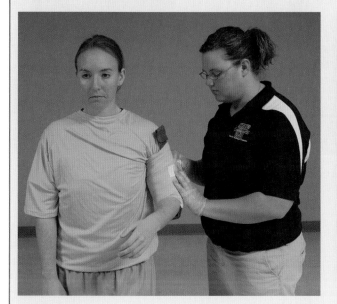

FIGURE 16.12

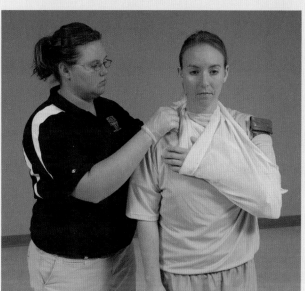

FIGURE 16.13

Shoulder Dislocations and Subluxations

Shoulder dislocations and subluxations are the most common dislocations experienced in athletics and can be classified as either anterior, posterior, or inferior dislocations, depending on the resting position of the humeral head. Shoulder dislocations of the **glenohumeral joint** occur because of poor congruency between the humeral head and glenoid fossa of the scapula.[3] When the shoulder is stressed, it relies on the static (ligaments) and dynamic (muscles) joint stabilizers to maintain proper humeral head position. When external forces applied to the shoulder joint exceed the limits of these stabilizers, the humeral head has no alternative other than to **translate** beyond its normal anatomical boundaries, thus resulting in an acute dislocation. Chronic dislocations share the same mechanism of injury as acute dislocations; however, they occur because of repeated episodes of traumatic or atraumatic injury (i.e., congenial laxity) which, over time, leads to greater instability of the static and dynamic stabilizers.[3]

Shoulder dislocations and instability often begin in adolescent athletes and progressively worsen as they become more active in sports.[19]

Anterior shoulder dislocations account for approximately 90% to 98% of all acute dislocations of the shoulder,[20] followed by posterior and inferior dislocations. Anterior dislocations result from direct and indirect forces applied to the shoulder. The most common mechanism of injury for anterior shoulder dislocations is a direct abduction or external rotation force applied to shoulder held in 90 degrees of abduction with full external rotation and 90 degrees of elbow flexion (i.e., 90-degree/90-degree position). Posterior dislocations occur when an athlete falls on an outstretched arm held in flexion, adduction, and internal rotation[17] or with a direct posterior force running longitudinally through the humerus (e.g., blocking in football). Inferior dislocations are rare and occur with an indirect or direct force, causing the humeral head to drop below the inferior rim of the glenoid fossa.

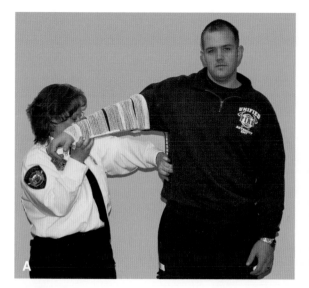
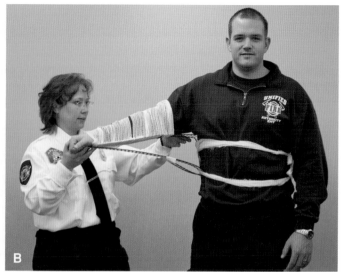

FIGURE 16.14   Ladder splint. (**A**) Create an "A" frame with the rigid ladder splint and (**B**) secure using roller gauze, cravats, or elastic bandages.

Clinically, a shoulder dislocation presents with obvious deformity, significant pain, unwillingness to move the limb, loss of shoulder joint function and the normal rounded contour of the deltoid muscle (i.e., flattened deltoid), awkward positioning of the shoulder while the athlete attempts to stabilize the joint (e.g., slight abduction and external rotation of the shoulder for an anterior dislocation and adduction and internal rotation for a posterior dislocation), swelling, and changes in the neurovascular status. Like humeral fractures, shoulder dislocations can

damage nerves and blood vessels in the area. The axillary nerve is most commonly affected with anterior shoulder dislocation; this results in loss of sensation over the lateral upper arm and muscle function of the deltoid.[20] Damage to the axillary artery is also possible if the joint spontaneously reduces or has been reduced incorrectly. Owing to the risk of neurovascular damage, it is recommended that the athlete be stabilized and immediately transported to the nearest medical facility. Initial immobilization of a shoulder dislocation is accomplished with a soft splint and a sling and swathe (Skill 16.6) and ladder splint (Fig. 16.14). A vacuum splint (Fig. 16.15), though, is the splint of choice for most athletic trainers because of its ability to readily conform to the joint (refer to application procedures in Chapter 15) and availability on the sidelines.

Elbow

Trauma to the elbow (distal humerus, radius, and ulna) occurs from a direct blow or compression force (i.e., landing on the elbow), indirect force such as falling on an outstretched hand with the elbow extended or flexed, or a rotational force,[13,21,22] resulting in fractures of the proximal radial shaft and head, proximal ulna, and supracondylar fractures of the distal humerus. The mechanism of injury and age of the individual will determine the type and extent of the trauma sustained. Clinically, the athlete will typically present with sudden pain, rapid swelling, joint deformity, loss of function, and muscle spasms (Table 16.2). As with trauma to the shoulder complex, a complete assessment of the neurovascular status should be completed before and after immobilization of the elbow joint because the neurovascular structures from the shoulder complex continue distally down the limb. Immobilization of an elbow fracture commonly requires the use of a posterior elbow splint in full extension (Skill 16.7)

FIGURE 16.15   Vacuum splint. Ensure that the Styrofoam beads are evenly spread out over the entire shoulder.

SKILL 16.6

Soft Splint with a Sling and Swathe

1. Stabilize and support the extremity.
2. Assess distal neurovascular status.
3. Reduction of the shoulder dislocation should be completed by trained medical professionals only.
4. Gently place the limb of the injured side across the athlete's chest. If moving the limb increases the pain, splint in the position found (Fig. 16.16).
5. Place some padding (e.g., pillow and/or blanket) between the limb and chest on the affected side (Fig. 16.16).

6. Support the limb and sling. Secure the sling at the forearm and tie the other end around the neck. The elbow should be bent and across the chest if possible (Fig. 16.16).
7. Secure the limb to the chest by applying a swathe, tying the knot on the uninjured side (Fig. 16.17). Place a gauze pad between the sling and swathe knots for comfort.
8. Reassess distal neurovascular status and document findings.

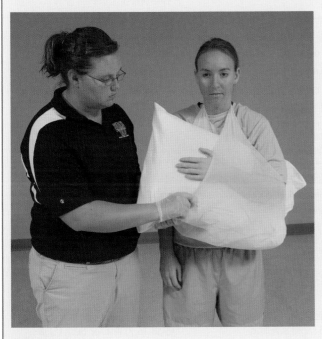

FIGURE 16.16

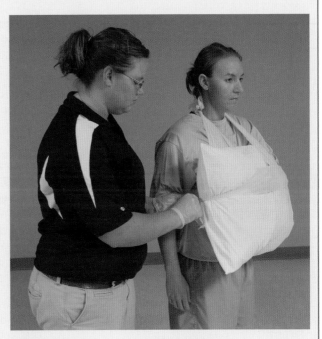

FIGURE 16.17

or flexion (Skill 16.8) or a vacuum splint (Skill 16.9) to stabilize the forearm and shoulder. Other immobilization techniques include a dorsal–volar splint and, when no gross deformity is present, a coaptation splint. When a triangular bandage is not available, consider pulling the shirt bottom-up and over the injured limb and use a safety pin to fix it at the correct height.

Elbow Dislocations

Like shoulder dislocations, elbow dislocations are classified according to the direction of movement of the radius and ulna (posterior, anterior, etc.) and are the second most commonly dislocated joint after shoulder dislocations[23] in all patients. Posterior elbow dislocations occur when the elbow is forced into hyperextension and the ulna's olecranon process impinges upon the humerus's olecranon fossa, forcing the forearm away from the distal arm, rupturing the

support structures, and driving the humerus in an anterior direction.[24] Anterior dislocations occur from a direct blow to the olecranon with a flexed elbow driving the olecranon forward in relation to the humerus. Elbow dislocations can also be classified according to the extent of the trauma to the joint. **Simple dislocations** are elbow dislocations without concomitant fractures about the elbow, whereas a dislocation and fracture about the elbow is known as a **complex dislocation** (e.g., elbow dislocation with a radial head fracture). A simple or complex dislocation may present with or without joint deformity, severe pain, snapping or cracking sensation, swelling, the inability to move the elbow through its normal range of motion, and changes in the neurovascular status.

If a simple or complex elbow dislocation is suspected, the athletic trainer must manage the injury carefully to limit damage to neurovascular structures such as the brachial

TABLE 16.2   Elbow Fractures and Immobilization Techniques

Injury	Mechanism of Injury	Signs and Symptoms	Immobilization Techniques
Radial neck fracture	Direct trauma (e.g., sporting equipment) FOOSH with the elbow partially flexed or fully flexed Rotation	Acute pain, tenderness and rapid swelling Paresthesia and/or loss of circulation due to neurovascular trauma Deformity and loss of or pain with supination and pronation and wrist flexion and extension	Posterior elbow splint in straight (Skill 16.7) and/or bent (Skill 16.8); sling and swathe Volar splint (Skill 16.12 and 16.13); sling and swathe Dorsolateral elbow splint (Skill 16.10); sling and swathe Dorsal–volar splint (Fig. 16.28); sling and swathe Vacuum splint (Skill 16.9)
Radial head fracture	Fall on an outstretched hand driving the radial head of radius into capitulum of humerus Concomitant elbow dislocation	Acute pain and tenderness directly over radial head Swelling over radial head Positive fat pad sign Crepitus or clicking over radial head with supination Typically no deformity, loss of motion	Posterior splint in flexion; sling and swathe Dorsolateral elbow splint; sling and swathe Sugar-tong splint (Skill 16.11); sling and swathe Vacuum splint (Skill 16.9)
Proximal ulnar fracture	Direct trauma (e.g., sporting equipment) Indirect trauma (e.g., FOOSH)	Acute pain tenderness, and rapid swelling Paresthesia and/or loss of circulation due to neurovascular trauma Deformity and loss of function	Posterior splint in flexion; sling and swathe Volar splint (Skill 16.12 and 16.13); sling and swathe Dorsolateral elbow splint; sling and swathe Dorsal-volar splint (Fig. 16.28); sling and swathe Vacuum splint (Skill 16.9)
Supracondylar humeral fracture	Commonly seen in children Extension injury • FOOSH Flexion injury • Direct trauma to the posterior elbow	Severe distal humerus pain, tenderness, and rapid swelling Paresthesia and/or loss of circulation due to neurovascular trauma Shortening of the arm, deformity, and loss of elbow function	Posterior elbow splint in straight (Skill 16.7) and/or bent (Skill 16.8); sling and swathe Coaptation splint; sling and swathe Dorsolateral elbow splint; sling and swathe Vacuum splint
Olecranon fracture	Direct trauma (e.g., landing on the elbow) Indirect trauma (e.g., contraction of triceps and brachialis) Concomitant ulnar shaft fracture	Severe pain and swelling over the olecranon process Paresthesia due to ulnar nerve damage Shortening of the arm and loss of elbow extension	Posterior splint in flexion; sling and swathe Dorsolateral elbow splint; sling and swathe Sugar-tong splint (Skill 16.11); sling and swathe Vacuum splint (Skill 16.9)

artery and ulnar and median nerves.[24,25] The ulnar nerve crosses the elbow's joint line medially and is relatively superficial. Damage to the ulnar nerve will result in numbness and tingling into the little finger. The median nerve crosses over the anterior elbow joint, following the same path as the brachial artery, and may become entrapped within the joint once the elbow is reduced. Changes in the neurovascular status such as a dismissed pulse, cold hand, numbness, or loss of distal limb function requires immediate medical attention to restore normal function. Immobilization of an elbow dislocation commonly requires the use of a rigid splint (Skill 16.10) or vacuum splint (Skill 16.9) to stabilize the joint in the position in which it was found.

SKILL 16.7

Posterior Elbow Splint: Straight Position

1. Stabilize and support the extremity.
2. Assess distal neurovascular status.
3. Using a 36-in. SAM Splint, begin by measuring the length of the splint from the axillary space to the metacarpophalangeal joint, using the uninvolved arm. Any extra distal material is folded back on itself.
4. Apply a C-curve down the length of the splint.
5. A reverse C-curve may be added for additional strength.
6. Using his or her arm as a model, the athletic trainer molds the splint to the extremity (Fig. 16.18).

7. Fill voids and protect bony prominences.
8. Further adjustments to the splint are made once the splint is applied.
9. Secure using the wrap of choice (e.g., elastic wrap, cravat, roller bandage) (Fig. 16.19). A second 9- or 18-in. oblique lateral A-frame splint may be added to the lateral aspect of the elbow for additional stability, or the limb may be secured to the body using—two or three swathes.
10. Reassess distal neurovascular status and document findings.

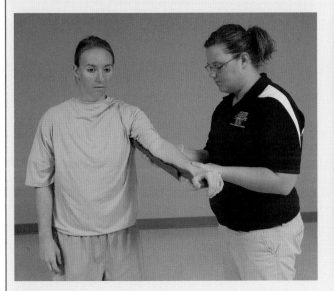

FIGURE 16.18

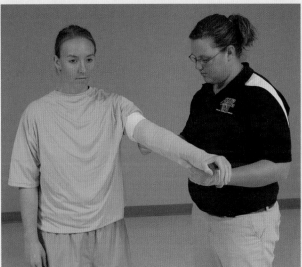

FIGURE 16.19

SKILL 16.8

Posterior Elbow Splint—Bent Position with Sling and Swathe

1. Stabilize and support the extremity.
2. Assess distal neurovascular status.
3. Using a 36-in. SAM Splint, begin by measuring the length of the splint from the axillary space to the metacarpophalangeal joint, using the uninvolved arm. Any extra distal material is folded back on itself.
4. Apply a C-curve down the length of the splint.
5. A reverse C-curve may be added for additional strength. Using his or her arm as a model, the athletic trainer molds the splint to the extremity (Fig. 16.20).

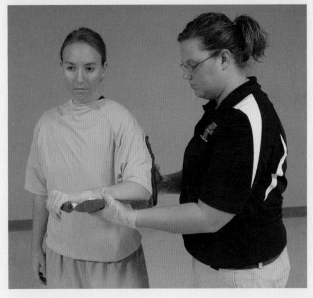

FIGURE 16.20

(Continued)

SKILL 16.8 *(Continued)*

Posterior Elbow Splint—Bent Position with Sling and Swathe (Continued)

6. Further adjustments to the splint are made once the splint is applied.

7. Fill voids and protect bony prominences.

8. The splint is secured using the wrap of choice (e.g., elastic wrap, cravat, roller bandage; Fig. 16.21).

9. Secure the limb to the chest by applying a swathe, tying the knot on the uninjured side (Fig. 16.22). Place a gauze pad between the sling and swathe knots for comfort.

10. Reassess distal neurovascular status and document findings.

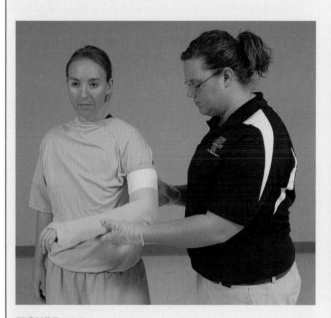

FIGURE 16.21

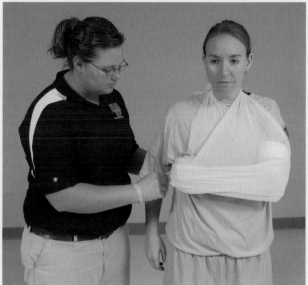

FIGURE 16.22

SKILL 16.9

Vacuum Splint

1. Stabilize and support the extremity. The ground can also act as the support.

2. Assess distal neurovascular status.

3. Move the uninvolved extremity away from the involved extremity.

4. Apply appropriate dressings to all wounds in and around the injury site if necessary.

5. Place the splint next to the athlete with the valve side down and evenly distribute the Styrofoam beads throughout the splint.

6. Continue to support and limit any excessive movement of the injured extremity as a second athletic trainer places the splint under the injury.

7. Position the splint so one strap is above and another below the suspected fracture site.

8. Wrap the splint around the injury and massage the beads to ensure that all voids are filled. If the splint does not conform easily to the injury, adjust the amount of air in the splint until the splint conforms appropriately (Fig. 16.23).

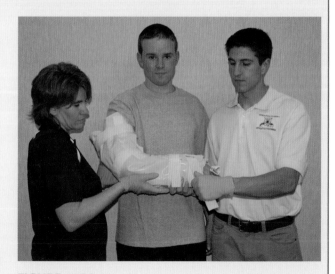

FIGURE 16.23

SKILL 16.9 *(Continued)*

Vacuum Splint *(Continued)*

9. Secure the splint, avoiding overlapping of the edges.
10. Attach the splint's vacuum pump to the coupling device and begin removing air (Fig. 16.24).

11. Disconnect the coupling device once the splint hardens.
12. Reassess distal neurovascular status and document findings (Fig. 16.25).

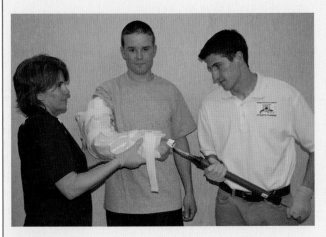

FIGURE 16.24

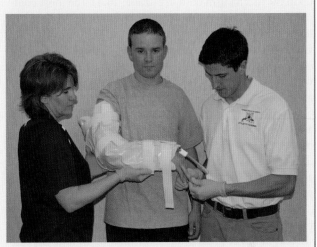

FIGURE 16.25

SKILL 16.10

Dorsolateral Rigid Splint for an Elbow Dislocation

1. Stabilize and support the extremity.
2. Assess distal neurovascular status.
3. Place a padded rigid splint with two cravats on an angle between the humerus and forearm on the anterior surface (Fig. 16.26).
4. Fill voids and protect bony prominences.
5. Using additional help to support the limb, grasp and secure the two tails of the cravat closest to the humerus, wrapping them around the humerus posteriorly so that one tail of the cravat is located on either side of the splint (Fig. 16.26).

6. Repeat for the other cravat.
7. Secure the extremity to the chest by applying a sling and swath for additional comfort and support (Fig. 16.27).
8. Place a gauze pad between the sling and swathe knots for comfort.
9. Reassess distal neurovascular status and document findings.

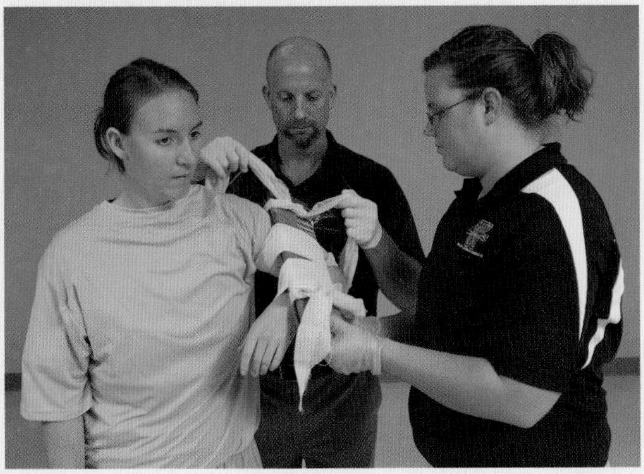

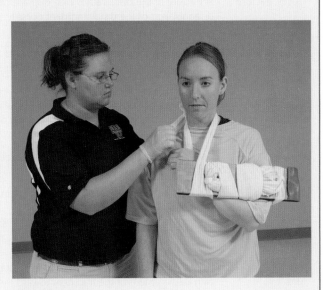

FIGURE 16.26

FIGURE 16.27

Forearm

The forearm is composed of the radial and ulnar shafts and reinforced by a dense band of fibrous tissue, which assists in transmitting forces applied to the radius to the ulna up through the humerus. A variety of fractures can occur to the radius and ulna, alone or in combination, depending upon the mechanism of injury (Table 16.3). The most common types of forearm trauma occur due to falls on an extended arm (e.g., slipping on ice or being tripped), direct violent blows to the forearm (e.g., being struck by sporting equipment or an opposing player), and/or a rotational force with an axial load, as seen in sports like wrestling and/or gymnastics.[26] The athlete's forearm position, particularly in cases with rotation and axial loading, determines the extent and type of trauma suffered.[26] Isolated ulnar fractures, for instance, can occur when excessive supination or pronation forces allow the ligamentous structures to remain intact and the ulna rotates beyond the tissues' normal elastic capabilities.[27]

Clinically, isolated fractures to the radius or ulna may present with pain, swelling over the fracture site, ecchymosis, and minimal to no gross deformity for an ulna fracture to minimal angulation of a radial shaft fracture.[27] **Longitudinal compression** through the wrist to the elbow will often create pain at the fracture site. A fracture involving both the radius and ulna presents with an angulation deformity, loss of wrist and/or elbow function, and false joint movement. Any change in the neurovascular status such as a dismissed radial pulse, cold hand, numbness, or loss of distal limb function requires immediate medical attention. Immobilization of radial and/or ulnar fractures commonly requires the use of a sugar-tong (Skill 16.11), volar (Skill 16.12), dorsal–volar (Fig. 16.28), rigid (Skill 16.13), air (when no gross deformity is present; Fig. 16.29), or vacuum splint to stabilize the wrist and elbow, followed by the application of a sling and swathe.

Wrist

Fractures

Trauma to the wrist and hand is often the result of a direct violent force, axial loading from FOOSH, rotational force, and/or repetitive movements. Injuries to the hand and wrist account for 3% to 9% of all athletic injuries[28] and 1.5% of all emergency room visits among the general population.[29] Among the carpal (wrist) bones, the scaphoid is the most commonly fractured (79%)[30,31]—and at the greatest risk for developing **avascular necrosis** due to the bone's poor vascular supply.[28] This is followed by the triquetrum (7% to 20%), trapezium (5%), hook of the hamate (2% to 4%), and lunate, pisiform, and capitate, fractures of which together account for approximately 3% to 4% of all carpal fractures.[28,32–35] Trapezoid fractures are very rare and account for 0.2% of carpal fractures.[35]

TABLE 16.3   Forearm Fracture Types

Name	Description	Mechanism of Injury
Barton's fracture	Break in the distal radius with volar (or dorsal) dislocation of the radiocarpal joint.	Fall on an outstretched hand
Colles' fracture	A fracture of the distal radius with displacement and/or angulation of the distal fragment dorsally. Also known as a "silver fork deformity."	Fall on an outstretched hand
Radial and ulnar epiphysial plate fractures	Fractures involving the epiphysis plate of the radius and/or ulna in a pediatric/adolescent patient.	Direct blow and fall on an outstretched hand
Essex-Lopresti fracture	Radial head fracture and an associated distal radi-oulnar joint dislocation attributed to tearing of the interosseous membrane.	Axial loading of forearm with arm pronated and elbow extended
Galeazzi fracture	Radial shaft fracture with dislocation of the distal radioulnar joint.	Direct blow and fall on an outstretched hand
Monteggia fracture	Fracture of the proximal ulna with dislocation of the head of the radius.	Direct blow and fall on an outstretched hand with forceful hyperpronation
Nightstick fracture	Isolated fracture of midshaft of ulna.	Direct blow, excessive supination or pronation
Smith's fracture	Reversed Colles' fracture; rupture of the distal radius with displacement of the fragment toward the palmar (volar) aspect.	Fall on an outstretched hand with the wrist flexed or direct blow with the wrist flexed

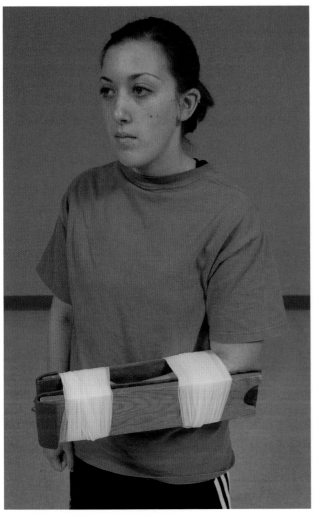

FIGURE 16.28 Dorsal–volar splint: Be sure padding is used when you are applying a rigid splint.

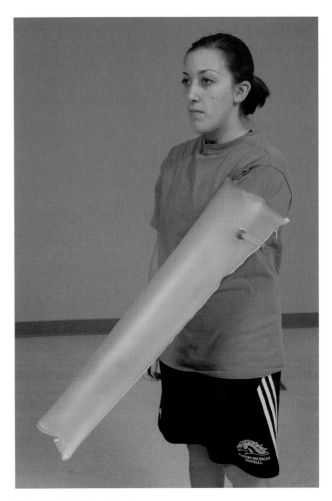

FIGURE 16.29 Air splint.

SKILL 16.11

Sugar Tong Splint

Immobilizing trauma to the radius and/or ulna is best accomplished using a sugar-tong splint.

1. Stabilize and support the extremity.
2. Assess distal neurovascular status.
3. A 36-in. SAM Splint is folded in half, creating two 18-in. halves.
4. To fit the splint correctly, place the folded splint around the elbow, running from the dorsal metacarpophalangeal joint to the proximal interphalangeal joint volarly. Any extra material should be folded over on the volar side (Fig. 16.30).
5. Fold a C-curve into the distal two thirds of the dorsal and volar halves of the splint.
6. Using your arm as a model, shape the splint to the approximate dimensions (Fig. 16.30).

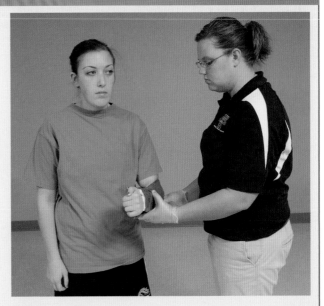

FIGURE 16.30

(Continued)

SKILL 16.11 *(Continued)*

Sugar Tong Splint *(Continued)*

7. Fill voids and pad any bony prominences, such as the radial styloid process, to avoid pressure points; fit to the athlete and secure using the wrap of choice (Fig. 16.31).
8. Secure the extremity to the chest by applying a sling and swath with the forearm in a slightly elevated position if comfortable (Fig. 16.32).

9. Place a gauze pad between the sling and swathe knots for comfort (Fig. 16.32).
10. Reassess distal neurovascular status and document findings.

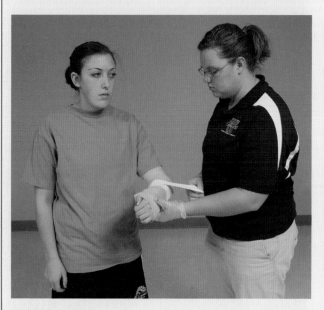

FIGURE 16.31

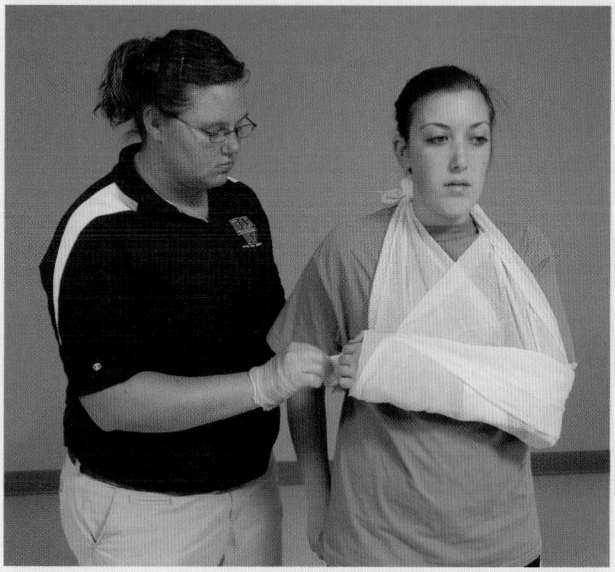

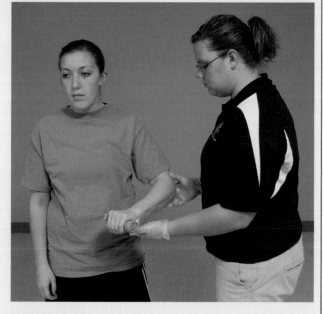

FIGURE 16.32

SKILL 16.12

Volar SAM Splint

1. Stabilize and support the extremity.
2. Assess distal neurovascular status.
3. Begin by folding a 24-in. SAM Splint in half so that one side is approximately 4 in. longer than the other.
4. Form a C-curve along the flat half of the splint (Fig. 16.33).

FIGURE 16.33

SKILL 16.12 *(Continued)*

Volar SAM Splint *(Continued)*

5. Using your arm as a model, mold the splint in the **position of function** (see Fig. 16.34) by rolling the longer half over for the athlete to grab.
6. The splint is applied from the distal palmar crease to the proximal forearm and secured using the wrap of choice (Fig. 16.35).
7. Fill voids and protect bony prominences.
8. Secure the extremity to the chest by applying a sling and swath with the forearm in a slightly elevated position if comfortable (Fig. 16.36).
9. Place a gauze pad between the sling and swathe knots for comfort.
10. Reassess distal neurovascular status and document findings.

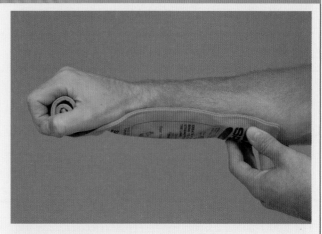

FIGURE 16.34

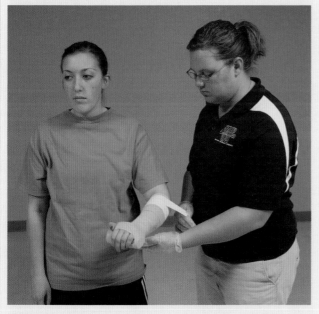

FIGURE 16.35

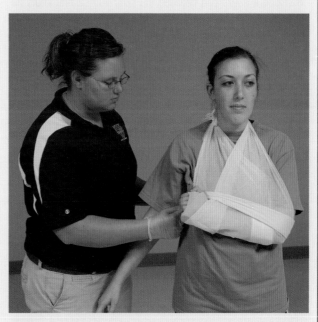

FIGURE 16.36

SKILL 16.13

Rigid Volar Splint

1. Stabilize and support the extremity.
2. Assess distal neurovascular status.
3. Place a padded rigid splint on the volar surface of the involved forearm (Fig. 16.37).
4. Place roller bandage in the hand so the hand assumes a position of function (Fig. 16.37). Secure the splint using the bandage of choice (e.g., elastic wrap, cravat, roller bandage) (Fig. 16.38).
5. When dealing with a trauma to the bone, be sure to immobilize the wrist to limit flexion and extension.
6. Fill voids and protect bony prominences.
7. Provide additional support by using a sling and swathe with the forearm in a slightly elevated position if comfortable (Fig. 16.39).
8. Place a gauze pad between the sling and swathe knots for comfort.
9. Reassess distal neurovascular status and document findings.

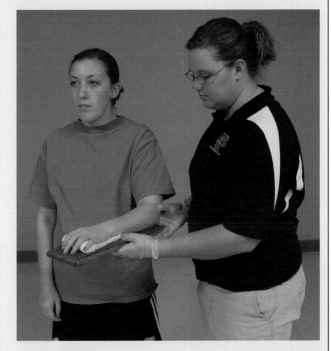

FIGURE 16.37

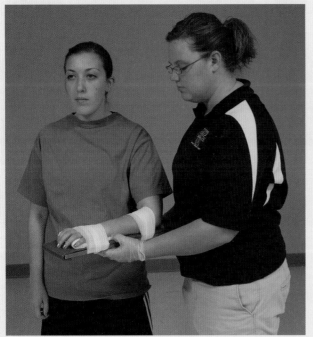

FIGURE 16.38

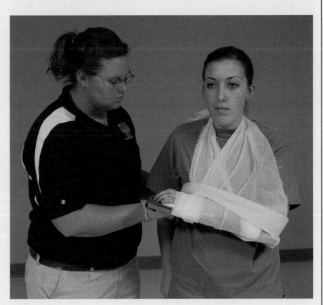

FIGURE 16.39

On physical examination, athletes generally complain of sudden pain and tenderness over the trauma site, swelling, ecchymosis, limited mobility, and/or complete loss of joint or hand function (e.g., making a fist). A further examination of the mechanism of injury and pain characteristics may help determine which carpal bone has been fractured. A scaphoid fracture occurs when an individual experiences FOOSH with the wrist extended at least 90 degrees and radially deviated 10 degrees,[30,36] or during hyperextension as the bone is compressed against the dorsal lip of the radius and the second row of carpal bones (Table 16.4). However, regardless of the specific type of fracture that has occurred, any painful, swollen, or deformed wrist should be immobilized and referred to the appropriate medical personnel for proper care and diagnostic imaging (i.e., radiographs, magnetic resonance imaging, computed tomography, bone scan) because some carpal fractures are not readily evident without this. Improper management of wrist fractures such as scaphoid and lunate fractures may lead to complications such as joint instability and arthritic degeneration.

Dislocations

The most commonly dislocated carpal bone is the lunate; this occurs when an individual experiences FOOSH or braces himself or herself as the wrist is forced into hyperextension (e.g., blocking in football).[21] This hyperextended position of the wrist causes the lunate to be squeezed out between the capitate and the radius. The displaced lunate moves in a volar direction, so that the lunate will characteristically lie at the front of the wrist and may rotate up to 90 degrees or more, so the lower concave articular surface faces forward[37] (Fig. 16.40). Clinically, dislocations present with swelling, loss of wrist function, numbness and tingling of the flexor muscles due to compression of the median nerve between the displaced lunate and flexor retinaculum, and a positive Murphy's sign (Fig. 16.41). Immobilization and immediate referral to the appropriate medical personnel

TABLE 16.4	**Carpal Fractures and Immobilization Techniques**		
Name	**Mechanism of Injury**	**Signs and Symptoms**	**Immobilization Techniques**
Scaphoid	FOOSH with wrist extended, hyperextension injury	Tenderness of the anatomical snuff box, pain with wrist extension and radial deviation	Volar splint (Skill 16.12) Radial gutter splint Vacuum splint (Fig. 16.42)
Lunate	Repetitive trauma with an insidious onset, direct blow	Tenderness along the lunate or at the radial carpal area, loss of grip strength	Volar splint Dorsal–volar splint (Fig. 16.28); sling and swathe Vacuum splint
Triquetrum	FOOSH with the wrist ulnarly deviated, direct blow to the dorsum of the hand	Tenderness along the proximal carpal row and pain with extension and ulnar deviation	Volar splint Ulnar gutter splint (Skill 16.14) Vacuum splint
Pisiform	Direct blow to the ulnar aspect of the wrist, forceful hyperextension, repetitive trauma	May present with volar pain and ulnar nerve palsy as a result of compression of the ulnar nerve	Volar splint Ulnar gutter splint Vacuum splint
Capitate	FOOSH resulting in forced extension of an ulnarly deviated or neutrally positioned wrist	Tenderness with direct palpation immediately proximal to the base of the third metacarpal	Volar splint Dorsal–volar splint Vacuum splint
Hamate	Direct blow, contact with a sport implement, and shearing force of the fourth and fifth flexor tendon	Occurs most often with fourth and fifth metacarpal base fractures. Volar tenderness along the ulnar border, pain with firm grasp/pressure, and ulnar nerve palsy as a result of compression to the ulnar nerve	Volar splint Ulnar gutter splint Vacuum splint
Trapezoid and trapezium	Direct blow to the dorsum of the hand or from a fall on a radially deviated closed fist	Painful and weak pinch; tenderness to direct palpation	Volar splint Dorsal–volar splint Radial gutter splint Vacuum splint

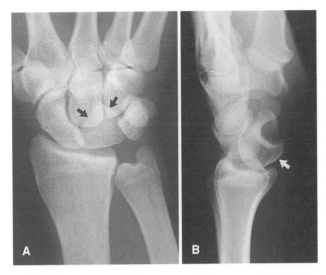

FIGURE 16.40 **A.** Dislocated lunate. **B.** The capitate and all other carpal bones lie posterior to lunate on right radiograph. (From Yochum TR, Rowe LJ. *Yochum and Rowe's Essentials of Skeletal Radiology*, 3rd ed. Philadelphia: Lippincott Williams & Wilkins, 2004.)

are necessary to avoid the risk of avascular necrosis and **osteoarthritis.**

Falling on an outstretched hand with a sufficient axial load to force the wrist into excessive hyperextension (beyond 100 degrees), ulnar deviation, and intracarpal supination results in a perilunate dislocation or fracture/dislocation. In this situation, the lunate maintains its normal position with respect to the distal radius while the remaining distal carpal bones displace posteriorly owing to a disruption of ligamentous structure of the carpal bones.[28] Athletes often present with diffuse pain during palpation associated with a common wrist sprain. They may present with significant swelling and decreased range of motion; joint deformity may not be noticeable.[28] Initial immobilization of a carpal fracture or dislocation can be accomplished with a volar splint (Skill 16.12), with the hand in the position of function; a rigid splint (Skill 16.13); a **gutter splint** (Skill 16.14); or a vacuum splint (Fig. 16.42). A 9-in. SAM Splint can be substituted for the 36-in. splint when only the wrist is being immobilized.

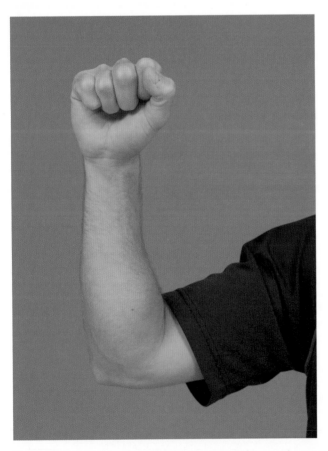
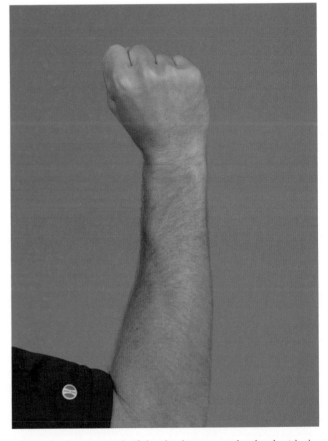

FIGURE 16.41 Murphy's sign. The examiner observes the position of the third metacarpal. If the third metacarpal is level with the second and fourth, then either a volar or dorsal displacement of the lunate is indicated.

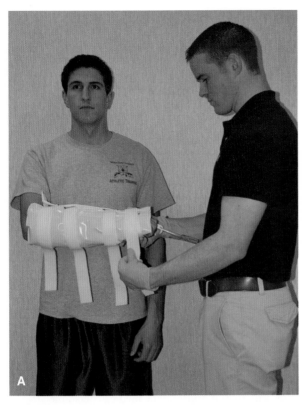

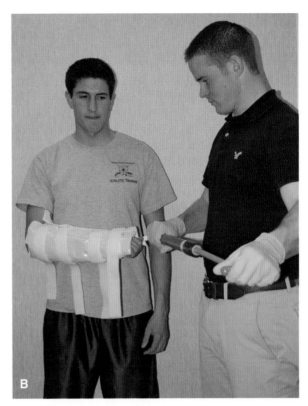

FIGURE 16.42 Wrist vacuum splint. **A.** Securing the splint. **B.** Evacuation of the air from the splint.

SKILL 16.14

Ulnar Gutter Splint

1. Stabilize and support the extremity.
2. Assess distal neurovascular status.
3. Begin by folding a 9-in. splint in half lengthwise.
4. Using your wrist as a model, mold the splint into the desired shape (Fig. 16.43).
5. Apply the splint to the ulnar border of the wrist from the distal interphalangeal joint to the proximal-mid ulnar shaft (Fig. 16.43).

6. Fill voids and protect bony prominences.
7. Secure using the wrap of choice (e.g., elastic wrap, cravat, roller bandage), filling voids and protecting bony prominences (Fig. 16.44).
8. Reassess distal neurovascular status and document findings.

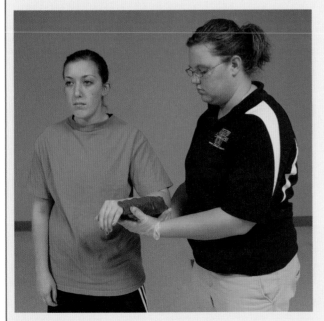

FIGURE 16.43

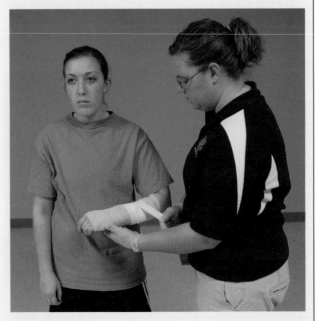

FIGURE 16.44

Hand and Finger Fractures and Dislocations

Metacarpal trauma is often the result of a direct violent force, such as being struck by an object (e.g., stick, ball, etc.), being stepped on, FOOSH, or striking an opponent or object.[38] Phalangeal fractures and dislocations occur from a wide variety of mechanisms including three-point bending, a direct blow, axial loading, and rotation and can result in a variety of fracture types.[39] One study examining fracture rates among collegiate athletes found that by location, fractures were most likely to occur at the hand[40] and that fractures to the fourth and fifth metacarpals were the most common of all metacarpal fractures.[19,30,38] Fractures of the fourth and fifth metacarpals occur from punching an immovable object such as the ground, wall, or another person with a closed fist and no boxing mitt.

Clinically, fractured metacarpals/fingers may be hard to recognize if an obvious deformity is not present. Frequently, an injury to the metacarpals/fingers will cause pain after the trauma and sometimes deformity at a joint (commonly a dislocation). A true fracture usually will be painful, but many times full active range of motion is possible. Swelling and redness of the hand and fingers may be present, with the fingers becoming very swollen and difficult to move. Any open finger fracture is considered a surgical emergency and requires prompt medical attention because of the risk of infection if it is not treated properly.[39] Management of

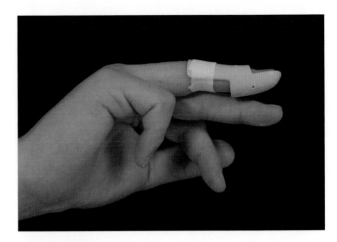

FIGURE 16.45 Stax splint.

finger dislocations and fractures should be to restrict the motion of the injured structures while allowing uninjured joints to remain mobile.[41] Open fractures or dislocations to the phalanges should be immediately dressed, splinted, and sent to the appropriate medical personnel regardless of the situation. Initial immobilization of a hand or finger commonly requires the use of an anatomical splint (see Fig. 15.13), rigid volar or dorsal splint (Skill 16.15), or commercial finger splint such as a Stax splint (Fig. 16.45).

SKILL 16.15

Dorsal Finger Splint

1. Stabilize and support the extremity.
2. Assess distal neurovascular status.
3. Place a padded rigid splint on the dorsal (Fig. 16.46) or volar surface of the involved finger.
4. Secure with tape (Fig. 16.47).
5. Reassess distal neurovascular status and document findings.

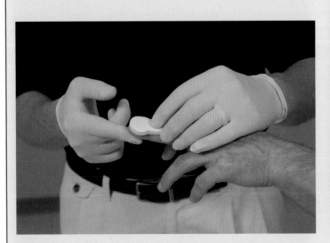

FIGURE 16.46

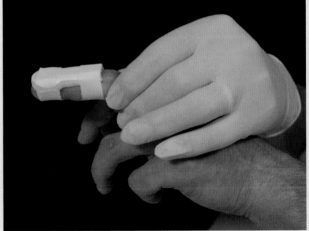

FIGURE 16.47

Ribs

Rib fractures occur as the result of a direct or indirect trauma to the chest, normally between the fourth and seventh ribs.[42] Rib fractures may also be induced by an outburst of coughing and sneezing.[43] Depending on the magnitude of the direct blow, a single rib fracture or multiple rib fractures can occur. If the fracture remains localized, with the soft tissue encasing the ribs, there is little concern for secondary damage to the lungs. However, when a fractured rib end pierces the casing, there is a risk that the rib may be forced into the **parietal pleura** and the lung itself. This increases the athlete's risk of developing a life-threatening intrathoracic injury (pneumothorax and **hemothorax**), which now requires immediate medical attention. In some cases, fractured ribs may be classified as a **flail chest.** This occurs when two or more ribs on the same side of the chest have been fractured in at least two places, resulting in chest wall instability and respiratory difficulties.

An athlete with a suspected rib fracture can experience several signs and symptoms. The treatment for a rib fracture is relatively simple. The goal is to stabilize the ribs and prevent any unwanted movement as well as to decrease the discomfort associated with the injury using an anatomical splint or a soft splint (see Skill 16.16).

Signs & Symptoms

Rib Fracture

- Tenderness on palpation, crepitus, and chest wall deformity
- Pain with compression of the sternum toward the spine
- Cyanosis and tachypnea
- Use of accessory muscles for ventilation
- Sharp pain when coughing or breathing
- Bruising or deformity of the chest
- Paradoxical chest wall excursion with inspiration with flail chest

The paradoxical movement occurs because the middle section of the rib between the two fracture sites moves in response to pressure changes, not intercostal muscle contractions.

ASSESSMENT OF THE LOWER EXTREMITY AND PELVIS

As in immobilization of the upper extremity and thorax, immobilization of the lower extremity and pelvis begins with the athletic trainer already having completed a scene survey and primary assessment, and having provided any necessary interventions. This is followed by completion of the secondary

SKILL 16.16

Rib Fracture Stabilization (Fig. 16.48)

1. Cut four or five strips of 1- or 2-in. adhesive tape (elastic bandages or cravats can be used as a substitute).
2. Make sure the tape strips are long enough to stretch from the athlete's sternum to the spine and that the cravats can be wrapped around the body. When using an elastic wrap, use a double 6-in. wrap.
3. Place one strip of tape directly over the fractured rib or ribs, running from the sternum and wrapping around the back to the spine. *Do not* place the adhesive tape around the entire chest. Wrap the cravat or elastic bandage around the chest.
4. Place the three or four additional pieces of tape (or cravats) on either side of the broken rib or ribs, running parallel to one another. In using an elastic wrap, be sure not to impede breathing.
5. Monitor the athlete breathing and document findings.

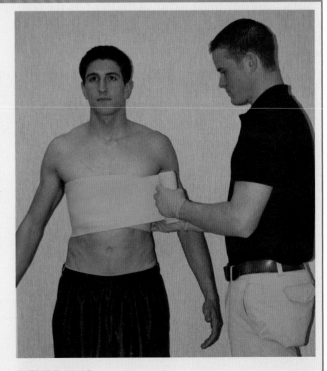

FIGURE 16.48

assessment: (a) physical assessment, (b) SAMPLE history, and (c) vital signs (Skill 16.1). As in the case of the upper extremity, not all lower extremity injuries are easily identified because of protective equipment and clothing. The general rule of thumb is to remove only necessary clothing and equipment according to the environment and severity of the injury and to activate the facility's EAP.

Neurovascular status should be assessed before and after the injury has been immobilized. The athlete's neurovascular status can be assessed by palpating the pulse of the dorsalis pedis or posterior tibial artery or assessing capillary refill. Sensation is assessed by stroking the tops of the metatarsals if the shoe is removed or by asking the athlete to if he or she can feel the athletic trainer touching the foot through the shoe. Motor testing is performed by asking the athlete to wiggle the toes or press down as though he or she were stepping on a gas pedal. A bilateral comparison of the extremities should be made.

Protective Equipment Considerations

To assess an ankle or foot injury adequately, it may be necessary to remove the athlete's shoe. This is accomplished by removing or cutting the shoelaces, opening the shoe, and pulling the tongue down to the toes (Fig. 16.49). The heel counter is then pulled away from the foot and then the shoe is slid up and off the foot as gently as possible, with assistance when possible.[1] In some instances, the athlete may elect to remove his or her own shoe. Ankle braces using Velcro or straps should be removed, following the manufacturer's directions. Ankle tape can be removed using a tape cutter on the side opposite the pain, beginning proximally and working distally along the plantar surface of the foot.[44] In the presence of a possible severe ankle fracture/dislocation, loosen the shoe or brace only enough to assess neurovascular status and then use the shoe as part of the splinting device.

An assessment of the lower leg, knee, or hip may require the removal of clothing and/or protective pads or braces. If it is necessary to cut away clothing to expose the area, cut away from the area, moving proximal to distal and following the clothing's seams. Knee injuries may require removal of the athlete's clothing in addition to removal of any prophylactic braces, sleeves, or padding (e.g., football pads).[44] Football pads can be removed by reaching under the anterior portion of the pants and grabbing the knee pad. While holding the kneepad firmly, the pant leg is pulled up and over the knee and kneepad and removed from the pocket. If the pants are extremely tight and attempts to remove the pad cause more pain, cut the pants.

To remove a hinged prophylactic knee brace, again grasp the anterior portion of the pant leg and remove the knee pad; then turn the pant leg so that the knee brace is exposed. Loosen the Velcro straps on the distal femur and proximal tibia. Grasp the medial and lateral hinges and lift the distal portion of the brace away from the quadriceps and slide the brace down toward the proximal tibia. If the athlete can flex the knee without discomfort, this may assist in loosening the proximal portion of the brace. Remove any additional undergarments (i.e., sleeves). If at any time removal of the pads or brace increases pain or begins to cause further injury, give up the attempt.

If other types of protective equipment are being used and they must be removed to gain access to an injury, do so with as little movement as possible. Athletic trainers should practice removing any unfamiliar pieces of protective equipment prior to the occurrence of an emergency situation.

IMMOBILIZING THE LOWER EXTREMITY AND PELVIS

Traumatic injuries to the lower extremity may result in anything from a fractured toe to a dislocated patella or hip. The type of injury sustained again depends on the mechanism of injury, location of force application, and force applied. This section outlines common types of skeletal trauma to the lower extremity and pelvis and the techniques for proper immobilization.

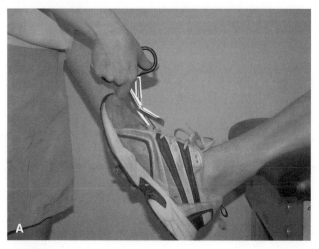
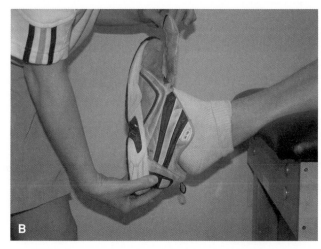

FIGURE 16.49   Athletic shoe removal. **A.** Using scissors or shears, cut along the laces. **B.** After pulling out the tongue, slide the heel counter down and away from the heel.

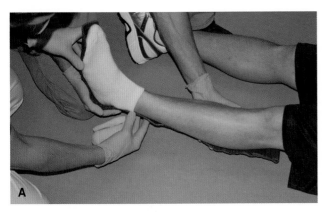

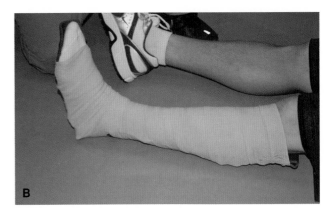

FIGURE 16.50 Posterior lower leg splint. **A.** Form the splint using a C-curve from the distal toes to the proximal tibia. **B.** Secure using an elastic wrap and check CSM.

Foot and Ankle

Trauma to the foot and ankle results from direct compression (i.e., stepping on another player, falling from a height, or dropping sporting equipment on the foot) or a combination of direct compression and an indirect or shearing force with or without the foot being firmly planted. For example, being kicked from behind with the foot firmly planted on the ground or forced inversion with the foot and ankle in plantarflexion is commonly seen with a **Jones fracture.** When falling from a height, the force of the impact can be transmitted up the involved extremity, resulting in trauma to the knee, thigh, pelvis, or lumbar spine; therefore, proper identification of the mechanism of injury is necessary to determine the extent of the injury.

Powell and Barber-Foss's[45] examination of selected high school sports injury rates found 7% to 42% of the injuries (in both boys and girls) sustained across sports occurred to the ankle and foot. Researchers also found that between 10% and 26% of the injuries sustained by professional soccer players occurred at the ankle and 7% at the foot.[46–49] Approximately 10% of all fractures involve the 26 bones of the foot and ankle.[50] An examination of amateur soccer players revealed that of the 122 injuries sustained, 9 (7%) were ankle fractures and 1 was a great toe dislocation (<1%).[51]

The extent of injury varies depending on the mechanism of injury, foot position (i.e., pronated, dorsiflexed, everted), direction of the force applied, and type of protective equipment or shoe worn by the athlete. For example, the lateral malleolus extends further distally, limiting the damage sustained to the deltoid ligament, but its position increases the risk of bony trauma when an excessive eversion force is applied to the ankle. The dome of the talus, which articulates with the tibia and fibula to form the ankle joint, is wider anteriorly than posteriorly; when the foot is forced in dorsiflexion or rotated, it increases the risk of talar trauma. Clinically, the athlete will present with sudden pain, swelling, possible joint deformity, loss of function, inability to bear weight, pain with ambulation or altered gait, and possible neurovascular compromise (Table 16.5). Initial immobilization of foot and/or ankle injuries can be accomplished with an ankle stirrup splint (Skill 16.17), Cadillac splint (Skill 16.18), posterior splint (Fig. 16.50), vacuum splint, box splint, buddy taping (Skill 16.19), sugar-tong splint, or soft splint (Skill 16.20), often with the shoe left in place.

TABLE 16.5	**Foot and Ankle Injuries and Immobilization Techniques**		
Injury	**Mechanism of Injury**	**Signs and Symptoms**	**Immobilization Techniques**
Phalangeal fracture	Axial load (i.e., jamming toe) Direct compression (i.e., dropping a weight)	Pain, swelling, ecchymosis, difficulty wearing footwear Antalgic gait when a great toe fracture is suspected	Buddy taping (Skill 16.19) Aluminum splint
Metatarsal fracture	Axial load (i.e., jamming toe) Direct compression (i.e., dropping a weight)	Deep pain, swelling, ecchymosis, difficulty wearing footwear Hesitance to bear weight and antalgic gait	Posterior splint (Fig. 16.50)
Acute Jones fracture	Inversion and plantarflexion force of the foot (e.g., tripping on a stair) and direct compression	Pain and tenderness within 1.5 cm distal to tuberosity of fifth metatarsal, difficulty with weight bearing, swelling, ecchymosis	Posterior splint (Fig. 16.50)

(Continued)

TABLE 16.5 Foot and Ankle Injuries and Immobilization Techniques *(Continued)*

Injury	Mechanism of Injury	Signs and Symptoms	Immobilization Techniques
Talar fracture	Varies depending on the location of the fracture (e.g., lateral talar dome fractures occur with a severe inversion and dorsiflexion force whereas medial talar dome fractures occur with a severe inversion and plantar-flexion force)	Tenderness and swelling over fracture site Pain on weight bearing or unable to bear weight Antalgic gait	Soft splint (Skill 16.20) Cadillac splint (Skill 16.18) Posterior splint Vacuum splint
Calcaneal fracture	High-energy axial load such as falling from a height or inversion and compression when an anterior process fracture occurs	Severe heel pain and tenderness over the fracture site Pain with ankle dorsiflexion Inability to bear weight	Soft splint Cadillac splint Posterior splint Ankle stirrup (Skill 16.17) Vacuum splint
Tarsal bone fracture (navicular, cuboid, cuneiform)	Varies depending on the location of the fracture and direction of force	Pain, swelling, ecchymosis, difficulty wearing footwear Hesitance to bear weight and antalgic gait	Soft splint Cadillac splint Posterior splint Ankle stirrup Vacuum splint
Phalangeal dislocation	Direct trauma (i.e., kicking an object)	Severe pain, swelling, deformity, loss of function, open wounds	Buddy tape Aluminum splint Posterior splint
Ankle fracture/dislocation	Axial load and direct compression (i.e., falling from a height) with the foot inverted or everted	Severe pain, swelling, deformity, changes in neurovascular status, loss of function, open wound	Ankle stirrup Cadillac splint Vacuum splint

SKILL 16.17

SAM Splint/Ankle Stirrup

Ankle stirrup splints are used to immobilize injuries to the distal tibia and fibula and ankle.

1. Stabilize and support the extremity.
2. Assess distal neurovascular status.
3. Pad the splint and/or bony areas to prevent local pressure.
4. Fold a 36-in. SAM Splint in half, creating a C-curve two thirds of the distance down each half. A reverse C-curve may be added for additional support.
5. Using your leg as a model, mold the splint around the extremity so that the medial and lateral malleoli are located in the middle of the splint. The ankle should be held in a neutral position if possible.
6. The splint is applied from the heel and gently molded to the distal tibia and fibula (Fig. 16.51).
7. Secure the splint using a wrap of choice (e.g., elastic wrap, cravat, roller bandage) (Fig. 16.52).
8. Beware of excessive pressure on the peroneal nerve when securing the splint.
9. Reassess distal neurovascular status and document findings.

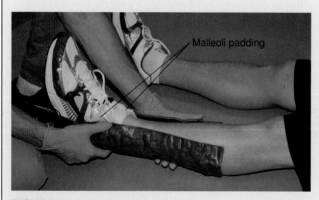

Malleoli padding

FIGURE 16.51

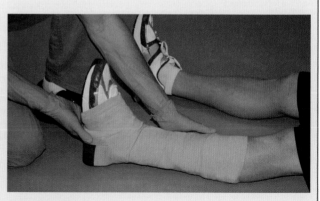

FIGURE 16.52

SKILL 16.18

SAM Splint: Cadillac

A Cadillac splint is used to immobilize injuries to the distal tibia and fibula, ankle, and foot and works when a neutral ankle position cannot be maintained.

1. Stabilize and support the extremity.
2. Assess the distal neurovascular status.
3. Pad splint and/or bony areas to prevent local pressure.
4. Fold a 36-in. SAM Splint in half, creating a U. Form a C-curve two thirds of the distance down each half of the splint.
5. Using your leg as a model, mold another 36-in. splint to form a posterior L splint from the toes to the popliteal fossa.
6. Apply the posterior splint L first from the toes to just distal to the popliteal fossa (Fig. 16.53), followed by the U splint centered over the axis of the tibia.
7. Mold the 36-in. U splint around the extremity so that the medial and lateral malleoli are located in the middle of the splint (Fig. 16.54).
8. Secure using a wrap of choice (e.g., elastic wrap, cravat, roller bandage) (Fig. 16.55). Beware of excessive pressure on the peroneal nerve when securing the splint if the splint goes that high.
9. Reassess distal neurovascular status and document findings (Fig. 16.55).

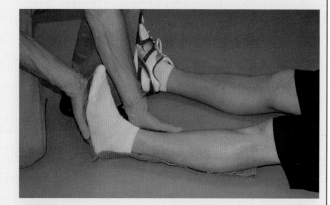

FIGURE 16.53

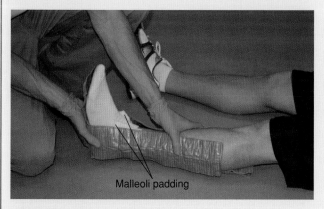

Malleoli padding

FIGURE 16.54

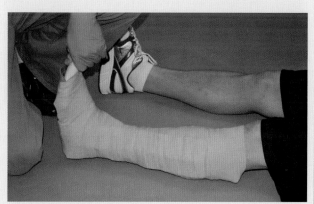

FIGURE 16.55

SKILL 16.19

Toe Buddy Taping

1. Stabilize and support the extremity.
2. Assess distal neurovascular status.
3. Pad the area to prevent local pressure if necessary.
4. Place gauze padding between the toes to prevent skin maceration (Fig. 16.56).

5. Tape toes together using 1/2-in. strips of adhesive tape (Fig. 16.57).
6. Expose the nail beds to avoid concealing rotational deformities.
7. Reassess distal neurovascular status and document findings.

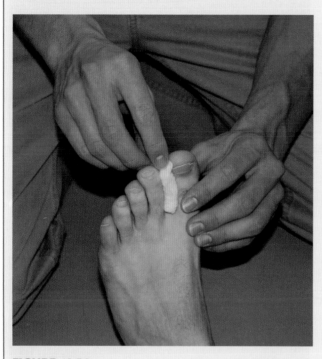

FIGURE 16.56

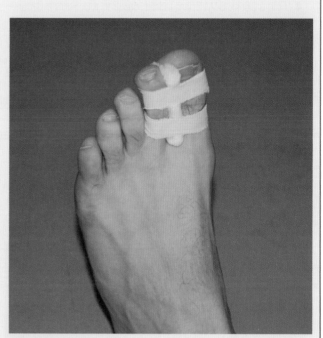

FIGURE 16.57

SKILL 16.20

Ankle Soft Splint

A soft splint can be used to immobilize injuries to the foot and ankle.

1. Stabilize and support the extremity.
2. Assess distal neurovascular status.
3. Prepare three cravats and slide them under the Achilles tendon.
4. Mold a pillow or rolled-up blanket around the injured ankle (Fig. 16.58).

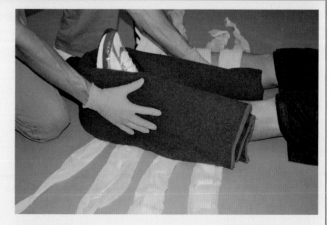

FIGURE 16.58

SKILL 16.20 *(Continued)*

Ankle Soft Splint *(Continued)*

5. Secure two cravats superior to the malleoli and secure a third cravat around the foot (Fig. 16.59).
6. Use additional cravats if warranted for greater support.

7. Reassess distal neurovascular status and document findings (Fig. 16.60).

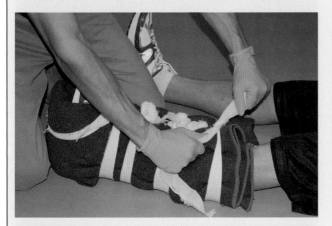

FIGURE 16.59

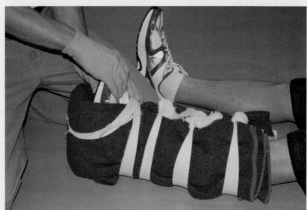

FIGURE 16.60

Tibia and Fibula

Trauma to the tibia and fibula is normally the result of a direct violent force applied to either bone, as in being kicked or tackled in soccer,[52] sliding in softball,[53] rotational forces (e.g., skiing), or an indirect trauma as seen in a **Maisonneuve fracture.**[54] Fractures and dislocations to the lower extremity have been reported as accounting for 6.2% and 1.5%, respectively, of all diagnosed sports- and recreation-related injuries in the United States.[55] Fractures of the tibia and fibula in one study accounted for 17.3% of all lower limb fractures among the United Kingdom's general population,[56] whereas half of the fractures sustained by amateur soccer players occurred to the tibia.[51]

Clinically, fractures of the proximal tibia present with significant soft tissue injury and swelling, because the anterior and medial aspect of the tibia lack adequate muscle bulk and subcutaneous tissue to protect skin and bone.[57] Such fractures involve the cartilage surface of the knee joint and may be displaced or nondisplaced. The proximity to the popliteal artery and tibial nerve also makes these structures vulnerable to injury[57] if the tibia is displaced. Tibial shaft fractures are the most common type of tibial fractures. Tibial shaft fractures often present with varying degrees of pain (usually severe), inability to bear weight, possible deformity, crepitus, and a laceration when the tibia is displaced and pierces the skin. Distal tibial fractures or tibial plafond fractures are fractures involving the weight-bearing surface of the distal tibia.[58] The individual may also present with swelling, tenderness at the fracture site, pain, inability to bear weight, and significant loss of ankle motion.

Fractures of the fibular shaft present with rapid swelling, tenderness, possible crepitus, loss of function and/or inability to bear weight, and pain during forced eversion and compression of the tibia and fibula (i.e., squeeze test).[13] Maisonneuve fractures are significant injuries involving the proximal fibula in association with a fractured medial malleolus or deltoid ligament disruption. They occur when an external rotation force is applied to the ankle and this force is carried through the **interosseous membrane** and exits the proximal fibula. If the foot is in a supinated position, the fibula often fails first.[59] Proximal fibular fractures present with pain and tenderness in addition to medial ankle pain, tenderness, swelling, and loss of function. A Pott's fracture is a bimalleolar fracture or fracture of the fibula near the ankle and fracture of the medial malleolus of the tibia and/or displacement of the medial ligament complex caused by lateral displacement of the foot.

Initial immobilization of tibia and/or fibula will be determined by the location of the trauma (e.g., tibial shaft fractures require stabilizing above and below the fracture site, whereas distal fibula fractures require stabilization of the ankle and knee joints), type, and extent of trauma. Various stabilization methods are available, including an anatomical/soft splint (Skill 16.21), rigid splint (Skill 16.22), long-leg box splint, vacuum splint (Skill 16.23), and SAM Splint.

SKILL 16.21

Lower Leg Anatomic/Soft Splint

1. Stabilize and support the extremity. The ground will act as the support.
2. Assess distal neurovascular status.
3. Move the uninvolved extremity away from the involved extremity.
4. Slide four cravats under the space behind the knee or ankle and maneuver two cravats so they are above knee and two below the knee, with one located near the ankle joint (Fig. 16.61).
5. Place the uninvolved extremity next to the involved one. Place a rolled-up towel or blanket between the legs for comfort and to ensure proper securing of the limb (Fig. 16.62).
6. Tie the four cravats snugly in place with the knots resting on the blankets (Fig. 16.62).
7. Reassess distal neurovascular status and document findings.
8. Place the athlete on a spine board for transport, using a six-person lift or scope stretcher.

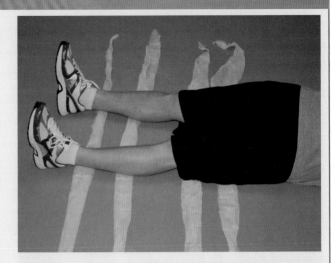

FIGURE 16.61

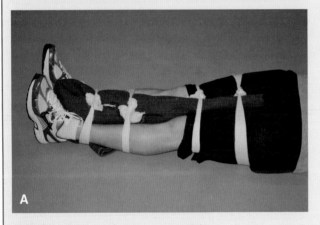

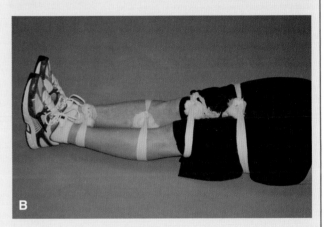

FIGURE 16.62   Soft (**A**); anatomic (**B**).

SKILL 16.22

Lower Leg Rigid Splint

1. Stabilize and support the extremity. The ground will act as the support.
2. Assess distal neurovascular status.
3. Move the uninvolved extremity away from the involved extremity.
4. Slide three or four cravats under the space behind the knee or ankle and maneuver one or two cravats so they are above the knee and one or two below the knee, with one located near the ankle joint (Fig. 16.63).

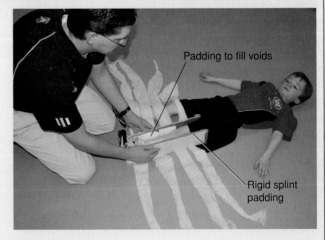

Padding to fill voids

Rigid splint padding

FIGURE 16.63

SKILL 16.22 *(Continued)*

Lower Leg Rigid Splint *(Continued)*

5. Place a padded rigid board on the lateral side of the involved extremity. Ensure that the board is of adequate length. Place a second padded rigid board on the medial side of the involved extremity. An alternative to the medial board is to bring the uninvolved extremity over as an anatomical splint. Be sure to fill any voids (Fig. 16.63).

6. Consider placing a rolled-up towel or blanket between the legs for comfort and to ensure proper securing of the limb.

7. Tie the cravats snugly in place with the knots resting on the board or blanket (Fig. 16.64).

8. Reassess distal neurovascular status and document findings.

9. Place the athlete on a spine board for transport using a six-person lift or scope stretcher.

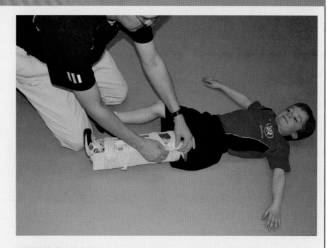

FIGURE 16.64

SKILL 16.23

Lower Leg Vacuum Splint

1. Stabilize and support the extremity. The ground will act as the support.

2. Assess distal neurovascular status.

3. Move the uninvolved extremity away from the involved extremity.

4. Apply appropriate dressings to all wounds in and around the injury site if necessary.

5. Place the splint next to the athlete with the valve side down, and distribute the Styrofoam beads throughout the splint evenly.

6. Continue to support and limit any excessive movement of the injured extremity as a second athletic trainer places the splint under the injury.

7. Position the splint so one strap is above and another below the suspected fracture site (Fig. 16.65).

8. Wrap the splint around the injury and massage the beads to ensure that all voids are filled. If the splint does not conform easily to the injury, adjust the amount of air in the splint until the splint conforms appropriately.

9. Secure the splint, avoiding overlapping of the edges (Fig. 16.65).

10. Attach the splint's vacuum pump to the coupling device and begin removing air.

11. Secure the splint by pressing the locking tab (Fig. 16.66).

12. Disconnect the coupling device once the splint hardens.

13. Reassess distal neurovascular status and document findings.

14. Place the athlete on a spine board for transport using a six-person lift or scope stretcher.

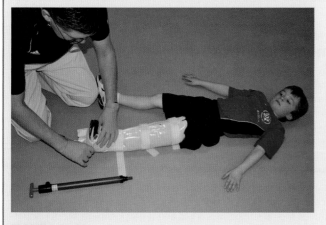

FIGURE 16.65

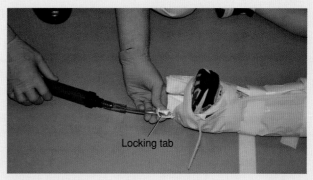

Locking tab

FIGURE 16.66

Knee

Trauma to the knee can result in a patellar fracture, dislocation, and/or subluxation and a knee dislocation and/or subluxation. Knee dislocations, typically considered rare traumatic events, occur in five main types (anterior, posterior, medial, lateral, and rotatory) and involve a significant force delivered to the knee.[60] Knee dislocations are further categorized as high-velocity or low-velocity dislocations. High-velocity dislocations occur during motor vehicle or motorcycle accidents and result in greater trauma to the soft tissue and vascular structures.[60,61] Low-velocity dislocations are normally seen in athletics and have a better prognosis than high-velocity dislocations.[62] Stannard et al.[61] found that high-energy mechanisms of injury were the cause of six dislocations related to athletics, compared with 106 dislocations resulting from some form of motor vehicle accident. Henrichs[60] suggests that the frequency of knee dislocations is unknown because they often reduce spontaneously and present as multiligament traumas. One of the main concerns of traumatic knee injury, particularly a knee dislocation, is the potential neurovascular damage to the sciatic and femoral nerves and popliteal artery. For further information on knee dislocations, see Henrichs.[60]

Other mechanisms of injury of traumatic knee trauma include direct impact (falling on the patella or direct force to the front of the leg), indirect trauma, such as sudden deceleration or forceful eccentric muscle contraction resulting in a severe pull of the patella or quadriceps tendon (e.g., patella fracture or patellar tendon avulsion), rotational force (e.g., patellar dislocation), or forceful hyperextension (e.g., knee dislocation).[66,67] A predisposition to an acute patellar dislocation may also be due to conditions such as increased Q-angle, patella alta, vastus medialis atrophy or insufficiency, femoral anteversion, genu valgum, and patellar hypermobility to name a few.[68,69] An acute lateral patellar dislocation stretches the medial **retinaculum** and patellofemoral ligament, which, when it heals, increases the length and de-

creases the substance of the supporting structures.[69] This insufficiency of the medial stabilizing structures increases patellar hypermobility and increases the risk of further patellar instability. Research has found that patients with a history of patellar instability had seven times higher odds of subsequent instability episodes than first-time dislocators.[70]

Various stabilization methods are available, including anatomical splints (Skill 16.24), rigid splints (Skill 16.25), long leg box splints, vacuum splints (Skill 16.26), and SAM Splints. If you suspect a knee dislocation, remember that this is a medical emergency; not only must the joint be immobilized above and below the dislocation, but also the athlete should be treated for shock and given immediate medical attention. Table 16.6 outlines the common mechanisms of injury, signs and symptoms, and possible immobilization choices for common skeletal trauma occurring about the knee.

Thigh and Pelvis

Trauma to the thigh and pelvis is often the result of a significant high-energy impact and may be associated with multiple system injuries such as trauma to the knee[71] as well as hemodynamic instability.[72] In athletics, femoral fractures and trauma to the pelvis are rare and occur due to direct (i.e., athlete-to-athlete contact) and indirect forces (e.g., rotational force when a skier falls or lands on an extended leg).[13] Among the general population, motor vehicle accidents (including vehicle–pedestrian), motorcycle accidents, and falls (e.g., elderly) appear to be common mechanisms of injury.[73–75]

Femoral Fractures

Femoral fractures in athletics are often due to a direct blow to the midthigh or rotational forces, resulting in isolated midshaft fractures. These fractures may be open or closed and are readily apparent because of the associated gross

Current Research

Possible Neurovascular Compromise after Knee Dislocation

The sciatic nerve is the largest posterior nerve, running the length of the lower extremity. As the nerve approaches the popliteal fossa of the knee, it diverges to form the tibial nerve (medially) and common peroneal nerve (laterally). The tibial nerve runs the length of the lower leg and innervates structures such as the gastrocnemius and soleus. The common peroneal nerve winds laterally just below the proximal head of the fibula. The nerve further branches to form the deep peroneal nerve (anterior tibialis) and superficial peroneal nerve (peroneus longus).

The popliteal artery, an extension of the femoral artery, also courses through the popliteal fossa and attaches proximally to the adductor hiatus; distally, it attaches to the soleus muscle. It too is vulnerable to injury because it is directly posterior to the knee[63] and tethered to the knee. Previous reports suggest that popliteal artery trauma occurs in 20% to 40% of knee dislocations.[64,65] Recent studies using selective **arteriography** to identify popliteal artery trauma found flow-limiting damage in only 7%[61] and 4%[63] of the cases identified. However, whether 4% or 40%, an athletic trainer in the presence of a possible traumatic knee injury (i.e., dislocation) should still be concerned about the possibility of substantial vascular trauma.

TABLE 16.6   Knee Injuries and Immobilization Techniques

Name	Mechanism of Injury	Signs and Symptoms	Immobilization Techniques
Patellar fracture	Falling onto the knee Direct blow to the knee Eccentric contraction of the quadriceps	Extra-articular swelling Retraction of the patella proximally Gross deformity and loss of function Inability to extend the knee against gravity	Vacuum splint (Skill 16.23) Rigid splint (Skill 16.22) Box splint Knee immobilizer:
Acute patellar dislocation	Direct contact to the medial patella Indirect from increased tension of the lateral musculature (quadriceps and iliotibial band)	Pain and swelling Snapping or popping sensation Gross deformity, flexed attitude of the knee Defect in patellar retinaculum once reduced May report a spontaneous reduction when attempting to straighten the leg	Prereduction • Vacuum splint • Rigid splint Postreduction • Vacuum splint • Rigid splint • Box splint • Knee immobilizer
Recurrent patellar dislocation/ subluxation	Direct contact to the medial patella Indirect from increased tension of the lateral musculature (quadriceps and iliotibial band)	Swelling and pain, but comparably less than with first time dislocations Tenderness under the medial patellar border Snapping or popping sensation Quadriceps atrophy Positive patellar apprehension test	Knee immobilizer
Patellar tendon avulsion	Indirect force caused a forceful eccentric contraction of the knee occurring from jumping, weight lifting, or stumbling	Sudden, sharp pain Proximally displaced patella, palpable defect Inability to extend the knee against gravity or bear weight on toe	Vacuum splint (Skill 16.23) Rigid splint (Skill 16.25) Box splint Knee immobilizer
Knee dislocation	Direct force to the anterior knee Excessive hyperextension Rotatory force The mechanism will vary for each classification (anterior, posterior, etc.), however, they will all involve a significant force delivered to the knee	Severe pain, swelling, and muscle spasms Deformity, shortening of the involved extremity, and loss of function Multidirectional ligamentous instability Diminished or absent neurovascular status	Prereduction • Vacuum splint • Anatomic/soft splint (Skill 16.21) • Rigid splint: Postreduction • Box splint • Rigid splint • Vacuum splint

SKILL 16.24

Knee Anatomic/Soft Splint

1. Stabilize and support the extremity.
2. Assess distal neurovascular status.
3. Move the uninvolved extremity away from the involved extremity.
4. Slide two to four cravats under the space behind the knee or ankle and maneuver one or two cravats so they are above knee and one or two below the knee, with one located near the ankle joint (Fig. 16.67).

5. Place the uninvolved extremity next to the involved one. Place a rolled-up towel or blanket between the legs for comfort and to ensure proper securing of the limb (Fig. 16.67).
6. Tie the cravats snugly in place with the knots resting on the blankets (Fig. 16.68).
7. Reassess distal neurovascular status and document findings.
8. Place the athlete on a spine board for transport using a six-person lift or scope stretcher.

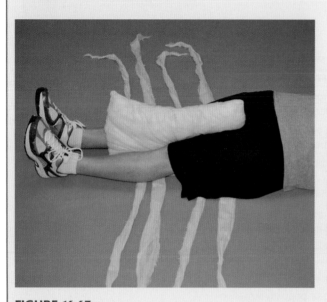

FIGURE 16.67

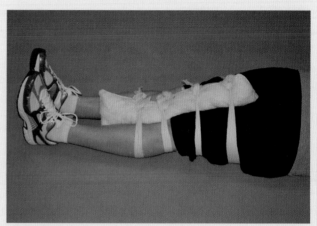

FIGURE 16.68

SKILL 16.25

Rigid Straight-Leg Splint

1. Stabilize and support the extremity.
2. Assess distal neurovascular status.
3. Move the uninvolved extremity away from the involved extremity.
4. Slide four cravats under the space behind the knee or ankle and maneuver two cravats so they are above knee and two below the knee (Fig. 16.69).
5. Using a second athletic trainer for support, raise the involved extremity high enough to slide a rigid board under it (Fig. 16.69). Place a padded rigid board on top of the cravats. Fill the void behind the knee (Fig. 16.70).

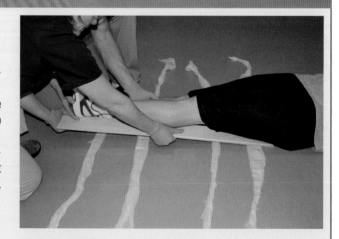

FIGURE 16.69

SKILL 16.25° *(Continued)*

Rigid Straight-Leg Splint *(Continued)*

6. Tie the cravats snugly (Fig. 16.70).
7. Place towels in the voids of the cravats for more support.
8. Reassess distal neurovascular status and document findings (Fig. 16.70).
9. Place the athlete on a spine board for transport using a six-person lift or scope stretcher.

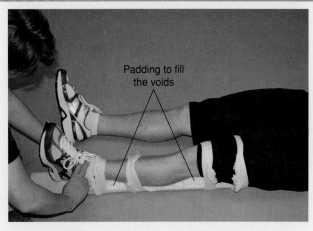

Padding to fill the voids

FIGURE 16.70

SKILL 16.26

Vacuum Splint

1. Stabilize and support the extremity.
2. Assess distal neurovascular status.
3. Move the uninvolved extremity away from the involved one.
4. Apply appropriate dressings to all wounds in and around the injury site if necessary.
5. Place the splint next to the athlete with the valve side down and distribute the Styrofoam beads throughout the splint evenly.
6. Continue to support and limit any excessive movement of the injured extremity as a second athletic trainer places the splint under the injury.

7. Position the splint so one strap is above and another below the suspected fracture site.
8. Wrap the splint around the injury and massage the beads to ensure that all voids are filled. If the splint does not conform easily to the injury, adjust the amount of air in the splint until the splint conforms appropriately (Fig. 16.71).
9. Secure the splint, avoiding overlap of the edges (Fig. 16.71).
10. Attach the splint's vacuum pump to the coupling device and begin removing air (Fig. 16.72).

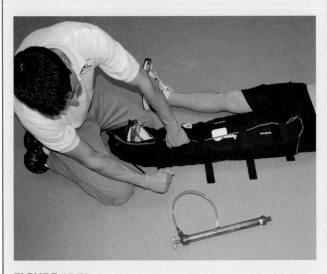

FIGURE 16.71

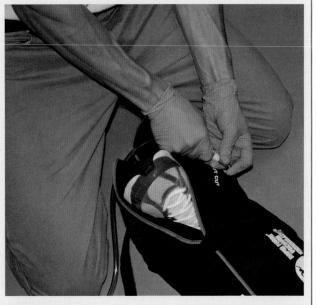

FIGURE 16.72

(Continued)

SKILL 16.26 *(Continued)*

Vacuum Splint (Continued)

11. Disconnect the coupling device once the splint has hardened.

12. Reassess distal neurovascular status and document findings (Fig. 16.73).

13. Place the athlete on a spine board for transport using a six-person lift or a scope stretcher.

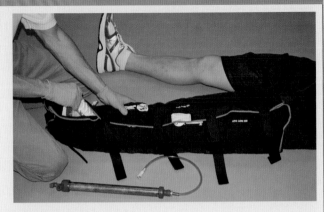

FIGURE 16.73

deformity of the bone, which presents with a shortened, externally rotated thigh. Clinically, femoral fractures present with severe pain, rapid swelling, and loss of limb function as well as severe quadriceps muscle spasms. Secondary neurovascular damage in the area is also possible. The femoral artery is often injured because of a displaced midthigh femoral fracture,[76] increasing the risk of hemorrhagic shock. Because of the risk of neurovascular damage and hemorrhagic shock, the athlete should be stabilized and immediately transported to the nearest medical facility. Immobilization of a femoral fracture is best accomplished using a traction splint; however, a simple rigid splint, padded board splint, or pillow may be just as effective[77] if a traction splint is unavailable.

Traction Splint   Traction splints are mechanical devices used on open (break in skin only) or closed midthigh factures[77,78] by securing the ankle and applying a distractive force with the proximal end of the splint secured or pressing against the pelvis. Traction splints are believed to stabilize the fracture, reduce blood loss, decrease quadriceps spasming and pain, and help maintain the patient's distal vascular supply.[77,79] Contraindications to the use of a traction splint include a dislocation of the hip and concomitant fracture/dislocation of the knee, tibia, fibula, and/or ankle.[77,78]

Application of a traction splint will vary according to the manufacturer's directions but generally requires two trained individuals, typically emergency medical technicians. The team should begin application of the traction splint by assessing distal neurovascular status, adjusting the length of the device against the uninvolved limb, applying manual traction, placing the splint and securing the straps and ankle hitch, taking up mechanical traction, attaching any remaining straps, and then reassessing distal neurovascular status (Fig. 16.74). Once the splint is secured, the athlete will have to be moved to a spine board for transportation. Proper

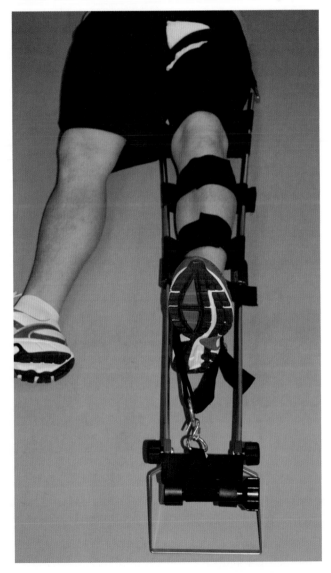

FIGURE 16.74   Hare traction splint. Application of a traction splint requires two well-trained athletic trainers.

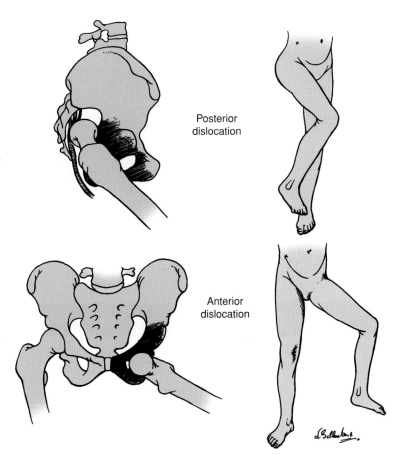

Posterior
dislocation

Anterior
dislocation

FIGURE 16.75 Hip dislocation. (From Mick CA. Initial management of fractures and joint injuries. In: Zuidema GD, Rutherford RB, Ballinger WF, eds. *The Management of Trauma.* Philadelphia: Saunders; 1985:673, with permission.)

training and practice are required to apply a traction splint. The athletic trainer should work with his or her local EMS system regarding training and should check with individual state laws and practice acts to determine whether the use of a traction splint is acceptable in his or her state.

Hip Dislocations

Hip dislocations in athletics occur from an indirect blow to hip joint when the foot is firmly planted and an internal rotation force is applied to the femur.[13] A direct blow causing a longitudinal force along the long axis of the femur when the hip is flexed 90 degrees and slightly adducted (e.g., falling on the knee) can result in a posterior hip dislocation as well as concomitant knee injuries due to the force on the knee. In fact, posterior hip dislocations are the most common type of dislocation. Dislocation and the rare fracture/dislocation have been reported in football,[80] rugby and skiing,[81] gymnastics,[82] and basketball.[83]

Clinically, a posterior hip dislocation will present with the classic sign of the hip held in a flexed, internally rotated, and adducted position (Fig. 16.75). This occurs because the femoral head is locked posterior to the acetabulum.[27] An anterior dislocation presents with the hip held in a partially

flexed, externally rotated, and abducted position with the femoral head palpable anterior to the femoral triangle. An athlete will complain of pain in the hip and groin, swelling, and loss of function. Secondary damage to the nerves and blood vessels, particularly the sciatic and femoral nerves, is also possible; therefore, a complete neurovascular examination should be conducted. Immediate transportation to appropriate medical care (reduction within 6 hours) is necessary to decrease the risk of avascular necrosis of the femoral head.[80,84] When immobilizing the hip dislocation, you must limit any excessive movement to prevent additional trauma and changes in neurovascular status. Immobilization of a hip dislocation can be accomplished using a vacuum splint or mattress or a soft splint and spine board (Fig. 16.76). It will require transport to the nearest medical facility for further evaluation and management.

Pelvic Fractures

As previously mentioned, pelvic fractures in athletics are rare, but when they do occur they are usually due to high-energy impact trauma, as in skiing or equestrian sports. Forces of great strength are necessary to disrupt the pelvis; therefore, when a pelvis fracture is suspected, concomitant

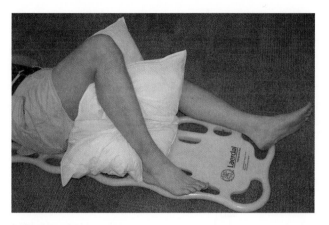

FIGURE 16.76 Stabilization of a hip dislocation using a soft splint.

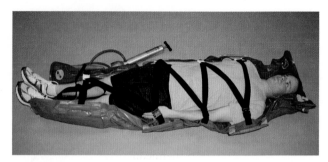

FIGURE 16.77 Vacuum mattress. A vacuum mattress is a more comfortable alternative to a spine board.

Scenarios

1. Seth, a high school football quarterback, is in the cocking phase of throwing when an opposing player strikes him from the side, driving his lateral right shoulder into the ground. He manages to get up but realizes that he is in significant pain. He grasps his involved elbow to support the joint and walks over to the sideline. Joel, the team's athletic trainer, begins evaluating the arm. He notes the pain and upward displacement of the clavicle. When Joel asks Seth to abduct his arm, he is unable to do so.

Identify the clinical diagnosis.
What type of immobilization technique should Joel use and how would he apply it?
What makes this case more challenging than dealing with a volleyball player with same clinical diagnosis?

2. Sally, a Division I volleyball player, attempts to block a ball during a match when she falls on her outstretched arm after misjudging her landing. She immediately begins to experience lateral elbow pain and tenderness over the proximal end of the radius. Nancy's evaluation of Sally's elbow reveals swelling over the radial head and clicking over the proximal radius with supination.

What is the clinical diagnosis? Describe how you would attempt to immobilize the joint.
Are than any alternative methods to immobilizing this injury?
What other type of trauma or injury might Nancy be concerned about?

3. Sam, a certified athletic trainer, is covering a men's recreational basketball league as a favor to his brother. During one of the games, a couple of the players get a little heated and begin fighting. Ted, a 23-year-old construction worker, goes to strike another player but misses, striking the wall behind him. He immediately grabs his hand. Sam already knows, based on the mechanism, what he is probably dealing with and brings over some of the splinting materials he will need.

Identify the clinical diagnosis and the common signs and symptoms of this injury.
What type of immobilization device would you recommend and why?

4. Toby, a college running back, is carrying the ball when he is tackled to the ground violently. Because he does not get up immediately, Shawn, the athletic trainer covering the event, goes to see what is wrong. His primary assessment is unremarkable. The secondary assessment, however, demonstrates tenderness and crepitus over the fourth and fifth ribs. Unsure whether the injury is a rib fracture or contusion, Shawn removes Toby from the game, immobilizes the ribs, and refers him to the emergency room for x-rays.

Discuss the most appropriate way to stabilize a rib fracture.
If Toby were to become cyanotic and tachypneic would referring him to the emergency room be appropriate? Why or why not?

5. While covering a high school ice hockey game, Shelia is summoned onto the ice for an injured player. She finds Kimberly, who is in severe pain, trying to stabilize her lower leg and ankle. Once Sheila finally calms her down, she begins gathering a SAMPLE history and determines the mechanism of injury to be direct contact and rotation to the lateral side of the ankle. A focused physical examination of the distal lower leg and ankle reveals tenderness over the distal fibula and medial ankle. Kimberly is unable to bear weight and is helped off the ice. Further evaluation reveals loss of ankle function, swelling, and pain with compression of the tibia and fibula.

Identify a possible clinical diagnosis and any possible concomitant injury.
Discuss the best method for evaluating this type of injury, given the sporting equipment.
If you were in Shelia's position, what immobilization technique would you use and why?

injuries such as neurological, thoracic, genitourinary, skeletal, and intra-abdominal injuries are also possible.[74,85] Given the risk of concomitant injury, possible disruption of major blood vessels protected by the pelvic ring, and the risk of venous bleeding from the fractured pelvis, it is no wonder that pelvic fractures are potentially life-threatening injuries. In fact, the morbidity risk of pelvis fractures is between 10% and 60%[85–87] and may require aggressive resuscitation and prehospital management to stabilize the athlete.

Clinically, a person with a pelvic fracture will complain of severe pain when the pubis or iliac crest is compressed; sacroiliac joint or groin pain; swelling over the bony prominences, pubis, perineum, or scrotum; inability to bear weight; and/or genitourinary dysfunction. Such a person may be hemodynamically unstable.[74,87] Traditional assessment procedures for a pelvic fracture include compression of the iliac crest in a downward and inward motion. However, Lee and Porter[77] suggest that this test is unreliable and increases the risk of further blood loss by disrupting blood clots. Furthermore, they suggest that if the athlete is unconscious, the pelvis *should not* be palpated for tenderness or instability; rather, it should immediately be immobilized.

Pelvic fracture will require immediate activation of EMS because most prehospital stabilization techniques require training above that of an athletic trainer. Prehospital immobilization of a pelvic fracture includes minimizing the number of examinations and examiners and stabilizing the pelvis. A pneumatic antishock garment or medical antishock trouser can be useful for stabilizing a pelvic fracture and redistributing blood from the limbs to the trunk.[88] Circumferential pelvic binders or sheets can also be used to stabilize the pelvis.[74,88] Once he or she is stabilized, logrolling the athlete onto a spine board for transport should be avoided because of the increased risk of pelvic disruption and dislodging blood clots.[74] A scoop stretch using a maximum 15-degree logroll angle should be used to place the athlete on a spine board or vacuum mattress for transport (Fig. 16.77).

WRAP-UP

Immobilization techniques used to stabilize skeletal trauma or any musculoskeletal injury vary depending upon the type of trauma sustained, clinical findings, available equipment, training, and an athletic trainer's EAP. In athletics, proper immobilization of an athlete is further complicated by protective equipment, which may need to be removed, using care to adequately assess and stabilize a bone or joint. Also complicating some situations is the rarity of the injury. Injuries such as pelvic fractures and/or hip dislocations do not occur often; however, when they do occur, athletic trainers must be prepared to manage these situations. Practicing the techniques described in this chapter at least once a year, most likely at the start of an athletic season or during

the annual review of the EAP, will allow athletic trainers to remain competent if presented with a trauma situation requiring emergency immobilization.

REFERENCES

1. Starkey C, Ryan J. *Evaluation of Orthopedic and Athletic Injuries,* 2nd ed. Philadelphia: F.A. Davis; 2002.
2. Kuzak N, Ishkanian A, Abu-Laban RB. Posterior sternoclavicular joint dislocation: case report and discussion. *Can J Emerg Med Care.* 2006;8(5):355–357.
3. Mazoue CG, Andrews JR. Injuries to the shoulder in athletes. *South Med J.* 2004;97(8):748–754.
4. Yeh GL, Williams GR Jr. Conservative management of sternoclavicular injuries. *Orthop Clin North Am.* 2000;31(2):189–203.
5. Cope R. Dislocations of the sternoclavicular joint. *Skeletal Radiol.* 1993;22(4):233–238.
6. Garreison RBI, Williams GR. Clinical evaluation of injuries to the acromioclavicular and sternoclavicular joints. *Clin Sports Med.* 2003;22:239–254.
7. Gleason BA. Bilateral, spontaneous, anterior subluxation of the sternoclavicular joint: A case report and literature review. *Mil Med.* 2006;171(8):790–792.
8. Hubble MW, Hubble JP. *Principles of Advanced Trauma Care.* Albany, NY: Delmar Thompson Learning; 2002.
9. Johns KL, Counselman FL. Evaluation and treatment of shoulder injuries. *Emerg Med.* 2001;33(8):20–40.
10. Beim GM. Acromioclavicular joint injuries. *J Athl Train.* 2000;35(3):261–267.
11. Rockwood C, Young D. Disorders of the acromioclavicular joint. In: Rockwood C, Matsen F, eds. *The Shoulder.* Philadelphia: Saunders; 1990:413–476.
12. Abbitt PL, Riddervold HO. The carpal tunnel view: Helpful adjuvant for unrecognized fractures of the carpus. *Skeletal Radiol.* 1987;6:45–47.
13. Gallaspy JB, May JD. *Signs and Symptoms of Athletic Injuries.* St. Louis: Mosby; 1996.
14. DeFranco MJ, Lawton JN. Radial nerve injuries associated with humeral fractures. *J Hand Surg.* 2006;31(4):655–663.
15. Ring D, Chin K, Jupiter JB. Radial nerve palsy associated with high-energy humeral shaft fractures. *J Hand Surg.* 2004;29(1):144–147.
16. Noaman HH. Microsurgical reconstruction of brachial artery injuries in displaced supracondylar fracture humerus in children. *Microsurgery.* 2006;26(7):498–505.
17. Daya M. Shoulder. In: Marx J, Hockberger R, Walls R, eds. *Rosen's Emergency Medicine: Concepts and Clinical Practice,* 6th ed. Philadelphia: Elsevier; 2006.
18. Perrin DH. *Athletic Taping and Bracing,* 2nd ed. Champaign, IL: Human Kinetics; 2005.
19. McFarland EG, Chronopoulos E, Kim TK. Upper extremity injuries in adolescent athletes. *Athl Ther Today.* 2002;7(6):13–17.
20. Baykal B, Sener S, Turkan H. Scapular manipulation technique for reduction of traumatic anterior shoulder dislocations: experiences of an academic emergency department. *Emerg Med J.* 2005;22:336–338.
21. Prentice WE. *Arnheim's Principles of Athletic Training: A Competency-Based Approach,* 13th ed. New York: McGraw-Hill; 2009.

22. Meredith RM, Butcher JD. Field splinting of suspected fractures: Preparation, assessment, and application. *Phys Sports Med.* 1997;25(10):29–39.

23. Paksima, Panchal A. Elbow fracture-dislocations: the role of hinged external fixation. *Bull Hosp Joint Dis Orthop Inst.* 2004;62(1 & 2):33–39.

24. Berg EE. Elbow dislocation with arterial injury. *Orthop Nurs.* 2001;20(6):57–59.

25. Kaminski TW, Power ME, Buckley B. Differential assessment of elbow injuries. *Athl Ther Today.* 2000;5(3):6–11.

26. McGinley JC, Hopgood BC, Gaughan JP, et al. Forearm and elbow injury: the influence of rotational position. *J Bone Joint Surg.* 2003;85-A(12):2403–2409.

27. Hartman JT. *Fracture Management: A Practical Approach.* Philadelphia: Lea & Febiger; 1978.

28. Rettig AC. Athletic injuries of the wrist and hand: Part I: traumatic injuries of the wrist. *Am J Sports Med.* 2003;31(6):1038–1048.

29. Chung KC, Spilson SV. The frequency and epidemiology of hand and forearm fractures in the United States. *J Hand Surg.* 2001;26(5):908–915.

30. Altizer L. Hand and wrist fractures. *Ortho Nurs.* 2003;22(3):232–239.

31. Simpson D, McQueen MM. Acute sporting injuries to the hand and wrist in the general population. *Scott Med J.* 2006;51(2):25–26.

32. Kouris GJ, Schenck RR. Carpal fractures. eMedicine. 2008. Available at http://emedicine.medscape.com/article/1238278-overview.

33. Akahane M, Ono H, Sada M, et al. Fracture of hamate hook: Diagnosis by the hamate hook lateral view. *Hand Surg.* 2000;5(2):131–137.

34. Rettig AC. Elbow, forearm and wrist injuries in the athlete. *Sports Med.* 1998;25(2):115–130.

35. Morhart M, Tredget EE, Jarman TA, Ghahary A. Hand, wrist fractures and dislocations. *eMedicine.* 2008. Available at http://emedicine.medscape.com/article/1285825-overview. Accessed June 25, 2010.

36. Weber ER, Chao EY. An experimental approach to the mechanism of scaphoid waist fractures. *J Hand Surg.* 1978;3A:142–148.

37. Adams JC. *Outline of Fractures: Including Joint Injuries.* London: Churchill and Livingstone; 1972.

38. Rettig AC, Ryan R, Shelbourne DK, et al. Metacarpal fractures in the athlete. *Am J Sports Med.* 1989;17(4):567–572.

39. Combs JA. It's not "just a finger." *J Athl Training.* 2000;35(2):168–178.

40. Hame SL, LaFemina JM, McAllister DR, et al. Fractures in the collegiate athlete. *Am J Sports Med.* 2004;32:446–451.

41. Leggit J, Meko C. Acute finger injuries: Part II. fractures, dislocations, and thumb injuries. *Am Fam Phys.* 2006;73(5):827–834.

42. Chase C, Turney SZ. Chest injuries. In: Fu FH, Stone DA, eds. *Sports Injuries: Mechanisms, Prevention, Treatment.* 2nd ed. Baltimore, MD: Lippincott Williams & Wilkins; 2001:1175–1184.

43. Roberge RJ, Morgenstern MJ, Osborn H. Cough fracture of the ribs. *Am J Emerg Med.* 1984;2(6):513–517.

44. Starkey C, Ryan J. *Evaluation of Orthopedic and Athletic Injuries.* 2nd ed. Philadelphia: F.A. Davis; 2001.

45. Powell JW, Barber-Foss KD. Injury patterns in selected high school sports: A review of the 1995–1997 seasons. *J Athl Train.* 1999;34(3):277–284.

46. Hagglund M, Walden M, Ekstrand J. Injury incidence and distribution in elite football: A prospective study of the Danish and the Swedish top divisions. *Scan J Med Sci Sports (Copenhagen).* 2005;15(1):21–28.

47. Ostojic SM. Comparing sports injuries in soccer: Influence of a positional role. *Res Sports Med.* 2003;11(3):203–208.

48. Walden M, Hagglund M, Ekstrand J. Injuries in Swedish elite football: A prospective study on injury definitions, risk for injury and injury pattern during 2001. *Scan J Med Sci Sports (Copenhagen).* 2005;15(2):118–125.

49. Sheppard C, Hodson A. Injury profiles in professional footballers. *SportEX Medicine.* 2006. Available at http://www.sportex.net/newsite/Common/articleDetail.asp?txtArticleID=463&txtDescription=title+contains%3A+%22Injury+profiles+in+professional+footballers%22&txtStartFrom=1. Accessed June 25, 2010.

50. Silbergleit R. Fracture, foot. *eMedicine.* 2010. Available at http://emedicine.medscape.com/article/825060-overview. Accessed June 25, 2010.

51. Goga IE, Gongal P. Severe soccer injuries in amateurs. *Br J Sports Med.* 2003;37:498–501.

52. Lenehan B, Fleming P, Walsh S, et al. Tibial shaft fractures in amateur footballers. *Br J Sports Med.* 2003;37:176–178.

53. Pollack KM, Canham-Chervak M, Gazal-Carvalho C, et al. Interventions to prevent softball related injuries: A review of the literature. *Inj Prev.* 2005;11:277–281.

54. Sproule JA, Khalid M, O'Sullivan M, et al. Outcome after surgery for maisonneuve fracture of the fibula. *Injury.* 2004;35:791–798.

55. Conn JM, Annest JL, Gilchrist J. Sports and recreation related injury episodes in the US population, 1997–1999. *Inj Prev.* 2003;9:117–123.

56. Kaye JA, Jick H. Epidemiology of lower limb fractures in general practice in the United Kingdom. *Inj Prev.* 2004;10:368–374.

57. Tejwani N, Achan P. Staged management of high-energy proximal tibial fractures. *Hosp Joint Dis.* 2004;62(1 & 2):62–66.

58. Norvell JG, Steele MS, Cooper TM. Fractures, tibia and fibula. *eMedicine.* 2009. Available at http://emedicine.medscape.com/article/826304-overview. Accessed

59. Lauge-Hansen N. Fractures of the ankle. III. Genetic roentgenologic diagnosis of fracutres of the ankle. *Am J Roentgenol Radium Ther Nucl Med.* 1954;71:456–471.

60. Henrichs A. A review of knee dislocations. *J Athl Train.* 2004;39(4):365–369.

61. Stannard JP, Sheils TM, Lopez-Ben RR, et al. Vascular injuries in knee dislocations: The role of physical examination in determining the need for arteriography. *J Bone Joint Surg Am.* 2004;86(5):910–915.

62. Shelbourne K, Porter D, Clingman J, et al. Low-velocity knee dislocation. *Orthop Rev.* 1991;20:995–1004.

63. Martinez D, Sweatman K, Thompson EC. Popliteal artery injury associated with knee dislocations. *Am Surg.* 2001;67(2):165–167.

64. Kaufman SL, Martin LG. Arterial injuries associated with complete dislocation of the knee. *Radiology.* 1992;184:153–155.

65. Merrill KD. Knee dislocations with vascular injuries. *Orthop Clin North Am.* 1994;25:707–713.

66. Adams N. Knee injuries. *Emerg Nurs.* 2004;11(10):19–27.

67. Enad JG. Patellar tendon ruptures. *South Med J.* 1999;92(6):563–566.

68. Dath R, Chakravarthy J, Porter KM. Patella dislocations. *Trauma.* 2006;8(1):5–11.

69. Cosgarea AJ, Browne JA, Kim TK, et al. Evaluation and management of the unstable patella. *Phys Sports Med.* 2002; 30(10):33.

70. Fithian DC, Paxton EW, Stone ML, et al. Epidemiology and natural history of acute patellar dislocation. *Am J Sports Med.* 2004;32(5):1114–1121.

71. Giannoudis PV, Roberts CS, Parikh AR, et al. Knee dislocation with ipsilateral femoral shaft fracture: A report of five cases. *J Orthop Trauma.* 2005;19(3):205–210.

72. Heetveld MJ, Harris I, Schlaphoff G, et al. Hemodynamically unstable pelvic fractures: Recent care and new guidelines. *World J Surg.* 2004;28(9):904–909.

73. Kobziff L. Traumatic Pelvic Fractures. *Orthop Nurs.* 2006;25(4): 235–241.

74. Lee C, Porter K. The prehospital management of pelvic fractures. *Emerg Med J.* 2007;24(2):130–133.

75. Heetveld MJ, Harris I, Schlaphoff G, et al. Guidelines for the management of haemodynamically unstable pelvic fracture patients. *ANZ J Surg.* 2004;74(7):520–529.

76. Burns KJ. Extremity and vascular trauma. In: Sheehy SD, Blansfield JS, Danis DM, et al. eds. *Manual of Clinical Trauma Care: The First Hour,* 3rd ed. St. Louis: Mosby; 1999:285–326.

77. Wood SP, Vrahas M, Wedel SK. Femur fracture immobilization with traction splints in multisystem trauma patients. *Prehosp Emerg Care.* 2003;7(2):241–243.

78. Lee C, Porter KM. Prehospital management of lower limb fractures. *Emerg Med J.* 2005;22:660–663.

79. Limmer D, O'Keefe MF, Grant HD, et al. *Emergency Care,* 9th ed. Upper Saddle River, NJ: Prentice Hall; 2001.

80. Giza E, Mithofer K, Matthews H, et al. Hip fracture-dislocation in football: A report of two cases and review of the literature. *Br J Sports Med.* 2004;38;2004:e17.

81. Mohanty K, Gupta SK, Langston A. Posterior dislocation of hip in adolescents attributable to casual rugby. *J Accident Emerg Med.* 2000;17:429.

82. Mitchell JC, Giannoudis PV, Millner PA, et al. A rare fracture-dislocation of the hip in a gymnast and review of the literature. *Br J Sports Med.* 1999;33:283–284.

83. Tennent TD, Chambler AF, Rossouw DJ. Posterior dislocation of the hip while playing basketball. *Br J Sports Med.* 1998;32:342–343.

84. Lam F, Walczak J, Franklin A. Traumatic asymmetrical bilateral hip dislocation in an adult. *Emerg Med J* 2001;18(6): 506–507.

85. Bassam D, Cephas GA, Ferguson KA, et al. A protocol for the initial management of unstable pelvic fractures. *Am Surg.* 1998;64(9):862–867.

86. Raafat A, Wright MJ. Current management of pelvic fractures. *South Med J.* 2000;93(8):760.

87. Frakes MA, Evans T. Major pelvic fractures. *Crit Care Nurse.* 2004;24(2):18.

88. Mohanty K, Musso D, Powell JN, et al. Emergent management of pelvic ring injuries: An update. *Can J Surg.* 2005;48(1):49–56.

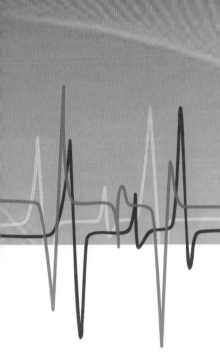

CHAPTER 17

Recognition and Management of Head and Spine Injuries

CHAPTER OUTCOMES

1. Identify the anatomy of the head and spine.
2. Identify common mechanisms of injuries associated with head and spine.
3. Identify the common signs and symptoms of head and spinal injuries.
4. Identify and describe the management procedures for application of cervical collars.
5. Identify and describe how to properly provide in-line stability of the head for a suspected neck/spine injury.
6. Identify and describe how to properly log roll an athlete.
7. Identify and describe the management procedures for securing an athlete to a spine board.
8. Identify and discuss types of emergency rescue equipment used for spinal injuries.
9. Determine when removal of protective equipment is warranted in spinal emergencies.
10. Identify and describe the specific procedures of protective equipment removal when necessary.

NOMENCLATURE

Avulsions: injuries in which a tendon or bone has torn away from its attached surface

Babinski reflex: flexion of the great toe and fanning of the other toes when the bottom of the foot is stroked, indicating damage to the nerve pathways

Brainstem: connection between the brain and the spinal cord

Burner: a traction or compression injury of the brachial plexus that causes a tingling/burning sensation of the affected shoulder/arm/hand area

Cerebellum: the lower back part of the brain, thought to control sensory and motor function

Cerebrum: the anterior part of the forebrain, divided into two hemispheres that account for approximately two thirds of total brain weight

Comminuted fracture: crushed or splintered bone

Decerebrate posture: rigid extension of the limbs as a result of brain injury

Decorticate posture: abnormal flexion of the extremities due to brain injury

Lamina: bony projection that extends dorsally and medially to form the pedicle

Lucid: aware

Meninges: membranous tissues in the brain consisting of three layers called the arachnoid, dura mater, and pia mater

Pedicle: bony projection from the bodies of the vertebrae

Priapism: painful erection in males, which may result from a groin injury

Sequelae: conditions resulting from an injury, disease, or trauma

Stinger: another name for a burner

Sulcus: a depression or fissure on the surface of the brain

BEFORE YOU BEGIN

1. What are the different types of bleeding in the brain?
2. What are the common signs and symptoms of a nerve injury to the brachial plexus?
3. What are common signs and symptoms of a concussion?
4. What are the steps for securing an athlete to a spine board?
5. What are some common steps required to remove a face mask in an emergency situation?
6. How should an athlete be stabilized while wearing a helmet?

Voices from the Field

The care of injuries to the head and spine is, and should be, of utmost concern for Athletic Trainers (ATs). Of all injuries encountered by ATs on a daily basis, head and spine injuries may not be the most common, but the catastrophic nature of these injuries requires proper emergency care for the best possible outcome.

When treating injuries to the head and spine, the AT may sometimes feel, or others may cause the AT to feel, that he or she is acting too conservatively. As a qualified health care professional, trained to act in these situations, it is up to the AT to put aside those feelings and protect the athlete. It is much better to say the athlete "probably could have played" than to say the athlete "should not have returned to play."

In addition to knowing and acting in accordance with the most current standard of care, the AT must always be prepared

to act both mentally and physically. The old saying "you play the game like you practice" should be heeded by all ATs. In other words, you must know what to do and you must physically and mentally practice on a regular basis, so when the unthinkable does occur, you are ready. You must be prepared to deal with what you think may happen in order to be prepared for what *will* happen. There is no room for error or mistakes when caring for head- or spine-injured athletes; their lives and livelihoods depend on your actions.

Patrick Sexton, EdD, ATC, CSCS
Undergraduate Athletic Training Program Director
Minnesota State University—Mankato

Some of the most severe sports injuries are injuries to the head and/or spine. Athletic trainers must be able to quickly recognize the signs and symptoms of a head or spine injury in order to properly care for and treat these injuries. Proper knowledge of securing and managing these conditions must be well rehearsed not only to prevent further damage but also to build confidence and experience when these emergency situations exist. Athletic trainers and other allied health professionals must also recognize that any head trauma can cause spinal trauma, and management of head trauma may be very similar to caring for spine injuries. In fact, according to the National Athletic Trainers' Association (NATA),[7] athletes who are suspected of having a head/neck or spine injury, diminished consciousness level, or neurological deficit should be managed properly and referred to appropriate medical facilities or personnel as quickly as

possible. In the event that an athlete must be transported because of such injuries, he or she should be properly secured to a spine board or an appropriate immobilization device. This chapter focuses on the common head and spinal injuries that may be prevalent in athletics and how these conditions should be managed in the emergency setting.

THE HEAD

Anatomy of the Head

The head is comprised of the skull and brain. The skull is made up of bones forming the protective structure of the brain and face; it can be divided into two sections: the cranium and the facial skeleton (Fig. 17.1). The cranial bones include the frontal, sphenoid, ethmoid, parietal, temporal, and occipital bones; the facial skeleton comprises the maxilla, mandible, nasal, and lacrimal bones. The outmost protective covering of the skull is the scalp.

This is a very resilient, highly vascular structure that functions to help absorb impact forces when a person is struck in the head.

The brain (Fig. 17.2), which lies underneath the skull, is composed of the **cerebrum, cerebellum,** and **brainstem**

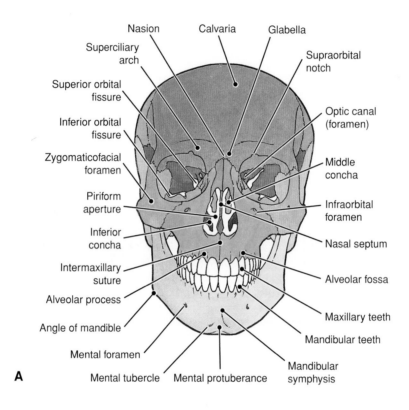

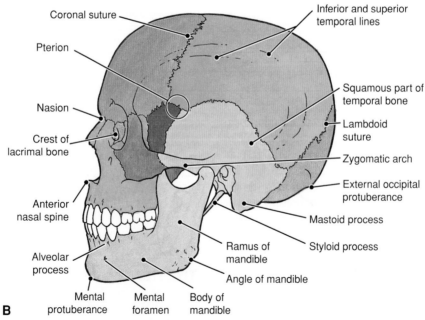

FIGURE 17.1   The skull. The whole of the skull is greater than the sum of its parts, but knowing the names of the parts is essential. **A.** Frontal view. **B.** Lateral view. (From Moore KL, Agur AMR. *Essential Clinical Anatomy,* 2nd ed. Baltimore: Lippincott Williams & Wilkins; 2002.)

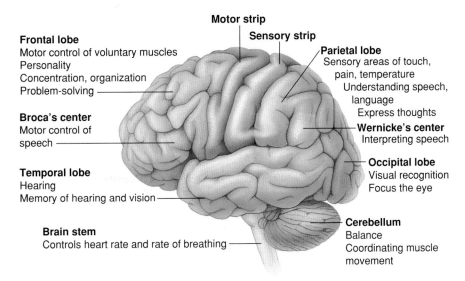

Motor strip

Sensory strip

Frontal lobe
Motor control of voluntary muscles
Personality
Concentration, organization
Problem-solving

Parietal lobe
Sensory areas of touch,
pain, temperature
Understanding speech,
language
Express thoughts

Broca's center
Motor control of
speech

Wernicke's center
Interpreting speech

Temporal lobe
Hearing
Memory of hearing and vision

Occipital lobe
Visual recognition
Focus the eye

Brain stem
Controls heart rate and rate of breathing

Cerebellum
Balance
Coordinating muscle
movement

FIGURE 17.2 Composition of the brain.

(midbrain, pons, and medulla). Cerebral hemispheres divide the cerebrum into right and left; they are separated by a longitudinal fissure. The cerebrum is responsible for voluntary muscular activities, sensory perceptions, and the higher brain functions, such as memory, learning, and emotions. The cerebellum controls the coordination of voluntary muscular motions, whereas the pons controls respiration and swallowing and the medulla controls functions such as heart rate, breathing, and blood pressure. Specific structures called **sulci** and fissures divide parts of the brain into four lobes (frontal, parietal, temporal, and occipital). When struck in the head, an athlete may present with signs and symptoms and/or deficits in function associated with the trauma to a particular lobe.

Surrounding the brain and spinal cord are special structures called the **meninges** (Fig. 17.3). Consisting of three layers, the meninges constitute a protective membrane. The outer layer is called the dura mater. It surrounds the entire brain and spinal cord and is separated from the outside cranial and skeletal bones by a thin space or cavity called the epidural space. Also located in the dura mater is the main arterial supply to the cranial bones and dura mater itself, called the meningeal artery. Located beneath the dura mater is a thin sheath called the arachnoid mater or, simply, arachnoid. The space between the dura mater and arachnoid is referred to as the subdural space. The arachnoid is a delicate structure named for its spiderlike filaments, which pass through the subarachnoid space to the pia mater. The innermost layer of the meninges is the pia mater, which attaches to the brain and spinal cord and follows the contours of the surface of the brain, projecting into the sulci and fissures. The space between the pia mater and arachnoid is called the subarachnoid space, in which the cerebrospinal fluid (CSF) is contained. The CSF is a clear, colorless fluid circulating between the ventricles of the brain and the central canal of the spinal cord. This watery fluid allows the brain to float and acts as a buffer against forces applied to the head externally.

Head Injuries

Any blow to the head can cause serious harm to the brain or spinal cord. In particular, a blow can disrupt the blood supply or cause damage to the brain tissue, such as a cerebral contusion. Forces to the head, such as hitting an object (e.g., falling to the ground), can cause an impact injury. In cases where this disrupts the meningeal arteries, blood can accumulate in the meningeal spaces in the form of a hematoma, causing serious brain injury. Blows to the head can be a result of either coup, contrecoup, shear, or rotational forces (Fig. 17.4). A coup injury to the head

Signs & Symptoms

Brain Injury

- Altered responsiveness or loss of consciousness
- Nausea and vomiting
- Pupils unequal or unresponsive/reactive to light
- Diplopia, visual impairments
- Memory loss or confusion
- Loss of balance
- Breathing irregularities
- Tinnitus
- Irritable or irrational behavior
- CSF in the ears (otorrhea) and nose (rhinorrhea)
- Hematoma formation around the eyes ("raccoon eyes") and behind the ears at the mastoid process (Battle's sign)
- Seizures

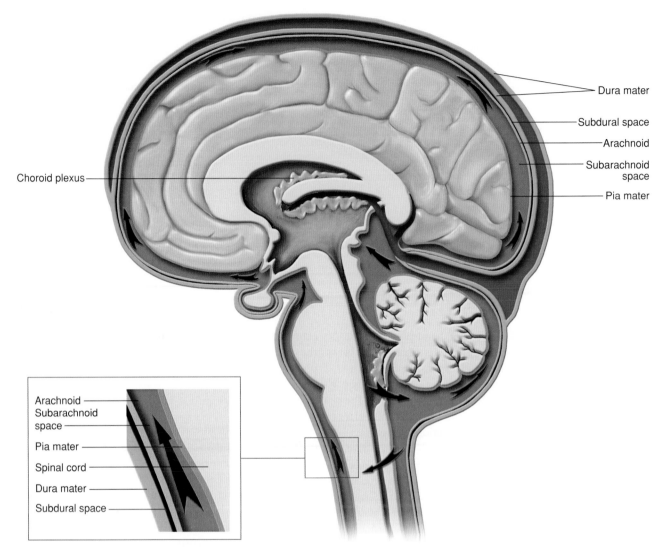

Choroid plexus

Dura mater

Subdural space

Arachnoid

Subarachnoid space

Pia mater

Arachnoid
Subarachnoid space
Pia mater
Spinal cord
Dura mater
Subdural space

FIGURE 17.3   The meninges. The arrows indicate the flow of cerebrospinal fluid. (Courtesy of Anatomical Chart Co.)

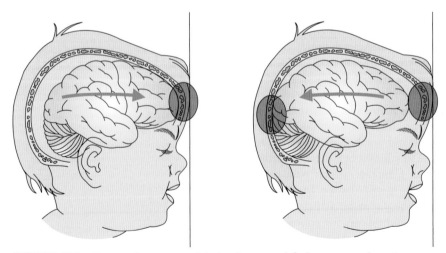

FIGURE 17.4   Coup and contrecoup injuries. Image on left demonstrates how, in a coup injury, a blow to the front of the skull results in an injury to the front of the brain. In a contrecoup injury (right), the brain recoils and strikes the posterior skull as well, injuring it twice. (LifeART image copyright (c) 2010 Lippincott Williams & Wilkins. All rights reserved.)

occurs at the site of impact, causing damage to the brain as it collides against the skull.[1] Coup injuries usually result when the brain accelerates to the point of impact at the skull, as when the stationary head is hit by a movable object. A contrecoup injury, where the moving head hits a stationary object, occurs on the opposite side of the point of contact. Here, the brain moves in the opposite direction and strikes the skull, producing damage away from the site of contact.[1] Contrecoup injuries are usually more severe than coup injuries.

Epidural Hematoma

An epidural hematoma results from a force or blow to the head causing a rip or tear in the meningeal arteries, usually from an acceleration/deceleration type of impact.[2] Blood accumulates quickly between the skull and the outside layer of the dura mater; this is often associated with a skull fracture. The athlete may initially report signs and symptoms of a mild concussion, which quickly subside. The athlete will then experience a **lucid** period with no symptoms of a head injury; this may last for hours or days.[2] However, as the arterial bleeding continues, the athlete may begin to experience severe neurological dysfunction, loss of consciousness, and, in the worst case, death.[3] Signs and symptoms include headache, dizziness, nausea, and dilation of the pupils. Progressive signs and symptoms include a gradual deterioration in the level of consciousness and neurological status and/or respiratory difficulties. Any athlete experiencing these signs or symptoms or suffering from a blow to the head should be referred to trained medical personnel for diagnostic procedures to check for bleeding.

Subdural Hematoma

Subdural hematomas occur more frequently than epidural hematomas and are usually a result from an acceleration/deceleration force to the head that disrupts the venous blood supply between the dura mater and the brain, within the subdural space.[2] Subdural hematomas are classified as either acute or chronic, depending on length of time since symptoms first appeared. In most cases, an athlete with an acute subdural hematoma will present with a headache, cloudiness of thought, neurological deficits (e.g., impairment of cranial nerve function), behavioral and motor changes, and loss of consciousness within 48 to 72 hours after injury.[3] Chronic subdural hematomas may not show signs for up to 3 weeks after injury because there is relatively little bleeding, which is insufficient to generate pressure within the subdural space, and also because the bleeding can migrate into the sulci and fissures of the brain.

Intracerebral Hemorrhage or Contusion

Any blow to the head causing an acceleration/deceleration mechanism of injury can damage the brain tissue, resulting in a hemorrhage contusion. An intracerebral hemorrhage is due to rupture of a vessel within the head; it can lead to an accumulation of blood within the area (contusion).

The contusion can be small and localized or may cover a large portion of the brain. Contusions can also occur from coup or contrecoup etiology. As with subdural hematomas, intracerebral contusions can take up to several days to manifest clinical signs and symptoms. As with other types of hematomas, the athlete may not experience any abnormal neurological symptoms initially but can develop neurological deficits and even coma if left untreated.

Skull Fractures

Blunt trauma, such as being hit by a ball or object to the head, may cause a skull fracture. This type of trauma can cause deformities of the skull such as (a) depressions of bone, (b) linear fractures of the skull, (c) **comminuted fractures** with bony fragments, and (d) a basal fractures at the base of the skull (Fig. 17.5). In addition, skull fractures can cause other symptoms or **sequelae**—such as headache, nausea, blood in the ear canal, blood accumulation around the eyes (raccoon eyes), and blood accumulation behind the ears (Battle's sign). In addition, CSF may be present in the ear canal or nose. Skull fractures are considered medical emergencies requiring immediate transportation of the athlete.

Concussions

A blow or injury to the head region can cause the athlete to suffer from a concussion. Concussions disrupt the normal physiological processes of the brain. They can be minimal or severe, depending upon the mechanism or extent of injury. Concussions are classified according to severity, and

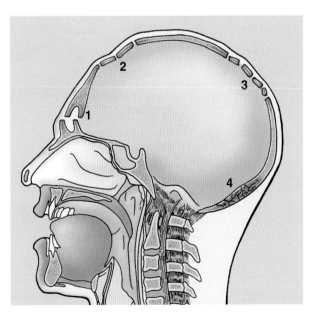

FIGURE 17.5 Types of skull fracture (medial view). **1.** Linear fracture. **2.** Depressed fracture. **3.** Comminuted fracture. **4.** Basilar fracture. (From Moore KL, Agur A. *Essential Clinical Anatomy*, 2nd ed. Philadelphia: Lippincott Williams & Wilkins; 2002.)

TABLE 17.1	Grades of Concussion[4]
Grading Scale	**Signs and Symptoms**
Grade 1	No loss of consciousness; post-concussion signs and symptoms (i.e., short-term memory, attention, concentration, memory processing) lasting less than 30 minutes
Grade 2	Loss of consciousness less than 1 minute, postconcussion signs and symptoms lasting more than 30 minutes but less than 24 hours
Grade 3	Loss of consciousness more than 1 minute, postconcussion signs and symptoms lasting more than 7 days

Signs & Symptoms

Concussion

- Confusion
- Amnesia
- Headache
- Fatigue
- Tinnitus
- Dizziness
- Nausea or vomiting
- Irritability
- Depression
- Sensitivity to light and noise
- Eating and sleeping disturbances
- Balance irregularities
- Vision irregularities
- Seizures
- Loss of consciousness
- Slurred speech
- Fluid emerging from the nose/ears

there are many different classification systems (see Table 17.1 for Cantu's system of classification). The signs and symptoms are varied, and the athletic trainer must distinguish the degree of severity. Concussions that result in a loss of consciousness are medical emergencies and may require emergency procedures, such as securing the athlete to a spine board or performing lifesaving procedures. Concussions may also cause brain damage that may develop over a longer period of time, resulting in emergency complications. Such long-term complications and life-threatening conditions may be due to postconcussion syndrome, which can occur after an athlete sustains a second head injury before the first injury has resolved. Concussion management is beyond the scope of this chapter, but the athletic trainer or allied health personnel must be aware of the complications that may arise from any injury to the head and be prepared for emergency situations.

Management of Head Injuries

If an athlete sustains a blow to the head, the athletic trainer may need to consider referring the athlete for medical evaluation and diagnostic testing (e.g., magnetic resonance imaging or computed tomography) to rule out intracranial bleeding, especially if the athlete lost consciousness at the time of head impact. When an athlete has sustained a blow to the head that may be severe enough to cause further harm, it is recommended that the athletic trainer follow the procedures for spinal management (Skill 17.1) discussed in this chapter to adequately secure and transport an athlete for medical referral. In addition, it is also prudent to assess for nerve damage (Table 17.2) in such athletes. Although some nerve dysfunction may not be severe enough to constitute a medical emergency, prolonged symptoms or complications may become emergency situations.

Scalp Injuries

Injuries to the scalp can include lacerations, contusion, **avulsions,** and abrasions (Fig. 17.6). Because the scalp

TABLE 17.2	Classification and Function of Cranial Nerves
Cranial Nerve	**Function**
I. Olfactory	Smell
II. Optic	Vision
III. Oculomotor	Eye movement and reaction to light, vision
IV. Trochlear	Lateral and inferior eye movement
V. Trigeminal	Mastication and facial sensation
VI. Abducens	Movement of the eye laterally
VII. Facial	Taste, facial expression
VIII. Vestibulocochlear	Hearing and equilibrium
IX. Glossopharyngeal	Swallowing, gag reflex, tongue sensation
X. Vagus	Speech, swallowing
XI. Accessory	Innervation of trapezius and sternocleidomastoid
XII. Hypoglossal	Movement of the tongue

SKILL 17.1

Skull and Brain Management

1. Any time you suspect a skull/brain injury, suspect a spinal injury.
2. Establish the athlete's level of responsiveness and initiate your emergency action plan.
3. Stabilize the head and neck.
4. Perform an initial assessment and care for any life-threatening conditions.
   a. Remember to use a jaw-thrust maneuver if a cervical spine injury is suspected, when breathing is compromised, or cardiorespiratory resuscitation is required.
   b. Control external bleeding.
5. Perform a physical assessment.
   a. Establish the presence of CSF if the athlete is bleeding from the nose or ears.
   b. Look for obvious signs of a skull deformity; never apply direct pressure to a soft spot on the skull.
   c. Examine the extremities for paralysis or loss of sensation.
   d. Check pupils for reaction (PEARL: pupils equal and reactive to light).
6. Check and care for shock.
7. If required, secure the athlete to a spine board.
8. Perform an ongoing assessment, watching for changes in level of responsiveness and vital signs. Consider using supplemental oxygen therapy.

has a rich blood supply, injuries to the scalp often cause heavy bleeding. A scalp injury, although not immediately life threatening, must be managed to minimize blood loss. Management includes identifying the type of injury and then controlling bleeding (Skills 17.2 and 17.3). Bleeding can be controlled by direct pressure over the injury with a clean or sterile cloth or gauze. If you suspect a skull fracture, *do not* apply direct pressure; direct pressure over a skull injury may cause bony fragments to depress into the brain. Instead, try to control bleeding by placing indirect pressure around the wound and putting a clean or sterile cloth or gauze over the site. Refer the athlete immediately to the appropriate medical personnel. If an object is impaled into the skull, do not remove it but stabilize the object with gauze or another appropriate device.

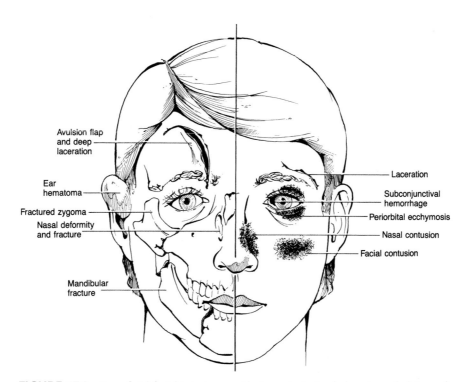

FIGURE 17.6 Superficial facial injuries provide important visual clues to underlying soft tissue and bony injuries. (From Harwood-Nuss A, Wolfson AB, Linden CH, et al. *The Clinical Practice of Emergency Medicine,* 3rd ed. Philadelphia: Lippincott Williams & Wilkins; 2001.)

SKILL 17.2

Immediate Care for Scalp Bleeding

1. Determine the extent of the injury and rule out possible skull fracture.
2. Place a clean or sterile cloth, bandage, or gauze directly over the injury.
3. Apply slight pressure to control bleeding.
4. Do not remove the cloth or gauze if it soaks through with blood; apply a new bandage, cloth, or gauze on top.
5. Secure with a pressure bandage (Fig. 17.7).

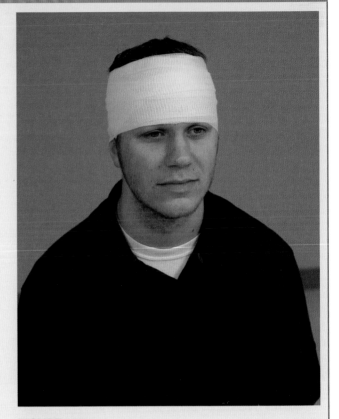

FIGURE 17.7

THE SPINE

Anatomy of the Spine

The spine consists of 33 bones, called vertebrae, which are grouped into five regions. There are 7 cervical, 12 thoracic, 5 lumbar, 5 sacral, and 4 coccygeal vertebrae. The sacral and coccygeal vertebrae, comprising the posterior portion of the pelvis, are fused together. All together, the vertebrae form the spinal column. Each spinal segment (Fig. 17.8) has specific bony properties causing them to vary in size and shape and allowing for different degrees of spinal movement. Each vertebra has a vertebral body or anterior portion; these anterior bodies progress in diameter and thickness from the cervical to lumbar regions (Fig. 17.9). Two bony structures, called the **laminae,** and **pedicle** form the vertebral arch. The pedicles extend from the vertebral body before connecting to the laminae, which are flatter bones. The arch creates a semicircular notch (vertebral foramen), which houses and protects the spinal cord.

SKILL 17.3

Immediate Care for an Impaled Object (see Chapter 14)

1. If you notice an impaled object, call emergency medical services immediately.
2. If the object is small enough, cut out a hole in a cup or use a shield or cone to cover the object. Avoid using a Styrofoam cup; it may crumble and break, causing further damage. If the object is too large, stabilize around the edges with sterile gauze or clothing if possible. Try not to touch the impaled object for risk of shifting and causing further damage.

3. Surround the cup or device with sterile gauze to stabilize.
4. Secure the cup with tape or self-adhesive bandage. Do not apply compression or downward pressure on the device for risk of pushing the object further into the tissue.

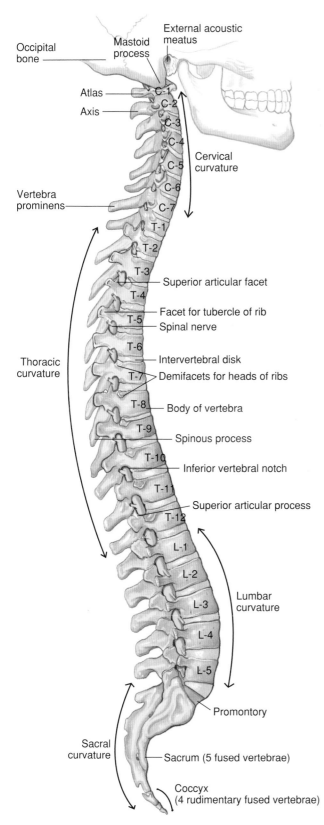

FIGURE 17.8. Vertebral column (sagittal view). (Courtesy of Anatomical Chart Co.)

Two transverse processes project from the pedicle and one spinous process projects posteriorly from the junction of the laminae. The spinous and transverse processes act as points of attachment for muscles and ligaments. Arising both superiorly and inferiorly from the laminae and pedicles are articular processes; these help to connect superior and inferior vertebrae, creating the intervertebral foramina. The intervertebral foramina are clinically significant because this is where the peripheral nerves exit the spinal cord.

The vertebral column has multiple joints that separate the vertebral bodies and allow movement and cushioning of the spinal column. The joint segments have specialized cartilaginous disks called intervertebral disks. Each intervertebral disk has a gelatinous inner portion, called the nucleus pulposus, and an outer ring portion, called the annulus fibrosus. There are no disks between the first and second cervical vertebrae or between the sacral and coccygeal fused vertebrae.

Common Mechanisms of Spinal Injury

Spinal injuries most commonly occur at the cervical level but can occur anywhere along the spinal column. They can occur during any sporting event but are most common in high-contact sports such as football and ice hockey or sports in which there may be contact with apparatuses, such as gymnastics or diving. The most common mechanism of injury to the spine include (a) axial loading (i.e., the head is driven caudally, or pushed downward); (b) excessive flexion or extension of the cervical vertebrae (head moving toward the chest or chin going up in the air); (c) rotation of the spinal column; or (d) excessive lateral bending (side bending) of the spinal column. Ruptures of the atlantoaxial or posterior longitudinal ligaments and disk herniations can also occur as a result of trauma to the spine. Injuries to the spine may range from no apparent complication to the loss of sensation and paralysis of the limbs or entire body.

Common Neurological Spinal Cord/Nerve Root Injuries

Injuries to the spinal cord or nerve roots often happen with bending or twisting motions of the head/neck and spinal column. Of particular interest is a condition called a **burner** or **stinger.** Burners or stingers affect the peripheral nervous system as a result of two common mechanisms: compressive forces or stretching/tensile forces. The first, or compressive force, occurs when the head and neck move into a posterolateral position, toward one side. The second, a tensile or stretching force, occurs when the arm and neck move in opposite directions. Burners or stingers often mimic spinal cord injuries, but the symptoms are usually transient. Burners or stingers must be differentiated from a spinal cord injury for proper management. A major difference is that burners or

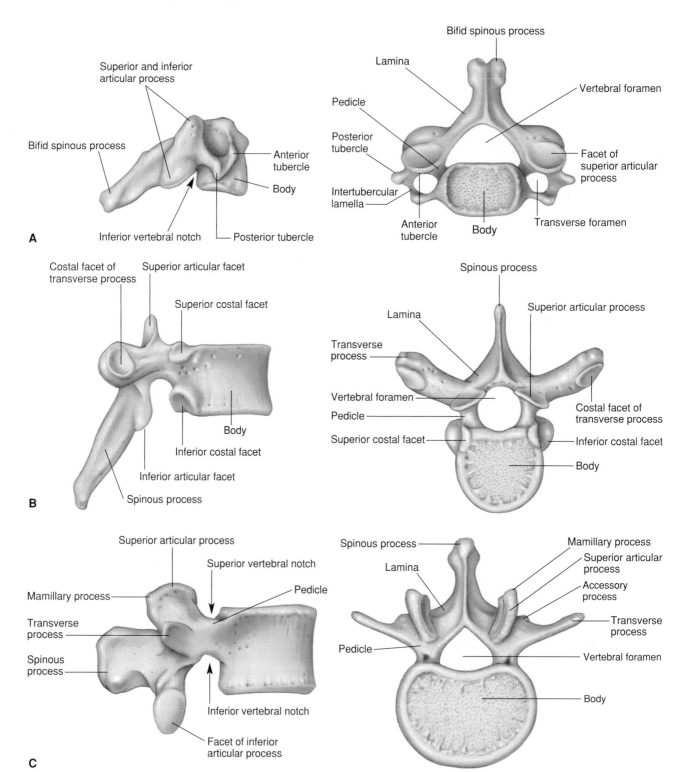

FIGURE 17.9 Vertebrae. **A.** Cervical. **B.** Thoracic. **C.** Lumbar. (Courtesy of Anatomical Chart Co.)

Signs & Symptoms

Burners and Stingers

- Burning sensation at the neck and upper limb on the affected side
- Muscle weakness
- Loss of grip strength on the affected side
- Numbness and tingling on the affected side
- Loss of motor function on the affected side

stingers present as unilateral upper extremity impairments (e.g., loss of muscle strength and sensation), which typically resolve quickly. Another distinction is that many of the athletes who have burners and stingers approach the medical staff after the injury has occurred, usually holding the affected arm.

Another type of neurological impairment is transient quadriplegia, a temporary paralysis of motor and sensory functions as a result of temporary restriction of blood flow to a section of the cervical spinal cord. Usually, the neck flexes upon contact, stretching the spinal cord and collapsing the blood vessels, or the neck extends, causing a narrowing and compression of the spinal cord.[5,6] The symptoms

Signs & Symptoms

Spinal Injury

- A mechanism of injury that compresses, distracts, or bends the spinal column excessively or from a direct blow to the vertebral column
- Tenderness anywhere on the spinal column
- Pain associated with extremity movement
- Pain when moving an extremity with no apparent injury
- Obvious spinal deformity
- Loss of sensation or tingling to the extremities, including toes and fingers
- Loss of extremity strength
- Unresponsiveness to reflex tests
- Injury to head or neck
- Urinary or fecal incontinence
- Breathing difficulties
- Unconsciousness or unresponsiveness
- **Priapism**
- **Decerebrate** or **decorticate** rigidity

associated with this mechanism are similar for a spinal cord injury, and the same management is used.

Assessment of a Spinal Injury

If the athletic trainer suspects a spinal injury, the first step is to determine whether the athlete is conscious followed by identification of any life-threatening conditions and initiation of the emergency action plan. If the situation is not immediately life threatening and vital signs are present, try to determine the mechanism of injury. Conduct a secondary assessment. Ask about any unusual sensations of the extremities or numbness and tingling. Inspect the area for any obvious deformity, discoloration, bruising, or swelling. Palpate the bony structures to feel for deformity (e.g., step-off deformity) or tenderness. Assess sensation by stroking the dorsal surfaces of the hands and feet and testing for the **Babinski reflex** (pathological reflex). Assess strength on each extremity by having the athlete wiggle his or her finger and toes, squeeze your hands, and push his or her toes against resistance. If, at the end of the assessment, you find any sign or symptom suggesting spinal trauma, immediately contact emergency medical services (EMS) and begin stabilization and immobilization procedures.

After determining the presence of life-threatening injuries, the athletic trainer should immobilize any athlete who is unconscious or is suspected of having a spinal injury (Skill 17.4). Immobilization procedures will vary based on the athlete's condition, protective equipment worn, and access to emergency medical supplies and equipment. In general, spinal injuries should be treated with manual cervical immobilization, application of a cervical collar if appropriate, and securing the athlete to some form of spine board. It takes time and practice to become proficient in these procedures, and multiple rehearsals are recommended.[7]

Stabilization of the cervical region requires manual immobilization before the application of a cervical collar or other protective equipment. Current guidelines recommend that the cervical spine be immobilized in a neutral position without applying traction.[7]

When the athlete has been immobilized, removal of any face mask or guard is recommended in order to gain access to the airway in case of breathing complications. Once the cervical spine is immobilized and any protective equipment covering the airway is removed, the athlete should be transferred to an immobilization device. If the athlete is wearing a helmet or shoulder pads, their removal is not essential. Application of a cervical collar is suggested before transferal to a spine board. Instructions for the application to a spine board and of a cervical collar are found in Skills 17.5 and 17.6. Transferal to a spine board may require a logroll or lift. When performing any of these maneuvers, maintain in-line stabilization (Skill 17.4). A 2003 study showed that there was less head movement with a lift and slide than with a logroll.[9]

SKILL 17.4

Spinal Care Stabilization, Logrolls, and Lifts

1. Any time you suspect a spinal injury, immediate activate EMS.
2. Stabilize the neck and check vital signs.
   A. Establish in-line stabilization of the head/neck.
      a. First, kneel behind the athlete (if supine).
      b. Place your fingers and thumb along the sides of the head to stabilize it.
      c. Move the head gently to a neutral position aligned with the spine.
      d. The head should be facing forward in line with the spine.
      e. Maintain head stabilization throughout the spine-boarding process until the head is secure on a back-board.
3. Logroll or use a lift to get the athlete onto a spine board.
   A. Prone logroll (requires four to five athletic trainers)
      a. Athletic trainer 1 stabilizes the head and neck using a cross-arm technique. Be sure that the athlete is rolled to the side opposite to the face (e.g., if the face is pointing to the left, roll to the right; Fig. 17.10).
      b. Place the spine board adjacent to the athlete (Fig. 17.10).
      c. Place the athlete's arms by his or her side (if wearing protective equipment) or place one arm over the head and the other arm to the side (Fig. 17.10).
      d. Place other athletic trainers at the athlete's shoulders, waist/thigh, and lower legs on one side to assist in log-rolling the athlete (Fig. 17.10).

   e. Each athletic trainer will reach over the athlete and grab the respective areas on the opposite side.
   f. Assign another athletic trainer to move the spine board into position.
   g. The athletic trainer at the head will give all of the commands to move and secure the athlete.
   h. On command, the athlete should be rolled toward the athletic trainers in a uniform fashion (Fig. 17.11).
   i. When the athlete is perpendicular to the ground (on his or her side), the spine board is slid behind the athlete at an angle (approximately 45 degrees; this helps to place the athlete on the middle of the board). If the athlete is in the prone position, the spine board must be slid between the athletic trainers and the athlete at an angle (Fig. 17.11).
   j. Slowly return the athlete to a supine position on the spine board (Fig. 17.12).
   k. If the athlete is not centered on the board, he or she will have to be readjusted by sliding on the command of the athletic trainer at the head.
   B. Supine logroll
      a. Athletic trainer 1 provides cervical stabilization (Fig. 17.13).

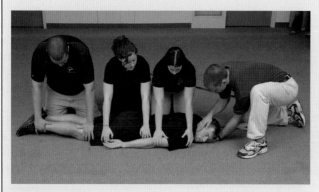

FIGURE 17.10

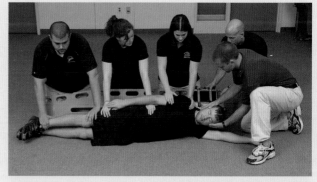

FIGURE 17.11

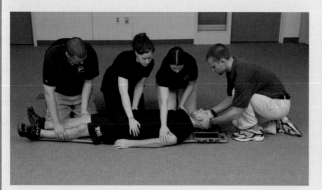

FIGURE 17.12

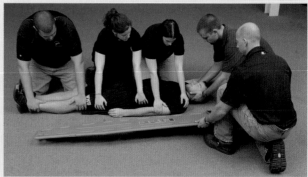

FIGURE 17.13

SKILL 17.4 *(Continued)*

Spinal Care Stabilization, Logrolls, and Lifts (Continued)

b. On one side of the athlete, athletic trainer 2 is positioned at the shoulder, athletic trainer 3 at the hips, and athletic trainer 4 at the legs (Fig. 17.13).

c. On the opposite side, the fifth athletic trainer should be ready with a spine board (Fig. 17.13).

d. On command from athletic trainer 1, athletic trainers 2, 3, and 4 roll the athlete toward themselves while athletic trainer 5 places the spine board at a 45-degree angle underneath the athlete (Fig. 17.14).

e. On command, the athlete is lowered onto the spine board (Fig. 17.15).

C. Person Lift (if athlete is wearing protective equipment) Larger athletes and athletes wearing protective equipment can be lifted onto a spine board using a six-person lift.

a. Have an athletic trainer stabilize the head/neck with the hands placed under the shoulder pads and the head resting on the athletic trainer's forearms (Fig. 17.16).

b. Place the other athletic trainers at the chest, pelvis, and legs, two on each side (Fig. 17.16).

c. All athletic trainers then slide their hands underneath the athlete (Fig. 17.16).

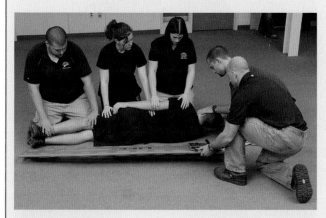

FIGURE 17.14

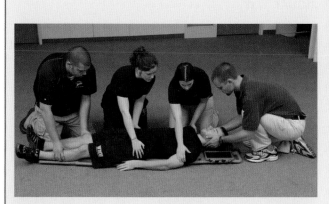

FIGURE 17.15

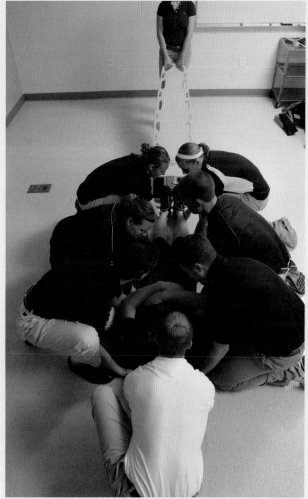

FIGURE 17.16

(Continued)

SKILL 17.4 *(Continued)*

Spinal Care Stabilization, Logrolls, and Lifts (Continued)

    d. The athletic trainer at the head gives verbal commands to lift the athlete.

    e. Lift the athlete approximately 6 in. off the ground in one smooth motion (Fig. 17.17).

    f. The spine board is then slid from the feet up to the head underneath the athlete (Fig. 17.17).

    g. Lower the athlete onto the spine board (Fig. 17.18).

4. Apply a rigid cervical collar if appropriate (see next section)

5. If an athlete is wearing a helmet and shoulder pads, a cervical collar may not be appropriate or fit properly. The application of towels or some other form of padding to help stabilize the head and neck is recommended. A cervical vacuum splint can be utilized in these situations.[8]

6. Secure the athlete to the spine board (Skill 17.6). Secure by placing straps at the pelvis, shoulder, legs, and head. Some spine boards have Helmet Huggers (Fig. 17.19) designed to stabilize the head of an athlete who is wearing a helmet on the backboard. Arms can be placed together on the body and fastened so that they do not fall while the athlete is being transported.

7. Any gaps between the security straps should be filled.

8. Reassess vital signs.

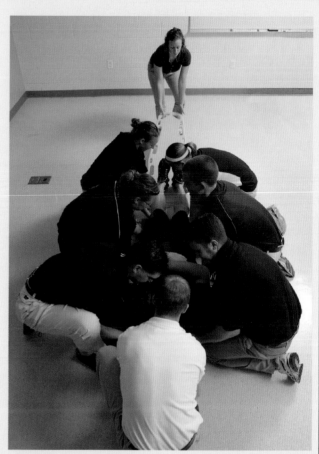

FIGURE 17.17

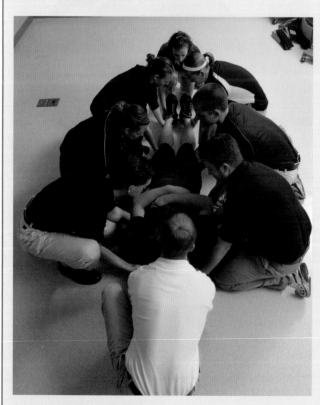

FIGURE 17.18

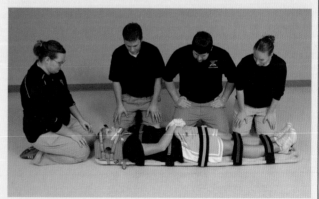

FIGURE 17.19

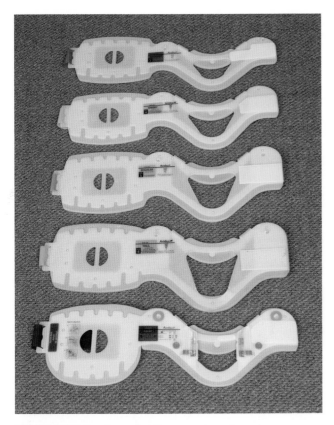

FIGURE 17.20   Cervical collars come in various sizes.

Cervical Collars

The purpose of a cervical collar is to limit flexion and extension as well as lateral and rotational movements of the head and neck. Cervical collars are applied to an athlete during the immobilization process with a spine board if you suspect any of the following: soft tissue damage to head/face/neck, blow to the head/neck or clavicular region of the chest, or other aspects of suspected spinal injury discussed previously.

Cervical collars come in various sizes (Fig. 17.20) and models. Selecting a cervical collar is dependent upon the length of the neck. The front height of the cervical collar should fit between the chin and the chest region at the sternal notch. The cervical collar should rest on the athlete's clavicles and help support the jaw. If properly fitted, the cervical collar should not stretch the neck, not support the chin, and not be too constricting.[10] The type of collar used in your setting will vary by preference; however, the sizing charts and measurements will vary by type of cervical collar. Whichever type of cervical collar is used, be cognizant of the sizing directions and methods and practice measuring fit for a cervical collar.

Applying a Cervical Collar

When applying a cervical collar, one athletic trainer must maintain in-line stabilization while another applies the cervical collar (Skill 17.5). Once the cervical collar is in place, the athletic trainer who is maintaining head alignment must still maintain head support. The cervical collar only helps stabilize the head and is not meant to fully support the head in neutral position. In situations where a cervical collar is not available or there are no individuals trained to apply one, applying a rolled towel or cloth that is taped or fastened to the spine board will help support the neck. However, as with cervical collar application, one athletic trainer must always maintain head support manually until the head is fully fastened onto a backboard.

Spine Boarding an Athlete

Backboards (or spine boards) usually come in two different types: short and long. Backboards are used for individuals who are suspected of having a spine injury or for individuals who are unconscious (assuming that a spinal injury is present). The short backboard is used for immobilizing an individual in a car or other situation where a long board cannot be applied. After securing the individual to a short board, he or she can be moved to another location and then secured to a long board for transportation. A vest-type extrication device can be used in such a situation. Although the specific application steps for short boards are beyond the scope of this chapter, in general, the steps include securing the chest/torso region, stabilizing the chest, applying a collar of the appropriate size, sliding a short board or wrapping a chest-type device around the individual, and securing the head to the board or device. The last steps are checking pulses and adjusting the tightness of the straps.

Long boards also come in different shapes and types of construction. Some long boards also have head immobilizers for added head/neck support. Other types of immobilization devices for the athlete with suspected spinal injuries include the Miller full-body splint and the vacuum mattress. The Miller full-body splint is a harness-type device with straps into which the athlete is fitted to help stabilize and immobilize any possible spinal injuries.

To secure an individual with a suspected spinal injury on a long board, follow the general guidelines in Skill 17.6. For more specific information on various procedures for spine-board stabilization, refer to the NATA Position Statement on Acute Management of the Cervical Spine-Injured Athlete.[7]

Another type of backboard that can be used is a vacuum mattress, which is composed of Styrofoam beads enclosed in a nylon covering, like vacuum immobilizers used for extremity injuries; it has wooden slats that run from head to toe. When air is suctioned out of the mattress, it becomes rigid, providing support and protection for an athlete with a spinal injury. A literature review comparing vacuum mattresses and spine boards showed that the vacuum mattress has comparable immobilization capabilities (see Skill 17.7 for application techniques) but also, more importantly, provides better comfort.[11,12]

SKILL 17.5

Applying a Cervical Collar

1. Remove any jewelry from the athlete and keep his or her hair away from the neck.
2. Place the head in neutral position, aligned with the spine, head up.
3. With your fingers, measure the distance between the top of the athlete's shoulders to the athlete's jaw line.
4. Use the value found in step 3 to find a collar of the same dimensions.
5. After measuring for fit, unfasten the cervical collar.
6. Place a collar of the appropriate size adjacent to the neck on one side and slide the back portion underneath the athlete's neck (Fig. 17.21).
7. Sliding up from the chest wall, align the chin piece of the collar to the athlete's chin. Make sure that the chin is supported (Fig. 17.22).

8. Fasten securely. If the chin section is not snug, you may need a smaller collar (steps 5 and 6 can be reversed for some collars) (Fig. 17.22).
9. Maintain head support throughout the entire process.

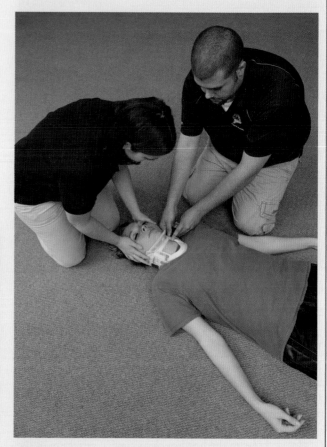

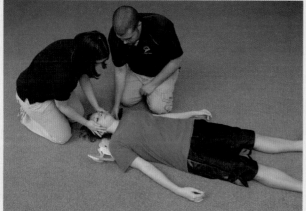

FIGURE 17.21

FIGURE 17.22

SKILL 17.6

Long Board Procedures

1. After application of a cervical collar (if indicated) and stabilization of the head (to be maintained throughout the process), place the backboard adjacent to the athlete (Fig. 17.23).
2. Have two to four athletic trainers kneel on the side of the athlete opposite the backboard; these athletic trainers will position themselves at the shoulder, waist, and knee levels (heavier athletes may require more athletic trainers at the torso level) (Fig. 17.23).

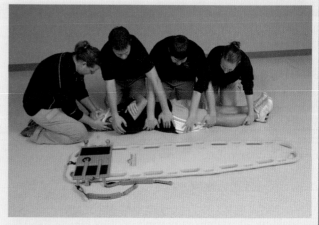

FIGURE 17.23

SKILL 17.6 *(Continued)*

Long Board Procedures (Continued)

3. The athletic trainers will reach across the athlete and gently pull the athlete toward themselves. The athletic trainer at the head (lead athletic trainer) (see Chapter 4, regarding lifting and moving patients for verbal commands and suggestions) gives all verbal commands (Fig. 17.24).

4. Once the athlete is on their side, usually the middle athletic trainer (waist level) reaches over the athlete and slides the backboard underneath the athlete as far as possible (or, if another athletic trainer is present, they can both slide the backboard) (Fig. 17.24).

5. In unison, the athletic trainers then slowly return the athlete onto the backboard (Fig. 17.25).

6. If the athlete is not in the center of the board, gently slide in unison.

7. Place padding in any void between the torso and the board to help stabilize and secure the athlete (Fig. 17.25).

8. Using the straps provided or other securing devices, secure the athlete to the board at the chest, waist, thigh, and knee levels. These straps should be snug without restricting circulation and secured to help prevent movement. Secure the athlete with the arms at the sides and the straps going underneath the arms. Place the arms on the body at waist level and secure with spider straps or other appropriate straps (Fig. 17.25).

9. If the backboard has a head immobilization device, secure the head to the backboard after securing the body. Using a bandage, adhesive tape, or the strap provided, wrap around the forehead of the athlete and secure. At this time, the athletic trainer at the head may release head stabilization. If the athlete is wearing a helmet, secure the helmet to the backboard with adhesive tape to make sure the head is properly stabilized and will not move or roll when lifted or when the spine board is tilted to the side (Fig. 17.26).

10. Check distal pulse and vital signs once the athlete is secured.

11. To transport, follow the steps in Chapter 6.

12. If the athlete vomits, the whole backboard can be logrolled to clear the airway without risk of further spinal trauma due to shifting body weight.

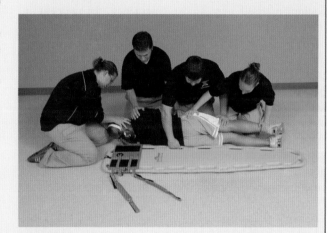

FIGURE 17.24

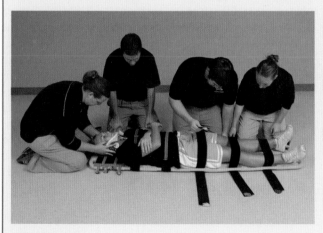

FIGURE 17.25

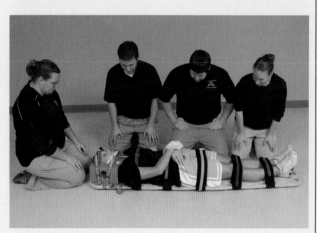

FIGURE 17.26

SKILL 17.7

Evac-U-Splint Air-Mattress® Technique

1. Place mattress next to the athlete with the athlete's shoulder aligned with the first buckle.
2. Logroll the athlete/lift onto the mattress.
3. Open the valve at the foot section to allow air to enter.
4. Attach the restraint straps (black and white buckles) in an alternate fashion from chest to feet.
5. Starting at the head, remove the slack between the buckles of all the straps.
6. Evacuate the air at the foot air valve.
7. Place red cap over the valve.

Protective Equipment

Many sports require the participants to wear protective equipment to prevent sports-related injuries or minimize their severity. Although beneficial for these purposes, the equipment itself may hinder emergency management in life-threatening situations. A particular issue is the removal of helmets, face masks, or other protective equipment in order to gain access to the airway or for spinal immobilization. The processes for removing such equipment should be part of any emergency action plan and all athletic trainers and other medical care providers must practice the removal of such equipment to be prepared in emergency situations. Although this chapter does not discuss removal of all the various types of protective equipment, it does outline some general guidelines and describes some of the protective equipment that is commonly used in the sports setting.

Face-Mask Removal

The NATA[7] recommends that when the athlete has a suspected spinal or possible head injury, the face mask (football or lacrosse) be removed immediately once a decision has been made to transport the athlete to the local medical facility. Removal of a face mask requires practice to perform the skills adequately and quickly in order to gain access to the airway while also limiting head movement (Skill 17.8). Specific football helmets, such as the Schutt (Skill 17.9) and Riddell, call for specific removal techniques based upon their design.

For example, the Riddell Revolution Speed Helmet (http://www.riddell.com) has specialized screws that attach the face mask to the helmet. Two screws are located at the top and one on each side. A pin device is inserted into the

screw, which pops off the screw without cutting or using a screwdriver (Skill 17.10).

In similar fashion, the Riddell Revolution IQ has clips that grasp the edges of the face mask and hold the face mask in place. Two of the screws are located at the top and one on each side. These screws are popped out using a pin device similar to that in the Riddell Revolution Speed Helmet.

Regardless of the type of helmet or manufacturer, athletic trainers who work with sports that require face masks should practice removal skills often and, most importantly, have tools or devices required for equipment removal readily available at all venues.

The specific tools used to remove a face mask vary but can include an FM Extractor, Trainer's Angel, Dremel tools, knives or scissors, pipe cutters, and pruning shears (Fig. 17.31). Screwdrivers, scalpels, or box cutters are not recommended by the NATA[7] because of the hardness of the plastic straps and difficulty of performing such procedures. In addition, although a screwdriver can be an effective means of removing a face mask,[16,17] the possibility of rusted or damaged screws or slipping of the screwdriver may make it difficult to use such a tool reliably.[13] However, a power screwdriver is more commonly used, thanks to the speed with which it can remove a screw. But it presents reliability issues, such as failure to hold a charge, not enough torque to remove a screw, or a drill bit that does not fit the screw on the face mask. It was found that the best device for removal a face mask is an anvil pruner (gardening tool),[13,14,18,19] but other research has shown that a combination of tools may be more suitable.[20] The NATA, based upon an extensive review of literature,[21] recommends that EMT shears should not be used for face-mask removal because of the time required to do so.

SKILL 17.8

Football Face Mask Removal (General Guidelines)

1. Have another athletic trainer stabilize the head/neck (Fig. 17.27).
2. Locate the plastic loop straps on the helmet.
3. Use an appropriate face mask removal tool to cut the straps from the face mask. The side loop straps should be removed first (Fig. 17.28).

4. Pressure may be needed and can be applied on the underside of the loop straps with your other thumb/finger (if using a T-nut).

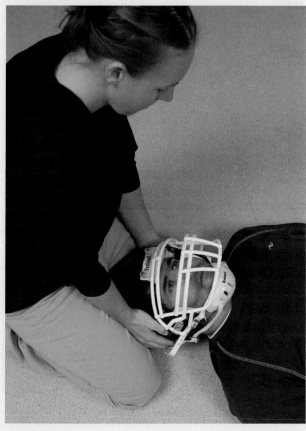

FIGURE 17.27

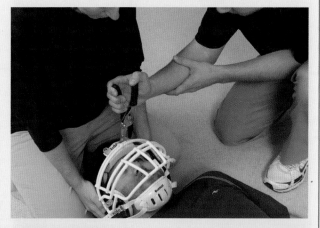

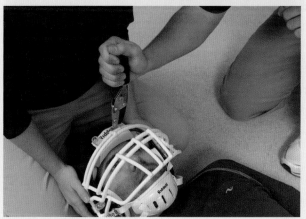

FIGURE 17.28

(Continued)

SKILL 17.8 (Continued)

Football Face Mask Removal (General Guidelines) (Continued)

5. Cut off all straps to totally remove the face mask. This provides better access to the airway and causes less head/neck or spine movement versus cutting the lateral straps and retracting the face mask (Fig. 17.29).[13,14]

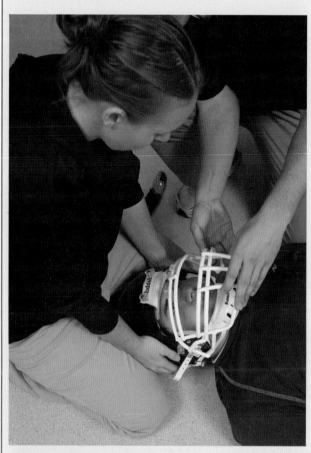
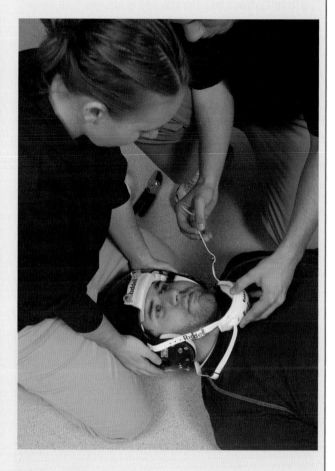

FIGURE 17.29

SKILL 17.9

Schutt Ion® Football Helmet Face Mask Removal

1. Use a pruner type of cutting device or the manufacturer's recommended cutting device.
2. Cut through the top and bottom of the retainer.
3. Cut the chinstraps that are looped through the face mask on the sides of the helmet.

4. Pull face mask forward, possibly moving it up/down or rotating it slightly to remove it from the side ports.[15]

SKILL 17.10 (see Fig. 17.30)

Using the Quick-Release Mounting System*

1. Use a small pointed object and depress the pin in the center of the Quick Release head.
2. After depressing the pin, pull the side clip directly away from the side of the helmet shell and remove both pins.
3. Using a loop strap removal tool, remove each top-mounted loop.
4. Remove the face mask by pulling it away from the athlete's face.

*From Riddell (2007). Emergency removal of Riddell Revolution Face Guards with side-mounted Quick Release Hardware.

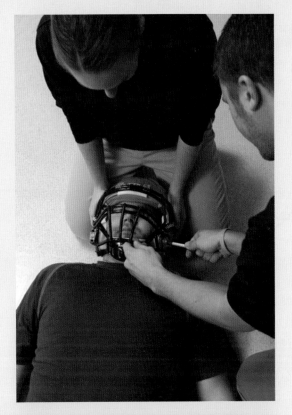

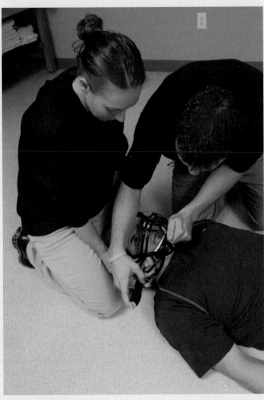

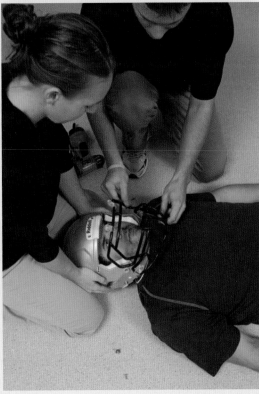

FIGURE 17.30

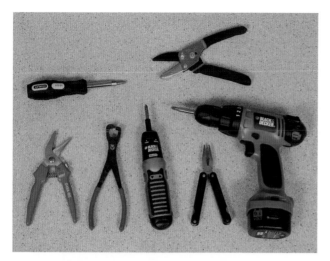

FIGURE 17.31   Tools that can be used to remove a face mask.

The type of face mask and helmet will determine the type of removal equipment needed. Specialized face mask clips require special removal tools, such as a screwdriver or a specialized pin device, to pop a clip out. Face masks for lacrosse helmets have shields or are attached to chin straps; a screwdriver is required to remove the clips because cutting the clip will not allow the face mask to be removed. The specific type of lacrosse helmet may require different facemask removal techniques (Skill 17.11; see Fig. 17.32, below). It should be noted that the protective equipment worn by lacrosse players has a different influence on neck position compared with helmets used in football and ice hockey and that the face mask is not easy to remove.[7] Lacrosse helmets have demonstrated statistically significant increases in cervical extension when worn and a statistically significant increase in cervical flexion when removed.[22] Sherbondy and colleagues[22] agree that a lacrosse helmet and shoulder pads should be left in place until

SKILL 17.11

Lacrosse Face Mask Removal*

Figure 17.32 shows the face masks listed below.

Brine Triumph Face Mask Removal

1. Remove entirely screws on either side of the face mask.
2. Remove the screw at the visor.
3. Remove the face mask/chin guard unit.

Brine Triad Face Mask Removal

1. Remove the screws on either side of the chin guard.
2. Remove the top center screw on the visor (may remove the other side screws on the visor to remove entire visor).
3. Remove the face mask/chin guard as one unit.

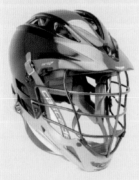

Brine Triumph Facemask

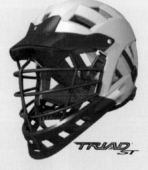

Brine Triad Facemask

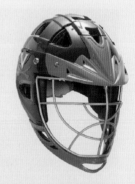

DeBeer Identity (Gait) Facemask

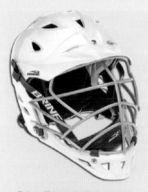

Cascade CPX, CLH2, PRO7, CS Facemask

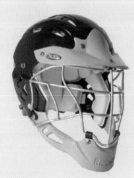

Onyx Riddell Facemask

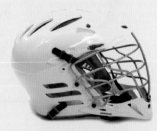

Warrior Viking Facemask

FIGURE 17.32

SKILL 17.11 *(Continued)*

Lacrosse Face Mask Removal* *(Continued)*

DeBeer Identity (Gait) Face Mask Removal

1. Remove the two top screws on the visor.
2. Remove the screw under the visor piece.
3. Using a cutting tool, cut the chin guard first layer on each side back as far as you can. Under the first layer of the chin guard, there is a recessed screw.
4. Remove the face mask/chin guard as one unit.

Cascade CPX, CLH2, PRO7, CS Face Mask Removal

1. Remove the two side screws with screwdriver or clip with cutting tool.
2. Remove the top screw at the visor with screwdriver/cut clip under visor.
3. Cut the chin guard at the back vent on both sides.

Onyx Riddell Face Mask Removal

1. Use a power screwdriver to remove the two side screws.
2. Remove the screw at the visor.

Warrior Viking Face Mask Removal

1. Remove the two screws on each side with a screwdriver.
2. The bottom screw must be removed to allow the chin guard to become released.
3. Remove the screw at the middle of the visor.

*Reprinted with permission, U.S. Lacrosse Sports Science and Safety Committee.[23]

---

they can be removed in a controlled environment such as the emergency department. However, according to Swartz et al.,[7] there have been no studies examining the motion created in the cervical spine during lacrosse helmet removal. Whichever type is used, the athletic trainer must practice removal techniques and have the appropriate tools.

Helmet Removal

Helmets for sporting events come in all sorts of shapes and sizes and are made of various materials. Their purpose is to protect the head and face. A properly fitted football helmet in addition to shoulder pads actually holds the head in neutral alignment[24,25]; therefore, removal of the helmet when the athlete is wearing shoulder pads can cause neck hyperextension[26] unless the shoulder pads are also removed. Additional head or neck movements when removing a football helmet can cause further damage if the athlete has a cervical spinal injury.[14] The helmet may be removed (Skill 17.12) only if it does not securely stabilize the head during immobilization, the athletic trainers cannot gain access to the airway, or if the helmet does not allow adequate immobilization during transportation. Other types of helmets not used in sports, such as motorcycle (Skill 17.13) or bicycle helmets (Skill 17.14), are often removed because of the variability in the fit, which may hinder spine-board immobilization.[10]

The NATA[27] recommends that the helmet be removed only after diagnostic images of the head/neck/spine are completed or when the airway is compromised and access cannot be gained with a helmet on. In cases of emergency, follow the steps in Skill 17.12 for football helmet removal. For lacrosse or other types of helmets, refer to the manufacturer's guidelines.

One of the challenges for athletic trainers working directly with ice hockey and lacrosse athletes is the fact that there are no established guidelines for the removal of ice hockey or lacrosse helmets in the event of cervical spine injury.[27] Therefore, athletic trainers must regularly practice face mask removal techniques using the athletes' equipment and the tools to which they will have access in the event of a cervical spine injury.

Shoulder Pad Removal

The shoulder pads worn by athletes help protect them from injury to the shoulder girdle region. However, they also are large enough to cause the athlete's torso to be elevated slightly when lying supine. If the athlete is not wearing a helmet, the neck can become extended. If a helmet must be removed, the shoulder pads must also be removed (Skill 17.15) to provide proper spinal alignment.[28] It is not recommend to remove the helmet or shoulder pads to transport an athlete; however, removal should be determined based upon the necessity of removing the helmet, access to the shoulder area, or in cases where the shoulder pads are not fitted properly and compromise spinal immobilization.

SKILL 17.12

Football Helmet Removal

1. One athletic trainer should stabilize the head/neck and helmet throughout the removal process (Fig. 17.33). Another athletic trainer then completes the following steps:
   a. Remove the chinstrap (Fig. 17.34).
   b. Remove the cheek pads or other accessible internal padding. Cheek pads can be removed by inserting a flat-bladed object (such as a tongue depressor) between the snaps and the helmet shell (Fig. 17.35).

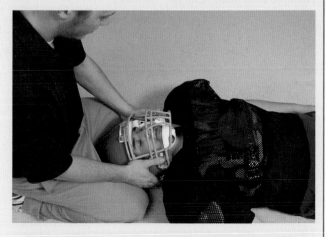

FIGURE 17.33

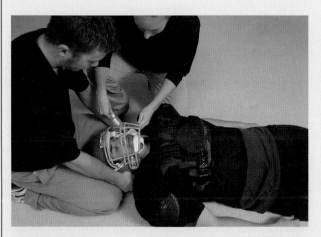

FIGURE 17.34

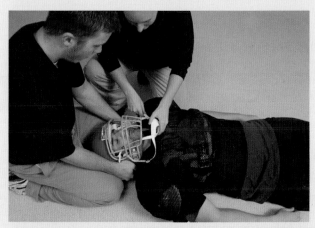

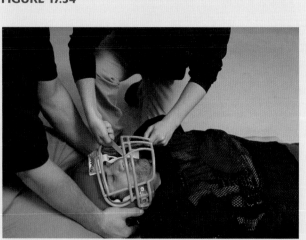

FIGURE 17.35

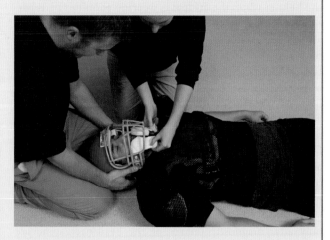

SKILL 17.12 *(Continued)*

Football Helmet Removal *(Continued)*

c. Deflate air padding at the external port if applicable (Fig. 17.36).

d. Slide the helmet off the occiput by first slightly rotating helmet forward. Do not spread apart the ear holes.

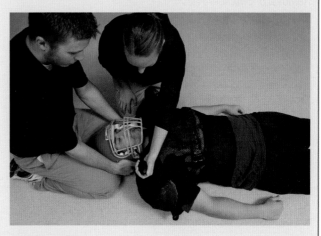

FIGURE 17.36

SKILL 17.13

Motorcycle Helmet Removal

1. One athletic trainer maintains stabilization by holding the bottom of the helmet and stabilizing the lower jaw with his or her fingers.

2. Another athletic trainer removes the chinstrap and eyeglasses, if any.

3. After chinstrap removal, the second athletic trainer stabilizes the mandible with one hand while the other hand reaches behind the neck and stabilizes the occiput, holding it securely.

4. The athletic trainer holding the helmet releases stabilization and begins to remove the helmet by pulling the helmet apart to clear the ears.

5. Avoid any backward tilting. If a full-face helmet is worn, slightly tilt it to move over the chin and nose.

6. After the helmet is removed, the first athletic trainer then stabilizes the head/neck by grasping the side of the head with the thumbs on the forehead and the fingers spread across the side of the head.

7. Apply a cervical collar if indicated.

SKILL 17.14

Bicycle Helmet Removal

1. One athletic trainer stabilizes the head by grasping the sides of the head with his or her thumbs on the maxillary region and fingers below the ears, avoiding any stabilization on the helmet itself.

2. Another athletic trainer then removes the chinstrap.

3. The second athletic trainer then removes the helmet by sliding it off the head, pulling apart at the ear sections to clear the ears.

4. Apply a cervical collar if indicated.

SKILL 17.15

Removal of Shoulder Pads[29]

1. Cut off the jersey or shirt from the torso and arms (Fig. 17.37).
2. Cut all shoulder pad straps and laces. Do not unbuckle or unstrap to avoid unnecessary movement (Fig. 17.38).
3. Remove neck rolls, collars, or other type of accessories.
4. After gaining access to the torso, another athletic trainer then stabilizes the head by placing his or her forearms on the athlete's chest and holding the maxilla and occiput; however, the athletic trainer should not be sitting on the athlete (Fig. 17.39).
5. Additional athletic trainers apply support to the sides of the athlete with their hands on the posterior thoracic region and other parts of the athlete, depending upon his or her size (Fig. 17.40).
6. The athlete is lifted (need enough athletic trainers) to remove the helmet and shoulder pads (Fig. 17.41).
7. The athlete is lowered.

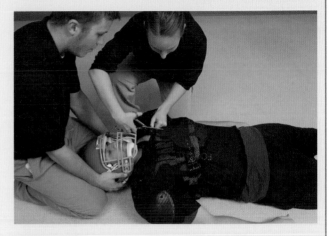

FIGURE 17.37

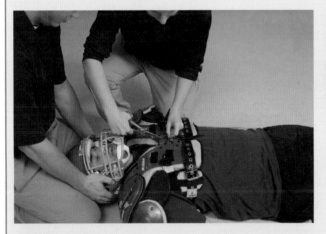

FIGURE 17.38

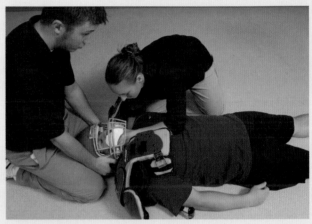

FIGURE 17.39

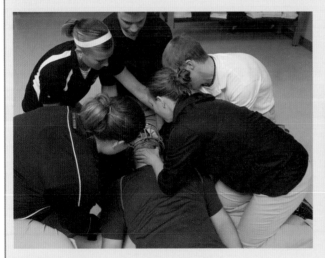

FIGURE 17.40

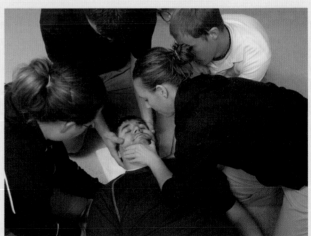

FIGURE 17.41

Scenarios

1. As an athletic trainer, you are covering a lacrosse game at your high school. During the match, two players collide; one player seems to be fine, while the other is still lying on the field. You approach the player and notice that he is unconscious. He is still wearing his lacrosse helmet and shoulder pads and is lying in the supine position.

   What do you do?

2. During a soccer match, two female players bang their heads together when trying to head the ball. Both fall down, but they get up after several seconds. One player initially seems to have difficulty walking toward you but then recovers after a few seconds. She reports that she has a headache. You assess her for a concussion and determine she has a mild, or grade 1, concussion and keep her out of the rest of the game. Later that night, she tells her roommate that her headache is getting worse and she is experiencing nausea. Her roommate calls EMS.

   What do you think happened?

3. A football player is hit during practice and is lying prone on the field. He is unconscious but is breathing. As the head athletic trainer, you summon several of your athletic training students to the scene. The athlete must be stabilized and spine-boarded.

   Who should stabilize the athlete?
   Which stabilization procedures should the head athletic trainer follow?

4. During a lacrosse game, one of your players sustains a severe injury. He is not breathing when you arrive on the field. You have a screwdriver and must remove the screws on his face mask. While you are trying to do so, one screw just spins in its socket.

   What do you do now?
   What types of tools should you have for such emergencies?

WRAP-UP

In this chapter, you were exposed to multiple injuries associated with head trauma that can lead to medical emergencies. The specific conditions and management steps for athletes suffering from concussions, including securing the athlete onto a spine board, were discussed. Protective equipment used in contact sports—such as helmets, face masks and shoulder pads, which help to protect an athlete from injury—can also lead to problematic issues for spinal mobilization and access to the airway. Multiple procedures for removal of the protective equipment were provided, including links to additional resources for other emergency management techniques. The information presented is not all-inclusive; it is the responsibility of the athletic trainer or allied health professional to become familiar with the procedures required to manage emergency situations that may arise in his or her particular sport or event.

REFERENCES

1. Morrison AL, King TM, Korell MA, et al. Acceleration-deceleration injuries to the brain in blunt force trauma. *Am J Forensic Med Pathol*. 1998;19(2):109–112.
2. Bailes JE, Hudson V. Classification of sport-related head trauma: A spectrum of mild to severe injury. *J Athl Train*. 2001;36(3):236–243.
3. Servadei F. Prognostic factors in severely head injured adult patients with epidural haematomas. *Acta Neurochir (Wein)*. 1997;139:272–278.
4. Cantu RC. Posttraumatic retrograde and anterograde amnesia: pathophysiology and implications in grading and safe return to play. *J Athl Train*. 2001;36(3):244–248.
5. Torg JS, Corcoran TA, Thibault LE, et al. Cervical cord neuroplaxia: classification, pathomechanic, morbidity, and management guidelines. *J Neurosurg*. 1997;87:843–850.
6. Torg JS, Naranja RJ Jr, Palov H, et al. The relationship of developmental narrowing of the cervical spinal canal to reversible and irreversible injury of the cervical spinal cord in football players. *J Bone Joint Surg Am*. 1996;78:1308–1314.
7. Swartz EE, Boden BP, Courson RW, et al. National athletic trainers' association position statement: Acute management of the cervical spine-injured athlete. *J Athl Train*. 2009;44(3):306–331.
8. Ransone J, Kersey R, Walsh K. The efficacy of the rapid form cervical vacuum immobilizer in cervical spine immobilization of the equipped football player. *J Athl Train*. 2000;35:65–69.
9. DelRossi G, Horodyski M, Powers ME. A comparison of spine-board transfer techniques and the effect of training on performance. *J Athl Train*. 2003;38(3):204–208.
10. Limmer D, O'Keefe MF, Dickinson ET. *Assessment of the Trauma Patient. Emergency Care*, 10th ed. Upper Saddle River, NJ: Pearson–Prentice Hall; 2005.
11. Ahmad M, Butler J. Spinal boards or vacuum mattresses for immobilization. *Emerg Med J*. 2001;18:379–380.
12. Luscombe MD, Williams JL. Comparison of a long spinal board and vacuum mattress for spinal immobilization. *Emerg Med J*. 2003;20:476–478.
13. Knox KE, Kleiner DM. The efficiency of tools used to retract a football helmet face mask. *J Athl Train*. 1997;32:211–215.
14. Kleiner DM. Face mask removal vs face mask retraction. *J Athl Train*. 1996;31(Suppl 2):32.
15. http://www.Schuttsports.com. Accessed 2008.
16. Decoster LC, Shirley CP, Swartz EE. Football face-mask removal with a cordless screwdriver on helmets used for at least one season of play. *J Athl Train*. 2005;40(3):169–173.

17. Gale SD, Decoster LC, Swartz EE. The combined tool approach for face mask removal during on-field conditions. *J Athl Train.* 2008;43(1):14–20.

18. Block JJ, Kleiner DM, Knox KE. Football helmet face mask removal with various tools and straps. *J Athl Train.* 1996; 31(Suppl 2):11.

19. Kleiner DM, Almquist JL, Hoenshel RW, et al. The effects of practice on face mask removal skills. *J Athl Train.* 2000;35(Suppl 2):S60.

20. Copeland AJ, Decoster LC, Swartz EE, et al. Combined tool approach is 100% successful for emergency football face mask removal. *Clin J Sport Med.* 2007;17:452–457.

21. Knox KE, Kleiner DM. The effectiveness of EMT shears for face mask removal. *J Athl Train.* 1996;31(Suppl 2):17.

22. Sherbondy PS, Hertel JN, Sebastianelli WJ. The effect of protective equipment on cervical spine alignment in collegiate lacrosse players [electronic version]. *Am J Sports Med.* 2006;34:1675–1679 from http://ajs.sagepub.com/cgi/content/abstract/34/10/1675.

23. US Lacrosse Sports Science and Safety Committee. Lacrosse Helmet Facemask/Chinguard Removal Hints for Certified Athletic Trainers 2008.

24. Feld F, Blanc R. Immobilizing the spine-injured football player. *J Emerg Med Serv.* 1987;12:38–40.

25. Patel MN, Rund DA. Emergency removal of football helmets. *Phys Sports Med.* 1994;22:57–59.

26. Waninger KN. On-field management of potential cervical spine injury in helmeted football players: Leave the helmet on! *Clin J Sports Med.* 1998;8:124–129.

27. Caswell SV, Deivert RG. Lacrosse helmet designs and the effects of impact force. *J Athl Train.* 2002;37:164–171.

28. Donaldson WF III, Lauerman WC, Heil B, et al. Helmet and shoulder pad removal from a player with suspected cervical spine injury: A cadaveric model. *Spine.* 1998;23:1729–1732, discussion 1732–1733.

29. National Athletic Trainers' Association consensus statements: Prehospital care of spine-injured athlete. 2001. http://www.nata.org/statements/consensus/NATAPreHospital.pdf. Accessed Feb 3, 2010.

FOR FURTHER RESEARCH AND INFORMATION

American College of Sports Medicine. Concussion (mild traumatic brain injury) and the team physician: A consensus statement. 2006.

National Athletic Trainers' Association Consensuses Statements: PreHospital care of spine-injured athlete. 2001. http://www.nata.org/statements/consensus/NATAPreHospital.pdf.

National Athletic Trainers' Association Position Statement: Head-down contact and spearing in tackle football. *J Athl Train.* 2004;39(1):101–111.

National Athletic Trainers' Association Position Statement: Management of sport-related. *J Athl Train.* 2004;39(3):280–297.

Swartz EE, Boden BP, Courson RW, et al. National Athletic Trainers' Association Position Statement: Acute management of the cervical spine-injured athlete. *J Athl Train.* 2009; 44(3):306–331.

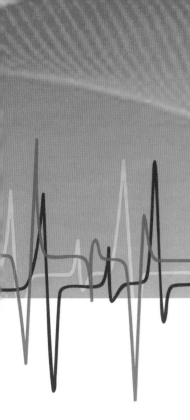

C H A P T E R · 18

Environmental Emergencies

CHAPTER OUTCOMES

1. Identify the effects of hyperthermia on performance.
2. Identify and recognize the signs and symptoms of an exertional heat stroke.
3. Properly care for and manage an individual who is suffering from an exertional heat stroke.
4. Identify and recognize heat cramps.
5. Properly care for and manage an individual who is suffering from heat cramps.
6. Identify the appropriate methods to prevent exertional heat illnesses.
7. Understand the rationale for environmental monitoring and testing of hydration status.
8. Identify and recognize frostbite.
9. Properly care for and manage an individual who is suffering from frostbite.
10. Identify and recognize hypobaric conditions.
11. Properly care for and manage an individual who is suffering from acute mountain sickness.
12. Identify and recognize lightning-related conditions.
13. Properly care for and manage an individual who has been struck by lightning.

NOMENCLATURE

Asystole: cessation of heart contraction or pumping; flatline

Convection: the transfer of heat to or from the body to a medium such as water or air. If the medium is cooler than body temperature, heat is lost. If the medium is warmer than body temperature, heat is gained

Core body temperature: the amount of heat deep within the body tissues, which must be measured rectally in exercising individuals

Evaporation: the vaporization of water into the air, as in sweat from the skin. The rate of evaporation depends primarily on the amount of water in the air, or the relative humidity. The higher the relative humidity, the less evaporation occurs. Evaporation also depends on the flow rate of air; a high flow rate encourages faster evaporation

Heat index: a combination of ambient temperature and relative humidity used by weather services to provide a measure of perceived heat; does not include radiant heat from the sun

Hyperthermia: core body temperature greater than normal and reaching dangerous levels around 40°C or 104°F, leading to end-organ damage

NOMENCLATURE *(Continued)*

Hyponatremia: also known as "water intoxication," where the sodium (salt) in the blood is too low (less than or equal to 130 mmol/L), often from dilution by too much water ingestion or excessive sodium loss from too much sweating (or both) without electrolyte replacement

Hypothermia: core body temperature below 35°C or 95°F, leading to frostbite and eventually asystole and death

Normothermia: normal core body temperature at rest, 37.0°C or 98.6°F, also called temperature homeostasis

Radiation: infrared or thermal heat generated from a heat source such as the sun and absorbed by the body

Sequelae: negative aftereffects of a condition

Thermoregulation: maintenance of a constant internal or core body temperature

Wet-bulb globe temperature (WBGT): the best measure of perceived heat stress on the body—includes a weighted calculation of ambient temperature (dry-bulb temperature), relative humidity (wet-bulb temperature), and radiant heat from the sun (black-globe temperature)

BEFORE YOU BEGIN

1. Why is it important to assess hydration status in athletes?

2. What are some signs and symptoms of an exertional heat stroke? How are the signs and symptoms different from those of heat exhaustion? How would you manage an athlete suffering from an exertional heat stroke?

3. Describe the steps you would take when managing a person suffering from a heat cramps.

4. What is the appropriate treatment for someone suffering from altitude sickness?

5. What resources can you identify that will provide information about the policies on postponing or canceling an athletic event because of lightning?

Voices from the Field

In my own experience, we have virtually eliminated heat illnesses, even in extreme environmental conditions. Because of the relationship we have built with our coaches, the athletic trainers are not adversaries, we are there to help the team. During preseason football, our team rarely practices in full pads and we follow the NCAA regulations for preseason practices. I think

it goes to show that with proper education and acclimatization, you can significantly diminish heat illnesses in football.

Brian Wong, ATC
Head Athletic Trainer for Football
University of Hawaii

HYPERTHERMIA

Exercise imposes a physiological stress that generates metabolic heat from active skeletal muscles, which must be dissipated to the environment through various processes. The body responds to the stresses it encounters in order to maintain a constant internal temperature at or near 37.0°C or 98.6°F (temperature homeostasis or **normothermia**).[1] Metabolic heat is generated by active skeletal muscles and can reach total energy expenditures 15 to 25 times that of heat expenditure at rest.[2] This level of work in active muscle cells is supported by redirecting blood away from the nonworking muscle tissues and organs and directing the blood toward the working skeletal muscle.[2,3] As much as 80% to 85% of total cardiac output is redirected to the active skeletal

muscles during maximal exercise.[4] Exercising in a hot, humid environment poses a thermoregulatory challenge to the body that requires compensatory adaptations to prevent a disruption of body temperature homeostasis.

Performing physical activity in a hot, humid environment is a challenge to the thermoregulatory system.[2,3] Regulating body temperature and maintaining an equal rate of heat gain versus heat loss requires a careful balance between internal and external environmental conditions. An increase in **core body temperature,** deep within the body tissues, above normal resting body temperature is known as **hyperthermia**[5] and can present a serious health threat. Understanding how the human body thermoregulates itself during exercise in a hot, humid environment is extremely important in preventing exertional heat illness.

Thermoregulation During Exercise

Body temperature regulation during exercise, or **thermo-regulation,** is required to maintain a constant deep core body temperature and prevent hyperthermia.[2,3] Maintaining a constant core body temperature requires a balance between the amount of heat lost and the amount of heat gained by the body. During exercise, the circulatory system works to transfer heat to the external environment. This transfer is accomplished by blood (primarily the water component), which has a high capacity for storing heat and easily dissipates this heat as it comes close to the surface of the body in the skin. Heat is generated inside the body by the metabolism of working skeletal muscles and is gained from the environment by thermal **radiation** from the sun. Heat loss from the skin occurs through **convection,** conduction, and evaporation. During exercise, however, evaporative heat loss is the primary mechanism utilized by the body.[3] **Evaporation** is the loss of heat through the process of changing sweat from a liquid phase to a gaseous phase, thus cooling the skin. Sweat losses vary from person to person, but sweat rates often range from 0.8 to 1.4 L/hr, depending on age, sex, exercise intensity, individual differences, environmental conditions, acclimatization, clothing, and baseline hydration status.[1,3] Evaporative heat loss contributes as much as 85% to 90% of all heat dissipated during exercise in a hot, dry environment.[2] However, as the relative humidity increases (Fig. 18.1), the amount of heat dissipated by evaporation of sweat from the skin decreases, creating a physiological challenge to the cardiovascular system to cool the body. The addition of protective equipment increases the cardiovascular strain, since it further impedes the evaporation of sweat from the skin (Fig. 18.2). Heat imbalance poses a threat to homeostasis and during exercise there is a careful balance between heat generated by active skeletal muscle and the ability of the sweat mechanism to provide evaporative cooling in the external environment.

Effects of Hyperthermia on Performance

An increase in core body temperature is commonly experienced during physical activity in hot, humid environments. Dehydration is not a prerequisite for hyperthermia; well-hydrated athletes are also subject to hyperthermia, although it is less likely in their case. Physical performance decreases in a number of ways when core body temperature is elevated above normal.

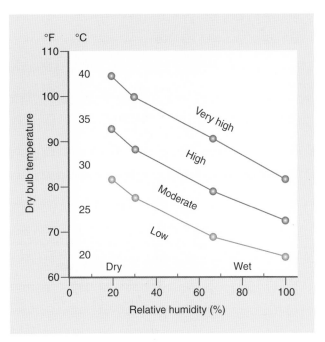

FIGURE 18.1 Chart showing risk of heat stress in terms of air temperature and relative humidity.[6] This graph may be used to approximate the risk of exercise in hot environments, but Figure 18.2 may be better suited for estimating heat-stroke risk when equipment is worn. (Data from the American College of Sports Medicine Position stand: the prevention of thermal injuries during distance running. *Med Sci Sports Exerc.* 1987;19:259–533.)

The central nervous system (CNS) consists of the brain and the spinal cord—two integral components of communication within the body during exercise. The neurological and mental functions are susceptible to high temperatures, observed through symptoms such as dizziness and confused behavior, usually observed during an exertional heat stroke (EHS).[5,6]

Brain temperature is an important factor affecting the coordination of motor activity. The temperature of the brain is determined by the balance between heat produced by cerebral energy turnover and the heat that is removed, primarily by cerebral blood flow.[8] Further, hyperthermia may cause central fatigue when a critical brain temperature is reached.[9] To reduce the risk of permanent brain and end-organ damage as a result of hyperthermia, appropriate management of exertional heat illnesses is essential.

Current Research

Core Temperature and Exercise

Research has shown that increases in core body temperature limit physical performance by causing premature fatigue,[7] presumably due to the effect of increased temperature on brain function.[5]

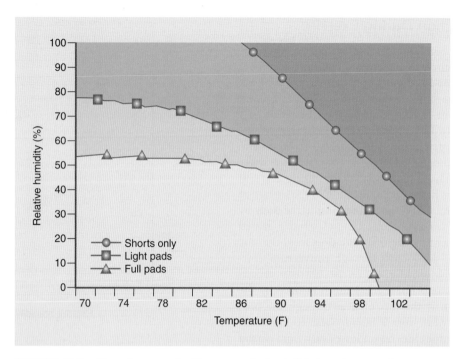

FIGURE 18.2   Chart showing risk of heat stress for football.[6] The risk rises with increasing heat and relative humidity. Fluid breaks should be scheduled for all practices and scheduled more frequently as the heat stress rises. *Add 5°F to temperature between 10 A.M. and 4 P.M. on bright, sunny days from mid-May to mid-September.* For the safety of the athletes, practices should be modified to reflect the heat-stress conditions. Conditions that fall into the *lightest pink area*: Regular practices with full practice gear can be conducted. Conditions that fall into the *second-lightest pink area*: Cancel all practices; practices may be moved into air-conditioned spaces or held as walk-through sessions with no conditioning activities. Conditions that fall into the *medium pink area*: increase rest-to-work ratio with 5- to 10-minute rest and fluid breaks every 15 to 20 minutes; practice should be in shorts only with all protective equipment removed. Conditions that fall into the *darkest pink area*: Increase rest-to-work ratio with 5- to 10-minute rest and fluid breaks every 20 to 30 minutes; practice should be in shorts with helmets and shoulder pads (not full equipment).

EXERTIONAL HEAT ILLNESSES: DESCRIPTION, IDENTIFICATION, AND MANAGEMENT

Exertional Heat Stroke

EHS is a risk for all athletes, particularly for those who train or compete in hot, humid conditions and especially when the heat and humidity are unexpectedly high or above the athlete's usual training and living conditions.[10] Classic, or nonexertional, heat stroke results from passive exposure to a high environmental temperature; however, EHS results from overloading or failure of the thermoregulatory system in response to intense exercise, usually in a hot environment.[11-13] EHS occurs when homeostatic thermoregulatory mechanisms fail, causing an elevation in core body temperature exceeding 40°C or 104°F.[1-13] Metabolic requirements of working muscle and cooling skin are exac-

erbated by temperature and humidity extremes, which can overwhelm the capacity to dissipate heat. Ultimately, heat production that exceeds heat dissipation leads the core temperature to rise dramatically, until dangerous hyperthermia exists.[11] Furthermore, EHS can progress to complete thermoregulatory system failure.[6,14,15] Table 18.1 describes the pathophysiology of EHS and the effects of overheating of organ tissues, such as multiorgan dysfunction syndrome or end-organ failure. Rapid reduction of body temperature with aggressive whole-body cooling is essential; otherwise EHS can be fatal, and those who do survive may sustain permanent neurologic damage.[10,15]

EHS can affect athletes involved in any sport, but it is more common in those who train outdoors, such as military recruits, distance runners, cyclists, and American football players. Any athlete performing heavy exercise can generate enough heat to rapidly overwhelm the body's ability to release heat into the environment, resulting in heat stress

TABLE 18.1   Pathophysiology of Exertional Heat Stroke in Each Major Organ System[4,10,11,16]

Body System Affected	Major Finding(s)
Central nervous system	Encephalopathy
Cardiovascular system	Myocardial injury, hemorrhagic complications such as disseminated intravascular coagulation (a bleeding disorder characterized by diffuse blood coagulation) with pronounced thrombocytopenia (decreased blood platelets)[14,17]
Muscular system	Rhabdomyolysis (destruction of skeletal muscle often associated with strenuous exercise)
Renal system	Acute renal failure
Respiratory system	Acute respiratory distress syndrome
Digestive system	Hepatocellular injury, intestinal ischemia or infarction, pancreatic injury

and extreme hyperthermia for which the body cannot compensate. EHS is most common among young athletes in apparent good health, most likely because members of this age group often participate in strenuous activity to which they are unaccustomed in high environmental temperatures.[10]

The primary finding that characterizes EHS is neurological dysfunction associated with an elevated core body temperature. The CNS is affected by increased core body temperature, resulting in neurological dysfunction, the characteristic sign of EHS. Failure to promptly recognize CNS dysfunction can lead to serious neurological depression, resulting in coma and eventually death (see the Signs & Symptoms box titled "Exertional Heat Stroke"). Without rapid whole-body cooling within minutes of collapse, failure to regain consciousness within 2 hours of collapse often points to a poor prognosis.

Management of Exertional Heat Stroke

EHS is a medical emergency; appropriate treatment strategies involve immediate reduction of core body temperature and restoration of homeostasis (Table 18.2).[6,11] The major factor determining patient outcome is the length of time that the body temperature remains hyperthermic. Therefore, immediate measures should be directed toward decreasing the core temperature to less than 38.9°C or 102.0°F as rapidly as possible.[13,15] Rectal core body temperature must be measured rapidly to correctly identify the condition as EHS and save the person's life with appropriate management (Fig. 18.3). Tympanic, oral, or axillary measurements are spuriously affected by peripheral (skin) and environmental temperatures and should never be used after exercise. Rectal temperature is a common procedure in the field in the military setting and at mass events such as marathons,

Signs & Symptoms

Exertional Heat Stroke[6,10,15,18,19]

Body System Affected	Signs and Symptoms
Thermoregulatory system	Rectal temperature ≥40°C or 104°F, sweating (although skin may be wet or dry at the time of collapse), and dehydration (not required)
Central nervous system	Altered mental status, neurological impairment, seizures, and coma
	Decreased visual acuity, impaired recent and remote memory, ataxic gait, and lethargy
Cardiorespiratory system	Hyperventilation/tachypnea, tachycardia, hypotension, also respiratory alkalosis and lactic acidosis
	Hemoconcentration (often associated with concomitant dehydration)
	Hypophosphatemia, hypercalcemia, and hyperproteinemia
Digestive system	Vomiting, diarrhea
Subjective report	Fatigue, flushing, chills, and alterations in personality (subtle)

TABLE 18.2	Decision-Making Factors in the Management of Exertional Heat Stroke[6,10-12,15,18-20]
Exertional heat stroke	A severe exertional illness characterized by central nervous system abnormalities and potential tissue damage resulting from elevated body temperatures; induced by strenuous physical exercise and increased environmental heat stress.
Signs and symptoms	• Increase in core body temperature, usually above 40°C or 104°F (measured rectally) when athlete falls ill • Central nervous system dysfunction, such as altered consciousness, coma, convulsions, seizures, confusion, disorientation, emotional instability, irrational behavior or decreased mental acuity, personality changes such as combativeness, irritability, emotional instability, confusion, hysteria, or apathy • Increased heart rate, decreased blood pressure or tachypnea • Nausea, vomiting, or diarrhea • Headache, dizziness, or weakness • Hot and wet, usually sweating • Dehydration
Treatment	• Aggressive and immediate whole-body cold-water immersion initiated within minutes. • Activate EMS; *cool first and transport second.* • Monitoring of vital signs until ambulance arrives.
Return-to-play strategy	Under direction of athlete's physician, should depend on the severity of the condition and include a gradual increase in the duration and intensity of exercise and in exposure to outdoor conditions (over days or weeks).[19]

where EHS is likely. Although it is not an entry-level athletic training proficiency at this time, athletic trainers should be prepared to measure rectal temperature in the event of an environmental emergency (see Skill 18.1). The athlete's airway, cardiorespiratory status, and core temperature should also be monitored continuously, and rapid, whole-body cooling should be started before emergency management services (EMS) arrive. Upon arrival of EMS, intravenous access should be obtained and the athlete rehydrated with normal saline or lactated Ringer's solution.[13,15]

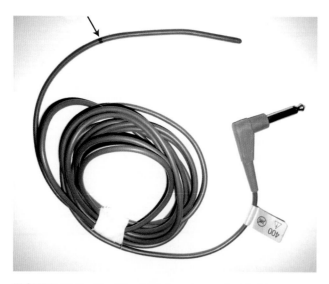

FIGURE 18.3 Flexible rectal thermistor—the ideal instrument for measuring a hyperthermic athlete's core temperature accurately in the field. The arrow points to the 10-cm insertion line.

Rapid Whole-Body Cooling

Effective heat dissipation depends on the rapid transfer of heat from the core of the body to the skin and from the skin to the external environment.[19] Therapeutic cooling techniques are, therefore, aimed at accelerating the transfer of heat from the skin to the environment without compromising the flow of blood to the skin. Aggressive and immediate whole-body cooling is the key to optimizing treatment. The duration and degree of hyperthermia may determine adverse outcomes. If untreated, hyperthermia-induced physiological changes that may be fatal can occur within vital organ systems (muscle, heart, brain, etc.).[19] Survival of the EHS athlete is dependent on rapid and effective whole-body cooling.

Because of superior cooling rates, immediate whole-body cooling (cold water immersion), approximately 5°C to 15°C or 41°F to 49°F, is the gold standard for immediate treatment of EHS and should be initiated within minutes after the incident (Fig. 18.4).[6,11,12,15,19,20] It is recommended to cool first and transport second if onsite rapid cooling is feasible and an athletic trainer is available. Tub immersion (Fig. 18.5A; see Skill 18.2 about the use of rapid whole-body cooling) or the very practical "taco method" (Fig. 18.5B), referring to the shape of the tarp, requires an unfolded tarp with the ends held by volunteers. The tarp or a tub should be filled with a sufficient mixture of ice and water to cover the body. The athlete must have all equipment and extra clothing removed; only enough clothing to ensure modesty should remain in place. The athlete is placed in the tub or tarp and the head is supported to maintain the airway and

Measuring Rectal Temperature

In the field, using a rectal thermistor to measure core body temperature in a hyperthermic individual is more accurate than using axillary, tympanic, oral, or temporal measurements. To measure rectal temperature during an environmental emergency, the following supplies will be needed:

- Flexible rectal thermistor, premarked with black marker or tape 10 cm from its end
- Latex thermistor sheath/cover or hospital-grade cleaner
- Lubricating gel
- Gloves

  1. Put on the gloves.
  2. Cover the end of the thermistor with a disposable sheath and lubricating jelly or water. Caution: too much jelly or water will cause the probe to slide out and give a false reading.
  3. If available, use towels or a sheet to drape from the waist and pull the athlete's shorts down to midthigh.
  4. Hold the thermistor at the premarked black line or tape with one hand.

  5. Use the other hand to shift one gluteal cheek to the side.
  6. Insert the thermistor up to the premarked line, which is at the 10-cm mark.
  7. Loop the rest of the thermistor in a "lasso" fashion and tuck it into the side of the shorts, pulling the shorts back into position around the waist with the thermistor plug easily accessible.
  8. Plug the thermistor end into the thermometer receiver.
  9. Do not remove the thermistor until the athlete recovers and returns to normal temperature. If transporting to the hospital, keep the thermistor inserted and send to the hospital with the athlete.
  10. To remove the thermistor, pull it out and, using a wet wipe, clean the last 15 cm of the probe. Put the thermistor into a hospital-grade cleaning solution such as Cidex to ensure complete decontamination. Rinse and dry thoroughly before returning the thermistor to its bag.
  11. Thoroughly wash your hands.

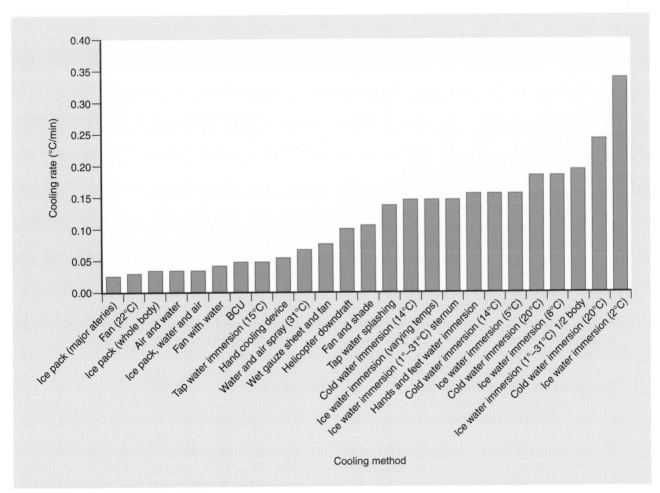

FIGURE 18.4 Rapid whole-body cooling.[21] Ice-water immersion offers the fastest cooling and must be used immediately if exertional heat stroke is suspected. This graph shows cooling rates in experiments with healthy hyperthermic athletes and individuals with heat stroke. (Adapted with permission from Casa, DJ, Armstrong LE, Ganio MS, et al. Exertional heat stroke in competitive athletes. *Curr Sports Med Rep.* 2005;4:309–317. Copyright © 2005 Current Medicine Group, LLC. Used with permission.)

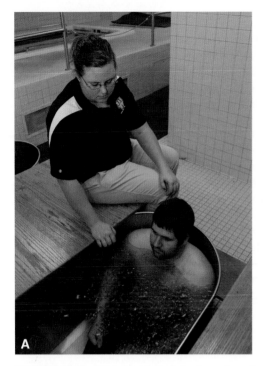
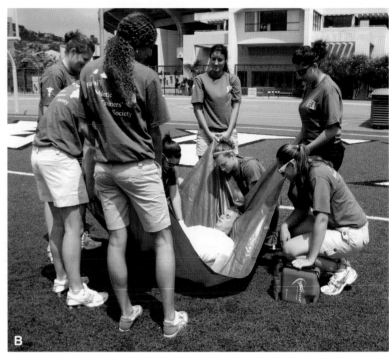

A

B

FIGURE 18.5 Methods of whole-body cooling. **A.** An ice bath. **B.** The "Taco" method can be used on the field.

SKILL 18.2

Procedures for Rapid Whole-Body Cooling[6]

To use rapid whole-body cooling, the following supplies will be needed:

- Tub, pool, or large tarp (6 × 8 ft)
- Two or three large coolers of ice water
- Eight large towels
- Blood pressure cuff and stethoscope
- Flexible rectal thermistor (if available)
- Automated external defibrillator (AED)

1. If feasible, measure the rectal temperature to differentiate between heat exhaustion and heat stroke. With heat stroke, rectal temperature is elevated (generally higher than 40°C [104°F]).

2. Assess cognitive function, which is markedly altered in EHS (see symptom list below). Athlete will still be sweating.

3. Lower the body-core temperature as quickly as possible. The fastest way to decrease body temperature is to remove the athlete's clothes and equipment and immerse the body (trunk and extremities) into a pool or tub of cold water (approximately 1°C to 15°C or 35°F to 59°F). *Aggressive cooling* is the most critical factor in the treatment of EHS. The following alternative field method ("taco" method) is also acceptable:

    a. Lay a tarp on the ground, preferably in the shade.

    b. Remove any equipment and extra clothing from the athlete.

    c. Place athlete onto the center of the tarp.

    d. Raise the athlete's head and the legs with the tarp beneath them. Maintain the elevation of the head and turn the head if vomiting occurs.

    e. Lift the corners of the tarp and pour ice water on the athlete; be sure it covers at least half of the body.

    d. If the athlete does not recover within a few minutes, continued cooling is needed. Wrap ice towels around the athlete to cover parts of the body not immersed in the ice water.

4. Monitor the athlete's vital signs and other signs and symptoms of heat stroke (see below) and have the AED nearby.

5. Monitor the temperature during the cooling therapy and recovery (every 5 to 10 minutes). Once the athlete's rectal temperature reaches approximately 38.3°C to 38.9°C (101°F to 102°F), remove him or her from the water to avoid overcooling.

6. If a physician is present to manage the athlete's medical care on site, then initial transportation to a medical facility may not be necessary; therefore, immersion can continue uninterrupted. If a physician is not present, aggressive first-aid cooling should be initiated on site and continued during EMS transport and at the hospital until the athlete is normothermic.

7. Activate EMS.

8. Monitor for organ-system complications for at least 24 hours.

    - During transport and when immersion is not feasible, other methods can be used to reduce body temperature: sponging with cool water and applying cold towels, or applying ice bags to as much of the body as possible.

    - In addition to cooling therapies, first-aid emergency procedures for heat stroke may include airway management.

    - Also, a physician may decide to begin intravenous fluid replacement.

Current Research

Core Temperature and Heat Exhaustion

Heat exhaustion is characterized by core body temperature less than 40°C or 104°F.[6]

to turn the head if vomiting occurs.[6] Monitor vital signs and remove the athlete from the water before shivering begins or when rectal temperature reaches approximately 38.3°C to 38.9°C (101°F to 102°F). In the absence of whole-body cold water immersion, an alternative is to apply cold water or ice to the skin of the entire body, using soaked ice towels or sheets, which are rotated or changed when no longer cool (see Fig. 18.5, step 6).[11,19] Fan and mist or evaporative cooling may be effective in some situations, but the cooling rates in actual EHS patients have not compared well (approximately half) with immersion or rotating towels, especially if used in humid conditions.[10] No cases of shock or adverse events have been reported when cooling a hyperthermic and otherwise healthy individual. Recovery of CNS function during cooling is a favorable prognostic sign and should be expected in the majority of patients who receive prompt and aggressive treatment.[19]

Heat Exhaustion

Exercise (heat) exhaustion is the inability to continue exercise and is associated with a combination of heavy sweating, dehydration, sodium loss, and energy depletion.[6,11,12,14,20] The inability to exercise is commonly associated with failure of the cardiovascular system to respond appropriately to the workload under high external temperatures and dehydration.[3] This common condition occurs most frequently in hot, humid environments.

Clinically, it is difficult to distinguish heat exhaustion from EHS without a direct measure of rectal temperature. However, in the absence of an accurate core body temperature, significant involvement of the CNS is the major distinguishing factor associated with EHS that is not present or present to only a minor degree in heat exhaustion. Other signs and symptoms of heat exhaustion are listed in Table 18.3.

TABLE 18.3	Decision-Making Factors in the Management of Exertional Heat Exhaustion[6,11,12,14,20]
Heat exhaustion	Heat exhaustion is a moderate illness, characterized by the inability to sustain adequate cardiac output, resulting from strenuous physical exercise and environmental heat stress.
Signs and symptoms	• Athlete finds it difficult or impossible to keep playing • Core body temperature <40.0°C or 104°F • Headache, loss of coordination, dizziness, or fainting, but lack of significant CNS involvement • Generalized malaise or weakness • Tachycardia and hypotension • Nausea, vomiting, anorexia, or diarrhea • Dehydration • Profuse sweating or pale skin • Stomach/intestinal cramps or persistent muscle cramps
Treatment	• Remove athlete from play and immediately move to shaded or air-conditioned area. • Remove excess clothing and equipment and have athlete lie comfortably with legs propped above heart level. • Cool athlete until rectal temperature is approximately 38.3°C or 101°F. • Monitor heart rate, blood pressure, respiratory rate, core temperature, and CNS status. • If athlete is not nauseated, vomiting, or experiencing any CNS dysfunction, treat as an EHS with cold-water immersion. • Rehydrate orally with chilled water or sports drink. If athlete is unable to take oral fluids, implement intravenous infusion of normal saline. • Transport to an emergency facility if rapid improvement is not noted with prescribed treatment.
Return-to-play strategy	• Athlete should be symptom-free and fully hydrated; recommend physician clearance; rule out underlying predisposing conditions; avoid intense practice in heat until at least next day.

Management of Heat Exhaustion

Full recovery occurs within a few hours with cessation of activity, replenishment of fluids, and rest in a cool environment. In the absence of rectal temperature, significant neurological impairment is the only major distinction between heat exhaustion and EHS, a serious medical emergency. Heat exhaustion and EHS exhibit similar signs and symptoms. Therefore, if the athletic trainer does not have access to rectal temperature and is unable to make a definitive diagnosis, it is recommended[6,12] to treat any significant heat-related illness as EHS with rapid whole-body cooling (see Skill 18.2).

Heat Cramps

Heat cramps are intense, involuntary, painful, sudden, spasmodic contractions of the skeletal muscles that occur during intense or prolonged exercise in the heat (Table 18.4). Considerable uncertainty exists in the literature regarding the etiology of heat cramps, primarily because the term "cramp" is used to indicate a variety of clinical features of muscles, leading to its use as an imprecise umbrella term that includes stiffness, contractures, and local pain. Although a usually benign and self-limiting problem, cramps can occur during exercise in the heat and can be extremely painful, involving multiple muscle groups. Individuals with sickle cell trait and others who are severely dehydrated with electrolyte imbalance may have severe cramps associated with more serious conditions such as myopathy, exertional rhabdomyolysis, and acute renal failure.[22]

Fatigue, sodium depletion, dehydration, and hyperthermia[23–25] seem to be involved in the development of heat cramps; their relative contribution to the etiology is uncertain. Heat cramps often occur near the end of long races (triathlons,[26] marathons[27]) or following repeated bouts of intense exercise with intermittent rest periods (football practice,[25,28] tennis match[29,30]). This pattern suggests that cramping may occur when an athlete has reached a point of dehydration or a depletion of adenosine triphosphate, resulting in an inability to meet the demands of exercising skeletal muscle.

Management of Heat Cramps

Usually, heat cramps are self-limiting, with the afflicted athlete unable to continue exercise. The condition usually resolves with rest, rehydration with electrolyte supplementation, massage, stretching the cramping muscle, and cold- or ice-water immersion of the affected extremity. For severe cramps affecting multiple muscle groups or whole-body cramping that does not respond to treatment, cold- or ice-water immersion is warranted and EMS should be activated. Upon arrival of EMS, intravenous rehydration and transportation to the hospital for follow-up blood testing is warranted.

Exertional Hyponatremia

Exertional hyponatremia is a plasma sodium concentration less than 130 mmol/L (normal is 135 to 146 mmol/L).[1,6,12,13,20,31] This condition is most commonly associated with long-duration, low-intensity events lasting 4 hours or more, often in the heat.[31] Also known as water intoxication, exertional **hyponatremia** is generally associated with repeated or prolonged exercise in hot environments, considerable sweating or the production of large amounts of salty sweat, following a low-sodium diet or consuming insufficient sodium, or rehydrating with inappropriate types or volumes of fluids for the athletic event. A combination of these etiological factors may result in sodium dilution,

TABLE 18.4	Decision-Making Factors in the Management of Heat Cramps[6,11,12,14,20]
Heat cramps	Heat cramps are intense, involuntary, painful, sudden, and spasmodic muscle contractions that occur in athletes who perform strenuous exercise in the heat. The specific mechanism is not well understood.
Signs and symptoms	• Intense pain (not associated with pulling or straining a muscle). • Persistent muscle contractions that continue during and after exercise.
Treatment	• Reestablish normal hydration status and replace some sodium losses with a sports drink or water. • Some additional sodium may be needed (especially in those with a history of heat cramps) earlier in the activity. • Light stretching, relaxation, ice, and massage of the involved muscle may help acute pain of a muscle cramp. • Intravenous fluids and transport to hospital may be necessary in severe case of heat cramps.
Return-to-play strategy	Athletes should be assessed to determine if they can perform at the level needed for successful participation.

which may detrimentally affect fluid balance. Excess water in the extracellular space or a large deficit in extracellular sodium concentration results in neurological disturbances that are often confused with signs and symptoms of heat stroke. Unrecognized or untreated exertional hyponatremia may result in CNS dysfunction, convulsions, cerebral edema, and death.[6,20,31] Athletic trainers should be aware of the recognition, evaluation, management, and prevention of this potentially life-threatening condition.

Athletes affected with exertional hyponatremia present with CNS dysfunction that may include disorientation, altered mental status, headache, vomiting, lethargy, and swelling of the extremities (hands and feet), pulmonary edema, cerebral edema, and seizures. This condition can be prevented by assessing hydration status and matching fluid intake with sweat and urine losses. The consumption of fluids and foods that contain sufficient sodium during prolonged exercise in the heat is essential to prevent hyponatremia.

Management of Exertional Hyponatremia

Recognizing the symptoms of exertional hyponatremia and making an accurate differential diagnoses between hyponatremia and EHS is essential. Since both conditions present primarily with CNS dysfunction, a thorough medical history and physical examination, including rectal temperature and a blood sodium measurement, are critical for making a definitive diagnosis. It is common for medical tents in large, mass sporting events such as marathons to have portable sodium analyzers available for this purpose.

Management of exertional hyponatremia is dictated by the severity of the condition or the magnitude of the symptoms. Because an accurate diagnosis is not always readily available, clinical suspicion of hyponatremia warrants rest, cooling, observation, and immediate transportation to the emergency department for observation and further evaluation.[33] Treatment of mild asymptomatic exertional hyponatremia when the athlete is medically stable and does not exhibit signs of cerebral edema includes transportation to the emergency department, observation for several hours, and fluid restriction while allowing spontaneous diuresis. Loss of consciousness or seizures are medical emergencies and EMS should be summoned immediately.[31,34] In cases of exertional hyponatremia, intravenous fluid therapy should be avoided until a physician's diagnosis has been made—including an assessment of body fluid balance, plasma sodium concentration, and rectal temperature—because of the risk of exacerbating unrecognized exertional hyponatremia.[31]

PREVENTION OF EXERTIONAL HEAT ILLNESS

Many cases of exertional heat illness (EHI) are preventable and can be successfully treated if properly recognized and appropriate medical care is provided in a timely manner (Fig. 18.6). The main objective of a sound emergency preparedness plan is to educate athletes, coaches, parents, and medical staffs alike on what can be done to avert EHS, heat exhaustion, and heat cramps. The athletic trainer should meet with the team, coaches, and parents to properly disseminate information on risk factors for EHI and strategies for its prevention.

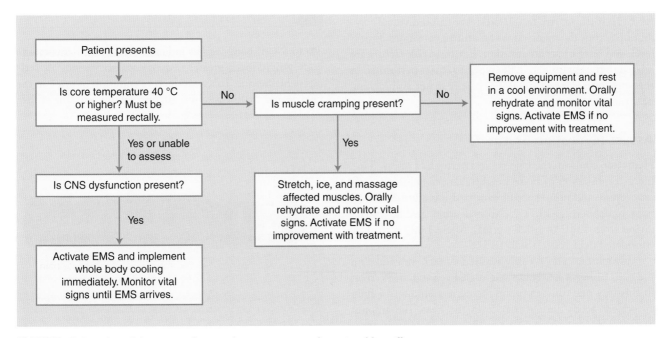

FIGURE 18.6 Clinical decision making in the management of exertional heat illness.

Breakout

There are various preventive strategies and recommendations for EHI.[6,15,20] These include the following:

1. Monitor individual hydration status by assessment of urine color and sweat rate.
2. Make sure that athletes maintain hydration status by checking urine samples before exercise for urine that is pale yellow or straw-colored.
3. Provide shade during breaks and increase rest-to-exercise ratio in red flag conditions or when WBGT is 23°C or 73°F (see Table 18.5).
4. Emphasize the importance of getting enough sleep and avoiding dangerous supplements while exercising in the heat.
5. Provide medical services with emergency equipment, including cold-water immersion for the treatment of EHI, available on site.
6. Ensure that preparticipation physical examinations have been completed, including specific questions regarding fluid intake, weight changes during activity, medication and supplement use, history of cramping/heat illnesses, and sickle cell trait.
7. Make sure that medical staff has the authority to alter work/rest ratios, practice schedules, amounts of equipment, and withdrawal of individuals from participation in sports based on environmental conditions and/or athletes' medical conditions.

Breakout

Both intrinsic and extrinsic risk factors are associated with exercise in hot, humid environments.[20]

Intrinsic Risk Factors

○ History of EHI
○ Inadequate heat acclimatization
○ Lower level of fitness
○ Higher percentage of body fat
○ Dehydration or overhydration
○ Presence of a fever
○ Presence of gastrointestinal illness
○ Salt deficiency
○ Inadequate meals/insufficient calorie intake
○ Skin condition (e.g., sunburn, skin rash, etc.)
○ Ingestion of certain medications (e.g., antihistamines, diuretics) or dietary supplements (e.g., ephedra)
○ Motivation to push oneself, or "warrior mentality"
○ Reluctance to report problems, issues, illness, etc.
○ Prepubescence

Extrinsic Risk Factors

○ Intense or prolonged (several hours) exercise with minimal breaks
○ High temperature/humidity/sun exposure
○ Inappropriate work/rest ratios based on intensity, WBGT, clothing, equipment fitness, and athlete's medical condition
○ Lack of education and awareness of heat illnesses among coaches, athletes, and medical staff
○ No emergency plan to identify and treat EHIs
○ No shade or rest breaks
○ Limited access to fluids before and during practice and rest breaks
○ Delay in recognition of early warning signs
○ Exposure to high heat/humidity (WBGT) in preceding days

EHIs can be best prevented by modifying activity depending on the extrinsic (environmental) risk factors and identifying intrinsic (nonenvironmental) risk factors that may predispose an individual to EHI. Intrinsic and extrinsic risk factors must be considered to accurately assess the risk for EHI. Intrinsic risk factors arise from an individual's hydration status, the medications an athlete consumes, fitness level, and level of acclimatization. Extrinsic risk factors are related to the environment, the type of activity performed in that environment, and amount of barrier materials blocking heat transfer from the skin.

Assess Hydration Status

Hydration status in the field is most accurately assessed using a combination of body-weight changes before and after exercise and urine-specific gravity using a urine clinical refractometer (Fig. 18.7).[6,13] Normal urine specific gravity ranges from 1.002 to 1.028 µg/mL, where 1.020 µg/mL is considered dehydrated (Skill 18.3).[6]

Hydration status is easily assessed by each individual on the basis of his or her body-weight changes and urine color; in this way one can determine the correct amount of fluid an athlete needs during exercise in the heat. The amount of sweat lost during exercise can easily be calculated using pre- and postexercise body-weight changes (Skill 18.4). A loss of

3% to 5% of body weight indicates significant dehydration; body-weight losses greater than or equal to 5% indicate serious dehydration.[6] To assess the concentration of urine in the field, instruct athletes to urinate into a white cup. The athlete

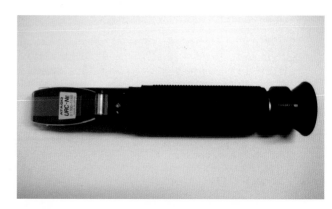

FIGURE 18.7 Clinical refractometer for measuring urine specific gravity. (From Atago Inc., Japan, Manufacturer's Instructions.)

SKILL 18.3

Using a Clinical Refractometer

Before using a clinical refractometer, check and adjust the instrument to calibrate it or put it on "zero setting" by opening the daylight plate and placing a few drops of distilled water on the face of the prism. Close the daylight plate gently. Adjust the scale into focus by turning the eyepiece. If the boundary line does not coincide with the 1.000 line or the 1.333 line, make an adjustment by turning the adjusting screw. *Do not* turn the scale adjustment screw excessively, since that may cause damage. Avoid excessive shock or dropping the instrument; keep it in its case. Use only lens paper to wipe the surface of the prism.

1. Place one or two drops of urine on the prism.
2. Close the plate gently. The sample must spread all over the prism surface.
3. Look at the scale through the eyepiece.
4. Read the scale where the boundary intercepts it.
5. Wipe the sample from the prism with a tissue and water.

can then observe the color of the urine, which indicates the concentration. In a well-hydrated condition, the urine should be pale yellow or straw-colored. Urine that is completely clear may indicate overhydration and a dangerous condition of hyponatremia. Urine that is darker in color, such as the color of apple juice, indicates a moderate level of dehydration; whereas urine that is very dark yellow or tinged with brown, such as a tea color, indicates severe dehydration. In addition to learning to estimate hydration status on the basis of urine color, sweat rate is easily measured by dry weighing before and after exercise in hot, humid conditions, using the steps outlined in Skill 18.4. Normal sweat rates vary considerably, but in hot, humid conditions, sweat rates can range from 0.5 to 1.5 L/hr and give an indication of how much fluid should be replaced during and after exercise to restore normal hydration.

Monitor Environmental Conditions

Since the external environment poses risks that contribute to the development of EHI, it is imperative to monitor environmental conditions. Individuals exercising an environment that is above skin temperature absorb heat from the environment. High ambient temperatures, relative humidity, air motion, and the amount of radiant heat from the sun or other sources contribute to EHI. High relative humidity inhibits evaporative heat loss, causing an increase in core body temperature. When the environmental temperature is above skin temperature, athletes begin to absorb heat from the environment and depend entirely on evaporation for heat loss.[17]

Environmental conditions are most commonly monitored by using a sling psychrometer (Fig. 18.8), which measures ambient temperature and relative humidity but does not account for the radiant heat of the sun. Many weather stations report these conditions as well as a combination of these conditions called the **Heat Index.** Unless a weather station is in close proximity, measure the conditions on site by using a sling psychrometer (see Skill 18.5). For best accuracy, the wet-bulb temperature should be read first and as quickly as possible because delay in reading may cause error. In addition, the wick must be kept clean, saturated with water, and whirled long enough to stabilize temperatures. Barometric pressure, misreading the scale, and other factors influence the determination

SKILL 18.4

Estimating Hydration Status Using Urine Color and Changes in Body Weight

1. Before exercise, the athlete should urinate into a white cup and completely empty his or her bladder. The color of the urine should then be assessed.
2. Wearing dry clothes, the athlete steps on the scale. Body weight is recorded in kilograms (kg) because it is easily converted to liters (1 kg = 1 L).
3. Record the start time of practice/exercise.
4. During practice, the athlete should drink from an individual bottle that has been weighed and should avoid spilling water or sharing it. If the athlete must urinate during exercise, the urine volume should be recorded. Record the volume in liters (L).
5. Record the end time of practice/exercise in hours (should be at least 1 hour).

6. After exercise, the athlete should remove sweat from the skin with a dry towel (or shower and dry thoroughly) and, after changing into the same dry clothes as before, step on the scale.
7. After weighing, the athlete should empty the bladder and urine color should again be examined.
8. Subtract the weight before exercise from the weight after exercise and add the volume of fluid consumed (if the athlete urinated during exercise, subtract that volume). Divide by the length of time exercised:

Percent change in body weight = [(weight before exercise − weight after exercise)/weight before exercise] × 100

Sweat rate = (weight before exercise − weight after exercise) + volume **of** fluid consumed/exercise duration (hours)

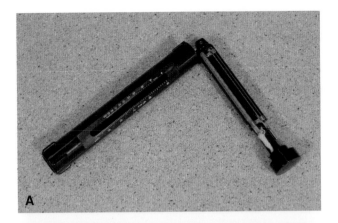

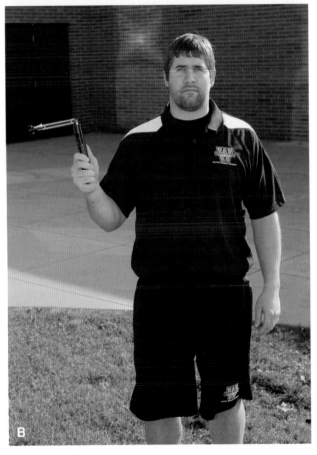

FIGURE 18.8 **A.** Sling psychrometer for measuring temperature and relative humidity (from Bacharach, New Kensington, PA, manufacturer's instructions.) **B.** After wetting the wick on the wet-bulb thermometer, fling the psychrometer into the air. Slide the body of the psychrometer inside the tub to read relative humidity from dry- and wet-bulb temperature.

of relative humidity negatively and may be sources of error. When **wet-bulb globe temperature (WBGT)** measures are not available, environmental heat stress can be estimated using a sling psychrometer or by charting the risk of exercise as shown in Figures 18.1 or 18.2.[6]

WBGT is the gold standard for monitoring environmental conditions in the field because it best simulates the

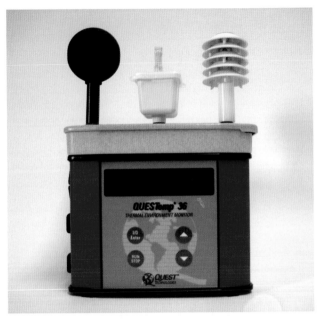

FIGURE 18.9 Wet Bulb Globe Temperature (WBGT) monitor for measuring heat stress. A thermal environment monitor internally calculates the WBGT for determining physiological response to heat stress and risk of exertional heat illness. The monitor must be set in a representative area on the field and allowed to adjust for at least 10 minutes before reading.

physiological response of the body in certain environmental conditions. WBGT is a weighted index that incorporates ambient air temperature, relative humidity, and the radiant heat of the sun (Fig. 18.9). The National Athletic Trainers' Association[6] and the American College of Sports Medicine[13] recommend using the WBGT to monitor environmental conditions to determine relative risk for EHI. For example, if the WBGT index is greater than 28°C or 82°F (black flag conditions), the event should be delayed, rescheduled, or moved into an air-conditioned space (Table 18.5).[6] Use of the WBGT index to modify activity in high-risk settings has virtually eliminated heat-stroke deaths in the military. When the WBGT is high to extreme, the risk of heat-related problems is greater the next day; this seems to be one of the best predictors of heat illness.[6]

HYPOTHERMIA

Physical activity occurs in a variety of environments, but emergencies occurring in cold-weather sports pose a special challenge to the athletic trainer. In cold-weather sports, body heat transfers from the body to the environment, allowing the body to regulate core temperature without excessive physiological strain. However, during cessation of physical activity in cold environments, often from exhaustion or fatigue, excessive heat loss occurs.[34] Cold stress is the physiological

SKILL 18.5

Procedures for Measuring Temperature and Relative Humidity Using a Sling Psychrometer

1. Be sure wick is wet and covers mercury (or red spirit) reservoir on the wet-bulb thermometer. Be sure the reservoir on the other thermometer is dry.
2. Pull the tube clear of the body so that the body can swivel.
3. Holding the tube, whirl the body two to three revolutions per second (120 to 180 rpm).
4. Continue whirling until temperatures stabilize (1½ minutes is usually ample).
5. Immediately read the wet- and dry-bulb thermometers; replace the body inside tube.
6. Set wet- and dry-bulb temperatures opposite each other on slide rule–type calculator scales, sliding the body into the tube as required.
7. Read percent relative humidity indicated by arrowhead on lower scale.

condition where heat is removed from the body faster than the body produces it, thereby decreasing body temperature (**hypothermia**).[35] Heat loss from the body occurs through four mechanisms: radiation, conduction, convection, and evaporation. The body is usually warmer than the environment, so that the net exchange of heat occurs from the body to the cooler environment. Heat loss by conduction involves the direct transfer of heat through a liquid, solid, or gas. If cooler air continuously replaces warmer air surrounding the body, heat loss increases by convection. Water evaporation from the respiratory passages and skin surface continually transfers heat to the environment.[34]

Hypothermia develops when net heat losses exceed net heat gain, causing core body temperature to decrease. The clinical definition of hypothermia is core temperature below 35°C (95°F), or approximately 2.0°C (3.5°F) less than normal body temperature.[36-38] Because of the serious nature of accidental hypothermia, it is imperative that the rectal temperature be accurately measured as soon as possible. However, this may not always be possible because of the environmental conditions and lack of instrumentation. The lowest core temperature reported in a survivor of accidental hypothermia is 13.7°C or 56.7°F, followed by 9 hours of resuscitation and stabilization, which led to good physical and mental recovery.[39] A hypothermic person, even in the most severe condition, should never be left for dead until aggressive and persistent resuscitation and rewarming efforts have been made.

Windchill

Monitoring the environmental conditions determines the relative risk of frostbite (Fig. 18.10). As air temperature decreases below freezing and with increasing wind speed, the risk of frostbite increases. Air temperature and wind speed are the primary determinants of relative risk[36] and are evaluated using the windchill temperature index value. This index integrates wind speed and air temperature to provide an estimate of the cooling power of the environment.[40] The windchill temperature index standardizes the cooling power of the environment to an equivalent air temperature for calm conditions. Windchill temperatures are grouped into frostbite risk zones based upon the period of time in which exposed cheek skin will freeze in more susceptible persons in the population, assuming that such individuals use standard cold-weather precautions, including gloves and proper clothing. Cheek skin was selected because this area of the body is typically not protected, and studies have determined that this area, along with the nose, is one of the coldest areas of the face. Wet skin exposed to the wind will cool even faster.[36] Since wind increases convective heat loss by disturbing the boundary layer of air that rests against the skin, it causes the skin to cool at a faster rate than if no wind were

TABLE 18.5 Wet-Bulb Globe Temperature Risk Chart[6]

WBGT	Flag Color	Level of Risk	Comments
<18°C or <65°F	Green	Low	Risk low but still exists on the basis of risk factors.
18–23°C or 65–73°F	Yellow	Moderate	Risk level increases as event progresses through the day.
23–28°C or 73–82°F	Red	High	Everyone should be aware of injury potential; individuals at risk should not compete.
>28°C or 82°F	Black	Extreme or hazardous	Consider rescheduling or delaying the event until safer conditions prevail; if the event must take place, be on high alert.

The WBGT can be measured with a WBGT meter. The calculation for the determination of WBGT is: WBGT = 0.7 (wet-bulb temperature) + 0.2 (black-globe temperature) + 0.1 (dry-bulb temperature).

Wind speed (in mph)	Actual temperature (°F)											
	50	40	30	20	10	0	−10	−20	−30	−40	−50	−60
	Equivalent chill temperature											
Calm	50	40	30	20	10	0	−10	−20	−30	−40	−50	−60
5	48	37	27	16	6	−5	−15	−26	−36	−47	−57	−68
10	40	28	16	3	−9	−21	−33	−46	−58	−70	−83	−95
15	36	22	9	−5	−18	−32	−45	−58	−72	−85	−99	−112
20	32	18	4	−10	−25	−39	−53	−67	−82	−96	−110	−124
25	30	15	0	−15	−29	−44	−59	−74	−89	−104	−118	−133
30	28	13	−2	−18	−33	−48	−63	−79	−94	−109	−125	−140
35	27	11	−4	−20	−35	−51	−67	−82	−98	−113	−129	−145
40	26	10	−6	−22	−37	−53	−69	−85	−101	−117	−132	−148
(Wind speeds greater than 40 mph have little additional effect)	**Little danger** (In less than 5 hrs with dry skin. Greatest hazard from false sense of security.)				**Increasing danger** (Exposed flesh may freeze within 1 minute.)			**Great danger** (Exposed flesh may freeze within 30 seconds.)				

FIGURE 18.10 Wind-chill chart recommended by the Department of the Army.[36] To determine the wind-chill temperature, enter the chart at the row corresponding to the wind speed and read right until reaching the column corresponding to the actual air temperature. (From Department of the Army. *Prevention and Management of Cold-Weather Injuries.* Washington, DC: Department of the Army, Technical Medicine Bulletin; 2005:1–94. http://www.usariem.army.mil/depcold/coldapd.htm. Accessed September 25, 2007.)

present. Wind will not cool the skin, or any tissue, below the ambient air temperature. Therefore, frostbite cannot occur if the air temperature is above 0°C or 32°F.[36,40]

COLD INJURIES: DESCRIPTION, IDENTIFICATION, AND MANAGEMENT

Although symptoms of hypothermia may differ among individuals, a decrease in body temperature results in clinical manifestations related to loss of effective thermoregulation, cellular dysfunction, ischemia, and edema. Hypothermia is generally classified into stages based on the severity and extent of physiological responses (Table 18.6). Clinical staging can be established by a nonmedical member of the rescue team at the rescue site, since it is not based on the measurement of rectal temperature.[41] Because there may be great individual variation in the observed clinical features, it is imperative that rectal temperature be accurately measured as soon as possible.[37] Predisposing factors for hypothermia include decreased heat production, increased heat loss, impaired thermoregulation, and renal failure.[35] Environment, clothing, anthropometric status, health status, gender, age, and exercise intensity collectively determine if exercising in the cold elicits additional physiological strain and injury risk beyond those associated with the same physical activity performed in temperate conditions.[42]

The acute care and treatment of cold injuries is similar to the rewarming process, which is a critical component of any management strategy for cold illnesses. Core temperature is considered a vital sign in the cold athlete; the vital

TABLE 18.6	Stages of Hypothermia Based on Core Body Temperature and Symptoms[36-38,41,42]	
Description*	**Core Body Temperature[38]**	**Clinical Stage[42]**
Mild hypothermia	35–33.0°C or 95.0–91.4°F	Stage I: alert, shivering athletes
Moderate hypothermia	32.0–29.0°C or 89.6–85.2°F	Stage II: drowsy, nonshivering athletes
Severe hypothermia	<28.0–24.1°C or 82.4–75.4°F	Stage III: unconscious athletes
	<24°C or <75.2°F	Stage IV: athletes without spontaneous breathing

*Based on the precise measurement of core body temperature.

Signs & Symptoms

Effects of Hypothermia on Body Systems[35,36,41,42]

Condition	Signs and Symptoms
Mild hypothermia	Athlete is alert and shivering
Musculoskeletal system	Maximal shivering, dysarthria (difficulty speaking)
Cardiovascular system	Increased blood pressure, tachycardia, cold diuresis (increased urine production)
Nervous system	Feeling cold, ataxia, exhibiting signs of apathy, amnesia, poor judgment, behavioral change, social withdrawal
Moderate hypothermia	Athlete is drowsy and not shivering
Nervous system	Cognitive/behavioral changes such as confusion or sleepiness, slurred speech, and a change in behavior or appearance
	Hyporeflexia, agitation, and hallucination
Respiratory system	Hypoventilation, respiratory acidosis, hypoxemia, aspiration pneumonia, and atelectasis (lung collapse)
Cardiovascular system	Hypotension, bradycardia, and prolonged QT intervals
	Blood becomes highly concentrated, with characteristics of hypercoagulability
Muscular system	Muscle rigidity and stiffness
Severe hypothermia	Athlete is unconscious and without spontaneous breathing
Nervous system	Areflexia, coma, and absent pupil responses
Respiratory system	Apnea
Cardiovascular system	Pulseless electrical activity, atrial fibrillation, ventricular fibrillation, and asystole
	Disseminated intravascular coagulation and bleeding
Muscular system	Rhabdomyolysis

signs should also include the "ABCDs": *A*irway, *B*reathing, *C*irculation, and *D*egrees. Rectal or esophageal temperature monitoring is the gold standard for measuring core body temperature in cold-stress athletes.[42] Obtaining core temperature is important and useful for assessing and treating hypothermia; however, it is difficult to obtain in the field and is tremendously variable among individuals' physiological responses at specific temperatures.[38]

Mild Hypothermia

Mild hypothermia is associated with transient physiological changes as well as a clinical presentation that includes physical and mental symptoms. The athlete may present with compromised fine and gross motor skills. Mental compromise includes impairment when completing both complex and simple tasks. Mildly hypothermic athletes have a good ability to rewarm without an external heat source.[38]

Management of Mild Hypothermia

The treatment of mild hypothermia primarily involves prevention of further heat loss. The athlete must be insulated from the ground, protected from the wind, wet clothing removed to eliminate evaporative heat loss, covered with a vapor barrier, and moved to a warm environment. If the

athlete is capable of swallowing and protecting the airway, provide the athlete with fluids containing carbohydrates to supply the energy necessary to continue shivering and replace energy stores.[38] Athletic trainers should passively

Breakout

When rewarming frozen tissue, the athletic trainer must be aware of several precautions:

- Avoid exposure to excessive heat, mechanical trauma, or any factor causing a loss of circulation.
- Avoid further tissue trauma, as by permitting the athlete to walk on injured feet or to rub of the affected tissue.
- Rewarming may be associated with other life-threatening factors, such as blood loss, which initially stopped when the tissue became frozen.
- Treat open blisters with a topical antibiotic and cover with sterile bandages to avoid infection.
- Avoid tobacco products, which can cause vasoconstriction and decrease blood flow to the injured area.
- Anyone with a peripheral freezing injury must be suspected of being hypothermic and be treated for hypothermia.

SKILL 18.6

Rewarming Frozen Tissue

The decision to rewarm a frostbite injury must be carefully thought out and should be based on the treatment of other injuries, the possibility of hypothermia, the possibility of refreezing, and the ease of evacuation.

1. Prepare a warm (98.0°F to 104.0°F) water bath. *Do not use hot water*, because local heat dissipation may be impaired and tissue injury could result.

2. Use a container that is large enough to accommodate the frostbitten tissue without allowing the tissue to touch the sides or bottom of the container.

3. Gently circulate the water around the affected tissue.

---

rewarm the athlete by applying heat to areas of high surface heat transfer such as the groin, axillae, and neck (see Skill 18.6).[38,41] If the athlete is stable, mild exercise may be performed to achieve active rewarming.[38]

Moderate Hypothermia

Moderate hypothermia involves a progression of the symptoms of mild hypothermia with physiological changes in the thermoregulatory system, including rapid cooling and the cessation of shivering.[35,41] The respiratory, cardiovascular, muscular, and nervous systems are affected and respond to the decreased body temperature (refer to the Signs & Symptoms box titled "Effects of Hypothermia on Body Systems"). Unconsciousness is likely to occur at 30.0°C or 85.2°F, the lowest point of the moderate hypothermia category.[35]

Management of Moderate Hypothermia

Moderate to severe hypothermia is a medical emergency necessitating maintenance of airway, breathing, and circulation as well as careful rewarming to increase core body temperature. Active external rewarming should be applied to the trunk rather than the extremities, because an "afterdrop" in core temperature may occur when blood supply to the cold periphery is recirculated to the core.[41] Although some have suggested withholding cardiopulmonary resuscitation, fearing precipitation of ventricular fibrillation, the athletic trainer should follow current guidelines for advanced cardiac life support for maintenance of cerebral blood flow.[41]

Severe Hypothermia

Severe hypothermia is characterized by changes in cardiac rhythms (refer to the Signs & Symptoms box titled "Effects of Hypothermia on Body Systems"). This stage of whole-body cooling requires immediate attention to rewarm and restore normal core body temperature.[35] Serious depression of the respiratory, cardiovascular, and nervous systems can result in a near-death state or death itself. Although life signs are almost impossible to discern at these temperatures, no one should be pronounced dead until an effort to rewarm has been made.[35] Hence the adage, "A person is not dead until they are warm and dead."[44]

Management of Severe Hypothermia

Rewarming a severely hypothermic athlete may be a passive or active process. Passive rewarming involves the use of blankets to cover the body and head; depending on shivering thermogenesis, the warming rate may be 0.5°C to 2.0°C per hour with this technique.[41] Active rewarming can be an external or internal process. Active external rewarming includes the use of heating blankets or a heated forced-air system. In a randomized trial involving 100 patients with minor trauma, of whom 80 had hypothermia, heating blankets warmed at a rate of 0.8°C per hour, compared with a temperature decrease of 0.4°C per hour with the use of wool blankets.[45] In another randomized trial[46] involving 16 adult patients with moderate or severe accidental hypothermia, rewarming rates were 1.0°C per hour faster with a forced-air system than with cotton blankets. In hypothermic athletes, the cold heart is prone to spontaneous ventricular fibrillation from any disturbance or movement.[38] Therefore, it is important to avoid unnecessary movement of the trunk and large joints to prevent the development of cardiac arrhythmias triggered by the flow of cold, peripheral blood to the irritable myocardium.[42]

For severe hypothermia or for circulatory arrest, invasive internal rewarming techniques are recommended.[41] If the athletic trainers have access to an AED and the device states that shocks are indicated, one set of three stacked shocks should be delivered. If the core temperature cannot be determined or is above 30°C (86°F), treat the athlete as normothermic. If the core temperature is below 30°C (86°F), discontinue use of the AED after the three shocks until the athlete's core temperature reaches normothermic level.[38]

Frostbite

Frostbite is the crystallization of fluids in the skin and subcutaneous tissue after exposure to subfreezing temperatures (0.6°C or 31.0°F).[47] This condition commonly affects the extremities of the nose, ears, cheeks, hands, and feet.[36] Frostbite is classified into four degrees, from superficial or "frost nip" to deep frostbite.[34,36,38,41] Skin exposed to cold air causes peripheral vasoconstriction that can significantly lower tissue temperature.[36] The first sign of frostbite is numbness

Signs & Symptoms

Four Degrees of Frostbite[35,36,39,41]

Condition	Signs and Symptoms
First-degree frostbite	Superficial freezing ("frostnip") of the skin and subcutaneous tissues, usually produced by a short-duration exposure to cold air or contact with a cold object.
Early signs	Pallor or erythema, edema, blistering, desquamation, transient tingling or burning sensation. The skin initially has a mottled blue–gray appearance, followed by a red appearance with thawing, and is hot and dry to the touch. Rewarmed skin often has clear blisters.
Prognosis	Swelling occurs within 2 to 3 hours of rewarming and may persist for 10 days.
	Desquamation of the superficial epithelium in 5 to 10 days, lasting up to 1 month.
Common sequelae	Paresthesia, aching, and necrosis of pressure points if the frostbite is on the foot. Increased sensitivity to cold and hyperhidrosis (excessive sweating).
Second-degree frostbite	Injury to the epidermis and superficial dermis.
Early signs	Skin appears gray–white and is cold and firm to the touch. There is little pain or loss of sensation, but the range of motion is decreased when skin is frozen.
Prognosis	Vesicles appear within 12 to 24 hours, forming an eschar (scab) when dry.
	Blisters must remain intact; if ruptured, care must be taken to avoid infection. As the vesicles dry, they slough pink granulation tissue, with no permanent tissue loss. Throbbing and aching pain persists for 3 to 10 days after injury.
Common sequelae	Hyperhidrosis often appears after the second or third week.
Third-degree frostbite	Freezing of the full dermis and into the reticular layer of the skin.
Early signs	Vesicles may be hemorrhagic, with generalized edema that abates after 5 to 6 days. The skin forms a black, hard, dry eschar; when the area of involvement finally demarcates, there is sloughing with some ulceration.
Prognosis	Burning, aching, throbbing, or shooting pain from to 5 days up to 4 to 5 weeks is common.
Common sequelae	Subfascial pressure increases and compartment syndromes are common. Hyperhidrosis and cyanosis appear late. Residual cold sensitivity is common.
Fourth-degree frostbite	Deep frostbite involving the entire thickness of skin and underlying tissue; may affect bones, joints, and tendons. No mobility in the frozen tissue.
Early signs	After rewarming, passive mobility returns but muscle function may remain poor. The skin has a deep cyanotic appearance with poor perfusion.
	Skin may have marked hemorrhagic blisters and anesthesia, followed later by hyperesthesia, ulceration, and gangrene.
	Favorable prognostic features include retained sensation, normal skin color, and clear rather than cloudy fluid in the blisters if present. Poor prognostic features include non-blanching cyanosis, firm skin, and dark, fluid-filled blisters.
Prognosis	Over several weeks, the tissue will slough. In rapidly frozen extremities or freeze–thaw–refreeze injuries, dry gangrene develops with mummification after 5 to 10 days. With slower freezing, demarcation takes much longer to occur, but is usually clear at 20 to 36 days. Some tissue damage is irreversible.
Common sequelae	Early surgical intervention is not indicated because there is a high propensity for tissue healing even in those cases where the original prognosis was poor.

Current Research

Hypothermia

During field management, it is more important to prevent hypothermia than to rapidly rewarm frostbite.[38,41]

in the periphery. The initial sense of cooling begins at skin temperatures approximately 82°F and pain appears at about 68°F; but as skin temperature falls below 50°F, these sensations are replaced by numbness.[36] The freezing point of skin is slightly below the freezing point of water because of the electrolyte content of the cells and extracellular fluid. Dry tissue typically freezes around 28°F, whereas wet skin freezes around 30°F because of the increased rate of heat loss.[36] Affected individuals often feel a "wooden" sensation in the injured area.[35,36]

Management of Frostbite

In the prehospital acute management of frostbite, nonadherent wet clothing should be removed. Local rewarming should begin only if refreezing will not occur in transit. Thawed tissue that refreezes almost always dies.[38] Avoid rubbing affected areas, as this procedure worsens tissue damage.[41] The management of freezing injuries in the field depends on many conditions, including the treatment of other injuries, the possibility of hypothermia, the possibility of refreezing, and the ease of evacuation.[38,41] Treatment of freezing injuries will follow some basic rules related to thaw–refreeze possibilities, rewarming, and other considerations.

Tissue that has thawed must not freeze again. If there is the possibility that tissue could be thawed and then refreeze, the tissue must not be allowed to thaw, since reformation of ice crystals will cause increased tissue damage. In addition, further trauma to frozen or injured parts must be avoided, including walking on injured feet and rubbing of the affected tissue. If the athlete must walk on a frozen extremity, he or she should do so without thawing the injury. This is a difficult decision, but it will decrease the chance of a freeze–thaw–refreeze injury as a result of mechanical trauma.[38,41]

Superficial frostbite, or frost nip, can be thawed at room temperature or against another individual's skin. Once the athlete is in a warm environment, insulative clothing must be removed from the area of frostbite, as it now serves to insulate the frozen part against rewarming. First-degree frostbite is easier to treat and results in less tissue damage than more severe frostbite, emphasizing the importance of early recognition of cold injuries.[38,41] Rewarming of frozen tissue requires avoiding exposure to excessive heat, mechanical trauma, or any factor causing a loss of circulation. Since the athlete's extremity is numb, he or she cannot determine if the temperature is too hot, so application of external heat using open flames, stovetops, hot air from vehicle exhaust, steam, or directly applied heat packs is not appropriate.[38,41]

If transport time to a medical facility will be 1 to 2 hours or less, the risks posed by improper rewarming or refreezing are greater than the risk of delaying treatment. If transport time will be more than 2 hours, frostbite often will thaw spontaneously, depending on the level of injury, exposure time, and activity level.

After rewarming, pain is significant, with initial sensations of an uncomfortable sense of cold, which may include tingling, burning, aching, sharp pain, and decreased sensation. The skin color may initially appear red; it then becomes waxy white. Peripheral temperatures in the hands and feet may be indicative of a generalized whole-body cooling, which may ultimately result in hypothermia.[36]

HYPOBARIA

Hypobaric environments involve low atmospheric pressure at high altitude. Many people live, work, and play at high altitude. Skiers (and athletes doing other snow sports), mountain climbers, hikers, and backpackers go to altitudes of 3,000 m or 9,840 ft to more than 8,000 m or 26,250 ft for recreation or competition (Fig. 18.11), and sudden ascents to high altitude without the benefits of acclimatization are common. The physiology of hypoxia provides the foundation of high-altitude medicine[48] and relates to environments where the partial pressure of oxygen (Po_2) is less than at sea level. High-altitude illness is common in people ascending to more than 2,500 m or 8,200 ft, especially if the ascent is rapid.[49] Altitude-related illness is rare at altitudes below 2,500 m, but it is common in individuals climbing to 3,500 m (11,480 ft) or more. Rapid gain in altitude is the primary causative factor, and slow ascent, allowing time for acclimatization, is the primary preventative factor.[49] The experience of climbers of Mt. Everest, at an altitude of 8,850 m or 29,030 ft, where the inspired Po_2 is less than 30% of its value at sea level, emphasizes the hypoxic insult of going to high altitude.[50,51]

High altitude affects the human body because of oxygen deprivation, but it can be influenced by other factors, such as severe cold, high winds, and intense solar radiation. The basic physiological mechanism of high-altitude illnesses is the low Po_2 in the inspired air (Fig. 18.11), which results from the reduced barometric or atmospheric pressure. The most deleterious effects of high altitude are greatly reduced by the process of acclimatization, the most important feature of which is hyperventilation caused by

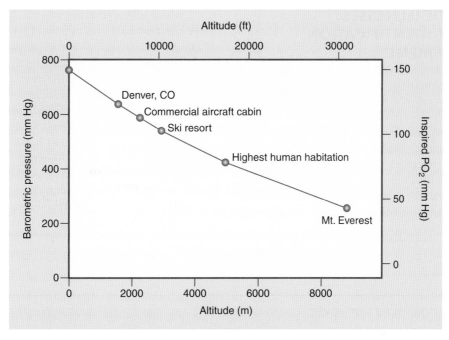

FIGURE 18.11 Relationship between altitude, barometric pressure, and inspired P_{O_2}.[51] Note that at an altitude of 5,000 m or 16,400 ft, the highest at which humans reside, the inspired P_{O_2} is only approximately half of the sea level value. On the summit of Mount Everest, at 8,850 m or 29,030 ft, the inspired P_{O_2} is less than 30% of the value at sea level. CO = Colorado. (From West JB. The physiologic basis of high-altitude diseases. *Ann Intern Med.* 2004;141:789–800.)

hypoxic stimulation of peripheral chemoreceptors. The risks of hypobaric illnesses can be reduced by using supplementary oxygen[51]; however, the likelihood of developing illnesses related to high altitude are dependent on the rate of ascent, the actual altitude reached, the altitude at which the individual sleeps, and individual susceptibility. Physical fitness is not protective, and exertion at altitude increases an individual's risk of developing a hypobaric illness. Table 18.7 describes definitions of altitude, examples, and associated physiological changes.[49]

TABLE 18.7	Definitions of Altitude, Examples, and Associated Physiological Changes[49]	
Altitude Definition	**Example**	**Physiological Changes**
Intermediate altitude 1,500–2,500 m or 4,900–8,200 ft	1,839 m or 6,035 ft (Colorado Springs, Colorado; location of U.S. Olympic Training Center)	Physiological changes detectable. Arterial oxygen saturation >90%. Altitude illness possible but rare.
High altitude 2,500–3,500 m or 8,200–11,480 ft	3,156 m or 10,355 ft (Alma, Colorado; highest town in the United States)	Altitude illness common with rapid ascent.
Very high altitude 3,500–5,800 m or 11,480–19,030 ft	5,100 m or 16,728 ft (Wenzhuan, Tibet; highest town on earth)	Altitude illness common. Arterial oxygen saturation <90%. Marked hypoxemia during exercise.
Extreme altitude >5,800 m or 19,030 ft	6,194 m or 20,320 ft (Mt. McKinley, in Denali National Park, Alaska; the highest peak in North America)	Marked hypoxemia at rest. Progressive deterioration despite maximal acclimatization. Permanent survival cannot be maintained.

HIGH-ALTITUDE ILLNESSES: DESCRIPTION, IDENTIFICATION, AND MANAGEMENT

The term *high-altitude illness* is used to describe the cerebral and pulmonary syndromes that can develop in unacclimatized persons shortly after ascent to high altitude. "Acute mountain sickness" and 'high-altitude cerebral edema" refer to the cerebral abnormalities; "high-altitude pulmonary edema" refers to the pulmonary abnormalities.[48] High-altitude illness is a growing concern in sports medicine with the increasing popularity of extreme sports, such as high-altitude mountain climbing, skiing, and snowboarding.[50]

Among elite endurance athletes, high-altitude illnesses have broad ramifications in prevention and management. A thorough understanding of the presentation, management, and prevention of high-altitude illness is necessary for the treatment of these athletes.[50] The incidence of illnesses arising from sports activities at high altitudes is increasing, as are their complications. Athletes are affected usually a short time after climbing to a new, higher altitude level to which their bodies are not acclimatized.[50] For most individuals, altitude-related illness is an unpleasant but self-limiting and benign syndrome, consisting chiefly of headache, anorexia, and nausea.[49] More severe symptoms include poor sleep, lassitude (weariness, debility, or fatigue), cough, dyspnea on exertion and at rest, ataxia, and mental status changes.[52] Without early recognition

Signs & Symptoms

Identification of Hypobaric Conditions[49-51]

Condition	Signs and Symptoms
Acute mountain sickness[46]	A collection of nonspecific symptoms associated with acute ascent to areas higher than 2,500 m or 8,200 ft
Symptoms	Headache, light-headedness, breathlessness, fatigue, weakness, insomnia, anorexia, nausea or vomiting
	Peripheral edema may be present
Onset	Usually within 2 to 12 hours of ascent to new altitude (but may occur sooner) and resolve over 1 to 3 days, provided that there is no further ascent
High-altitude pulmonary edema	Potentially fatal condition in altitudes above 3,000 m or 9,842 ft
Signs and symptoms	Dyspnea with exercise progressing to dyspnea at rest, weakness, lethargy, and poor exercise tolerance
	Tachycardia and tachypnea, mild pyrexia, and crepitations (crackles) detectable by auscultation
	Dry cough at first, progressing to a cough that produces frothy, bloodstained sputum; also, often, dependent edema
	Progresses to severe dyspnea and frank pulmonary edema, with coma and death following
Onset	Usually within 2 days of ascent to new altitude
High-altitude cerebral edema	A rare but potentially very serious condition associated with ascents above 4,500 m or 14,760 ft, usually preceded by acute mountain sickness; may lead to coma and death
Signs and symptoms	Headache, nausea and vomiting, disorientation, confusion; also possible mood changes or hallucinations; seizures less common
	Papilledema (swelling and protrusion of the blind spot of the eye), retinal hemorrhages, or even hemiparesis
	Focal neurological signs may occur
	Progressive deterioration in consciousness level, proceeding to coma and death
Onset	2 to 4 days within ascent to new altitude
	Prodromal symptoms of early mental impairment or a change in behavior, which may be ignored by athletes and their companions. Ataxia, a common early feature that may be disabling, is often the last sign to disappear during recovery

and treatment, high-altitude illness can progress to cerebral or pulmonary edema, which can be fatal.[49] The morbidity and mortality associated with high-altitude illness are significant and unfortunate, given that they are preventable. Athletic trainers working with those climbing to a high altitude must be familiar with the early symptoms, prompt and appropriate treatment, and proper preventative measures.[53] There are three major high-altitude illnesses: acute mountain sickness, high-altitude pulmonary edema, and high-altitude cerebral edema, as well as many other less important conditions.

In the field, an athletic trainer may be called to the aid of a severely ill or unconscious athlete. As a rule, illness occurring at high altitude, particularly in an unconscious athlete, should be attributed to the altitude until proven otherwise.[52] When available, an appropriate history will go far to determine the nature and severity of the condition. The athlete will almost certainly have some respiratory signs, and it can be difficult to know if the underlying illness is high-altitude pulmonary or cerebral edema; however, this matters little, as the pragmatic management is the same: oxygen administration, pharmacological intervention, and hyperbaric treatment if available—and, most importantly, descent as soon as possible. The treatment of altitude-related illness is to stop further ascent and, if symptoms are severe or getting worse, to descend.[49–51] Oxygen, medications, and other treatments such as a pressure chamber for altitude illness should be viewed as adjuncts to aid descent. Descent of even a few hundred meters may be lifesaving, using whatever means are necessary in the shortest amount of time.[49] Under no circumstances should a person with worsening symptoms of high-altitude illness delay descent.[52]

Hyperbaric treatment is accomplished with some variation of a portable pressure chamber, or Gamow bag, originally invented by Dr. Igor Gamow at the University of Colorado. The bag is an air-impermeable chamber that completely encloses the athlete and is inflated to a significant pressure above ambient atmospheric pressure in order to simulate a physiological "descent."[49,54] A chamber pressure of 2 psi is equivalent to a decrease in altitude of 2,000 m. This commonly used portable hyperbaric pressure chamber can be used for simulated descents when a climber cannot be moved.[50] The bag is a bright-red coated nylon fabric cylinder with a long zipper to allow entry with small clear windows for viewing in/out of the chamber. The athlete is placed completely within the bag, the zipper is sealed shut, and the bag is inflated with the foot pump. Two pop-off pressure valves set to 2 psi (not adjustable) start to hiss when maximum pressure is reached; this prevents overpressurization of the bag. Ventilation is accomplished while the athlete is inside by continuously pumping (about once every 5 seconds) to flush fresh air through the bag and prevent the buildup of CO_2.[54] The portable hyperbaric chamber may be claustrophobic, and lying down in it may worsen orthopnea (difficulty in breathing that occurs when lying down and is relieved upon changing to an upright position). Despite these problems, the chamber remains popular and is carried by many larger expeditions.[49]

Acute Mountain Sickness

Acute mountain sickness is very common in people who ascend from near sea level to altitudes higher than approximately 3,000 m or 9,840 ft, but it may occur at altitudes as low as 2,000 m or 6,560 ft. This condition (refer to the Signs & Symptoms box titled "Identification of Hypobaric Conditions") is characterized by fatigue, weakness, nausea, vomiting, dizziness or light-headedness, and difficulty sleeping, although nonspecific symptoms may be attributed to other conditions, especially by people who are anxious to stick to a preplanned schedule.[49,50] Typically, symptoms begin within hours of ascent, but the condition is generally self-limiting and most of the symptoms disappear after several days. The precise pathogenesis of acute mountain sickness is not understood, but hypoxia is likely to be a major factor, although respiratory alkalosis may also play a role.[51]

Management of Acute Mountain Sickness

Treatment of acute mountain sickness (Table 18.8) by oxygen or descent is usually not required,[51] because resting at the

TABLE 18.8 Treatment of Altitude Illnesses[49,50]

Mild acute mountain sickness	• Rest days, relaxation; consider descent • Aspirin, ibuprofen, antiemetics or acetazolamide
Severe acute mountain sickness High-altitude cerebral edema	• Descent, evacuation, oxygen • Pressure bag to facilitate descent • Dexamethasone
High-altitude pulmonary edema	• Descent, evacuation, oxygen • Pressure bag to facilitate descent • Nifedipine
Altitude illness, type unknown	• Descent, evacuation, oxygen • Pressure bag to facilitate descent • Dexamethasone, nifedipine

same altitude often relieves the symptoms and most athletes will improve without treatment at the same altitude within 24 to 48 hours.[49] However, severe or prolonged acute mountain sickness responds well to descent.[51] Medications such as aspirin, acetaminophen, or ibuprofen may relieve headache, while a physician may prescribe acetazolamide (a diuretic) 250 mg three times per day, which is helpful in relieving symptoms, as is dexamethasone, 4 mg four times per day, if the condition is severe. The athletic trainer may administer over-the-counter analgesics and antiemetics, which may reduce headache and nausea in mild acute mountain sickness.[51] The main principles of treating acute mountain sickness are to stop further ascent, to descend if symptoms do not improve or deteriorate over 24 hours, and to descend urgently if signs of high-altitude pulmonary edema or high-altitude cerebral edema appear.[51]

High-Altitude Pulmonary Edema

High-altitude pulmonary edema is a potentially fatal condition that typically occurs 2 to 4 days after ascent to altitudes above 3,000 m (refer to the Signs & Symptoms box titled "Identification of Hypobaric Conditions"). With normal ascent rates, the incidence is low; but as ascent rate increases, particularly to elevations above 4,500 m or 14,760 ft, the incidence increases.[51] High-altitude pulmonary edema is also seen in residents of high altitudes who travel to a lower altitude and then return; this is termed "reascent high-altitude pulmonary edema." Considerable individual variability exists, with people who have once developed high-altitude pulmonary edema being more likely to develop it again.[51] Athletes with high-altitude pulmonary edema tend to have lower oxygen saturations than unaffected people at the same altitude, but the degree of desaturation by itself is not a reliable sign.[49] High-altitude pulmonary edema may be preceded by acute mountain sickness, but this is not always the case.[51]

Management of High-Altitude Pulmonary Edema

Descent is the mainstay of treatment of high-altitude pulmonary edema (Table 18.8), with a descent of even a few hundred meters often being of benefit.[49] Supplemental oxygen and hyperbaric therapy should be utilized if available. A physician may prescribe nifedipine (a coronary vasodilator), which is effective in preventing and treating high-altitude pulmonary edema in affected individuals (10 mg orally initially, then a 20 mg slow-release preparation every 12 hours).[49] The primary management of high-altitude pulmonary edema is the provision of oxygen support, pharmacological intervention, and, if possible, immediate descent to provide hyperbaric therapy until evacuation to a medical facility is possible.[49,50]

High-Altitude Cerebral Edema

High-altitude cerebral edema is a rare but potentially very serious condition in people ascending above 4,500 m.[51]

High-altitude cerebral edema is usually preceded by acute mountain sickness and may lead to coma and death. Early recognition of prodromal symptoms (refer to the Signs & Symptoms box titled "Identification of Hypobaric Conditions") of early mental impairment or a change in behavior is essential for survival. Clinical signs include ataxia—a common early feature that may be disabling and is often the last sign to disappear during recovery, and a progressive deterioration in consciousness level proceeding to coma and death. Focal neurological signs may occur; but, in the absence of other signs and symptoms of cerebral edema, these should prompt consideration of other diagnoses. Severe illness caused by high-altitude cerebral edema may develop over a few hours, especially if the prodromal signs are ignored or misinterpreted, and such illness may be accompanied by high-altitude pulmonary edema.[49]

Management of High-Altitude Cerebral Edema

As with other high-altitude illnesses, the cardinal rule in the treatment of high-altitude cerebral edema is descent to a lower altitude as quickly as possible (Table 18.8).[51] Delay may be fatal.[49] If descent to a lower altitude is not feasible because of the remote situation, oxygen, if available, and a portable hyperbaric chamber should be used.[49] A physician may prescribe dexamethasone; the suggested dose is 8 mg initially followed by 4 mg every 6 hours; this will usually relieve some symptoms, making evacuation easier.[49,50] Athletes with high-altitude cerebral edema sometimes recover very rapidly after descent to a lower altitude.[51] Even with descent, recovery may be delayed, and good supportive care is essential.[49]

LIGHTNING-RELATED CONDITIONS: DESCRIPTION, IDENTIFICATION, AND TREATMENT

Athletes involved in outdoor sports are subject to various weather hazards, including lightning-related conditions. About one third of lightning-related injuries occur during recreational or sports activities.[55,56] Lightning-related deaths far outweigh the number of deaths from any other natural disaster.[56] Fortunately, only about 10% of people who are struck by lightning are killed, leaving 90% with various degrees of disability.[55] It is important for athletic trainers to be aware of existing knowledge and current recommendations regarding lightning safety in order to most effectively protect athletes from the dangers of lightning.[57] On average, lightning causes more casualties annually in the United States than any other storm-related phenomenon except floods. Although 90% of those injured survive, they may have permanent **sequelae** and disability. Many of these people incur injuries or are killed by lightning because of misinformation and inappropriate behavior during thunderstorms.[58]

TABLE 18.9   Determining Risk of Lightning-Related Injury[58,60]

Flash-to-bang method	• An observer begins counting when a lightning flash is sighted. • Counting is stopped when the associated bang (thunder) is heard. • Divide this count by 5 to determine the distance to the lightning flash (in miles). For example, a flash-to-bang count of 30 seconds equates to a distance of 6 mi (9.66 km).
The "30–30 rule"	• Easy to remember and applies to the warning time before the storm and the time that should be waited before resumption of activities. • If the time delay between seeing the flash (lightning) and hearing the bang (thunder) is less than 30 seconds, all individuals should be in or seeking a safer location.[62]

Lighting detection methods have been developed to warn of pending strikes; however, these may prove to be inaccurate and may give both athletes and staff a false sense of security.[57] Several different methods are currently being used in the sports medicine setting to detect lighting. Inexpensive handheld lightning detectors have become widely accessible in recent years and claim to prevent lightning injuries and deaths by tracking the speed and paths of thunderstorms.[59] Unfortunately, the performance of most handheld lightning detection products has not been independently or objectively verified.[57] In addition to the questionable reliability of these devices, there is evidence that handheld lightning detectors do not trace lightning accurately, do not detect weak and/or infrequent strikes, and are used improperly. Handheld lightning detectors may provide a false sense of confidence, as they fail to detect all lightning strikes.[57] This evidence is of major concern, as many athletic trainers who are responsible for the safety of athletes rely heavily if not solely on the handheld lightning detector as their method of detecting lightning strikes. In situations termed "bolts out of the blue," the first lightning strike to an area can directly strike a person. In these situations, handheld lightning detectors are ineffective because the athlete will have no warning before he or she is instantaneously struck.[57]

Several organizations have recommendations for determining the risk of a lightning strike during a thunderstorm. The Lightning Safety Group[58] and the National Athletic Trainers' Association,[60] recommend that handheld lightning detectors should only complement the use of the "flash-to-bang" method or the "30-30 rule" (Table 18.9).[57,58,60] Both methods are based upon a period of 30 seconds or less in which all individuals should already be inside or should immediately seek a safe structure or location.[58,60] The 30-30 rule, or 30-second rule, is a compromise between an inordinately short flash-to-bang count of 10 to 15 seconds and a flash-to-bang count of 50 seconds (or the most conservative rule of all, which is leaving the athletic site at the first sign of lightning activity or sound of thunder).[61] Generally speaking, if an individual can see lightning or hear thunder, he or she is already at risk. Louder or more frequent thunder indicates that lightning activity is approaching, thus increasing the risk for lightning injury or death.[58] Unfortunately, these methods of ranging lightning have limitations primarily related to the difficulty of associating the proper thunder to the corresponding flash. It is probably better to recommend seeking safer shelter when the first lightning is seen or the first thunder heard, or "If you can see it, flee it; if you can hear it, clear it."[58] Regardless of the method used, sound judgment and common sense are the hallmarks of effective lightning-related injury prevention.

Identification of Lightning-Related Injuries

A lightning strike on the field of play or into the stands can result in multiple injuries (Table 18.10). These may result directly from the voltage itself, from the trauma of being

TABLE 18.10   Pathophysiology of Lightning-Related Injuries[59,60,62,64,65]

Permanent sequelae	• Cardiac arrest, respiratory arrest, cyanosis, chest trauma secondary to blast injury, anoxic brain damage (related to delay in resuscitation) • Loss of consciousness, intense headaches, ringing in the ears, dizziness, nausea, vomiting, and other postconcussive symptoms • Seizures, subdural and epidural hematomas, transitory paralysis • Blunt trauma, contusions, fractures, cutaneous burns
Additional findings	• Hyperirritability, sleep disturbances, distractibility, confusion, amnesia, and other short-term memory deficits • Ocular problems (detached retina, blurred vision, hyphemas, fixed and dilated pupils), anterior compartment syndrome, internal organ damage, ruptured tympanic membrane

SKILL 18.7

Procedures for Management of Lightning-Related Injury [60]

Observe the following basic first-aid procedures when treating athletes struck by lightning:

1. Survey the scene for safety. Ongoing thunderstorms may still pose a threat to emergency personnel responding to the situation.
2. Activate the local emergency management system and bring an AED to the location.
3. Move the athlete carefully to a safer location if necessary.

4. Evaluate and treat for apnea and asystole; use AED if needed.
5. Evaluate and treat for hypothermia and shock.
6. Evaluate and treat for fractures.
7. Evaluate and treat for burns.
8. All persons involved in the emergency action plan should maintain current cardiopulmonary resuscitation and first-aid certification.

---

thrown back from the site of contact, or from extreme muscular contractions of various muscle groups in the body.[63] Athletes who have been struck by lightning have various degrees of disruption in many of their organ systems. In many ways, the results of a lightning accident resemble those of an electrical injury. The most immediate and disastrous sequela is cardiac arrest. Lightning acts as a massive direct-current countershock that depolarizes the entire myocardium at once, resulting in ventricular **asystole**.[64]

Lightning delivers a large amount of direct electrical current, often more than a million volts. This can result in respiratory arrest from an insult to the CNS and asystole from the direct current delivered to the cardiac tissue.[63] Resistance to the flow of electricity is graded depending on the type of tissue. The order from least resistance to greatest is as follows:

> Nerve → blood vessels → muscle → skin → tendon → fat → bone

The resistance of skin is affected by moisture, cleanliness, thickness, and vascularity. Since the flow of electrical current is inversely proportional to resistance, those tissues with the least resistance are most prone to serious injury.[62]

The ultimate degree of injury in lightning-related trauma depends on the amount of current, the time of passage, and the resistance of the specific tissue.[59] Although the only acute cause of death from lightning injury is cardiac arrest, the anoxic brain damage that can occur if the person is not rapidly resuscitated can be devastating. Even for the survivor who did not sustain a cardiac arrest, permanent sequelae can include brain injury,[60] among other major complications (Table 18.10). In addition to primary neurological lesions as a direct result of the electrical shock in athletes who have been struck by lightning, neurological lesions secondary to cardiac arrest and consequent falling can occur.[59]

Management of Lightning-Related Injuries

During an active thunderstorm, the athletic trainers may be placing themselves in significant danger of lightning injury, particularly if the athlete is located in a high-risk area

(e.g., mountain top, isolated tree, open field). Because it is relatively unusual for those who survive a lightning strike to have major fractures or internal injuries unless they have suffered a fall or been thrown a distance, the athletic trainer must decide whether evacuation from a high-risk area to an area of lesser risk is warranted; therefore, he or she should not be afraid to move the athlete rapidly if necessary. If the athlete is not breathing or has no pulse, normal advanced cardiac life support protocols should be followed. If it is decided to move the athlete, a few quick breaths should be administered before the person is moved. In situations that are cold and wet, putting a protective layer between the athlete and the ground may decrease hypothermia, which can further complicate resuscitation.[58,65]

It is most important to realize that people injured by lightning can recover fully after being apneic and asystolic if they are resuscitated and supported (Skill 18.7).[63,65] If the athlete's respiratory status can be supported, often the CNS will recover and reinitiate respiration. If the circulatory system can be supported with cardiopulmonary resuscitation, the intrinsic electrical activity of the heart may restart organized cardiac contractions. It is often said that triage principles are reversed in the case of lightning injuries, as those who appear dead with no respirations or pulse are the ones who are treated aggressively first.[63] Most athletes survive their encounter with lightning, especially with timely medical treatment. Individuals struck by lightning do not carry a charge, and it is safe to touch them to render medical treatment. Although the proximate cause of death is cardiac arrest at the time of the strike, anyone who has signs of life is highly likely to survive. Fixed, dilated pupils should not be used to establish death.[58] The prehospital care provided by the athletic trainer in the field can save the life of an athlete. All lightning-related injuries should be treated as medical emergencies by activating EMS and rendering care immediately.

WRAP-UP

Environmental illnesses and injuries are preventable, but the athletic trainer must be prepared to recognize, care for, and manage environmental emergencies. Exertional heat

Scenarios

1. Jameel, a 16-year-old African American football player, is carried into your athletic training clinic by his coaches. The coaches explain that they were conducting preseason conditioning drills outside, on the artificial turf, when Jameel collapsed. Since this was only the third day of conditioning after the summer break, the coaches were pushing him hard throughout the drills. When he collapsed, they knew that they had to bring him to you. He is semiconscious now with intervals of stupor and combativeness; he is sweating and breathing heavily.

   Based on Jameel's presentation and your initial physical exam, what conditions would you include in your differential diagnosis? Why? What steps will you take in managing Jameel's condition? What are the return-to-play criteria for Jameel?

2. You are covering a track-and-field meet on a sunny late spring afternoon. During the last event of the meet, an athlete limps toward you holding his hamstring and complains of a painful muscle cramp.

   What condition do you suspect? Why? What steps will you take in managing the athlete's condition?

3. You are traveling with your track team to Colorado Springs. On the first day of training, a long-distance runner approaches you out of breath and complaining of a headache and light-headedness that he first noticed starting the night before.

   What condition do you suspect the athlete has? What steps will you take in managing this condition?

4. You are the head athletic trainer covering a home soccer game. As the game starts, you notice large dark clouds coming toward the field. As the storm comes closer, you see lightning and, 15 seconds later, you hear thunder.

   Based on the 30-30 rule, how far away is the lightning? What steps will you take to alert the officials and evacuate the field? What emergency situations must you be prepared to handle?

illnesses such as heat stroke or an environmental emergency such as a lightning strike can create a unique challenge for the athletic trainer in that rapid identification and management can save a life. The athletic trainer must be vigilant in preventing environmental emergencies and stay current with the best evidence so he or she can implement appropriate management strategies when caring for athletes with environmental illnesses or injuries.

REFERENCES

1. Armstrong LE, ed. *Exertional Heat Illness.* Champaign, IL: Human Kinetics; 2003.
2. Noakes TD, Myburgh KH, Plessis JD, et al. Metabolic rate, not percent dehydration, predicts rectal temperature in runners. *Med Sci Sports Exerc.* 1991;23:443–449.
3. Powers SK, Howley ET. *Exercise Physiology: Theory and Application to Fitness and Performance,* 5th ed. New York: McGraw-Hill; 2004.
4. Laughlin MH, Korthius R. Control of muscle blood flow during sustained physiological exercise. *Can J Appl Sport Sci.* 1987;S-12:775–835.
5. Hancock PA, Vasmatzidis I. Effects of heat stress on cognitive performance: The current state of knowledge. *Int J Hyperthermia.* 2003;19:355–372.
6. Binkley HM, Beckett J, Casa DJ, et al. National Athletic Trainers' Association Position Statement: Exertional Heat Illnesses. *J Athl Train.* 2002;37(3):329–343.
7. McLellan TM. The importance of aerobic fitness in determining tolerance to uncompensable heat stress. *Comp Biochem Physiol.* 2001;128:691–700.
8. Cheung SS, McLellan TM. Comparison of short-term aerobic training and high maximal aerobic power tolerance to uncompensable heat stress. *Aviat Space Environ Med.* 1999; 70:637–643.
9. Nielsen B, Hales JR, Strange S, et al. Human circulatory and thermoregulatory adaptations with heat acclimation and exercise in a hot, dry environment. *J Physiol.* 1993;460:467–485.
10. Roberts WO. Exertional heat stroke: Life-saving recognition and onsite treatment in athletic settings. *Rev Bras Med Esporte.* 2005;11(6):329e–332e.
11. Knochel JP, Reed G. Disorders of heat regulation. In: Narins RG, ed. *Maxwell & Kleeman's Clinical Disorders of Fluid and Electrolyte Metabolism,* 5th ed. New York: McGraw-Hill; 1994:1549–1590.
12. Casa DJ. Exercise in the heat. II. Critical concepts in rehydration, exertional heat illnesses, and maximizing athletic performance. *J Athl Train.* 1999;34(3):253–262.
13. Armstrong LE, Epstein Y, Greenleaf JE, et al. American College of Sports Medicine position stand: Heat and cold illnesses during distance running. *Med Sci Sports Exerc.* 1996;28(12):i–x.
14. Armstrong LE, Maresh CM. The exertional heat illnesses: A risk of athletic participation. *Med Exerc Nutr Health.* 1993;2:125–134.
15. Casa DJ, Roberts WO. Considerations for the medical staff in preventing, identifying, and treating exertional heat illnesses. In: Armstrong LE, ed. *Exertional Heat Illnesses.* Champaign, IL: Human Kinetics; 2003:169–195.
16. Casa DJ, Armstrong LE. Heatstroke: a medical emergency. In: Armstrong LE, ed. *Exertional Heat Illnesses.* Champaign, IL: Human Kinetics; 2003:29–56.
17. Bouchama A, Knochel JP. Heat Stroke. *N Engl J Med.* 2002; 346(25):1978–1988.
18. McDermott BP, Casa DJ, Yeargin SW, et al. Recovery and return to activity following exertional heat stroke: Considerations for the sports medicine staff. *J Sports Rehabil.* 2007;16: 163–181.
19. Armstrong LE, Lopez RM. Return to exercise training after heat exhaustion. *J Sport Rehabil.* 2007;16:182–189.
20. Casa DJ, Almquist J, Anderson S, et al. Inter-Association Task Force on Exertional Heat Illness consensus statement. *NATA News.* 2003;6:24–29.

21. Casa, DJ, Armstrong LE, Ganio MS, et al. Exertional heat stroke in competitive athletes. *Curr Sports Med Rep.* 2005;4:309–317.

22. Parisi L, Pierelli F, Amabile G, et al. Muscular cramps: proposals for a new classification. *Acta Neurol Scand.* 2003;107:176–186.

23. Bergeron MF. Exertional heat cramps. In: Armstrong LE, ed. *Exertional Heat Illnesses.* Champaign, IL: Human Kinetics; 2003:91–102.

24. Jung AP, Bishop PA, Al Nawwas A, et al. Influence of hydration and electrolyte supplementation on incidence and time to onset of exercise-associated muscle cramps. *J Athl Train.* 2005;40:71–75.

25. Stofan JR, Zachwieja JJ, Horswill CA, et al. Sweat and sodium losses in NCAA football players: A precursor to heat cramps? *Int J Sport Nutr Exerc Metab.* 2005;15:641–652.

26. Sulzer NU, Schwellnus MP, Noakes TD. Serum electrolytes in Ironman triathletes with exercise-associated muscle cramping. *Med Sci Sports Exerc.* 2005;37(7):1081–1085.

27. Maughan RJ. Exercise-induced muscle cramp: A prospective biomechanical study in marathon runners. *J Sport Sci.* 1985;4:31–34.

28. Bergeron MF, McKeag DB, Casa DJ, et al. Youth football: Heat stress and injury risk. *Med Sci Sports Exerc.* 2005;37:1421–1430.

29. Bergeron MF. Heat cramps: Fluid and electrolyte challenges during tennis in the heat. *J Sci Med Sport.* 2003;6:19–27.

30. Bergeron MF. Heat cramps during tennis: A case report. *Int J Sport Nutr.* 1996;6:62–68.

31. Cleary MA, Casa DJ. Hyponatremia: Considerations for the athletic trainer. Featured article. *Athl Ther Today.* 2005;10:61–66.

32. Speedy DB, Noakes TD, Kimber NE, et al. Fluid balance during and after and Ironman triathalon. *Clin J Sport Med.* 2001;11:44–50.

33. Garigan TP, Ristedt DE. Death from hyponatremia as a result of acute water intoxication in an Army basic trainee. *Mil Med.* 1999;3:234–238.

34. McArdle WD, Katch FI, Katch VL. *Essentials of Exercise Physiology,* 2nd ed. Philadelphia: Lippincott Williams & Wilkins; 2000.

35. Castellani JW, Young AJ, Ducharme MB, et al. American College of Sports Medicine position stand: Prevention of cold injuries during exercise. *Med Sci Sports Exerc.* 2006;38:2012–2029.

36. Department of the Army. Prevention and management of cold-weather injuries. Washington, DC: Department of the Army, Technical Medicine Bulletin; 2005:1–94. From: http://www.usariem.army.mil/depcold/coldapd.htm. Accessed September 25, 2007.

37. Danzl DF, Pozos RS. Accidental hypothermia. *N Engl J Med.* 1994;331:1756–1760.

38. State of Alaska. *Cold Injuries Guidelines.* Juneau, AK: Section of Community Health and EMS; 2003.

39. Gilbert M, Busund R, Skagseth A, et al. Resuscitation from accidental hypothermia of 13.7°C with circulatory arrest. *Lancet.* 2000;355:375–376.

40. Quayle RQ, Steadman RG. The Steadman wind chill: An improvement over present scales. *Am Meteorological Soc.* 1998;13:1187–1193.

41. Biem J, Koehncke N, Classen D, et al. Out of the cold: Management of hypothermia and frostbite. *Can Med Assoc J.* 2003;168:305–311.

42. Brugger H, Durrer B, Adler-Kastner L, et al. Field management of avalanche victims. *Resuscitation.* 2001;51:7–15.

43. Rennie DW. Tissue heat transfer in water: Lessons from the Korean divers. *Med Sci Sports Exerc.* 1988;20:S177–S184.

44. Auerbach PS. Some people are dead when they're cold and dead. *JAMA.* 1990;264:1856–1857.

45. Kober A, Scheck T, Fulesdi B, et al. Effectiveness of resistive heating compared with passive warming in treating hypothermia associated with minor trauma: A randomized trial. *Mayo Clin Proc.* 2001;76:369–375.

46. Steele MT, Nelson MJ, Sessler DI, et al. Forced air speeds rewarming in accidental hypothermia. *Ann Emerg Med.* 1996;27:479–484.

47. Armstrong LE, Epstein Y, Greenleaf JE, et al. American College of Sports Medicine position stand: Heat and cold illnesses during distance running. *Med Sci Sports Exerc.* 1996;28(12):i–x.

48. Hackett PH, Roach RC. High-altitude illness. *N Engl J Med.* 2001;12(2):107–114.

49. Barry PW, Pollard AJ. Altitude illness. *Br Med J.* 2003;326;915–919.

50. Weil WM, Glassner PJ, Bosco JA. High-altitude illness and muscle physiology. *Bull Hosp Jt Dis.* 2007;65(1):72–77.

51. West JB. The physiologic basis of high-altitude diseases. *Ann Intern Med.* 2004;141:789–800.

52. Rodway GW, Hoffman LA, Sanders MH. High-altitude-related disorders–Part I: Pathophysiology, differential diagnosis, and treatment. Heart Lung. 2003;32(6):353–359.

53. McGuire NM. Monitoring in the field. *Br J Anesthesia.* 2006;97(1):46–56.

54. Gamow bag. Wikipedia.org. From http://en.wikipedia.org/wiki/Gamow_bag. Accessed September 28, 2007.

55. Cooper MA. Medical aspects of lightning. National Weather Service. http://www.lightningsafety.noaa.gov/medical.htm. Accessed September 28, 2007.

56. López RE, Holle RL. Demographics of lightning casualties. *Semin Neurol.* 1995;15(3):286–295.

57. Roeder WP, Vavrek RJ, Lushine JB. Lightning Safety for Schools: An update. 10th Symposium on Education. *Am Meteorological Soc.* 2001. From: http://www.lightningsafety.noaa.gov/pdfs/LSSchools.pdf. Accessed on September 29, 2007.

58. Zimmermann C, Cooper MA, Holle RL. Lightning safety guidelines. *Ann Emerg Med.* 2002;39(6):660–665.

59. Cherington M. Lightning injuries. *Ann Emerg Med.* 1995;25:4.

60. Walsh KM, Bennett B, Cooper MA, et al. National Athletic Trainers' Association position statement: Lightning safety for athletics and recreation. *J Athl Train.* 2000;35:471–477.

61. Bennett BL. A model lightning safety policy for athletics. *J Athl Train.* 1997;32(3):251–253.

62. Cwinn AA, Cantrill SV. Lightning injuries. *J Emerg Med.* 1985;2:379–388.

63. Delaney JS, Drummond R. Mass casualties and triage at a sporting event. *Br J Sports Med.* 2002;36:85–88.

64. Clore ER, House MA. Prevention and treatment of lightning injuries. *Nurse Pract.* 1987;12:37–45.

65. Cooper MA. Emergent care of lightning and electrical injuries. *Semin Neurol.* 1995;15:268–278.

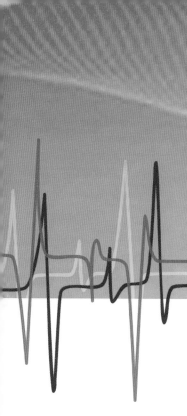

CHAPTER 19

General Medical/ Sudden Illness

CHAPTER OUTCOMES

1. Identify the two major classifications of diabetes mellitus.

2. Recognize the signs, symptoms, and complications of diabetes mellitus.

3. Identify the appropriate blood glucose levels in a diabetic individual.

4. Recognize the rationale for blood glucose and urine monitoring.

5. Recognize and manage the complications of diabetes, which include ketones, hyperglycemia and hypoglycemia, and hyperosmolar hyperglycemic nonketotic syndrome.

6. Identify and recognize the different types of seizures.

7. Explain how to properly care for and manage an individual who is suffering from a seizure attack.

8. Identify and recognize the different types of stroke and their management.

9. Identify a transient ischemic attack as well as dizziness, syncope, and presyncope conditions; also outline their causes and management.

NOMENCLATURE

Aneurysms: a ballooning or widening of a portion of an artery, which can cause it to rupture

Autoimmune: the failure of the body to recognize its own *self*, resulting in an immune response against its own cells and tissues

Electroencephalogram: a recording of the ongoing electrical activity in the brain

Embolus: something that travels through the bloodstream and becomes lodged in a vessel to block it

Endolymph: fluid in the labyrinth of the inner ear

Gestational diabetes: high blood glucose seen in women during pregnancy

Glycosylated hemoglobin (HbA1c): the average plasma glucose concentration over a long period of time

Hyperglycemia: high blood sugar or glucose

Hypoglycemia: low blood sugar or glucose

Insulin: hormone produced by the pancreas to facilitate the uptake of glucose into cells

Kussmaul breathing: an abnormal deep breathing pattern seen in individuals with metabolic acidosis

NOMENCLATURE *(Continued)*

Polydipsia: increased thirst

Polyphagia: increased hunger

Polyuria: frequent urination

Postprandial: after eating a meal

Thrombosis: formation of a clot within a blood vessel

Type 1 diabetes: an autoimmune disease that destroys the insulin-producing beta cells of the pancreas

Type 2 diabetes: the most common form of diabetes, in which the body does not produce enough insulin or there is insulin resistance

Vertigo: a sensation of spinning or swaying while the body is stationary

BEFORE YOU BEGIN

1. Why is it important to monitor the glucose values of an athlete?

2. What are some signs and symptoms of hypoglycemia, and how would you conduct the medical management of a hypoglycemic athlete?

3. Describe the appropriate steps when managing a person suffering from a seizure attack.

4. Describe some conditions that may cause an athlete to experience dizziness or have fainting spells.

5. What sources can you identify that will provide information about the care and treatment of stroke?

Voices from the Field

Successful management of sudden illness requires a rapid and sound response. The athletic trainer must be able to recognize the signs and symptoms of life-threatening injuries or those that may result in permanent impairment so that the appropriate care can be administered without delay. A thorough understanding of the etiology of the illness will help the certified athletic trainer understand the relevant signs and symptoms and the progression of the illness leading to a medical emergency. Sudden illnesses like stroke may offer a sign, such as a transient ischemic attack, which is a warning to the informed athletic trainer that a major stroke is likely. With diabetic emergencies, it is not enough to know the consequences of the illness but also the more sudden onset of illness that occurs when the condition is mistreated with too much insulin. Recognition of the signs of insulin shock will lead the certified athletic trainer to a course of sugar ingestion that will provide drastic recovery.

It is crucial that these important skills for the recognition and management of sudden illness are taught by both faculty and clinical instructors and understood by students in athletic training education programs. All competencies and proficiencies are important, but those dealing with sudden illnesses that are potentially life threatening should be emphasized. To provide this crucial care under tremendous pressure, certified athletic trainers must work with great confidence. Gaining this confidence begins in the classroom with this textbook but must continue with guided clinical experiences where the student is allowed to become gradually more involved in emergency care under the watchful eye of an approved clinical instructor.

Bill Holcomb, PhD, ATC, LAT, CSCS*D
Associate Professor
Department of Kinesiology
University of Nevada, Las Vegas

DIABETES

According to the American Diabetes Association, approximately 20.8 million individuals in the United States have diabetes, but approximately 6.2 million are not aware that they have this condition.[1] Of the two major types of diabetes, approximately 5% to 10% individuals diagnosed have **type 1 diabetes** with the majority of the remaining individuals having **type 2 diabetes.** During pregnancy, women can develop **gestational diabetes,** which affects roughly 135,000 individuals (or 4% of pregnant women) each year.[1] Gestational diabetes is a temporary form of insulin resistance that occurs during pregnancy during the second and possibly the third trimester. In most cases, women who develop gestational diabetes have no history of diabetes. Women diagnosed with gestational diabetes have an increased risk of developing type 2 diabetes.[1]

A revised classification system, based upon glucose values, has been developed to identify individuals at risk for diabetes, called prediabetes. Prediabetes is defined as blood glucose levels higher than normal but not high enough for a diagnosis of type 2 diabetes. It has been estimated that 57 million individuals have prediabetes, beyond the more than 20 million with diabetes.[1]

TABLE 19.1 Blood Glucose Values for Adults

Glucose Test	Glucose Values
HbA1c	<7.0%
Preprandial glucose (before a meal)	90 to 130 mg/dL (5.0 to 7.2 mmol/L)
Postprandial glucose (after a meal)	<180 mg/dL (<10.0 mmol/L)

Diabetes is a condition in which the body cannot regulate blood glucose or "blood sugar." There are several mechanisms for this, ranging from beta-cell destruction in the pancreas to cellular insulin resistance. In type 1 diabetes, the body fails to produce **insulin** because of an **autoimmune** pathology, resulting in the destruction of beta cells.[2] This limits the effectiveness of food metabolism so that exogenous insulin is required to sustain life.

Type 2 diabetes can occur at any age, including adolescence. It is increasing in prevalence recently, usually affecting older individuals. Type 2 diabetes stems from insulin resistance or failure of the pancreas to produce enough insulin.[3–6] With insulin resistance, tissues do not readily absorb glucose, and levels of glucose in the bloodstream begin to rise, creating the condition called **hyperglycemia.** In a person with prediabetes, the level of hyperglycemia gradually increases, so that such individuals rarely notice symptoms before the disease becomes obvious.[1,7,8] Most individuals with type 2 diabetes are obese, and obesity has been shown to correlate with some form of insulin resistance.[9] A strong genetic link may also be associated with type 1 diabetes.

Blood Glucose and Urine Monitoring

Diabetics are encouraged to monitor their blood glucose levels on a regular basis, regardless of how they are classified, to help prevent complications such as nerve, kidney, eye, and blood vessel damage. Glucose levels, under normal conditions, are 90 to 130 mg/dL (Table 19.1). For normal individuals, 2-hour **postprandial** (after meals) glucose concentrations should be below 180 mg/dL.

To determine whether an individual has diabetes, a fasting plasma glucose test is recommended, especially if signs and symptoms of diabetes are observed, by using self-monitored blood glucose (SMBG) equipment (Fig. 19.1 and Skill 19.1). Although most diabetics use SMBG equipment, clinicians and physicians usually assess glucose concentrations over time using **glycosylated hemoglobin** (HbA1c) levels. HbA1c is an indicator of average glycemic control for a period of 2 to 3 months. Normal HbA1c values for a nondiabetic individual range from 4% to 6%. HbA1c is the preferred test because it is least affected by daily fluctuations in blood glucose.[10]

The values obtained during routine monitoring serve as a guide for the athlete on how their condition is being controlled. Over time, the athlete with diabetes will become more aware of how foods and exercise affect glucose levels. The records of glucose monitoring should be shared not only with the athletic trainer but also with the athlete's primary care physician on a regular basis. In addition, alterations or values that are out of the ordinary should be reported to the physician for treatment strategies.

Ketones

The metabolism of fatty acids produces a by-product called ketones. Without adequate insulin, fatty acids are metabolized and used by the cells as an alternate energy source instead of glucose. As ketones accumulate in the blood, the blood becomes more acidic, resulting in ketoacidosis. Although ketoacidosis gradually develops over time, moderate or large amounts of ketones can be harmful for the body, possibly leading to coma and death. Testing for ketones is a simple process, using specialized strips that are placed in the urine (Skill 19.2). Ketones should be checked whenever blood glucose is more than 240 mg/dL or when the person is sick from a cold or flu. One should never exercise when large amounts of ketones are present or when blood glucose is high because the body then has a more difficult time using available glucose energy sources.

Signs and symptoms of ketoacidosis include hyperglycemia, thirst, excess urination, fatigue, blurred vision, nausea, muscular stiffness, flushed face, dry skin and mouth, a rapid and weak pulse, and low blood pressure. Athletes may also experience respirations that are deep and sighing in order to blow out excess ketones. This respiration technique is often called **Kussmaul breathing** and the breath often has a fruity odor.

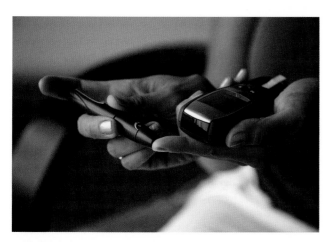

FIGURE 19.1   Example of equipment for the self-monitoring of blood glucose.

SKILL 19.1

Testing for Blood Glucose

Be sure to follow the manufacturer's guidelines when using SMBG equipment.

1. Select a blood glucose meter that is suitable to your needs.
2. Wash hands, forearms, or thigh (depending upon meter used) thoroughly; use an alcohol prep as a final cleaning step.
3. Use the lancet (or spring-loaded device) to obtain a drop of blood; wipe away the first drop of blood.

4. Stick the side of your fingertip by your fingernail.
5. Place drop of blood on the testing strip.
6. Place testing strip into the meter.
7. After a few seconds, a readout will appear, providing a blood glucose reading.

Hypoglycemia

Hypoglycemia is a condition of low blood sugar that is potentially life threatening. Usually, hypoglycemia is caused by excess amounts of insulin, skipping meals, or exercising excessively. In most cases, blood glucose levels below 50 mg/dL are considered to be associated with hypoglycemia. Signs and symptoms of hypoglycemia can occur suddenly. Therefore, it is very important to monitor an individual who has diabetes.

Treatment of Hypoglycemia

To avoid hypoglycemia, athletes should monitor their glucose levels regularly, eat snacks if necessary, and learn glucose responses to food and exercise. In addition, all insulin-dependent athletes should carry at least 15 to 20 g of carbohydrates (such as glucose tablets—up to three of them, or glucose gel), ½ cup of fruit juice, table sugar, ½ cup of low-fat milk, or other forms of carbohydrate (Skill 19.3). After ingesting glucose of any type, the athlete should wait for approximately 15 or 20 minutes and then check blood glucose again. If the blood glucose is still low or symptoms of hypoglycemia persist, more glucose must be consumed.

In severe cases, an athlete can lose consciousness from low blood sugar (insulin shock). This occurs when there is too much insulin or not enough glucose (hypoglycemia) or both. Signs and symptoms of insulin shock include tremors, lack of coordination, and changes in level of consciousness. If the athlete loses consciousness, immediate medical treat-

ment is indicated (Skill 19.4). One particular measure to increase glucose levels is the injection of glucagon, a treatment that must be prescribed by a physician, who will also instruct the athlete how to use it. Glucagon should also be readily available for people with diabetes and their family members, friends, and athletic trainers who work with them. Each member should be instructed on the indications and administration of glucagon if needed.

In some instances, an athlete may experience hypoglycemic unawareness. In this condition, athletes may lose consciousness unexpectedly. Although not common, this usually affects diabetics who have had the disease for many years, those who suffer neuropathy, those who control their glucose within a very limited range, or those who are taking certain heart or blood pressure medications.

Hyperglycemia

Hyperglycemia (high blood sugar) occurs when there is not enough insulin in the body or when the body cannot effectively utilize insulin. It can occur in athletes with either type 1 or 2 diabetes, even in the presence of insulin. The signs and symptoms of hyperglycemia include elevated blood glucose, glucose in the urine, frequent urination **(polyuria),** increased thirst **(polydipsia),** increased appetite **(polyphagia),** and warm dry skin. Hyperglycemia can lead to ketoacidosis (diabetic coma) because the body cannot use glucose and instead relies on fats for energy (as mentioned in the discussion of ketones, above). If the athlete does experience ketoacidosis, immediate medical referral is necessary.

SKILL 19.2

Testing for Ketones

1. Use a clean container to sample urine.
2. Purchase ketone strips.
3. Place the strip in the container of urine (can pass the strip through the urine stream).
4. Shake excess urine off the strip.

5. Wait for the strip to change color (instructions included with the strips will indicate the duration).
6. Compare the color of the strip with the color chart on the strip bottle/container.

Signs & Symptoms

Hypoglycemia

- General weakness
- Drowsiness
- Confusion
- Dizziness
- Hunger
- Headaches
- Irritability
- Sweating (cool and moist skin)
- Dilated pupils
- Possible tachycardia
- Possible loss of consciousness
- Seizures
- Possible coma

Treatment of Hyperglycemia

Hyperglycemia can be treated in various ways: by diet, exercise, and the use of oral hyperglycemic agents. During and after exercise, skeletal muscle cells can readily take up glucose without the presence of insulin. This uptake can last as long as 10 to 12 hours after exercise. However, exercise should be delayed when glucose levels exceed 240 mg/dL because high glucose levels indicate insulin deficiency and the possible presence of ketones. Conversely, athletes who have normal glucose levels prior to exercise increase their chance of developing hypoglycemia. Those with normal glucose levels should be instructed to ingest 10 to 20 g of carbohydrates prior to exercise or to decrease the dose of insulin (if on insulin therapy) or oral hyperglycemic agents to prevent hypoglycemia. Although hyperglycemia is not life threatening, the condition should be treated appropriately (Skill 19.5). Therefore, regular communication and referral, as appropriate, to a physician is required in the management of athletes with diabetes.

If insulin is required and the athlete is physically able to administer it, help him or her with the procedure. Injection sites vary, but usually include the arms, thighs, abdomen, or buttocks. If the athlete has a prefilled insulin pen, follow same procedures for insulin injection but omit the drawing up of the insulin from the vial (first 3 steps in Skill 19.6). An athlete may have an insulin pump, which are prefilled and programmed to deliver insulin on a preset basis. If the athlete should require more insulin, refer to properly trained medical personnel. Procedures to follow when injecting insulin are found in Skill 19.6.

Hyperosmolar Hyperglycemic Nonketotic Syndrome

Hyperosmolar hyperglycemic nonketotic syndrome (HHNS) occurs when the glucose levels in the blood and urinary output increase because the excess glucose is being excreted. Initially, urination is frequent, but it can gradually diminish and change color (grow darker) as a result of dehydration. Although HHNS affects older people, those with type 1 diabetes and type 2 diabetes, it is more frequent in the latter. HHNS may take several days to weeks to fully develop; thereafter, it can lead to seizures, coma, and eventually death. If you suspect that an athlete is experiencing HHNS, immediately refer him or her to the proper medical personnel.

SEIZURES

Seizures stem from sudden, electrical discharges affecting the central nervous system; they may cause changes in behavior. Typically, seizures have three distinct phases—a beginning, middle, and end; however, these phases are dependent upon the person. Usually, at the beginning, many individuals experience a warning sign, or aura, that a seizure is coming. This may include having a partial seizure, headache, feeling of uncertainty, or other symptom. During the middle phase, some symptoms of a partial seizure may escalate to a more complex seizure. A complex seizure is defined as a seizure that affects part of the brain, impairing consciousness or producing a convulsion. The end phase is the period during which the individual's brain transitions back to a normal state, often termed the postictal ("after seizure") stage. Depending upon the severity of the seizure, this phase can last anywhere from a few seconds to hours, during which the individual's awareness of the surroundings will gradually improve.

SKILL 19.3

Treatment of Athletes Suffering from Hypoglycemia (Conscious)

1. Look for Medical Alert tags.
2. Maintain airway, breathing, and circulation.
3. Ask questions about history (food, insulin, oral medications).
4. Treat for shock.
5. Administer oral glucose, milk, fruit juice, or other form of carbohydrate (unless the airway is compromised).
6. Seek medical referral if the condition does not improve.

SKILL 19.4

Treatment of Athletes Suffering from Hypoglycemia (Unconsciousness)

1. Look for Medical Alert tags.
2. *Do not* inject insulin.
3. *Do not* give food or fluids by mouth.
4. Inject glucagon if trained to do so.
5. Maintain airway, breathing, and circulation.
6. Seek medical attention immediately.

SKILL 19.5

Treatment of Hyperglycemia

1. Obtain medical history and vital signs.
2. Check for Medical Alert identifications.
3. Perform a blood glucose check (if applicable to athletic training licensure/state guidelines).
4. Determine if the athlete has taken his or her medications (insulin or oral); if not, such an athlete should be instructed to follow the prescribed medical guidelines.
5. Refer the athlete to medical personnel if medication is required (if none are on hand) or if vital signs become compromised.

SKILL 19.6

Insulin Injection

1. Sterilize the site and the mouth of the vial with an alcohol pad.
2. Roll the insulin vial between the palms of your hands to mix the insulin.
3. Draw the appropriate amount of insulin into the syringe.
4. Pinch up the injection site to create a firm surface.
5. Quickly insert the needle into the site and inject the insulin.
6. Remove the syringe.
7. Release the skinfold.
8. Apply an alcohol swab or gauze/cotton ball to the site to prevent leakage.

Signs & Symptoms

Hyperosmolar Hyperglycemic Nonketotic Syndrome

- Blood glucose more than 600 mg/dL
- Decreased sweating
- Confusion
- Weakness on one side of the body
- Extreme thirst (may disappear over time)
- Fever
- Loss of vision
- Warm dry skin
- Sleepiness
- Hallucinations

Signs & Symptoms

Warning Signs of Possible Seizure

- Dizziness
- Headache
- Nausea
- Smells
- Numbness
- Panic/fear
- Unusual taste
- Visual abnormalities
- Unusual feelings
- Light-headedness
- Tingling
- Sounds

Signs & Symptoms

Seizure

- Confusion
- Convulsions
- Difficulty talking
- Drooling
- Loss of consciousness
- Eyes rolling up
- Incontinence
- Visual abnormalities
- Tremors
- Staring
- Sweating
- Increased heart rate
- Increase respirations
- Biting of the tongue
- Teeth clenching or grinding

Types of Seizures

There are several types of seizures, usually classified as primary generalized and partial seizures. Primary generalized seizures are associated with bilateral electrical discharges in the brain, whereas partial seizures are associated with electrical discharge in one specific area of the brain (Tables 19.2 and 19.3). Diagnosis of the different types of seizures depends upon electrical activity and diagnostic tests, such as the **electroencephalogram** (EEG).

Management of Seizures

In most cases, athletes who suffer from seizures will already have notified their immediate medical staff and athletic trainers of their condition, the medications used, and the proper treatment or precautions. However, there may be instances where seizures occur because of a traumatic brain injury or a severe sports-related injury. If you encounter an individual who is having a seizure, follow the appropriate steps required to ensure the safety and protection of the athlete (Skill 19.7)

TABLE 19.2   Seizures: Primary Generalized Types and Definitions

Absence seizures	Classified as brief episodes of staring (up to 20 seconds); may also be called petit mal. Awareness and responsiveness are impaired and most individuals do not know that they have had a seizure. Seen in children between ages 4 and 14, with 70% of cases resolved by age 18.
Atypical absence seizures	Classified as a seizure lasting less than 20 seconds (range from 5 to 30 seconds) characterized by a stare or associated with blinking or brief automatic movements of the mouth or hands. Begin in childhood, are usually easily controlled with medication, and are outgrown by approximately 75% of children. Most children affected have below-average intelligence as well as other types of seizures.
Myoclonic seizures	Classified as brief, shocklike jerks of a muscle or muscle group. Usually begin during childhood but can occur at any age.
Atonic seizures	Classified as a sudden loss of muscle tone; may cause the head to nod or drop, eyelids may droop, or there may be loss of leg strength (falling down if standing). The individual usually does not lose consciousness. Lasts less than 15 seconds.
Tonic seizures	Classified as an increase in muscle tone with stiffening of the body, arms, or legs. Occur most often during sleep; however, if the individual is standing, he or she will often fall. Usually lasts less than 20 seconds.
Clonic seizures	Classified as rapidly alternating contraction and relaxation of a muscle, which cannot be stopped by restraining or repositioning the arms or legs. These seizures are rare.
Tonic–clonic seizures	Classified as a loss of consciousness, falling, stiffening, and jerking; previously called a grand mal seizure. Individuals may bite the tongue or cheek and may turn blue in the face. Bladder or bowel control may be compromised. Consciousness returns slowly, and the person may be drowsy, confused, agitated, or depressed. Usually lasts from 1 to 3 minutes.

TABLE 19.3   Partial Seizures: Types and Definitions

Simple partial seizures	Classified as seizures that affect a part of the brain without loss of consciousness, usually lasting less than 2 minutes. Classified into subcategories (motor, sensory, autonomic, psychic) depending upon the type of experience.
Complex partial seizures	Classified as seizures that begin in the temporal or frontal lobes and then spread to other brain areas, which can affect alertness or awareness (the person may not be aware that anything happened). May be associated with "automatisms," which are purposeless actions (picking at clothes or the air). Individuals may also repeat words or phrases, laugh, scream, or cry.
Secondarily generalized seizures	Classified as seizure that become generalized (both sides of the brain) after a partial seizure has begun. Can affect people of all ages who have partial seizures.

Epilepsy

Epilepsy is a disorder that is often characterized by transient but recurrent disturbances of brain function, which may or may not result in loss of consciousness or abnormal behavior.[11] Epilepsy is also known as a seizure disorder, since it is a result of excessive discharge of electrical activity within the nervous system, with resultant changes in behavior. However, the term "epilepsy" does not indicate a specific type or degree of severity. It has been estimated that approximately 3 million Americans have been treated for epilepsy during the past 5 years,[12,13] and it seems to affect men more than women. Epilepsy can occur at any age, and it can be controlled with medications in approximately 70% of adolescents and adults who are newly diagnosed. Severe head injury is the most common known cause of epilepsy in young adults; strokes, tumors, and traumatic injuries are more frequent causes in middle-aged adults, although there are other risk factors as well. Management of an individual who is having an epileptic seizure is the same as management of any seizure (see Skill 19.7).

SKILL 19.7

Management of Seizures

1. Remain calm and check for Medical Alert identification (if applicable).
2. Remove potential dangers (equipment, desks, chairs, etc.) surrounding the individual to prevent contact or further harm.
3. Loosen any restrictive clothing.
4. Record the length of time the seizure lasted.
5. Do not restrain the athlete.
6. Do not place anything in the athlete's mouth, including water, medications, food, or anything else during the seizure.
7. If the seizure lasts longer than 5 minutes, contact emergency medical services.
8. After the seizure, place athlete on his or her side (the HAINES position; Fig. 19.2) unless the person is fully alert; this will prevent aspiration in case of vomiting.
9. Maintain the airway and administer oxygen if the athlete is cyanotic.
10. If the athlete suffered any injuries during the seizure, treat accordingly.
11. If there is any suspicion that the athlete's spine may have been damaged during the seizure, immobilize him or her and refer immediately.
12. Be empathetic to the needs and emotions of the athlete and remain with him or her until full recovery.

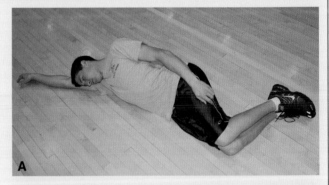

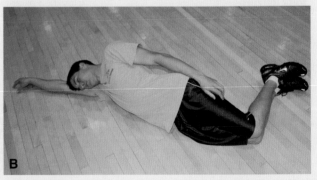

FIGURE 19.2   **A.** HAINES position. **B.** Modified HAINES position.

STROKE

Stroke is the third leading cause of death in the United States and the chief cause of disability in adults.[14] A stroke is a condition in which a blood clot blocks an artery or vessel, interrupting the blood flow to an area within the brain; or there may be an aneurysm that is causing bleeding within the brain and disrupting the brain's blood supply. The diminished or blocked blood flow causes cellular death (ischemia), affecting brain function. Depending upon the region of the brain, normal physiological function can be altered or lost, including speech, body movements, and memory. The extent of injury or loss of function relates to the amount of damage incurred. This can range from a temporary loss of speech and weakness of an arm or leg to permanent paralysis. In most cases, the individual will experience warning signs pointing to the possibility of a stroke.

Types of Strokes

There are several different types of stroke, depending upon how the clot develops or enters the brain. A stroke in which a clot disrupts or clogs the blood supply to the brain is called an ischemic stroke and is further subdivided into two types: embolic and thrombotic. An embolic stroke is caused by a blood clot that forms somewhere in the body (usually the heart) and travels through the bloodstream to the brain (this type of clot is referred to as an **embolus**). A thrombotic stroke is a blockage to one or more of the arteries of the brain **(thrombosis).** These blood clots can happen as the result of fatty deposits and cholesterol in the vessels.

Another type of stroke is called hemorrhagic, which is due to the breakage of a vessel in the brain. This type of stroke is most commonly associated with high blood pressure and cerebral **aneurysms** and is further divided into two categories. A subarachnoid hemorrhage occurs when an aneurysm breaks in a large artery within or near the subarachnoid

Signs & Symptoms

Stroke

- Sudden numbness or weakness of face, arm, or leg
- Sudden confusion
- Trouble speaking
- Visual abnormalities in one or both eyes
- Dizziness
- Loss of balance or coordination
- Headache without a known cause

lining of the brain; an intracerebral hemorrhage or stroke occurs with bleeding from vessels within the brain.

Management of Stroke

If an athlete is experiencing any of the above symptoms or other signs associated with a possible stroke, the athletic trainer or other medical personnel can use the FAST approach (face, arms, speech, and time) to determine if the person is actually experiencing a stroke. To begin, ask the athlete to smile and look for any drooping or other abnormal conditions on one or both sides of the face (face). Ask the athlete to raise and lower both arms and look for unequal or drifting of one arm downward (arms). Ask the athlete to repeat a sentence and look for words that are slurred and for improper recall of a sentence (speech). Finally, if the athlete is experiencing any of these symptoms, refer to a medical facility immediately (time). If a stroke is suspected, immediate medical referral is required so that the athlete may receive proper diagnostic tests and medications to identify and potentially lessen the severity of the stroke.

Transient Ischemic Attack

A transient ischemic attack (TIA) is commonly referred to as a "ministroke." In most cases, TIAs seldom cause permanent brain damage but serve as warning signs of a stroke, indicating that medical referral is needed. It has been estimated that approximately 5% of individuals who suffer from a TIA will have a stroke within 2 days[14,15] and 11% within 90 days. TIAs are most often caused by lack of blood flow to the brain or a clot that blocks blood flow to the brain. Symptoms of a TIA include sudden numbness or weakness of the face, arms, or legs (especially on one side of the body), confusion, difficulty speaking, visual abnormalities, difficulty with walking and balance, and dizziness. Immediate management of a TIA is the same as for stroke; however, once a TIA has been diagnosed, medical therapy and lifestyle changes (diet and exercise) are generally required. In

Breakout

Risk Factors for Epilepsy

- Seizures occurring in the first month of life
- Abnormalities in brain structure at birth
- Serious brain injury or lack of oxygen to the brain
- Infections of the brain (i.e., meningitis)
- Stroke
- Cerebral palsy
- Family history of epilepsy
- Drug use (i.e., cocaine)

the case of an arterial blockage, surgery to open the arteries is usually prescribed.

DIZZINESS

Dizziness is described as light-headedness, feeling faint, and weakness or loss of balance. Dizziness is usually classified into the following categories or groups: (a) vertigo, (b) disequilibrium without vertigo, (c) presyncope, and (d) psychophysiological dizziness.[16,17] **Vertigo** (an illusory sensation of motion or spinning) results from a disruption of the inner ear (vestibular system), which senses movement and changes of head position. It is commonly caused by rapid changes in motion, as in riding on a roller coaster or in a boat, car, or airplane. Dysequilibrium is imbalance without vertigo, whereas presyncope refers to the light-headedness that occurs before fainting (from reduction of blood flow). Psychophysiological dizziness is described as a floating or internal spinning sensation that worsens with feelings of anxiety, stress, or fatigue.

Dizziness associated with vertigo is often diagnosed as benign paroxysmal positional vertigo (BPPV). BPPV is an intense, brief episode of vertigo associated with changes in the position of the head, usually from debris that becomes trapped into the canals of the inner ear.[18] Inflammation of the inner ear (acute vestibular neuronitis or labyrinthitis) can cause vertigo that may persist for several days, often associated with nausea and vomiting. Often, the individual is incapacitated and requires bed rest until the condition clears.

Ménière's disease is an excessive buildup of fluid in the inner ear, characterized by episodes of vertigo lasting 30 minutes to an hour, ringing in the ears (tinnitus), and fluctuating hearing loss.[19,20] The increasing pressure in the semicircular canals is due to increases in the volume of **endolymph,** which can last for hours. Individuals with Ménière's disease usually complain of pressure in the head, headache, nausea, hearing loss, nystagmus, and tinnitus lasting from minutes to hours and usually lie down until the attack subsides. These episodes undermine the person's quality of life.[20] The exact cause of Ménière's disease is still under investigation, but viral and immunologic factors seem to be the most likely suspects.

Breakout

Conditions that May Cause Dizziness
- Noncancerous growths
- Brain tumors
- Alcohol or drug use
- Cardiac Insufficiencies
- TIA
- Low blood pressure
- Hypoglycemia
- Anemia

Treatment of dizziness depends on the causes, symptoms, and severity. In most cases, having the individual sit or lie down until the dizzy spell passes is appropriate; but if symptoms worsen, occur more frequently, or are of unknown or uncertain cause, medical referral is required. For athletes who do have a form of vertigo, vestibular rehabilitation and exercises for postural control and stability are required along with medication.[21]

Syncope and Presyncope

Syncope is a brief loss of consciousness followed by a spontaneous recovery that usually lasts for only a few seconds. Presyncope is defined as feeling faint and light-headed without loss of consciousness. Syncope and presyncope can be caused by a drop in blood pressure (orthostatic hypotension) or hypovolemic conditions, such as blood loss or from dehydration, inadequate output of blood from the heart, loss of balance, inner ear problems, sensory disorders, medications, anxiety, and hyperventilation. Many individuals have warning signs before experiencing syncope. The signs and

Breakout

For further research on diabetes, stroke, or epilepsy, refer to the following Web sites:

The American Diabetes Association
http://www.diabetes.org
Diabetic Journals (Diabetes, Diabetes Care, Clinical Diabetes, and Diabetes Spectrum)
http://www.diabetesjournals.org
International Diabetes Federation
http://www.idf.org
National Stroke Association
http://www.stroke.org
Epilepsy Advocate
http://www.epilepsyadvocate.com/
Cleveland Clinic
http://www.clevelandclinic.org/

Signs & Symptoms

Dizziness

- Spinning or moving (vertigo)
- A loss of balance
- Nausea
- Light-headedness
- Faintness
- Weakness
- Blurred vision after quick head movements

Scenarios

1. One of your soccer players, standing on the sideline during practice, becomes disoriented and falls to the ground. This player has a medical history of seizure activity and is on medication to control the frequency and severity of such events, although she will have an episode from time to time. Because you already know about her medical history, you are aware of her condition; however, you have never seen her have an episode and you have no experience with seizure management.

   Because the athlete has already collapsed to the ground and is beginning her seizure episode, what would you do at this point?

2. During a district wrestling meet at your high school, a wrestler become unresponsive while waiting for his match. A team member approaches you, informing you of the wrestler's condition, and both of you quickly respond. As you approach, you see him sitting with his head and back against a wall. He is dazed and confused and answers your questions with long delays. You notice that he has cool, moist skin, dilated pupils, and a fast heart rate. The team member informs you that the wrestler is diabetic but does not know when he last ate or took insulin.

   What do you do?

3. An elderly athlete is performing his rehabilitation in your clinic. He suddenly starts to feel uncoordinated, has some trouble speaking, and feels ill. His rehabilitation activity at the time was Thera-Band arm curls, so you rule out exertional illnesses. Taking into account his age, you suspect a possible cerebrovascular accident.

   What is a quick way to access any cerebrovascular accident? What should you do for this athlete?

4. A cross-country athlete begins to feel dizzy after a run. You provide fluids, monitor her activity, and keep her relaxed. After about 10 minutes, she feels better, with no symptoms of dizziness. During the next several practices, she suffers from the same response after running. Vital signs appear to be normal, but you cannot find other conditions/symptoms to help you to determine the cause.

   What could be her condition and what should you do?

---

symptoms are very similar to dizziness but will also include chest palpitations, tachycardia, bradycardia, headache, lightheadedness, nausea, weakness, and sweating. Management of syncope and presyncope is the same for anyone experiencing dizziness. If an individual suffers from syncope, especially before, during, or after exercise, medical referral is warranted.

WRAP-UP

This chapter is intended as an introduction of common general medical conditions or illnesses that may be encountered in the career of the athletic trainer and that may require emergency medical management. In these events, immediate recognition of the signs and symptoms and prompt referral may lessen the severity of such episodes.

REFERENCES

1. American Diabetes Association http://www.diabetes.org/main/application/commercewf. Accessed October 17, 2009.
2. Atkinson MA, Maclaren NK. The pathogenesis of insulin dependent diabetes. *N Engl J Med*. 1994;331:1428–1436.
3. DeFronzo RA, Sherwin RS, Kraemer N. Effect of physical training on insulin action in obesity. *Diabetes*. 1987;36:1379–1385.
4. Reaven GM, Bernstein R, Davis B, et al. Nonketotic diabetes mellitus: Insulin deficiency or insulin resistance? *Am J Med*. 1976;60:80–88.
5. Rice B, Janssen I, Hudson R, et al. Effects of aerobic or resistance exercise and/or diet on glucose tolerance and plasma insulin levels in obese men. *Diabetes Care*. 1999;22(5):684–691.
6. Wing RR, Blair EH, Bononi P, et al. Caloric restriction per se is a significant factor in improvements in glycemic control and insulin sensitivity during weight loss in obese NIDDM patients. *Diabetes Care*. 1994;17:30–36.
7. Fujimoto WY, Leonetti DL, Kinyoun JL, et al. Prevalence of complications among second-generation Japanese-American men with diabetes, impaired glucose tolerance or normal glucose tolerance. *Diabetes*. 1987;36:730–739.
8. Harris MI. Impaired glucose tolerance in the U.S. population. *Diabetes Care*. 1989;12:464–474.
9. Bogardus C, Lillioja S, Mott DM, et al. Relationship between degree of obesity and in vivo insulin action in man. *Am J Physiol*. 1985;248:E286–E291.
10. Bunn HF. Nonenzymatic glycosylation of protein: Relevance to diabetes. *Am J Med*. 1981;70:325–330.
11. Engel J. A proposed diagnostic scheme for people with epileptic seizures and with epilepsy: Report of the ILAE Task Force on classification and terminology. *Epilepsia*. 2001;42(6):796–803.
12. Epilepsy Foundation. Epilepsy and Seizure Statistics. http://www.epilepsyfoundation.org/about/statistics.cfm. Accessed May 12, 2010.

13. Epilepsy.com. Homepage. Available at http://www.epilepsy. com. Accessed May 12, 2010.

14. National Stroke Association. Homepage. http://www.stroke. org/. Accessed May 12, 2010.

15. National Stroke Association. Stroke Rapid Response™ Prehospital Education Training. http://www.stroke.org/site/ PageServer?pagename=EMS. Accessed May 12, 2010.

16. Dieterich M. Dizziness. *Neurologist.* 2004;10:154–164.

17. Karatas M. Central vertigo and dizziness: Epidemiology, differential diagnosis, and common causes. *Neurologist.* 2008; 14(6):355–364.

18. Bhattacharyya N, Baugh RF, Orvidas L, et al. Clinical practice guideline: Benign paroxysmal positional vertigo. *Otolaryngol Head Neck Surg.* 2008;139:S47–S81.

19. Hanley K, O'Dowd T, Considine N. A systematic review of vertigo in primary care. *Br J Gen Pract.* 2001;51:666–671.

20. Gates GA. Ménière's disease review 2005. *J Am Acad Audiol.* 2006;17:16–26.

21. Mira E. Improving the quality of life in patients with vestibular disorders: The role of medical treatments and physical rehabilitation. *Int J Clin Pract.* 2008;62:(1): 109–114.

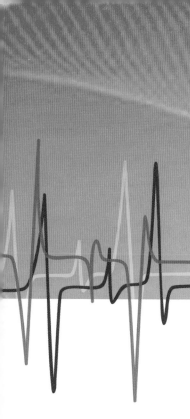

CHAPTER · 20

Allergic Reactions and Poisons

CHAPTER OUTCOMES

1. Identify the basic principles of how an allergen causes an allergic reaction.
2. Identify some of the common causes of allergies and allergic reactions by the body.
3. Provide an example of an appropriate emergency management response to someone suffering from anaphylaxis.
4. Identify the step-by-step procedures for epinephrine administration.
5. Identify the different types of poisons obtained from plant contact and how to provide proper management for adverse reactions.
6. Identify the signs and symptoms of common insect, scorpion, and spider bites and stings and understand how to provide appropriate first-aid management to individuals who suffer from allergic reactions.
7. Identify the causes and management steps for individuals suffering from exercise-induced anaphylaxis.
8. Describe and identify allergic reactions to latex in the athletic training setting.
9. Describe how to manage individuals who are having breathing difficulties caused by asthma.
10. Describe the steps involved in using asthma inhalers to treat the restriction of airflow caused by asthma.
11. Identify the types of medications used when treating and managing asthma.
12. Identify the four types of poisons (injection, inhaled, absorbed, ingested), their signs and symptoms, and their proper management.

NOMENCLATURE

Activated charcoal: an odorless, tasteless, nontoxic black powder that, when ingested, absorbs almost any toxic substance or poison

Allergen: a substance (bacteria, chemical, food, drug, etc.) that can cause an allergic reaction

Allergic reaction: a response, ranging from itchiness to a life-threatening condition, by the body's immune system to an allergen

Anaphylaxis: a serious allergic reaction to an allergen

Angioedema: swelling underneath the skin as opposed to on the surface of the skin

NOMENCLATURE *(Continued)*

Contaminate: to infect by contact

Dermatitis: inflammation of the skin

Diplopia: double vision

Dysphagia: difficulty swallowing

Epinephrine: hormone or neurotransmitter utilized by the sympathetic nervous system in the body's "fight-or-flight" response

Erythematous: characterized by erythema (redness of the skin)

Hemotoxic: causing blood poisoning

Hyperesthesia: increased sensitivity to touch

Loxoscelism: condition produced by the bite of a spider, usually a gangrenous reaction at the bite site

Neurotoxic: poisonous to a nerve or nerve tissues

Neurotoxin: a substance that causes damage to nerves

Oleoresin: a mixture of oil and resin from plants

Pallor: a pale color of the skin, especially of the face

Papules: a solid elevation of the skin with no visible fluid, may vary in size

Postprandially: after a meal

Pruritus: an itchy sensation due to a dermatologic condition

Ptosis: drooping of the eyelids

Rhinitis: irritation of the nose, causing a runny nose or inflammation of the nasal areas

Urticaria: commonly called hives; characterized by red, itchy, raised bumps on the skin

Vasodilatation: widening of the blood vessels

BEFORE YOU BEGIN

1. What are some of the most common poisons found in the athletic training setting?

2. What are some of the steps an athletic trainer would follow for treating an athlete who has poison ivy?

3. What types of allergic reactions may require the use of an EpiPen?

4. What is exercise-induced anaphylaxis?

5. How should an athlete use a metered-dose inhaler for an asthma emergency?

Voices from the Field

Athletic trainers are responsible for recognizing and responding to many situations encountered in this profession. Our educational backgrounds have taught us to deal with a variety of emergency situations by developing policies and procedures in the athletic training room. Our preparation for recognizing these potential-life threatening situations begins with acquiring information during the preparticipation examination at the beginning of each year to adequately manage a critical situation. An allergic reaction is an often overlooked condition that must be identified almost immediately in order to determine the proper treatment. An **allergic reaction** is simply the body's way of responding to an attack on the immune system. Allergies are commonplace, and there are many different types, such as allergies to food, insect bites, animals, medicine, latex/rubber, and other seasonal allergies.

Athletic trainers have been known to be proactive and informed in a variety of situations, and coaches as well as administrators have relied upon their expertise in providing the appropriate planning and implementation of an emergency action plan in the event of a medical emergency. Our exposure to allergic reaction is not limited to student athletes, since many of our athletic departments host summer athletic camps for youth. We are the initial contact for the coaches, parents, and campers for the management of athletic injuries and other related problems. Often we are not informed of any ongoing medical conditions, and allergies happen to be most common malady treated during summer camp. Although allergies are common, they can become life-threatening because they have the potential to precipitate anaphylactic shock. Under a physician's guidance, we have the ability to administer a dose of epinephrine (using the EpiPen) once someone exhibits signs of anaphylactic shock. Emergency management is an important responsibility of the athletic trainer, who must remain aware of the potential danger posed by such situations.

Kyle Blecha, MS, ATC
Head Athletic Trainer
Western Michigan University
Kalamazoo, MI

This chapter discusses the various environmental factors—including poisons, insect bites, and asthma allergens—that may cause an allergic reaction. In most cases, such allergic reactions are minimal, but they can become severe and/or life-threatening, requiring immediate medical attention. Therefore, as you read through this chapter, be aware of the steps and management strategies for the specific type of allergic reaction or poison presented.

ALLERGIC REACTIONS

Before discussing the specific management procedures, the definition and understanding of how the body reacts to an **allergen** must be discussed. An allergen is any type of substance that can cause an allergic reaction. An allergic reaction is the body's response to an allergen, ranging from a simple itch or rash to breathing difficulties and death. If the response is severe, it is often classified as **anaphylaxis** or anaphylactic shock. Anaphylaxis is usually associated with sudden systemic **vasodilatation** and a drop in blood pressure (often referred to as hypotension). In certain cases, fluid will accumulate in the lungs and will depress the function of the alveoli, obstruct the airway, and cause respiratory distress or failure. These symptoms can also lead to shock.

Signs & Symptoms

Common Allergic Reactions

- Red skin
- Raised blotches on the skin
- Itchy skin
- Swelling of the eyes, face, hands and feet, tongue, or neck
- Warm skin
- Tingling
- Tightness of chest
- Cough
- Difficulty breathing
- Hoarseness
- Wheezing
- Increased heart rate
- Runny nose
- Altered mental status
- Nausea
- Stridor
- Decrease in blood pressure
- Headache
- Vomiting
- Watery eyes

Signs & Symptoms

Anaphylactic Shock

- Decreased blood pressure
- Rapid pulse
- Cool skin
- Moist skin
- Pale color

The causes of allergic reactions are multifactorial, including insect bites, food, medicines, pollutants, and irritants. Insect stings from bees, wasps, or yellow jackets may cause an allergic reaction due to the venom. Many of the foods we eat—including nuts, eggs, milk, and shellfish—can also cause allergic reactions. One of the most common causes of allergic reactions aside from food is exposure to plants that produce pollens or oils—such as poison ivy, oak, and sumac—which cause an irritating rash and itching. Many environmental pollutants can cause difficulty breathing, as can exposure to irritants such as latex, especially in the athletic training setting, where latex gloves are often used to limit the contact and exposure to blood-borne pathogens. Finally, medicines may cause allergic reactions, especially antibiotics, but the listing of types and specific reactions is beyond the scope of this chapter. Instead, the athletic trainer must be aware that allergies to medicines do exist; a detailed medical history and consultations with pharmacists and physicians may limit their adverse effects.

Recognizing the signs or symptoms is the first step in the proper management of any allergic reaction. Exposure to an allergen may cause minimal discomfort, but it can also be life threatening, leading to anaphylactic shock. Treatment can be as simple as removing the allergen, washing the affected area thoroughly, or administering **epinephrine** (Skill 20.1).

Exercised-Induced Anaphylaxis

An allergic reaction as a result of exercise is called exercise-induced anaphylaxis. This can be caused by a variety of exercises, including walking, running, bicycling, skiing, soccer, basketball, volleyball, dancing, and swimming.[1,2] Exercise-induced anaphylaxis is also possibly related to the ingestion of foods (i.e., seafood, wheat, cheese, celery, eggs) and medicines (i.e., nonsteroidal anti-inflammatory drugs [NSAIDs], aspirin).[2,3]

In some cases, increases in physical activity will cause **urticaria,** or "hives", and hypotension. Urticaria is characterized by white or sometimes **erythematous** plaques that can change in size or coalesce to form "wheals."[4] Urticaria is produced by capillary vasodilation with fluid flowing into the superficial layers of the dermis.

SKILL 20.1

Anaphylaxis

1. Assess vital signs.
2. Determine if the athlete is suffering from an allergic reaction. If so, remove the allergen or remove the athlete from the allergen if possible.
3. If the allergic reaction is due to direct contact with a plant, immediately wash the area with soap and water.
4. If the athlete does not have a known allergy to insect bites/stings and has been bitten, remove any visible stinger and apply ice.

5. If the athlete has a known allergy to insect bites/stings and has been bitten, administration of epinephrine may be necessary, along with supplemental oxygen.
6. If the athlete goes into shock, follow the procedures listed for treatment of shock in Chapter 13. Contact emergency medical services or refer immediately to a medical facility if the symptoms progressively become worse, the athlete has difficulty breathing (compromised airway), or the athlete demonstrates an altered mental status.

The pathology of exercise-induced anaphylaxis is still speculative but is thought to be due to vasoactive mediators released by mast cells (histamine, leukotrienes, and prostaglandins).[1] Symptoms include a chocking sensation, warmth, fatigue, itching, nausea, headache, wheezing, pruritus, dizziness, syncope, and gastrointestinal distress, which typically occur about 10 minutes after exercise and can last up to 4 hours. Many times, exercise-induced anaphylaxis is associated with exercise in hot and humid or cold weather, after the ingestion of food or drugs, or in women before and during menstruation.

If an athlete develops exercise-induced anaphylaxis, try to maintain his/her airway, provide epinephrine if warranted based upon symptoms, and seek medical referral immediately. Epinephrine administration should be made upon physician referral or recommendation when anaphylaxis occurs.

Prevention of exercise-induced anaphylaxis includes modifying the exercise regimen by decreasing its intensity and/or duration; avoiding exercise in hot, humid environments; and delaying the initiation of exercise at least 4 to 6 hours **postprandially.** Avoidance of NSAIDs may be warranted, or delaying exercise for 4 to 6 hours after ingesting an NSAID.[1,5] Finally, athletes who suffer from exercise-induced anaphylaxis should exercise with a partner and carry a self-injectable epinephrine device when exercising.

Epinephrine Administration

Epinephrine (also called adrenalin) is a hormone found in the body that helps to constrict blood vessels, thus increasing blood pressure and heart rate; it also dilates the bronchioles to improve breathing. In the athletic training setting, where it may be necessary to administer epinephrine in emergency situations, this drug may be found in bee-sting kits, EpiPens (Fig. 20.1), and anaphylaxis kits. The administration of epinephrine is relatively easy, but it should only be done if the athlete is suffering from anaphylaxis—that is, if the athlete is presenting with difficulty breathing, symptoms of shock, low blood pressure, diarrhea, itching, swelling, and loss of bladder control. The administration of epinephrine to an athlete who does not require it can cause severe reactions such as increased heart rate, **pallor,** dizziness, headache, nausea, excitability, and even death; therefore, a health history of athletes at risk is paramount, and epinephrine should be used only under the supervision of a physician.

The most common way to administer epinephrine is via a preloaded autoinjector such as the EpiPen (Skill 20.2). Commonly, an EpiPen containing 0.3 to 0.5 mg of epinephrine is used for adults; 0.15 to 0.3 mg is used for infants and children who weigh less than 66 pounds.

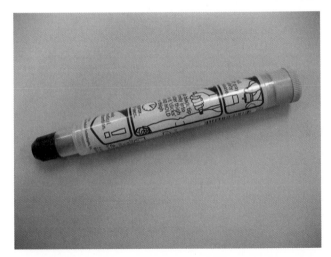

FIGURE 20.1 EpiPen. (From Long B, Hale C. *Athletic Training Exam Review.* Baltimore: Lippincott Williams & Wilkins; 2010.)

SKILL 20.2

EpiPen Administration (http://www.epipen.com)

1. Be sure that the athlete is suffering from anaphylaxis and is in shock.
2. Remove the cap and pull the safety release off the EpiPen.
3. Place the tip of the EpiPen on the outside of the athlete's thigh (lateral side) halfway between the knee and hip. Clothing, if any, should be removed from the site.
4. Push or swing (jab) the EpiPen firmly against the thigh at a 90-degree angle until the autoinjector activates (clicks).
5. Hold the EpiPen in place for at least 10 seconds until all the medication is delivered.
6. Monitor the athlete's vital signs.
7. Treat for shock.
8. Refer to a medical facility or licensed medical personnel if symptoms worsen.
9. Dispose of the EpiPen in a sharps container.

POISONING

In the athletic training setting, there are various potential poison hazards, including medications, to which an athlete, athletic trainer, or client may be exposed. There are four specific routes of poisoning: ingestion, inhalation, injection, and absorption. Each route will have different management outcomes; therefore, a quick review of these routes and the relevant treatments is provided below.

Ingested Poison

An ingested poison is a contaminant (i.e., liquid, solid that is chewed, medication) (Fig. 20.2) administered by mouth.

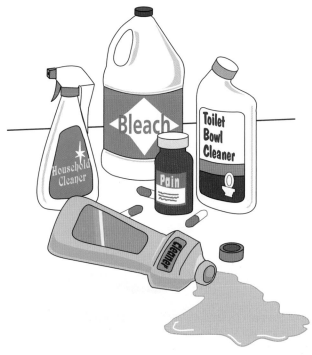

FIGURE 20.2 Ingested poison.

Sometimes, ingested substances will cause only minimal discomfort; at other times, the ingested materials can cause death. The first step when managing an ingested poison is determining what was taken, how much was taken, and when it was taken. This will help the athletic trainer decide how to best treat the situation, whom to call, and whether transport to a medical facility is required. Since there are unlimited types of ingestible poisons, the best way to determine the appropriate management is to call the Poison Control Center (PCC). The PCC is open 24 hours a day, 365 days a year, staffed by physicians, nurses, pharmacists, and other trained medical personnel who can assist in the identification of the type of poison and the appropriate treatment steps. Each state has a toll-free number, which should be posted in all athletic training facilities for quick reference.

In addition, the athletic trainer must examine the person for signs and symptoms of poisoning, such as nausea, abdominal pain, vomiting, diarrhea, mouth odors, physical damage at the mouth, difficulty breathing, and confusion. These signs and symptoms can be used by the PCC to determine treatment. If possible, find out how much the athlete weighs. That figure is often used when determining therapy (Skill 20.3).

Based upon the type of poison, it may be pertinent to provide the athlete with **activated charcoal** (Fig. 20.3). This substance helps to prevent the absorption of certain types of ingested poisons. The charcoal binds to the poison and makes the poison inert; however, activated charcoal should be given only to athletes who are fully aware of their surroundings, can swallow, and have ingested a noncaustic poison. Usually, a dose of about 1 g/kg of body weight is recommended.

Inhaled Poisons

Inhaled poisons are more difficult to manage because many times the gases or fumes are difficult to identify or see. Many inhaled poisons come from fumes of cleaning supplies that are often found in the athletic setting. If you suspect that an

SKILL 20.3

Management of Ingested Poison

1. Try to determine what poison was ingested/inhaled/injected.
2. Monitor vital signs.
3. Contact the PCC or local trained medical personnel and provide the following: description or type of poison ingested, time ingested, amount ingested, weight of the athlete.
4. Provide activated charcoal if so advised by PCC or medical personnel.
5. Provide supplemental oxygen if applicable.
6. Transport to medical facility if required.

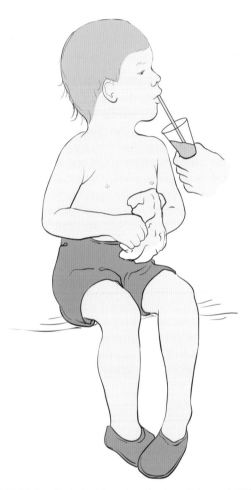

FIGURE 20.3   Oral administration of activated charcoal. (LifeART image copyright © 2010 Lippincott Williams & Wilkins. All rights reserved.)

athlete has inhaled a poison, look for signs and symptoms such as difficulty breathing, coughing, headaches, dizziness, confusion, altered mental status, or loss of consciousness. The athletic trainer should never approach a scene if he or she suspects a poison that is airborne; instead, emergency personnel should be contacted. The athlete should be removed from the scene only if the scene is safe. Treat the athlete by examining his or her vital signs, controlling for shock, delivering supplemental oxygen, and referring him or her to a medical facility (see Skill 20.3).

Injected Poisons

Athletic trainers may encounter athletes who have injected themselves with illegal chemicals or substances for pleasure or to harm themselves. In other instances, an injected poison can come from an insect or snake sting or bite (described further on in this chapter). In either case, the major signs and symptoms include pain and/or soreness at the injection site, dizziness, vomiting, nausea, altered mental status, variable consciousness, shivering, and fever. The goal for the athletic trainer is to manage these conditions in similar fashion as with other poisons (Skill 20.3).

Absorbed Poisons

Last, poisons can be absorbed through the skin or cell membranes and cause serious health consequences (see Fig. 20.2). Depending upon the type of poison, the skin itself can be irritated or severely damaged; underlying vessels and tissues can also be damaged, especially if contact is made with acids. Absorbed poisons usually manifest themselves with redness

SKILL 20.4

Treatment for Absorbed Poisons

1. Remove the athlete from any poison contact.
2. Remove clothing around the site of contact.
3. Flush the body area with copious amounts of water.
4. If the eyes came in contact with a poison, flush them with clean water for at least 20 minutes. Be careful not to flush the **contaminated** eye into the noncontaminated eye.
5. Call emergency personnel or the PCC.

Signs & Symptoms

Poisons from Plant Sources

- Redness, red bumps
- Intense itching
- **Pruritus**
- **Papules**
- Blisters

Breakout

Rupture of a blister does not cause spreading of the rash; only exposure to the actual oil can spread the poison to other areas of the body.

of the skin, possible burns at skin contact, itching, and difficulty breathing. If you suspect that an athlete has been poisoned by contact with a hazardous substance, make sure that the scene in a safe and follow the guidelines in Skill 20.4.

POISON IVY, OAK, AND SUMAC

Poisons can also come from plant sources (Fig. 20.4). Although not an immediate threat to life, contact with poison plants can cause allergic dermatitis. The poison from ivy and oak comes from direct or indirect contact with the sap or oil found in the leaves, stems, and roots, called **oleoresin.** This is a known allergen for many individuals, and typical symptoms appear 24 hours after exposure. Usually, these symptoms resolve within 2 weeks of contact. Management can include washing the area with soap and water immediately after contact as well as removal and washing of clothing to avoid recontamination. For rashes that are moderate, calamine lotion or Burow's solution work well to alleviate discomfort. Topical steroids, such as hydrocortisone cream, work well if administered before any blistering develops. Antihistamines, such as Benadryl, will help alleviate itching. If the rash becomes severe, a physician may prescribe an oral steroid, such as prednisone. In some instances, poisons from plant sources can lead to anaphylaxis, and proper medical referral may be needed.

INSECT BITES AND STINGS

Sooner or later, everyone will come in contact with an insect (i.e., yellow jackets, honeybees, bumble bees, fire ants) (Fig. 20.5) that can bite or sting. It is often an uncomfortable experience, painful, shocking to the athlete, and can lead to

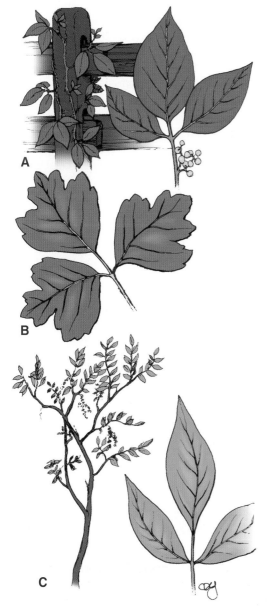

FIGURE 20.4 **A.** Poison ivy (*Rhus radicans*). **B.** Poison oak (*Rhus toxicodendron*). **C.** Poison sumac (*Rhus vernix*).

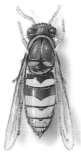
Yellow jacket

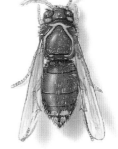
Hornet

FIGURE 20.5 Yellow jackets and hornets, which belong to the order Hymenoptera, are responsible for many cases of insect allergy each year. (Courtesy of Anatomical Chart Co.)

SKILL 20.5

Insect Sting Management

1. If stung, determine if the stinger is present in the skin. If so, remove it by any means as quickly as possible, with your fingernail, forceps, tweezers, pieces of a card, or even a scalpel blade; do not touch the stinger with your fingers or swipe across it.
2. Wash the area thoroughly.
3. Try not to scratch or rub the skin; doing so may allow dirt to enter the site and cause an infection.
4. If the athlete is not allergic to the sting, apply a topical steroid or antihistamine to reduce the inflammation.
5. Apply a cold compress to help decrease pain.
6. If an athlete develops severe symptoms (difficulty breathing, shock, chest tightness) or is stung in the mouth or throat, seek medical attention and administer epinephrine (via EpiPen) if indicated.
7. Monitor the stung site closely for several days and look for signs of infection (increased redness, tenderness, pus).

severe allergic reactions. Most stings are inflicted by wasps, bees, or ants. Only the females sting, and they usually do so only if threatened, injured, or otherwise disturbed. The stingers deliver venom that causes the nerve endings on the skin to perceive pain. The body reacts to a sting by increasing blood flow and releasing antibodies to dissipate the venom. Areas of the body that are stung usually develop redness, itchiness, and possibly swelling. When an athlete is stung for the first time, the symptoms may be more pronounced as the body develops specific antibodies to fight the venom.

Honeybees have a stinger that is barbed and remains in the skin (a honeybee can sting only once; wasps, on the other hand, can sting multiple times). If an athlete is stung by a honeybee, it is recommended to remove the stinger as soon as possible to prevent all the venom from being released into the body. Removal with your fingernail, forceps, tweezers, pieces of a card, or even a scalpel blade may suffice, but grasping the stinger may inject more venom into the site.[6] It has been estimated that it takes approximately 45 to 60 seconds for all of a honeybee's venom to be delivered. Refer to Skill 20.5 for the management of insect stings.

A small percentage of the population is allergic to insect stings and may develop anaphylaxis. The venom from the sting circulates throughout the body, combines with antibodies, and attaches to mast cells on vital organs, resulting in a release of histamine and other chemical substances. These cause the blood pressure to drop and increase fluid leakage into the lungs. Symptoms associated with anaphylaxis include shock, dizziness, tightness in the chest, laryngeal blockage, and difficulty breathing. If an athlete experiences anaphy-

laxis, administration of epinephrine is warranted. Systemic toxicity can develop from multiple stings; in such a case, immediate referral to a medical facility will be required.

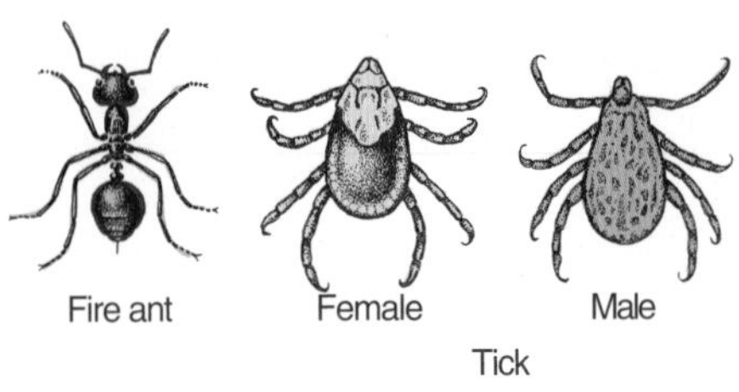

Bites by ants and ticks (Fig. 20.6) can also cause discomfort, and symptoms can range from a local redness to an allergic reaction. Bites from fire ants (located in the southern and western United States) release a venom that consists of alkaloids,[6] and the area bitten on the skin produces a lesion that is usually arc-shaped. Ticks do not produce venom but can carry Lyme disease, which may be detected by examining for a red rash than enlarges over time, fatigue and headaches, muscle and joint pain, fever, numbness and tingling of an extremity, or memory changes. A tick found on the body should be removed (refer to Skill 20.6 for tick removal). Bites from other pests—such as mosquitoes, chiggers, gnats, and fleas—can cause slight irritation but usually do not produce an allergic reaction. Bites from these pests can be treated with calamine lotion and topical anesthetics to relieve discomfort.

SPIDER BITES

Various types of spiders are found throughout the United States. Most spider bites cause little if any harm. However there are two specific species of spiders than inject venom: the brown recluse, found mostly in the Midwest and South, and the black widow, which is found in all 48 contiguous states (Fig. 20.8). The brown recluse causes a skin reaction known as **loxoscelism,** and its venom can also lead to a systemic reaction.[6] Symptoms include itching, redness, swelling, pain and blistering at the bite site, nausea, and, in severe cases, vomiting and/or muscle pain.

A bite from the black widow spider causes sharp pain, sometimes more perceptible than that caused by a bite from the brown recluse. Locally, the skin will become red, with swelling; most athletes will notice two fang marks at the bite site.[8] Severe reactions can occur, such as abdominal cramping, dizziness, headaches, vomiting, increased heart rate, and restlessness. Treatment for black widow spider bites is the same as for bites from the brown recluse (Skill 20.7).

Fire ant   Female   Male

Tick

FIGURE 20.6   Ants and ticks can be dangerous.

SKILL 20.6

Tick Removal[7]

1. Grab the tick as close to the skin as possible with blunt, angled forceps (Fig. 20.7).
2. Pull up on the tick. If the tick is locked into place, you will feel pressure on the skin. Do not twist or jerk the tick; this may cause the tick's mouth to break off and remain in the skin.
3. Once the tick has been removed, wash the area thoroughly, especially if the mouth breaks off.
4. Apply antiseptic ointment or cream to the area.
5. *Do not* squeeze the tick's body; use petroleum jelly, a lit match, or alcohol to kill.

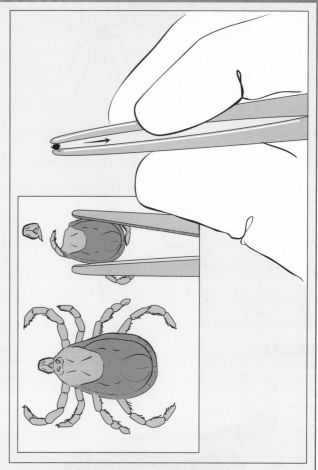

FIGURE 20.7 (LifeART image copyright © 2010 Lippincott Williams & Wilkins. All rights reserved.)

SCORPION STINGS

About 40 different species of scorpions are found in the United States (Fig. 20.9). Most individuals will not be exposed to or stung by a scorpion, but those who are stung will find it to be a very painful experience. Scorpions (depending upon the species) can release a potent **neurotoxin** that causes pain and **hyperesthesia,** muscle spasms, excessive salivation, fever, slurred speech, tachycardia, and respiratory distress.[6] Some species of scorpions have venom that causes signs and symptoms similar to bee stings, and their bites can be managed in similar fashion. If stung by a scorpion, follow the basic management steps for insect bites (Skill 20.5). If

SKILL 20.7

Management of Spider Bites

1. Try to identify the type of spider. Most spider bites are not harmful.
2. Wash the area thoroughly.
3. To relieve discomfort, apply the following:
   a. Ice pack
   b. Topical analgesics
   c. Topical antibiotics (if the wound becomes infected)
4. If the bite is large or becomes necrotic or infected, general wound cleaning may be necessary.
5. Athletes who develop allergic reactions or anaphylaxis need medical referral.

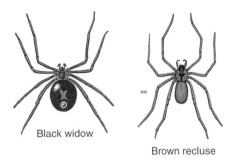

FIGURE 20.8 Bites from brown recluse spiders and black widow spiders can be life-threatening.

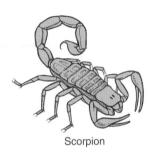

FIGURE 20.9 A scorpion bite can be life-threatening.

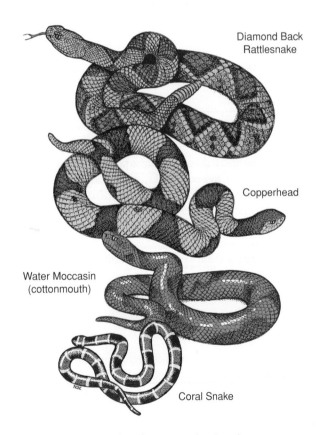

FIGURE 20.10 Rattlesnakes, copperhead snakes, water moccasins, and coral snakes are poisonous snakes found in North America. (Neil O. Hardy, Westpoint, CT.)

Signs & Symptoms

Snake Bite[9]

- Pain (burning, bursting, throbbing)
- Weakness
- Swelling and edema
- Numbness
- Increased heart rate
- Vomiting
- Ecchymosis
- **Ptosis**
- **Diplopia**
- **Dysphagia**
- Sweating
- Difficulty breathing

symptoms worsen, management may include the application of a tourniquet, antihistamines, and possibly corticosteroids administered by a professional health care provider.

SNAKE BITES

Snakes found commonly in the United States include rattlesnakes, copperheads, cottonmouths (often referred to as pit vipers because of the small heat-sensitive pits between their eyes and nostrils), and coral snakes (Fig. 20.10). The venom from a snake can be **hemotoxic** or **neurotoxic.** Pit vipers in particular have venom that is neurotoxic. If one is bitten by a pit viper, two fang marks with concurrent swelling are usually the hallmark signs. The seriousness of the side effects depends upon the type of snake, the location of the bite, the amount of venom injected with the bite, and the overall health, age, and size of the person.

If one is bitten by a snake, it is important to identify markings on the snake to help determine the snake's species, which may be useful for medical personnel; however, do not try to capture the snake. Careful management and medical referral are indicated (Skill 20.8). Often, a wide constriction band can be fabricated and placed proximal to the bite site to restrict only the superficial venous and lymphatic flow. The constriction band is left in place until medical personnel remove it during care. Sucking the venom or blood from the site has not been shown to be beneficial.[10,11] Immediate referral to a medical facility, where antivenin therapies may be initiated, and calling the PCC is recommended.

LATEX ALLERGY

In the athletic setting, barriers such as latex gloves (Fig. 20.11) are often used to help prevent the spread of blood-

SKILL 20.8

First Aid for Snake Bite

1. Immediately identify the snake if this can be done safely.
2. Reassure the athlete.
3. Limit the athlete's activity.
4. Remove tight-fitting or restrictive clothing.
5. Immobilize the body part with a splint or sling (movement can increase the movement of venom into the bloodstream).
6. Apply a constriction band to reduce blood flow if appropriate.
7. Do not elevate an extremity that has been bitten.
8. Refer the individual to a medical facility and call the PCC.

borne pathogens and contact with them. Many individuals may report a skin rash or allergy to latex, with a prevalence rate of 5% to 10% in the general population.[12] Latex is manufactured from the milky sap of the rubber tree. During this process, a donning powder (cornstarch) is added, which may be a precursor to latex sensitivity, along with the proteins that are found in latex.[13] Because of the possibility of contact allergies with latex gloves, the Centers for Disease Control and Prevention recommend that gloves be powder-free or that oat starch instead of cornstarch should be used as the powder. The use of latex-free alternatives is common; however, the latex-free gloves sometimes cause a delayed hypersensitivity reaction, lack the preferred feel, and are not biodegradable.[14] In addition to latex gloves, latex can be found in other products, such as Band-Aids, clothing and shoes, condoms, balloons, and various kinds of sporting equipment.

Reactions to latex can be categorized as irritant contact **dermatitis,** allergic contact dermatitis, or an immediate hypersensitivity reaction. The most common adverse reaction is irritant contact dermatitis (which is a nonallergic type of reaction) characterized by itchy, dry skin as well as cracks and fissures in the skin as a result of abrasion from repetitive use. Allergic contact dermatitis is pri-

marily caused by the additives used in making the latex. Symptoms include a red rash, itching, or blisters (similar to poison ivy) that occur up to 24 hours after exposure. Immediate allergic reactions are more severe forms of allergy to latex; they can lead to urticaria, **angioedema**, rhinitis, nausea, vomiting, and anaphylaxis. Urticaria, as explained previously, occurs with contact to latex proteins that causes a hypersensitivity reaction of the skin, with red wheals, usually about 1 hour after exposure. Angioedema can occur with localized nonpitting swelling, usually in the lips, face, larynx, trunk, or limbs. If such a reaction occurs in the larynx, closure of airways may ensue, which is life-threatening. Allergic **rhinitis** is characterized by nasal congestion, sneezing, and watery eyes. If severe, a reaction to latex can cause anaphylaxis (Skill 20.9).

ASTHMA

Asthma is defined as an inflammatory disorder of the airways that can cause airway hyperresponsiveness, which may lead to wheezing, breathlessness, chest tightness, and coughing. Breathing difficulty results from constriction of the airways due to chemical mediators such as histamine, tryptase, prostaglandins, and leukotrienes.[15-18] Causes of asthma are multifactorial and can include exercise or environmental factors, such air pollution, smoke, or the presence of allergens from animals, cockroaches, mold and fungal spores, chlorine, and pollens.[19-27]

Whether asthma is caused by exercise or other factors, management remains more or less the same. A family

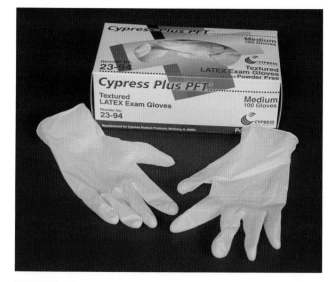

FIGURE 20.11   Latex gloves.

Signs & Symptoms

Asthma

- Coughing
- Wheezing
- Dyspnea
- Chest tightness and/or pain
- Feeling tired or weak

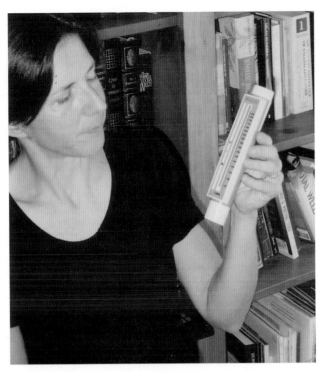

FIGURE 20.12 Peak flow meters measure the highest volume of airflow during a forced expiration (*left*). Volume is measured in color-coded zones (*right*): the green zone signifies 80% to 100% of personal best; yellow, 60% to 80%; and red, less than 60%. If peak flow falls below the red zone, the athlete should take the appropriate actions prescribed by his or her health care provider.

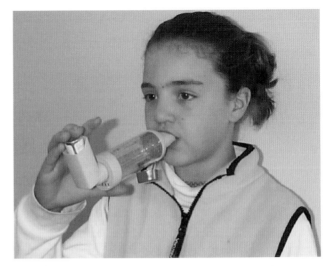

FIGURE 20.14 Multidose inhaler use with spacers. (From Nettina SM. *Lippincott Manual of Nursing Practice,* 9th ed. Philadelphia: Wolters Kluwer Health; 2010.)

history and health history questionnaire must be completed for athletes suspected of having asthma or reported to be having difficulty breathing. Asthma screenings, via laboratory tests, are recommended for positive medical histories; recording of the baseline of peak expiratory flow (PEF) using a peak flow meter (Fig. 20.12) is also recommended (Skill 20.10).

An asthma management plan must be developed for the athletic training setting in order to deal with asthma emergencies (Skill 20.11). The use of medications to relieve chest tightness and open the airways should be discussed with each asthmatic athlete and proper inhalation techniques reviewed and demonstrated.

The use of a medicated inhaler is often the best way to reduce the severity of an asthma attack (Skills 20.12 and 20.13).

Although there are several varieties of inhalers, they are usually either of two types: metered-dose (Fig. 20.13) and dry-powder inhalers. Metered-dose inhalers use a specific amount or measured dose of a medication, which is propelled forcefully into the mouth or spacer. Some metered-dose inhalers have a counter on the unit to notify the user of how many doses remain, but most have only a short canister of medication with no indication of the amount that is left. Other options that can be used with these inhalers are spacers, which help to deliver the medication to the lungs. A spacer is a short tube (4 to 8 in.) that extends from the mouthpiece of the inhaler (Fig. 20.14). When the inhaler is

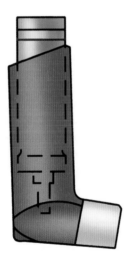

FIGURE 20.13 Metered-dose inhaler (handheld). (From *Nursing Procedures.* 4th ed. Ambler, PA: Lippincott Williams & Wilkins, 2004.)

SKILL 20.9

Management of Latex Allergy

1. Remove the exposure risk (latex glove).
2. Wash the area thoroughly.
3. Apply a topical corticosteroid if applicable and recommended by medical personnel.
4. Refer immediately if symptoms worsen.

SKILL 20.10

Using a Peak Flow Meter

1. Stand up or sit straight.
2. Place indicator at the zero mark.
3. Take a deep breath.
4. Place your mouth over the mouthpiece and close your lips around it.
5. Blow out as fast and forcibly as possible.
6. Remove the peak flow meter from your mouth and record the number represented by the indicator.
7. Repeat two more times.
8. Use the highest value.

SKILL 20.11

Management of Asthma

1. First, cease all exercise or move the athlete into a filtered, well-ventilated environment (if environmental irritants are the suspected causes of the attack).
2. Measure PEF with a peak flow meter (if applicable).
3. If PEF is low, or 15% of baseline measurements, have the athlete take two puffs of his or her prescribed rescue inhaler.
4. Monitor airway and breathing for several minutes.
5. Measure PEF and administer additional puffs if needed.
6. If symptoms worsen, refer the athlete to a medical facility immediately.

SKILL 20.12

Proper Use of a Metered-Dose Inhaler

1. Shake the inhaler to mix the medication.
2. Remove the cap.
3. Attach a spacer tube if desired.
4. Keep your head erect.
5. Exhale normally.
6. Close your mouth around the mouthpiece/spacer tube.
7. Breathe in slowly while activating the inhaler. Keep breathing even after activation until your lungs are comfortably full of air.
8. Remove the inhaler from your mouth.
9. Hold your breath for 10 seconds.
10. Exhale slowly.

SKILL 20.13

Proper Use of a Dry-Powder Inhaler

1. Dry-powder inhalers are activated by different methods. Refer to the user's manual to determine how to assemble the inhaler and activate the medication.
2. After step 1, hold the inhaler away from your mouth and gently breathe out. Do not blow into the inhaler.
3. Close your lips around the mouthpiece of the inhaler.
4. Inhale rapidly and deeply for a full breath and hold up to 10 seconds.
5. Resume normal breathing.
6. If applicable, remove the medicated capsule from the inhaler.
7. Throw away the used capsule.

Scenarios

1. You are working as an athletic trainer at a collegiate field hockey game on a fall afternoon. The field is located off campus about a mile from the athletic training room. During stretching, one of your players is stung by a bee. She does not immediately report to you, but after 5 minutes, her arm, where she was stung, is swelling rapidly. When she approaches holding her arm, you notice swelling and redness. She looks frightened, tells you she was stung, and does not recall the last time, if ever, she was stung by a bee.

   What steps should you take to manage this situation?

2. As a staff athletic trainer, you are showing prospective freshmen how to care for wounds. Part of your instructional procedures is the application and removal of gloves that are used as barriers to blood-borne pathogens. During practice, one of the freshmen, after removing the gloves, notices that his skin in the area that was covered by the gloves has become red. His redness then progresses to itchiness.

   What should steps should you take to deal with this situation?

3. During preseason physicals, a health history of one of your athletes suggests symptoms of asthma. You decide, in consultation with the team physician, to conduct a screening to confirm your suspicion of asthma and assess lung function. After testing, you have baseline values for the athlete.

   If the athlete were to suffer from an asthma attack in the future, how would these baseline values, particularly PEF rate, be used for management?

4. The cross-country team recently ran in fields and sparse woods near your high school. After practice, one of your female cross-country runners reports to the athletic training room, saying that she found a bug attached to the skin of her upper leg. You indentify the bug as a tick. The tick appears to be clamped to the skin quite securely.

   How would you go about removing the tick and how would you treat the bite area once it had been removed?

---

activated, the medication travels through the tube, extending the time during which the medication is inhaled. The second type of inhaler is a dry-powder inhaler, which does not use a propellant but is activated by the user's forceful breaths or inhalations, pulling the dry powder into the lungs.

The types of medications used with inhalers vary, but they can be classified into several groups. Short-acting bronchodilators (in rescue inhalers) are used for immediate relief of asthma symptoms. Long-acting bronchodilators provide relief of symptoms that lasts for many hours. Only the short-acting bronchodilators are used in emergency situations; the use of long-term controls—although helpful in decreasing the severity of attacks and also likely to decrease sustained exacerbations—are not useful for immediate breathing emergencies.

For more formal recommendations for the prevention of asthma, its diagnosis and management, and medications used to treat it, refer to the National Athletic Trainers' Association position statement.[28]

WRAP-UP

The information given in this chapter should provide the athletic trainer with the necessary skills and knowledge to effectively manage reactions to various poisons, venoms, and allergic reactions to environmental conditions found in the athletic training setting. The management steps focus on airway monitoring, injection of epinephrine (where applicable), or ingestion of activated charcoal. Many cases of anaphylaxis will require referral to appropriate and qualified medical personnel during these emergencies. Managing the body's reaction to the information provided in this chapter

is relatively easy, but the athletic trainer should realize that an individual can suddenly progress into a life-threatening situation; therefore, close monitoring is warranted.

REFERENCES

1. Castells MC, Horan RF, Sheffer AL. Exercise-induced anaphylaxis (EIA). *Clin Rev Allergy Immunol.* 1999;17:413–424.
2. Shadick NA, Liang MH, Partridge AJ, et al. The natural history of exercise-induced anaphylaxis: Survey results from a 10-year follow-up study. *J Allergy Clin Immunol.* 1999;104:123–127.
3. Fukutomi O, Kondo N, Agata H, et al. Abnormal responses of the autonomic nervous system in food-dependent exercise-induced anaphylaxis. *Ann Allergy.* 1992;68:438–445.
4. Hosey RG, Carek PJ, Goo A. Exercise-induced anaphylaxis and urticaria. *Am Fam Physician.* 2001;64(8):1367–1372.
5. Castells MC, Horan RF, Sheffer AL. Exercise-induced anaphylaxis. *Curr Allergy Asthma Rep.* 2003;3(1):15–21.
6. Kemp ED. Bites and stings of the arthropod kind-treating reactions that can range from annoying to menacing. *Postgrad Med.* 1998;103(6):88–90.
7. Gammons M, Salam G. Tick removal. *Am Fam Physician.* 2002;66(4):643–645.
8. Zukowski CW. Black widow spider bite. *J Am Board Fam Pract.* 1993;6(3):279–281.
9. Juckett G, Hancox JG. Venomous snakebites in the United States: Management review and update. *Am Fam Physician.* 2002;65(7):1367–1374.
10. Stewart ME, Greenland S, Hoffman JR. First-aid treatment of poisonous snakebite: Are currently recommended procedures justified? *Ann Emerg Med.* 1981;10:331–335.
11. Wingert WA, Chan L. Rattlesnake bites in southern California and rationale for recommended treatment. *West J Med.* 1988;148:37–44.

12. Ahmed DD, Sobczak SC, Yunginger JW. Occupational allergies caused by latex. *Immunol Allergy Clin North Am.* 2003; 23:205–219.

13. Huber MA, Terezhalmy GT. Adverse reactions to latex products: Preventive and therapeutic strategies. *J Contemp Dent Pract.* 2006;7(1):97–106.

14. Yip E, Cacioli P. The manufacture of gloves from natural rubber latex. *J Allergy Clin Immunol.* 2002;110(2 Suppl):S3–S14.

15. Wenzel SE, Westcott JY, Smith HR, et al. Spectrum of prostanoid release after bronchoalveolar allergen challenge in atopic asthmatics and in control groups. An alteration in the ratio of bronchoconstrictive to bronchoprotective mediators. *Am Rev Respir Dis.* 1989;139:450–457.

16. Persson CG. Role of plasma exudation in asthmatic airways. *Lancet.* 1986;2:1126–1129.

17. Djukanovic R, Wilson JW, Britten KM, et al. Quantitation of mast cells and eosinophils in the bronchial mucosa of symptomatic atopic asthmatics and healthy control subjects using immunohistochemistry. *Am Rev Respir Dis.* 1990;142:863–871.

18. Koshino T, Arai Y, Miyamoto Y, et al. Mast cell and basophil number in the airway correlate with the bronchial responsiveness of asthmatics. *Int Arch Allergy Immunol.* 1995;107:378–379.

19. Woodfolk JA, Luczynska CH, De Blay F, et al. Cat allergy. *Ann Allergy Asthma Immunology.* 1992;69:273–275.

20. Croner S, Kjellman N-IM. Natural history of bronchial asthma in childhood: a prospective study from birth to 14 years of age. *Allergy.* 1992;47:150–157.

21. Sarpong SB, Karrison T. Season of birth and cockroach allergen sensitization in children with asthma. *J Allergy Clin Immunol.* 1998;101:566–568.

22. Kuster PA. Reducing the risk of house dust mite and cockroach allergen exposure in inner city children with asthma. *Pediatr Nurs.* 1996;22:297–303.

23. Platt SD, Martin CJ, Hunt SM, et al. Damp housing, mould growth, and symptomatic health state. *Br Med J.* 1989;298: 1673–1678.

24. Potter PC, Juritz J, Little F, et al. Clustering of fungal-allergen specific IgE antibody responses in allergic subjects. *Ann Allergy.* 1991;66:149–153.

25. Bar-Or O, Inbar O. Swimming and asthma. *Sports Med.* 1992;14:397–405.

26. Suphioglu C, Singh MB, Taylor P, et al. Mechanism of grass-pollen induced asthma. *Lancet.* 1992;339:569–572.

27. D'Amato G, Spieksma FT, Liccardi G, et al. Pollen-related allergy in Europe. *Allergy.* 1998;53:567–578.

28. Miller MG, Weiler J, Baker R, et al. National Athletic Trainers' Association position statement: Management of asthma in athletes. *J Athl Train.* 2005;40(3):224–245.

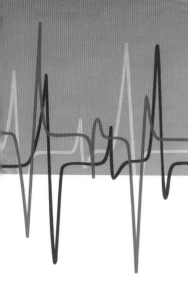

Note: Page numbers followed by *f* and *t* indicate figures and tables.